Academic Lifestyle Medicine

There is no longer any serious doubt that what individuals do in their daily lives profoundly impacts their short- and long-term health, quality of life, and risk of developing chronic diseases. Despite overwhelming evidence in this area, physicians often feel inadequately prepared to discuss these issues with their patients. This results from the relative lack of education for physicians in these components of lifestyle medicine. Authored by renowned cardiologist and lifestyle medicine researcher Dr. James Rippe and lifestyle medicine education and behavioral medicine expert Dr. Beth Frates, *Academic Lifestyle Medicine: A Curriculum for Medical Educators* blends state-of-the-art information on the robust medical literature supporting lifestyle medicine with an innovative approach to medical education.

This book starts with an extensive discussion of the robust evidence that underlies the major components of lifestyle medicine including physical activity, nutrition, weight management, substance abuse and addiction, sleep, and positive connections to others. This information is then linked to how this evidence can be used to lower the risk of chronic diseases such as heart disease, diabetes, cancer, metabolic syndrome, brain health, cognitive function, and many other health issues. The authors then provide a specific framework for applying the principles of lifestyle medicine to all stages of medical education—from undergraduate to graduate training and continuing medical education. Additional specialty topics include the evidence supporting lifestyle medicine practice to ensure healthy aging, the unique lifestyle challenges for women, and how lifestyle medicine applies to healthy habits amongst children and families. Other topics include how lifestyle medicine components interact with planetary health, health equity, and advocacy across numerous professional and regulatory groups.

A volume in the *Lifestyle Medicine Series*, this book is a must-read for physicians wishing to understand the robust academic foundations of modern lifestyle medicine practice. It also provides an authoritative guide for physicians who are tasked with preparing the next generation of physicians in lifestyle medicine.

Lifestyle Medicine
Series Editor
James M. Rippe, MD
Professor of Medicine, University of Massachusetts Medical School

Led by James M. Rippe, MD, founder of the Rippe Lifestyle Institute, this series is directed to a broad range of researchers and professionals consisting of topical books with clinical applications in nutrition and health, physical activity, obesity management, and applicable subjects in lifestyle medicine.

Increasing Physical Activity
A Practical Guide
James M. Rippe, MD

Manual of Lifestyle Medicine
James M. Rippe, MD

Obesity Prevention and Treatment
A Practical Guide
James M. Rippe, MD and John P. Foreyt, PhD

Improving Women's Health Across the Lifespan
Michelle Tollefson, MD, Nancy Eriksen, MD and Neha Pathak, MD

Lifestyle Nursing
Gia Merlo, MD and Kathy Berra, MSN

Integrating Lifestyle Medicine in Cardiovascular Health and Disease Prevention
James M. Rippe, MD

Lifestyle Medicine for Prediabetes, Type 2 Diabetes, and Cardiometabolic Disease
Michael A. Via, MD and Jeffrey Mechanick, MD

Empowering Behavior Change in Patients: Practical Strategies for the Healthcare Professional
Beth Frates, PhD and Mark Faries, MD

Lifestyle Psychiatry
Through the Lens of Behavioral Medicine
Gia Merlo, MD and Christopher P. Fagundes, PhD

Lifestyle Nutrition
Eating for Good Health by Lowering the Risk of Chronic Diseases
James M. Rippe, MD

Lifestyle Medicine and the Primary Care Provider
A Practical Guide to Enabling Whole Person Care
Ron Stout, MD, Dan Reichert, MD and Rebecca Kelly, PhD

Geriatrics, Lifestyle Medicine and Healthy Aging
A Practical Guide
Susan M. Friedman, MD

Academic Lifestyle Medicine
A Curriculum for Medical Educators
James M. Rippe, MD and Beth P. Frates, MD

For more information, please visit: www.routledge.com/Lifestyle-Medicine/book-series/CRCLM

Academic Lifestyle Medicine

A Curriculum for Medical Educators

James M. Rippe, MD and Beth Frates, MD

CRC Press
Taylor & Francis Group
Boca Raton London New York

CRC Press is an imprint of the
Taylor & Francis Group, an **informa** business

Designed cover image: Shutterstock

First edition published 2027
by CRC Press
2385 NW Executive Center Drive, Suite 320, Boca Raton FL 33431

and by CRC Press
4 Park Square, Milton Park, Abingdon, Oxon, OX14 4RN

CRC Press is an imprint of Taylor & Francis Group, LLC

Library of Congress Control Number: 2026937203

ISBN: 9781041048091 (hbk)
ISBN: 9781041037958 (pbk)
ISBN: 9781003630043 (ebk)

DOI: 10.1201/9781003630043

Typeset in Times
by codeMantra

"To our families whose love and support make it all worthwhile."

Contents

Preface

Academic Lifestyle Medicine A Curriculum for Medical Educators

We are proud to offer a new evidence-based curriculum for physicians at every level of medical training. The need to summarize evidence and place it in an actionable curriculum is both timely and vitally important.

There is no longer any serious doubt that daily habits and actions profoundly impact both short- and long-term health and quality of life. This concept is supported by overwhelming medical and scientific literature. Literally thousands of studies provide strong evidence that regular physical activity, healthy nutrition, maintenance of a healthy body weight, not smoking cigarettes, reducing stress, getting healthy sleep, and having positive interactions with other individuals all significantly lower the risk of chronic diseases. These are the cornerstones of the new field of "lifestyle medicine."

Despite overwhelming evidence in support of the power of these daily habits and actions, mainstream medical practitioners have been largely absent from the table when it comes to a deep understanding of these issues and counseling their patients in these areas. Since the publication of the 1st edition of the multi-authored academic textbook edited by one of us (JMR) with the eponymous name *Lifestyle Medicine* in 1999, which named the field "lifestyle medicine" in the academic literature, the field has experienced exuberant growth! The American College of Lifestyle Medicine (ACLM), which was founded utilizing materials from Dr. Rippe's textbook, has now expanded to over 13,000 members, making it the fastest-growing health care organization in the world. The *American Journal of Lifestyle Medicine,* also edited by Dr. Rippe, has over 25,000 subscribers, and in the year 2024, it experienced over 325,000 downloads of full-length articles.

Lifestyle medicine has become a truly international movement. In fact, the World Health Organization (WHO) has launched a major campaign to combat non-communicable diseases (NCDs), which the WHO states result in over 74% of all annual mortality. One of us (JMR) observed the phenomenal growth of lifestyle medicine firsthand when giving an opening keynote address to a lifestyle medicine conference in China in November 2023. His address was viewed virtually by over 2.5 million individuals! Lifestyle medicine represents the cornerstone of the nationwide "Healthy China" initiative. Over 100 hospitals in China have now joined in this effort. When Dr. Rippe gave the opening keynote address on "Lifestyle Medicine and the Prevention of Heart Disease" at an academic symposium as part of a lifestyle medicine conference in Beijing in 2024, over 2.8 million individuals attended virtually!

Despite this robust growth, physicians practicing in mainstream medical environments have been largely absent from discussions. This is despite the fact that the evidence that supports lifestyle medicine is fundamental to the consensus expert guidelines from virtually every prestigious panel on metabolic disease. These consensus guidelines have been developed to provide the evidence base for the risk reduction and treatment of conditions ranging from heart disease and diabetes to cancer and obesity, utilizing lifestyle measures. The guidelines have also provided robust evidence in areas such as physical activity and healthy nutrition. Thus, while lifestyle medicine serves as an umbrella combining much of the evidence, the underlying scientific rationale has been present at the highest level of mainstream medicine for decades.

Perhaps it is not surprising that so few physicians practice or are even aware of the field of lifestyle medicine. For example, fewer than 20% of medical schools have nutrition courses, and only 14% of individuals who graduate from medical school feel that they have adequate nutritional knowledge. In Dr. Rippe's own discipline (cardiology), it is shocking that 90% of cardiologists report that they do not have adequate nutrition knowledge to provide expert counseling in this area. It is noteworthy, however, that 95% of cardiologists feel that nutrition counseling is important and would welcome more information in this area!

In the area of physical activity, it is shocking that only 9% of medical schools have academic offerings in this area. Thus, it is not surprising that a recent survey of 175 primary care physicians revealed that only 12% were aware of physical activity recommendations from the American College of Sports Medicine (ACSM). Furthermore, an evaluation of 51 internal medicine residents reported that while 88% felt confident in their knowledge of the benefits of exercise, only 25% could demonstrate adequate knowledge that would be useful for patient counseling.

The fundamental basis of this book and the embedded curriculum is to summarize robust evidence that supports the concepts behind lifestyle medicine and place it in the context of detailed scientific evidence. Our goal is also to educate physicians about how to apply this information in their practices. Our curriculum attempts to respond to the low levels of physician education in the areas of physical activity, nutrition, weight management, etc., and to address the strong interest from practicing physicians to provide more information in this area in the form of an actionable curriculum.

The need for this type of curriculum is urgent. For example, in a recent survey of 1,000 physicians, only 13.5% agreed or strongly agreed that they were adequately trained to discuss the area of nutrition with their patients. However, a significant majority (78.4%) stated that additional training in nutrition would help them provide clinical care in the prevention of cardiovascular disease. We hope and intend to provide this training. We believe that physicians will be receptive to this message. For example, when physicians have been asked to rate the importance of various therapies in the area of cardiovascular disease (CVD) on a scale of 1–10 (with 10 being the most important), respondents rated nutrition at 8.1+2.05 and physical activity at 8.2+1.56. Both of these results were higher than statins (7.8+2.11).

Unfortunately, the areas of physical activity and nutrition are de-emphasized at every level of medical education. Among medical students, the four years spent in medical school result in plummeting interest in these areas. In one study, 72% of entering medical students reported nutritional counseling to be highly relevant, but only 46% did in their final year.

We recognize that the lack of training in nutrition, physical activity, and other components of lifestyle medicine can also reflect the fact that physicians are not tested in these areas on standard examinations. For example, there is not a single question on nutrition or physical activity on the Internal Medicine Boards, which all internal medicine residents must pass in order to practice either internal medicine or move on to a subspecialty. Despite this lack of emphasis in medical schools, most physicians are eager to learn more in the areas that comprise lifestyle medicine and would welcome further education in these areas, provided that it is based on high-level evidence. That is what we intend to accomplish in this book and with this curriculum.

As co-editors of this book, we both have in-depth knowledge and experience in lifestyle medicine and education and represent prestigious medical schools. One of us (JMR) is Professor of Medicine at UMass Chan Medical School and has been tasked with developing a comprehensive curriculum in lifestyle medicine. The other (BPF) is Associate Professor of Medicine (part-time) at Harvard Medical School and has developed multiple lifestyle medicine educational materials for diverse audiences at this institution. We are both committed, passionate, and knowledgeable in the area of the linkages of high-level clinical evidence and how to educate physicians in this area.

Our book starts with an Introductory chapter which provides an overview of the robust and persuasive academic evidence base for lifestyle medicine. This book is then divided into four major parts. Part 1 surveys the vast amount of high-level evidence supporting each of the various components of each of the seven components of lifestyle medicine. Part 2 then links this evidence to specific metabolic conditions, demonstrating how it can be utilized to prevent and treat the various chronic diseases. Part 3 provides a new medical education pathway and curriculum for physicians at every level of training. This curriculum provides detailed evidence specifically for medical professionals to support the health-related benefits of each part of the curriculum and provides a detailed pathway for its dissemination. Part 4 provides supplementary material on topics such as the relationship between individual health and planetary health. Part 4 also provides strategies for advocating lifestyle medicine in medical institutions, government agencies, and the public at large.

The educational materials provided in our *Academic Lifestyle Medicine: A Curriculum for Medical Educators* book are the first academic, clinically oriented educational materials in lifestyle medicine for practicing physicians and physicians in training. This information is strongly linked to consensus statements from major professional organizations and is also linked to the recently published 4th edition of Dr. Rippe's *Lifestyle Medicine* textbook (CRC Press, 2024).

We also present the first curriculum to specifically align with the knowledge and skills of the Accreditation Council for Graduate Medical Education Core Competencies framework. Our curriculum is also the first lifestyle medicine framework to address medical education across the spectrum of undergraduate medical education, graduate medical education, and continuing medical education. We emphasize teaching strategies along with robust medical science and evidence for each pillar.

Each chapter in Part 3 will have a separate section demonstrating how the principles of lifestyle medicine can be efficiently and effectively taught to medical professionals at each level of training.

Our goal throughout the book and the embedded curriculum has been to combine the practical application of lifestyle medicine principles and practices with the high level of evidence that physicians require in order to feel comfortable with the underlying credibility of the lifestyle medicine components and provide them with a framework and specific tools to convey these principles to their patients. Our intent has been to not only encourage mainstream medicine physicians to understand the profound evidence behind lifestyle medicine but also encourage individuals who are currently practicing lifestyle medicine to have a deeper, evidence-based understanding of the enormous evidence supporting lifestyle medicine. We believe that this will underscore the fact that lifestyle medicine is as evidence-based as any other aspect of mainstream medical practice.

James M. Rippe, MD
Professor of Medicine
UMass Chan Medical School

Beth Frates, MD
Associate Professor of Medicine (Part-time)
Harvard Medical School

Acknowledgments

We are grateful for the many individuals who have contributed to and influenced our thinking about the interaction between academic medicine, lifestyle, and health. We believe that there is an important opportunity to continue to underscore the academic evidence base that supports lifestyle medicine and embed it more specifically into the mainstream of American medicine.

Textbook writing and editing are collaborative efforts and involve the input from many individuals. Numerous individuals have contributed to our thinking in the area of not only academic medicine but also its particular and specific role in lifestyle medicine. Furthermore, many individuals have contributed to our thinking about how lifestyle medicine can be integrated into medical education. We believe there is an opportunity to expand lifestyle medicine into the academic sphere of medicine in a more overt way. That is, in essence, why we have developed this book and focused on the academic evidence behind lifestyle medicine and in the embedded curriculum.

Dr. Rippe's long-term Editorial Director, Beth Grady, continues to play a very important role in major writing and editing projects that emerge from his research organization. This book is one of over 62 books that Beth has managed that has been generated through Rippe Lifestyle Institute. Beth also provides editorial direction to two academic journals where Dr. Rippe serves as the Editor in Chief (The *American Journal of Lifestyle Medicine* and the *Journal of Intensive Care Medicine*). She also plays a major role in two academic textbooks: *Lifestyle Medicine* (4th edition, CRC Press, 2024) and *Irwin and Rippe's Intensive Care Medicine* (9th edition, 2023). Beth blends excellent editorial skills with an exceptional work ethic. She remains calm and has an unfailing sense of good humor, which is essential to make these complex and difficult projects possible. In addition, she coordinates with hundreds of physicians in multiple fields across all branches of medicine on a regular basis.

The office staff at RLI also play a critical role in all of the publishing projects. These include Dr. Rippe's Executive Assistant, Carol Moreau, who coordinates his schedule and travel plans and has also word-processed many chapters in this book. The Editorial Office Assistant at RLI, Deb Adamonis, plays multiple and diverse roles and assists in numerous complicated daily tasks to execute diverse projects. In addition, Deb tracked down thousands of academic references in the current book. The RLI Chief Financial Officer, Wendy Graves, manages the financial processes to ensure that our projects move forward smoothly.

The Rippe Lifestyle Institute research team continues to play important roles and provides insights to clarify thinking on various aspects of lifestyle medicine and its key components such as physical activity, plant-forward nutrition, weight management, risk factor reduction, avoiding risky substances, and maintaining positive relationships with other individuals.

Developing a book in the area of medical education, which we hope and believe will play a role at UMass Chan Medical School and Harvard Medical School, has required the enthusiastic support of multiple individuals. Dr. Rippe, in particular, wishes to acknowledge the strong institutional support from Dr. Terence Flotte, the Dean of UMass Chan Medical School, and Dr. David McManus, the Chairman of the Department of Medicine. Dr. Frates specifically wishes to thank and acknowledge multiple individuals who have helped this project at Harvard Medical School, including Dr. Bernard Chang, the Dean of Undergraduate Medical Education at HMS, and Dr. George Daley, the Dean of Harvard Medical School.

The outstanding editorial team at Taylor & Francis Group/CRC Press plays a vital role in all the books in the *Lifestyle Medicine Series*. Randy Brehm, Senior Editor, has been an important supporter of lifestyle medicine in general and the multiple books that have been published through CRC Press, including the 2nd, 3rd, and 4th editions of Dr. Rippe's major academic textbook *Lifestyle Medicine* and Dr. Frates' book on promoting behavior change. Randy has also been a strong supporter of the *Lifestyle Medicine Series* in which the current volume resides.

Tom Connelly coordinated all aspects of the publication process and provided day-to-day assistance on multiple issues related to each chapter. Tom is a true pleasure to work with. He is detail oriented and maintains a positive and helpful attitude throughout the arduous process and final publication of all books in the *Lifestyle Medicine Series*, including this one.

Marsha Hecht, Production Editor at the Taylor & Francis Group, oversaw all aspects of the production of this book with great expertise. Bryan Moloney, Project Manager, and the team at Deanta Global have managed the day-to-day production in preparing our manuscript with great skill.

We would also like to thank and single out the Ardmore Institute for Health for providing generous grant support, which partially funded the writing of this book and the research behind it. In particular, the CEO of the Ardmore Institute for Health, Dr. Ron Stout, has offered many important insights and continued support and guidance in the whole area of lifestyle medicine and how it can serve as a toolbox for whole person care.

Finally, we are very grateful for the support of our families, including Dr. Rippe's wife, Stephanie Hart Rippe, and his wonderful daughters, Hart, Jaelin, Devon, and Jamie, who continue to support him through the arduous process of writing a major textbook as well as his other professional responsibilities, which he juggles along with his family life. Beth Frates' husband, Jim, and her two sons also play a critical role in supporting her diverse academic interests in the area of lifestyle medicine.

If there are errors or omissions in *Academic Lifestyle Medicine: A Curriculum for Medical Educators*, the responsibility is ours. If there is any credit due to the project, it belongs to the numerous people who have made and continue to make substantial contributions to our knowledge and performance along the way and bring great joy to our lives.

James M. Rippe, MD
Worcester, Massachusetts

Beth Frates, MD
Boston, Massachusetts

About the Authors

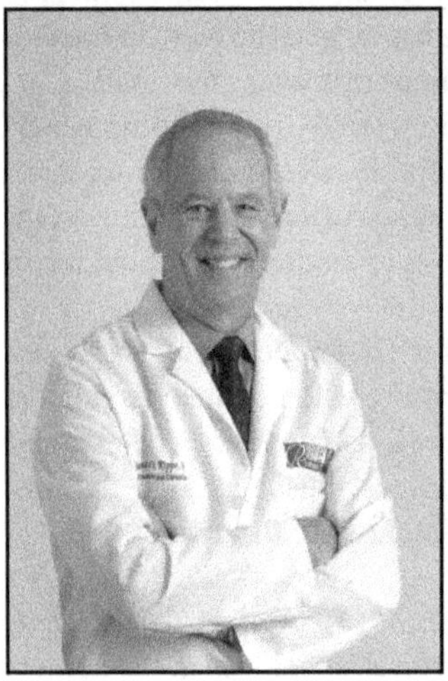

James M. Rippe, MD, is an honors graduate of Harvard College and Harvard Medical School with postgraduate training at Massachusetts General Hospital and the University of Massachusetts Medical School. He is currently the Founder and Director of the Rippe Lifestyle Institute and Professor of Medicine (Cardiology) at the UMass Chan Medical School.

Over the past 30 years, Dr. Rippe has established and run the largest research organization in the world exploring how daily habits and actions impact short- and long-term health and quality of life. This organization, Rippe Lifestyle Institute (RLI), has published hundreds of papers that form the scientific basis for the fields of lifestyle medicine, risk factor reduction, and high-performance health. Rippe Lifestyle Institute also conducts numerous studies every year on physical activity, nutrition, and healthy weight management. Dr. Rippe has written over 500 academic papers and abstracts and written or edited 62 books, including 39 for health care professionals and 23 for the general public.

Dr. Rippe is the editor of the major academic textbook in lifestyle medicine with the eponymous name *Lifestyle Medicine* (4th edition, CRC Press, 2024). The first edition of this textbook, which was published in 1999, named the field "lifestyle medicine" in the academic literature. Dr. Rippe is the editor-in-chief of the *American Journal of Lifestyle Medicine,* the only academic journal in lifestyle medicine. Dr. Rippe is also the editor-in-chief of the *Lifestyle Medicine Series,* which is a series of smaller, single-topic books. Currently, 13 books have been published in this series with four more anticipated in the next 18 months. Dr. Rippe is also the senior editor of the major intensive care medicine textbook in the United States (*Irwin and Rippe's Intensive Care Medicine*), which is now in its 9th edition.

Dr. Rippe has won numerous awards for his work and publications. Two of his books on fitness walking won American Health Magazine Book Awards, and he was one of ten Healthy American Fitness leaders named by the President's Council on Physical Fitness and Sports. He won Lifetime Achievement Awards from the International Dance, Exercise Association, and the Lifestyle Medicine University. He also received the Annual Trail Blazer Award from the American College of Lifestyle Medicine in 2024.

A lifelong and avid athlete, Dr. Rippe maintains his personal fitness with a regular walk, jog, swimming, and weight training program. He holds a black belt in karate and is an avid windsurfer, skier, and tennis player. He lives outside of Boston with his wife, television news anchor, Stephanie Hart, and their four children, Hart, Jaelin, Devon, and Jamie.

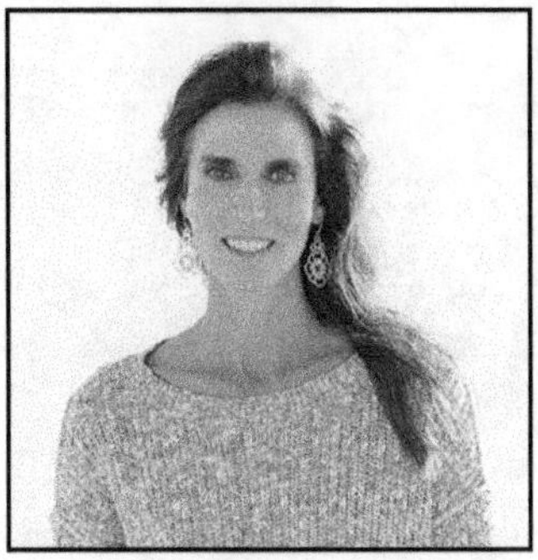

Beth Frates, MD, is a trained physiatrist and a health and wellness coach, with expertise in Lifestyle Medicine. She has received several teaching accolades from Harvard Extension School and Harvard Medical School, where she is an associate professor, part-time. Most recently, in spring 2025, Dr. Frates received the Petra Shattuck Excellence in Teaching Award.

Dr. Frates is one of the first women to be recognized as a Fellow of the American College of Lifestyle Medicine, and she is a pioneer in lifestyle medicine. In 2008, Dr. Frates created the first Lifestyle Medicine Interest Group at Harvard Medical School. In 2014, she developed and taught a bachelor's and master's level Lifestyle Medicine curriculum at the Harvard Extension School, which is still one of the most well-received courses offered at the school. In 2017, Dr. Frates was selected to be one of four item writers for the American Board of Lifestyle Medicine's inaugural exam for certification in this specialty. She was voted President of the American College of Lifestyle Medicine in August 2020. Dr. Frates served as President until November 2024 and now serves two years as Immediate Past President.

Dr. Frates co-authored *The Lifestyle Medicine Handbook: An Introduction to the Power of Healthy Habits*, which was ranked in the top 20 by Book Authority for medical books released in 2018. To accompany the syllabus and handbook, she also co-created *Lifestyle Medicine 101*, a full bachelor's- and master's-level curriculum with 12 modules of material, including PowerPoints for each week and a teacher's manual. Dr. Frates has made this resource free, and it is accessible through the ACLM website. In addition, Dr. Frates co-authored *The Teen Lifestyle Medicine Handbook*, published in October 2020, which, when paired with the Teen Curriculum consisting of a teacher's manual and 12 PowerPoint decks, can be used to teach and empower middle school and high school students to adopt and sustain healthy habits. In 2023, Dr. Frates co-authored *The Lifestyle Medicine Pocket Guide* and co-edited the book *Empowering Behavior Change in Patients*. Most recently, in June 2024, she co-edited the book *Essentials of Clinical Nutrition in Healthcare*.

Dr. Frates has created and implemented a 12-step wellness program, PAVING the Path to Wellness™ for patients and providers. Most recently, she co-authored the book *PAVING the Path to Wellness Workbook: A Guide to Thriving with a Healthy Body, Peaceful Mind and Joyful Heart*. In addition, Dr. Frates has her own Lifestyle Medicine consulting/coaching practice where she sees patients 1:1 and in groups.

1 Overview of the Evidence Base for Academic Lifestyle Medicine

1.1 INTRODUCTION

Robust evidence supports the linkage between the fundamental tenets of lifestyle medicine and their role in lowering risk, and, in some instances, assisting in the treatment of chronic disease (1,2).

This evidence base is supported by literally thousands of studies and is incorporated into the evidence-based guidelines of virtually every metabolic disease expert panel for both children and adults (see the next section).

In addition, the World Health Organization (WHO) has launched a major strategy on daily habits and actions as key components of its initiative to combat non-communicable diseases (NCDs) (3). The WHO states that 74% of all mortality each year comes from NCDs.

While most physicians generally know that strong evidence exists for exercise, nutrition, weight management, and other components of lifestyle medicine, many are unaware that this evidence has now been combined into a field named "lifestyle medicine."

It is a source of great chagrin for both of us that so few physicians have embraced the evidence supporting the major components of lifestyle medicine. Physicians have adopted the mantra that we practice "evidence-based medicine." The enormous evidence that supports the daily lifestyle habits and actions comprising lifestyle medicine, and their impact on health, is sadly underappreciated and underutilized in mainstream medicine. The purpose of this book, and the embedded curriculum, is to provide physicians with the robust evidence that underlies lifestyle medicine. This evidence will serve as the foundation for the curriculum, which is geared toward multiple levels of physician education.

Unfortunately, the failure to fully embrace this evidence has significant adverse impacts on patient care. For example, in the area of nutrition, studies have indicated that only 21% of patients feel they receive adequate nutritional advice from their physician (4). It is not surprising that physicians do not actively counsel their patients in this area, as there is very little training in medical school, residency, or fellowship in nutrition and exercise. In fact, less than 20% of medical schools offer a nutrition course (5) and only 14% of individuals who graduate from medical school feel they have adequate nutritional knowledge (6). In the field of cardiology, it is shocking that 90% of cardiologists feel they do not have adequate nutritional knowledge (7). The good news, however, is that 95% of cardiologists feel that nutritional counseling is important and try to share it with their patients.

The area of physical activity shows shockingly similar abysmal results. Only 9% of medical schools have any course offerings in physical activity (8). It is not surprising then, that in one survey of 175 primary care physicians, only 12% were aware of the recommendations of the American College of Sports Medicine (ACSM) related to physical activity (9). Another survey of 51 internal medicine residents reported that 88% felt confident in their knowledge of the benefits of exercise, yet only 25% demonstrated adequate knowledge that would be useful in patient counseling (10).

All of these unfortunate results reflect that there is inadequate education among physicians within the multiple evidence-based pillars of lifestyle medicine. This inadequate education does

DOI: 10.1201/9781003630043-1

not reflect a lack of interest on the part of medical students and physicians. For example, in a recent survey of 1,000 physicians, only 13.5% agreed or strongly agreed that they were adequately trained to discuss nutrition with their patients (11). A significant majority (78.4%), however, felt that additional training in nutrition would help them provide better clinical care for the prevention of cardiovascular disease.

Interestingly, when physicians were asked to rate various therapies for CVD on a scale of 1–10 (with 10 being the most important), they rated nutrition at 8.1+2.05 and physical activity at 8.2+1.06. Both of these were higher than statins 7.8+2.11!

Unfortunately, the lack of education in lifestyle practices and habits persists through residency and fellowship. For example, over 90% of cardiologists report receiving minimal education in physical activity and nutrition during their fellowship training. Only 8% describe themselves as having "expert" knowledge in nutrition (7). This is despite the fact that in 2013, the Practice Guidelines released by the American Heart Association (AHA) and the American College of Cardiology (ACC), which were entitled the "AHA/ACC Guideline on Lifestyle Management to Reduce Cardiovascular Risk" (12) recommended nutritional counseling as a key component of the practice of cardiology. Moreover, the evidence-based guidelines issued by the ACC and AHA, both for lipid management (13) and for the detection and treatment of high blood pressure (14), strongly recommend dietary intervention as a key component for managing these CVD risk factors.

Some organizations have now started to train physicians and other health care professionals in the area of lifestyle medicine. For example, the American College of Lifestyle Medicine (ACLM) has developed educational materials for medical schools, residencies, and fellowships to help fill the gaps in physician knowledge in this area (15). Moreover, the Academy of Geriatrics, the American College of Preventive Medicine, the American Academy of Pediatrics, the American Academy of Orthopaedic Surgeons, and the American Psychiatric Association have all issued statements encouraging their members to address physical activity as well as other components of lifestyle medicine. Both of us are lifelong exercisers and strongly support these efforts!

In the area of nutrition, the Food is Medicine initiative, which has been sponsored by the National Institutes of Health (NIH), Robert Wood Johnson Foundation, and other organizations provides hope that we can make headway in educating physicians in nutrition (16). In the area of physical activity, the Exercise is Medicine (17) initiative, sponsored by the ACSM, provides another area where physician education is occurring at a higher level.

The evidence base provided by Dr. Rippe's *Lifestyle Medicine* textbook (4th edition, CRC Press, 2024) offers a wide range of scientific proof supporting the concepts behind lifestyle medicine based on the expert advice of over 325 contributors (1). Moreover, the *American Journal of Lifestyle Medicine* (also edited by Dr. Rippe) has over 25,000 subscribers and, in 2024, had over 325,000 downloads of full-text articles (18). These are current efforts to enhance physician knowledge about the robust and wide-ranging evidence base behind lifestyle medicine.

1.2 THE RELATIONSHIP OF LIFESTYLE MEDICINE AND GUIDELINES FOR THE PREVENTION AND TREATMENT OF THE METABOLIC DISEASE

The concept of lifestyle medicine was designed to provide an umbrella for physicians with an opportunity to review multiple areas of guidelines in one convenient place. It is important to emphasize, however, that the individual guidelines themselves upon which the lifestyle medicine pillars are based contain very strong evidence supporting the tenets of lifestyle medicine. These guidelines and scientific statements, which have been promulgated over the last 20 years by expert consensus panels, consistently recommend regular physical activity, proper nutrition, weight management, avoidance of risky substances, stress reduction, and healthy sleep to lower the risk of chronic disease or assist in its treatment.

These foundational guidelines span a wide range of organizations and consensus statements in the area of metabolic disease. They include multiple statements from the ACC/AHA, the Institute of Medicine, the American Diabetes Association (ADA), the Dietary Guidelines for Americans 2020–2025 (DGA 2020–2025), the Physical Activity Guidelines for Americans 2018 (PAGA 2018), guidelines from the American Academy of Pediatrics (AAP), the American Cancer Society (ACS), the American Stroke Association (ASA), and many others (19). Some of these guidelines are listed in Table 1.1.

The critical underlying point is to emphasize that the field of lifestyle medicine did not invent any of these concepts. Rather, lifestyle medicine serves as an umbrella framework, bringing evidence-based guidelines from prestigious organizations and panels together in one convenient place for physicians. The underlying robust evidence behind lifestyle medicine emanates from virtually every authoritative panel and organization that has promulgated guidelines for either the reduction or treatment of metabolic disease.

TABLE 1.1
Examples of Consensus Statements from Expert Panels in Various Metabolic Diseases That Emphasize Lifestyle Medicine Principles and Practices

- JNC VIII Guidelines for Hypertension, Prevention and Treatment
- ACC/AHA Guidelines for the Prevention, Detection, Evaluation, and Treatment of High Blood Pressure 2018
- NCEP (ATP IV) Guidelines for Blood Cholesterol
- Institute of Medicine Guidelines for Obesity Treatment
- ACC/AHA Scientific Consensus Statement of the Treatment for Blood Cholesterol
- Guidelines from the American Diabetes Association for the Management of Diabetes
- Dietary Guidelines for Americans 2020–2025
- American Heart Association Nutrition Implementation Guidelines
- Guidelines from the American Academy of Pediatrics for the Prevention and Treatment of Childhood Obesity
- Guidelines from the American Academy of Pediatrics for the Treatment of Pediatric Blood Pressure
- Guidelines from the American Academy of Pediatrics for the Treatment of Lipids
- Guidelines from the American Heart Association and the American Academy of Pediatrics for the Prevention and Treatment of the Metabolic Syndrome
- American Heart Association Strategic Plan for 2020
- Joint Statement from the American Heart Association and the American Cancer Society for the Prevention of Heart Disease and Cancer
- Presidential Advisory from the AHA and the American Stroke Association
- AHA/ACC/TOS Guideline for the Management of Overweight and Obesity in Adults
- ACS/ADA/AHA Scientific Statement on Preventing Cancer, Cardiovascular Disease and Diabetes
- Physical Activity Guidelines Advisory Committee Report of 2018
- The AHA/ACC Guidelines for the Management of Blood Cholesterol
- Adult Treatment Panel from the Expert Panel on Detection, Evaluation, and Treatment of High Blood Cholesterol in Adults
- 2013 AHA/ACC Guideline on Lifestyle Management to Reduce Cardiovascular Risk
- Recommendations for Cardiovascular Health and Disease Surveillance for 2030 and Beyond: A Policy Statement from the American Heart Association
- 2021 American Heart Association (AHA) Scientific Statement on Dietary Guidance to Improve Cardiovascular Health
- The AHA Guidelines for Detection, Evaluation, and Treatment of High Blood Pressure
- World Health Organization Executive Summary for the Non-Communicable Disease Initiative

Examples of the Use of Lifestyle Medicine Principles and Practices in Expert Consensus Statements in Metabolic Disease.

Source: Adapted from Rippe JM (ed), *Lifestyle Medicine*, 4th ed, CRC Press, Boca Raton) FL, 2024. With permission.

1.3 EVIDENCE SUPPORTING THE BENEFIT OF POSITIVE LIFESTYLE FACTORS TO REDUCE THE RISK OF CHRONIC DISEASE

As already indicated, what individuals do in their daily lives has enormous power to impact their health either positively or negatively. Thus, the pillars of lifestyle medicine have been chosen because they contain the highest level of evidence supporting the power of daily habits and actions to reduce the risk of chronic disease. Each of these factors will be listed as a separate chapter in the first section of this book and subsequently combined in the second section of this book to underscore how they act synergistically to lower the risk and/or assist in the treatment of various chronic diseases. These lifestyle factors include the following:

- Physical Activity
- Healthy Nutrition
- Weight Management
- Avoidance of Risky Substances
- Stress Reduction
- Healthy Sleep
- Positive Interactions with Other People

Let's take a brief look at each of these. Each of these will be discussed in depth in individual chapters in Part 1 of this book.

- *Physical Activity*: Regular physical activity has been demonstrated to reduce the risk of CVD, type 2 diabetes, metabolic syndrome, obesity, and certain forms of cancer (20). This message is supported by an enormous body of evidence assembled in the Physical Activity Guidelines Advisory Committee Scientific Report 2018 (21). In addition, physical activity has been shown to prevent or minimize excessive weight gain, lower the risk of dementia, improve other aspects of cognitive function, and promote healthy sleep.
- *Healthy Nutrition*: Healthy nutrition plays multiple roles in reducing the risk of chronic disease (22). For example, there is strong evidence for the role of healthy nutrition in reducing the risk of CVD, diabetes (T2DM), obesity, cancer, and many other conditions. Guidelines for healthy nutrition have been promulgated by multiple organizations including the DGAs 2020–2025, the AHA (23), the ADA (24), and the Academy of Nutrition and Dietetics (AND) (25), among others. These guidelines are consistent in recommending increased consumption of fruits and vegetables, whole grains, fish, non-fat or low-fat dairy, legumes, and nuts. Furthermore, the guidelines uniformly recommend reduction in red meat, processed meats, refined grains, sugar-sweetened foods, and saturated and trans fats. In contrast, recent evidence has shown that the typical American diet is inflammatory and contributes to multiple diseases that are united by the underlying etiology of inflammation.
- *Weight Management*: In many ways, overweight and obesity represent quintessential lifestyle diseases. Unfortunately, the United States is undergoing an epidemic of overweight and obesity. Over 72% of all adults in the United States are either overweight or obese (26). Obesity was once thought to be mostly a cosmetic issue. Fat cells (adipocytes) were once thought to function basically as passive storage cells for extra fat. Now adipocytes have been clearly shown to produce multiple inflammatory factors.
- *Avoiding Addictive Substances*: Avoiding tobacco products and excessive consumption of alcohol are key components of the WHO initiative to combat non-communicable diseases (27). Opioids and cannabis overuse also represent ongoing or emerging threats to people's health both in the United States and worldwide.
- *Stress Reduction*: Recent data have shown that over 30% of individuals in the United States suffer from enough stress in their daily lives to hinder their performance at work or at

home (28). Multiple mind/body therapies are available to assist in the treatment of stress. These will be outlined in Chapter 5.

- *Healthy Sleep*: Sleep has frequently not been recognized as a potent risk factor underlying chronic disease. There are over 100 different sleep disorders (29). Perhaps the most prominent is obstructive sleep apnea, which is responsible for 20%–40% of all hypertension. Sleep problems are associated with 30%–40% of all CVD. This is such an important topic that the AHA recently added sleep to its mantra of "Life's Essential 8." This is a framework for simple steps that people can utilize in their daily lives to lower their risk of heart disease.
- *Positive Interactions with Others*: There has been a recent increase in research in the area of the health-promoting power of positive relationships with other people. The former US Surgeon General Vivek Murthy has, in fact, written a Surgeon General's Advisory and a book focused on this. Dr. Murthy has cited evidence that loneliness represents a risk factor as potent as obesity or smoking half a pack of cigarettes per day (30).

1.4 WHAT IS LIFESTYLE MEDICINE?

One of us (JMR) had the privilege of naming the field of "lifestyle medicine" in 1999 in the academic literature with the first edition of his eponymously titled book *Lifestyle Medicine*. Lifestyle medicine was defined in this book as "the discipline of studying how daily habits and practices impact the prevention and treatment of disease often in conjunction with pharmaceutical or surgical therapy to provide an important adjunct to overall health" (31).

While there have been a number of subsequent frameworks and definitions basically utilizing this concept, it is clear that the field is going to coalesce around the term "lifestyle medicine." For example, the AHA changed the name of one of its councils from the "Council on Nutrition, Physical Activity and Metabolism" to the "Council on Lifestyle and Cardiometabolic Health" in 2013 (32). In addition, also in 2013, the AHA and ACC issued guidelines entitled "Guideline for Lifestyle Management to Reduce Cardiovascular Risk." Multiple organizations including the American Academy of Family Practice (AAFP), the American College of Preventive Medicine (ACPM), and others, have adopted lifestyle medicine as the rubric under which recommendations about the power of daily habits and actions are promulgated. Importantly, the ACLM has been formed and is the fastest-growing health care organization in the world, now reaching over 13,000 members (12).

Despite the robust growth of lifestyle medicine as outlined above, the field is still relatively unknown among mainstream physicians. In fact, one of us (JMR) gave a grand rounds presentation to a group of 500 physicians at a major teaching hospital, and only a handful had ever heard of lifestyle medicine. A series of lectures given by one of us (JMR) to internal medicine residents indicated that only 5% had ever heard of the concept of lifestyle medicine.

We hope that by generating the evidence-based curriculum found in this book, we will engage and educate mainstream medical practitioners in ways that will lead them to utilize the powerful modalities of lifestyle medicine to enhance the health of their patients.

1.5 LINKAGE BETWEEN LIFESTYLE MEDICINE PREMISES AND PRACTICES AND REDUCTION OF RISK OF CHRONIC DISEASE

As already indicated, robust evidence exists linking the daily habits and actions that form the pillars of lifestyle medicine to reduced risk of chronic disease. This issue will be discussed in detail through the lens of each of the pillars of lifestyle medicine in Part 1 of this book. In Part 2 of this book, we will take an in-depth look at many of the chronic diseases where lifestyle medicine habits and practices, when used in combination, have been shown to lower risk factors or assist in treatment. These diseases include coronary heart disease (CHD), T2DM and pre-diabetes, cancer, obesity, metabolic syndrome, cognitive decline and Alzheimer's disease. In addition, in Part 2, we will provide an in-depth analysis of how these issues relate to individuals over the age of 65, children, and women. In Part 3 of this book, we embed this information in an evidence-based curriculum for physicians at all levels of training.

1.6 THE ROLE OF PHYSICIANS IN PRESCRIBING LIFESTYLE MEDICINE MODALITIES

We hope that the evidence-based curriculum we have developed will provide physicians with the tools that they need in order to prescribe lifestyle medicine modalities and practices to their patients. A large number of physicians already exists who are utilizing the framework of lifestyle medicine as the core organizing principle for their practice. We recognize, however, that for many physicians practicing in mainstream medicine, this is not likely to occur. Rather, we hope that individuals in mainstream medicine will initially adopt at least one or two of the pillars of lifestyle medicine and focus on those issues in their counseling of patients, with the goal of ultimately expanding this concept to include all seven pillars. Good places to start would be either physical activity or nutrition.

In Part 2 of this book, we will provide not only an in-depth look at how daily lifestyle habits and practices impact the reduction of risk and treatment of various chronic diseases, but in addition, we will provide a section at the end of each chapter offering specific recommendations for how physicians can counsel patients in these areas in as little as five minutes.

We hope that by utilizing the curriculum found in Part 3 more physicians will engage in counseling patients in the area of lifestyle medicine modalities and practices. As already indicated, only 40% of physicians are currently engaged in this type of counseling (33). This is clearly a missed opportunity since between 70% and 75% of patients see their primary care physician on at least an annual basis. Moreover, there is also strong evidence that physicians who adopt these habits and actions in their own lives are more likely to counsel their patients in these areas. We also hope that an added benefit of the curriculum we present in this book will provide physicians with the impetus to adopt some, or preferably many, of the pillars of lifestyle medicine in their own lives.

Enormous data exist concerning the benefits that a combination of lifestyle medicine practices and habits can bring to reduce the risk of both heart disease and diabetes. For example, in the Nurses Health Trial (34), which is an ongoing study of over 110,000 largely female nurses, individuals who adopted five simple practices, namely: 30 minutes of physical activity on at least five days per week, healthy nutrition including increased consumption of fruits, vegetables, and whole grains, weight management (BMI between 19 and 25 kg/m^2), not smoking cigarettes, and, most controversially, consuming one alcoholic beverage a day, lowered their risk of heart disease by 83% and the risk of diabetes by 91%. The US Health Professionals Study (largely male physicians) has shown very similar results for males (35).

It is interesting to note that adoption of only one of these positive lifestyle habits and actions cut the risk of heart disease and diabetes by 50%. Sadly, only 5% of nurses, physicians, and other health care workers in these two major studies adopted all five of these habits and practices. We hope that the curriculum we present here will encourage physicians and other health care workers to adopt more positive habits in their own lives. Not only will their own health benefit, but it will also increase the likelihood that they will utilize this information in their counseling of patients.

1.7 THE NEED FOR AN EVIDENCE-BASED CURRICULUM IN LIFESTYLE MEDICINE

Some organizations have begun to develop educational materials for health care providers who are already deeply committed to lifestyle medicine. These curricula, while important, have a fundamentally different emphasis than what we intend to accomplish with this book and curriculum.

We hope and believe that by expanding and categorizing the profound evidence behind lifestyle medicine, more mainstream physicians will be motivated to understand what lifestyle medicine is all about and utilize at least portions of it in their daily practices. This is the major strategy behind the curriculum presented in this book.

1.8 CONCLUSIONS

It is clear that many physicians in mainstream medicine are either not familiar with the field of lifestyle medicine or are not utilizing the power of these modalities in their daily practices. The good news is that many physicians have already strongly indicated that they would welcome and benefit from more education in these areas and are seeking convenient ways to obtain this knowledge. It is important to understand that these individuals will be motivated largely through an understanding of the strong health-promoting evidence that lies behind lifestyle medicine. In addition, they will need tools to encourage them to adopt counseling strategies in these areas within the context of busy clinical practices. An added benefit is that physicians who utilize this curriculum will also benefit from the health-promoting effects of adopting these habits and strategies in their lives and thereby substantially improve their own health.

REFERENCES

1. Rippe JM. *Lifestyle Medicine* (4th ed). Boca Raton, FL: CRC Press, 2024.
2. Rippe JM. Lifestyle medicine: the health promoting power of daily habits and practices. *Am J Lifestyle Med.* 2018;12(6):499–512. Epub 2019/02/21.
3. World Health Organization on Non-Communicable Diseases. https://www.who.int/news/item/17-10-2018-who-launches-active-a-toolkit-for-countries-to-increase-physical-activity-and-reduce-noncommunicable-diseases. Accessed October 22, 2024.
4. Rippe JM. Physician education and lifestyle medicine: a key to the future. *Am.J Lifestyle Med.* 2024;0(0).
5. Frates B. The evolving state of nutrition education. *Am J Lifestyle Med.* 2023;17(6):759–761.
6. Nestle M, Baron RB. Nutrition in medical education: from counting hours to measuring competence. *JAMA Intern Med.* 2014;174(6):843–844.
7. Devries S, Agatston A, Aggarwal M, et al. A deficiency of nutrition education and practice in cardiology. *Am J Med.* 2017;130(11):1298–1305.
8. Rippe JM. The role of physicians in promoting and prescribing increases in physical activity. In Rippe JM (ed.) *Lifestyle Medicine* (4th ed). Boca Raton, FL: CRC Press, 2024.
9. Walsh JM, Swangard DM, Davis T, et al. Exercise counseling by primary care physicians in the era of managed care. *Am J Prev Med.* 1999;16(4):307–313.
10. Rogers LQ, Gutin B, Humphries MC, et al. Evaluation of internal medicine residents as exercise role models and associations with self-reported counseling behavior, confidence, and perceived success. *Teach Learn Med.* 2006;18(3):215–221.
11. Kushner RF, Van Horn L, Rock CL, et al. Nutrition education in medical school: a time of opportunity. *Am J Clin Nutr.* 2014;99(5 Suppl):1167S–1173S.
12. Eckel RH, Jakicic JM, Ard JD, et al. 2013 AHA/ACC guideline on lifestyle management to reduce cardiovascular risk. *Circulation.* 2014;129(25_suppl_2):S76–S99.
13. Grundy SM, Stone NJ, Bailey AL, et al. 2018 AHA/ACC/AACVPR/AAPA/ABC/ACPM/ADA/AGS/APhA/ASPC/NLA/PCNA guideline on the management of blood cholesterol: a report of the American College of Cardiology/American Heart Association Task Force on Clinical Practice Guidelines. *J Am Coll Cardiol.* 2019;73(24):e285–e350.
14. Whelton PK, Carey RM, Aronow WS, et al. 2017 ACC/AHA/AAPA/ABC/ACPM/AGS/APhA/ASH/ASPC/NMA/PCNA guideline for the prevention, detection, evaluation, and management of high blood pressure in adults: executive summary: a report of the American College of Cardiology/American Heart Association Task Force on Clinical Practice Guidelines. *Hypertension.* 2018;71(6):1269–1324.
15. American College of Lifestyle Medicine. https://lifestylemedicine.org/. Accessed October 22, 2024.
16. FoodisMedicine.https://odphp.health.gov/our-work/nutrition-physical-activity/food-medicine.Accessed October 22, 2024.
17. ACSM Exercise is Medicine. https://www.exerciseismedicine.org/. Accessed October 22, 2024.

18. *The American Journal of Lifestyle Medicine*. https://journals.sagepub.com/home/ajl. Accessed October 22, 2024.
19. Rippe JM. Preface. In Rippe JM (ed.) *Lifestyle Medicine* (4th ed). Boca Raton, FL: CRC Press, 2024.
20. Rippe JM. Lifestyle strategies for risk factor reduction, prevention, and treatment of cardiovascular disease. *Am J Lifestyle Med*. 2019;13(2):204–212.
21. Physical Activity Guidelines Advisory Committee. 2018 Physical Activity Guidelines Advisory Committee Scientific Report. Washington, DC: U.S. Department of Health and Human Services, 2018.
22. U.S. Department of Agriculture and U.S. Department of Health and Human Services. U.S. Department of Agriculture and U.S. Department of Health and Human Services. Dietary guidelines for Americans, 2020–2025 (9th ed). December 2020. DietaryGuidelines.gov. https://www.dietaryguidelines.gov/resources/2020-2025-dietary-guidelines-online-materials.
23. Lichtenstein AH, Appel LJ, Vadiveloo M, et al. 2021 dietary guidance to improve cardiovascular health: a scientific statement from the American Heart Association. *Circulation*. 2021;144(23):e472–e487.
24. American Diabetes Association. Lifestyle management: standards of medical care in diabetes 2019. *Diabetes Care*. 2019;42(Suppl. 1):S46–S60.
25. The Academy of Nutrition and Dietetics. https://www.eatright.org/. Accessed October 23, 2024.
26. National Center for Health Statistics. United States, 2016: With Chartbook on Long-term Trends in Health. Hyattsville, MD: National Center for Health Statistics, 2017.
27. World Health Organization. Global Non Communicable Disease Compact 2020–2030. https://www.who.int/initiatives/global-noncommunicable-diseases-compact-2020-2030.
28. Ramchandani S, Loiselle E, Proszynski J, et al. Behavioral approaches to manage stress. In Rippe JM (ed.) *Lifestyle Medicine* (4th ed). Boca Raton, FL: CRC Press, 2024.
29. Office of Disease Prevention and Health Promotion. Sleep Health. US Department of Health and Human Services. Washington, DC: Sleep Health, Healthy People, 2020.
30. Murthy V. *Together: The Healing Power of Human Connection in a Sometimes Lonely World*. New York: Harper, 2020.
31. Rippe JM. *Lifestyle Medicine*. London: Blackwell Science, Inc., 1999.
32. American Heart Association. https://www.heart.org/. Accessed October 22, 2024.
33. US Preventive Services Task Force. Behavioral counselling in primary care to promote a healthy diet: recommendations and rationale. *Am J Prev Med*. 2023;24(1):93–100.
34. Liu S, Stampfer MJ, Hu FB, et al. Whole-grain consumption and risk of coronary heart disease: results from the Nurses' Health Study. *Am J Clin Nutr*. 1999;70:412–419.
35. Chiuve SE, McCullough ML, Sacks FM, et al. Healthy lifestyle factors in the primary prevention of coronary heart disease among men: benefits among users and nonusers of lipid-lowering and antihypertensive medications. *Circulation*. 2006;114(2):160–167.

2 Physical Activity

2.1 INTRODUCTION

We open Part 1 on the evidence behind the various pillars of lifestyle medicine with a discussion of physical activity. We start with this for a number of reasons.

Among the various important practices that individuals can perform in their lives, perhaps no single lifestyle habit or practice is more powerfully associated with improved long-term health and quality of life than regular physical activity. An enormous and compelling literature exists that has been generated over the past several decades relating moderate or vigorous physical activity to reduced risk of developing chronic disease (1,2). Regular physical activity also significantly improves quality of life and sleep. In addition to reducing the risk of chronic disease, regular physical activity also plays a very important role in the treatment of chronic disease (see Figure 2.1).

In this chapter, we will focus specifically on the known health benefits of physical activity. We will revisit this again in somewhat less depth in the second section of this book, when we talk about the various combinations of lifestyle medicine modalities for specific chronic diseases. In that context, regular physical activity will be linked to proper nutrition, weight management, avoiding tobacco, etc., with an overall approach to lowering the risk of chronic disease.

Numerous professional organizations have issued guidelines supporting the multiple health benefits of regular physical activity. These include the American Heart Association (AHA) (3,4), the American Academy of Pediatrics (AAP), the American Diabetes Association (ADA) (5), and the Physical Activity Guidelines for Americans 2018 (PAGA 2018) (1), as well as many others. In addition, regular physical activity is the cornerstone of the recommendations for both Healthy People 2020 (6) and Healthy People 2030 (7).

The benefits of regular physical activity extend throughout the lifespan and are also very important for the reduction of risk and treatment of various chronic diseases. Many organizations have

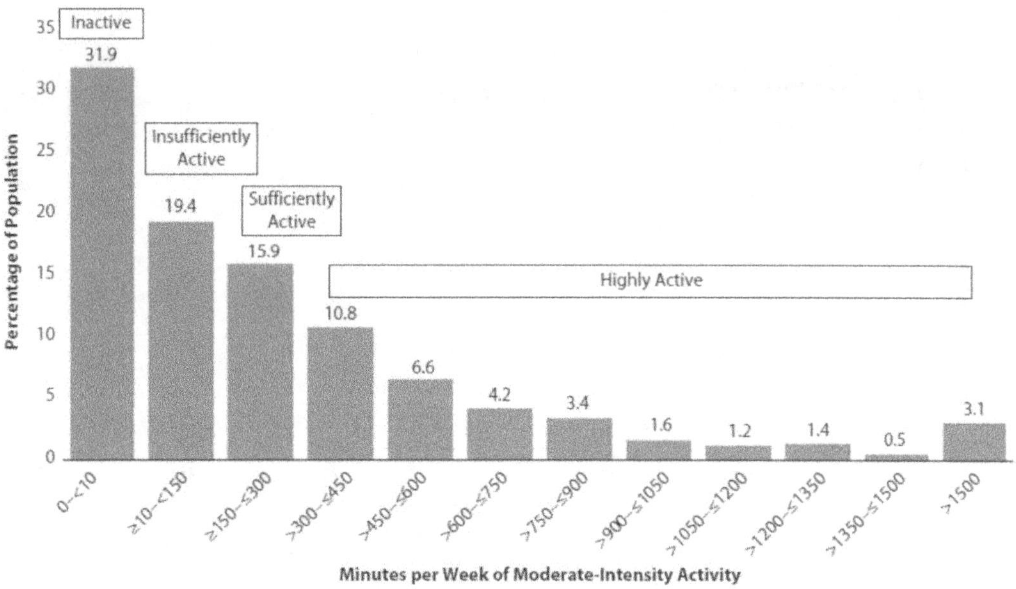

FIGURE 2.1 Distribution of moderate-to-vigorous physical activity.

DOI: 10.1201/9781003630043-2

played significant roles in advancing the understanding of the field of physical activity. These include the American College of Sports Medicine (ACSM) (8), the American College of Lifestyle Medicine (ACLM) (9), as well as the AHA, ADA, and many others.

While the evidence supporting the health benefits of regular physical activity is profound, the medical community has been slow to embrace this concept as an important component of regular healthcare and counseling. It is estimated that less than 40% of physicians regularly counsel their patients on the importance of regular physical activity (10). This clearly is a missed opportunity, since over 70% of people see their primary care physician on at least an annual basis.

The American public has also been slow to embrace the habit of regular physical activity. The Centers for Disease Control (CDC) estimates that fewer than 25% of adults in the United States meet the recommended levels of physical activity (11). These recommendations include 30 minutes of moderate-intensity physical activity on five days per week (accumulating 150 minutes of moderate-intensity physical activity per week) or 75 minutes of vigorous physical activity per week. In addition, and often ignored, all of these organizations also recommend two or three sessions of musculoskeletal strength training per week for reasons that we will discuss later on in this chapter.

For all of these reasons, it is important that physicians recommend physical activity to all patients, even those with chronic illnesses where some modifications may be necessary. In Part 3 of this book, we will outline the best ways to perform brief counseling sessions to emphasize physical activity for all patients.

2.2 CURRENT LEVELS OF PHYSICAL ACTIVITY IN THE UNITED STATES

As already indicated, only 25% of adults in the United States obtain the recommended amount of physical activity to yield health benefits according to the CDC. This can be further segmented into what levels of physical activity various percentages of the population achieve. As documented in the PAGA 2018, over 30% of the adult population is very inactive, and another 25% are insufficiently active (1). These data are depicted in Figure 2.2.

The PAGA 2018 also summarizes the recommendations with the simple phrase "Some is better than none" to underscore that inactivity exerts health hazards and to encourage everyone to be more active. Thus, the major target is to get those people who are truly inactive to be more active.

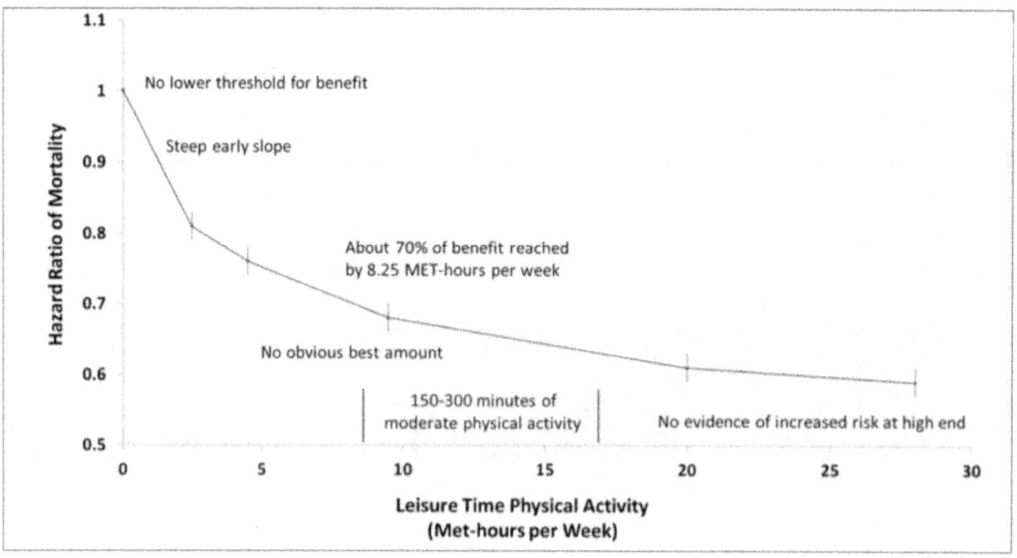

FIGURE 2.2

2.3 THE RELATIONSHIP BETWEEN MODERATE AND VIGOROUS PHYSICAL ACTIVITY AND CHRONIC DISEASE

Enormous data support the concept that individuals who are physically active decrease their risk of multiple chronic diseases, which will be described later in this chapter. Regular physical activity can also assist in the treatment of a variety of chronic diseases. Some of the benefits of regular physical activity can occur after a single bout of exercise; others require consistent physical activity throughout the lifespan. It is important to understand that the benefits of physical activity can occur in very young children, as young as three years old, and continue to individuals over the age of 65. Some of the multiple benefits of physical activity related to health benefits are documented in the PAGA 2018 Scientific Report.

In addition to lowering the risk of chronic diseases, there is a robust relationship between regular physical activity and improved quality of life. Individuals who are physically active experience less anxiety, depression, and stress and, in general, feel and sleep better. All of these benefits contribute to an improved quality of life and also promote longevity. There are so many benefits of regular physical activity that some investigators have likened it to a "polypill" that contributes to virtually every aspect of health. Thus, the recommendation for physicians to counsel patients on increased physical activity represents one of the most important and evidence-based modalities in all of lifestyle medicine.

2.4 PHYSICAL ACTIVITY AND CHRONIC DISEASES

2.4.1 Cardiovascular Disease

Hundreds of studies show that regular physical activity significantly reduces the risk of both cardiovascular disease (CVD) and all-cause mortality. Numerous organizations, including ACSM, AHA, ACLM, and PAGA 2018, all recommend 150 minutes of moderate-intensity physical activity per week as well as two to three strength-training sessions per week to substantially lower the risk of all-cause mortality (1–5). This recommendation is depicted in Figure 2.2.

While minor additional reductions in mortality can occur in individuals who engage in physical activity over 150 minutes per week, the additional benefit in terms of reduction in all-cause and cardiovascular mortality is very small. The important concept depicted in this figure emphasizes that sedentary individuals derive important benefits even with relatively small amounts of physical activity. This is depicted on the left-hand side of the graph which shows that there is no lower threshold for benefit and that there is a "steep early slope." Indeed, sedentary individuals who begin to exercise only 30 minutes per week achieve a 20% reduction in risk of cardiovascular disease.

When individuals who are physically active are compared for risk of CVD with sedentary individuals, sedentary individuals are at 150%–240% higher risk (1,12). Thus, a sedentary lifestyle essentially doubles the risk of CVD. This is the same increased risk that individuals accept if they smoke a pack of cigarettes a day. Unfortunately, about 12% of adults in the United States still smoke a pack of cigarettes a day (13). With inactivity, however, we have a risk factor generating comparable risk for CVD to that of smoking a pack of cigarettes a day and five or six times as prevalent!

It is obvious that helping individuals who are highly inactive become more active yields enormous benefits. In addition, regular physical activity lowers the risk of adult weight gain. Physical activity also represents a powerful modality for controlling blood pressure. In addition to lowering the risk of hypertension, physical activity decreases the risk of stroke and heart failure.

For all of these reasons, it is important for physicians to counsel patients on physical activity. This is one of the reasons why we have given it such prominent emphasis in our curriculum. Unfortunately, at the current time, physicians have typically not emphasized the role of regular physical activity in reducing the risk of CVD. In fact, in one survey of 175 primary care physicians, only 12% were aware of the physical activity recommendations from ACSM and PAGA 2018 (14).

2.5 PHYSICAL ACTIVITY AND DIABETES, PRE-DIABETES, AND THE METABOLIC SYNDROME

Physical activity is one of the cornerstones of diabetes and pre-diabetes care, along with proper nutrition and weight management (15). The ADA recommendations for physical activity are similar to those of PAGA 2018.

The ADA recommends that each physical activity session should be at least 10 minutes, with the goal of 30 minutes per day. Recent data, however, have now demonstrated that even shorter bouts of physical activity interspersed throughout the day can also yield significant reductions in diabetes (T2DM) and assist in its treatment. Individuals with T2DM should also be encouraged to reduce sedentary activities. Good data show that sedentary activity is associated with an increased risk of diabetes.

The ADA recommends that medical providers should obtain a history of cardiovascular risk factors in individuals with T2DM prior to recommending a program of physical activity and should customize a physical activity regimen for individual needs. We will emphasize this in our physical activity recommendations. Individuals should start slowly and gradually increase the amount of physical activity if they have been sedentary. Proper footwear is particularly important in individuals with diabetes because of the risk of potentially developing foot ulcers from ill-fitting shoes.

It should also be stressed that physical activity plays an important role in reducing the risk of pre-diabetes turning into T2DM. The Diabetes Prevention Program (DPP) (16) and the Da Qing Study (17), as well as the Finnish Diabetes Prevention Study (18), all showed significant reduction in progression to T2DM in individuals with pre-diabetes who engage in regular physical activity and lost 5–7 pounds. In the DPP, these modalities reduced the risk of pre-diabetes advancing to T2DM by 58%. It is also important to note that 80% of individuals over the age of 70 have pre-diabetes. Several studies, however, have now suggested that only 9% of these individuals will proceed to develop diabetes over a seven-year period. Nonetheless, these recent studies have underscored the importance of regular physical activity in individuals with both pre-diabetes and T2DM.

2.6 PHYSICAL ACTIVITY, WEIGHT GAIN, AND OBESITY

It is now estimated that 73% of adults in the United States are either overweight (body mass index ≥25, ≤30 kg/m^2), or obese (body mass index ≥30 kg/m^2), or severely obese (body mass index ≥35 kg/m^2) (19). Regular physical activity by itself is not highly effective for acute weight loss. However, regular physical activity has been shown in multiple studies to reduce the likelihood of initial weight gain and is critically important for long-term maintenance of weight loss. Thus, regular physical activity represents a very important adjunct to therapy for individuals who are even at a healthy weight and wish to lower their risk of gaining weight and potentially developing overweight or obesity and, certainly, provides a key long-term strategy for individuals who are overweight or obese.

2.7 PHYSICAL ACTIVITY AND CANCER

A number of cancers have been linked to an inactive lifestyle. Moreover, physical activity has been shown to play an important and positive role in lowering the risk of many cancers and also helping in their treatment (19). The PAGA 2018 Scientific Report greatly expanded the literature on a number of cancers where strong evidence exists that increased physical activity can play multiple positive roles. These include cancers of the gastrointestinal tract, some that are endocrine-associated and many others. Because of this information, every clinician should discuss and prescribe physical activity to cancer patients for the entire spectrum of their treatment. Physicians should not only include counseling relative to reducing the risk of developing many cancers but also discuss the benefits of physical activity in all phases of cancer prevention and treatment with all patients.

Many physicians are not aware that regular physical activity can reduce the likelihood of developing cancer, despite knowing that lifestyle is related to preventable cancers, which include such modalities as tobacco use, alcohol intake, diet, obesity, and behaviors that expose individuals to oncogenic viruses. The various lifestyle issues related to both the prevention and treatment of cancers will be discussed in more detail in the next two sections of this book.

2.8 WOMEN'S HEALTH, INCLUDING PREGNANCY

Abundant evidence exists that regular physical activity represents a critically important lifestyle behavior for women throughout their lifespan. Multiple guidelines from prestigious organizations, including the AHA, ACSM, PAGA 2018, and the American College of Obstetrics and Gynecology (ACOG), all recommend 30 minutes of moderate-intensity physical activity on most days of the week with an overall goal of accumulating 150 minutes of moderate-intensity physical activity per week (20).

These recommendations are based on numerous studies that show that women who engage in regular physical activity can reduce the risk of a variety of chronic diseases, including heart disease (21). Many physicians still are not aware that heart disease causes more deaths in women than breast cancer. In one study, women who engaged in exercise for 1.5 hours or more a week reduced their risk of heart disease by 30% (22). Moreover, regular physical activity is critically important for healthy pregnancies and for reducing weight or eliminating the extra weight gained following pregnancy (23). These issues will be discussed in more detail, along with other lifestyle factors, in Part 2 of this book.

2.9 BRAIN HEALTH AND COGNITION

Regular physical activity has been demonstrated to improve cognition and lower the risk of various forms of dementia, including Alzheimer's disease (24). This fact was emphasized in PAGA 2018 and further underscored in the Presidential Advisory from the AHA and the American Stroke Association (ASA), both of which recommended increased physical activity as a key modality for improving cognition and overall brain health. In addition, regular physical activity has been clearly shown to improve sleep and reduce feelings of anxiety and depression in healthy people as well as those who have affective symptoms.

The AHA/ASA Presidential Advisory entitled "Optimizing Brain Health" included physical activity as a key recommendation (24). It is important to emphasize that physical activity throughout a lifespan lowers the risk of cognitive decline and dementia. In fact, the only proven modality to lower the risk of Alzheimer's disease is lifelong physical activity. There are multiple theories as to why lifelong physical activity lowers the risk of cognitive decline, but it may be based on the concept of "cognitive reserve." There is also evidence that regular physical activity reduces inflammation, which is another theory for why it reduces the risk of Alzheimer's disease.

2.10 PHYSICAL ACTIVITY IN YOUTH

Physical activity guidelines for children are very important. Physical activity during childhood can start a lifelong habit (25). The PAGA 2018 guidance recommended regular physical activity for children as young as three years and onward (1). Multiple benefits accrue to children becoming involved in regular physical activity, including lowering the risk of heart disease and reducing the risk of weight gain. In addition, regular physical activity has been demonstrated to improve bone health. Muscular fitness, cognitive function, and respiratory fitness are also improved in individuals ages six through seventeen through regular physical activity.

While the curriculum in this book is focused on adults, oftentimes they will ask questions about children, so we will include at least some information about children. The PAGA 2018 document recommends 60 minutes daily of moderate-intensity physical activity for children. Thus, it is a higher recommendation than for adults.

2.11 PHYSICAL ACTIVITY IN OLDER ADULTS

Physical activity should be a priority throughout the lifetime. Multiple benefits for older adults can be derived from regular physical activity (26). Individuals in this age group are particularly susceptible to and worried about cognitive decline and dementia, both of which have been shown to be reduced in individuals who participate in regular physical activity. In addition, regular physical activity decreases the likelihood of falls and fall-related injuries. A comprehensive physical activity program should also include muscular strength and balance and flexibility exercises in addition to aerobic activities. These will all be included as recommendations later in this chapter. It may be necessary to slightly modify physical activity recommendations for people over the age of 65, particularly if they have previously been sedentary.

2.12 PHYSICAL ACTIVITY IN INDIVIDUALS WITH CHRONIC CONDITIONS

By the time an individual reaches the age of 65, they have an 80% chance of having a chronic condition (19). It may be necessary to modify recommendations for physical activity for individuals who have chronic conditions. Nonetheless, regular physical activity in individuals who have chronic conditions can be very beneficial and should be recommended with whatever appropriate modifications are relevant to the individual's particular chronic condition.

2.13 OVERCOMING SEDENTARY BEHAVIOR

Recently, there has been an increased emphasis on research into health risks of sedentary behavior. It is currently estimated that children and adults spend on average 7.7 hours per day (55%) of waking time in sedentary pursuits (1). Perhaps the most common sedentary pursuit is screen time, either on a computer or watching television. Individuals who have seven hours or more of sedentary occupations or lifestyle will particularly benefit from increased physical activity.

2.14 THE ROLE OF PHYSICIANS IN PROMOTING PHYSICAL ACTIVITY

Physician recommendation has been regularly shown to be the most powerful motivator for people changing various aspects of their lifestyle, including physical activity. Physicians are a trusted source of information (27). Thus, physician recommendation can play a very important role not only in physical activity, but also in multiple other positive lifestyle behaviors, including weight management, proper diet, and avoidance of tobacco. Thus, it is particularly important for physicians to play an active role in these areas. Conversely, if a physician does not discuss physical activity and make recommendations in this area, patients may have the misperception that physical activity is not important. Thus, for multiple reasons, it is important that physicians recommend regular physical activity.

With lifestyle medicine, it is beneficial if the physician who is counseling the patient is also working toward reaching the physical activity guidelines and at least trying to include more movement into his or her own life. Physicians who perform regular aerobic activity are more likely to counsel on it, and physicians who perform strength training are more likely to counsel on it, which we have known for a quarter of a century (28).

2.15 EVALUATING PATIENTS FOR INCREASED PHYSICAL ACTIVITY

Guidance from both PAGA 2018 and the AHA recommends that basically healthy people can begin a program of moderate-intensity physical activity without a formal medical evaluation. This is particularly important since PAGA 2018 emphasizes the importance of removing barriers to get people started on physical activity. There are, however, some instances where evaluation by a physician who is knowledgeable about physical activity can be helpful for both the safety and benefits of patients. This is particularly true for older or sedentary individuals, or individuals who have T2DM or a history of CVD. These decisions are beyond the scope of the current book and curriculum but should be undertaken based on the expertise of each physician.

2.16 GETTING STARTED

The PAGA 2018 makes the important statement that, when it comes to physical activity, "Some is better than none." The PAGA 2018 and ACSM both recommend that clinicians have a discussion about physical activity with every patient and make it as easy as possible for individuals to become physically active.

An excellent way to start this discussion is to utilize a two-question questionnaire supported by the US National Physical Activity Plan and the Exercise is Medicine (EIM) initiative from ACSM (29). These tools used for discussion were developed by Stanford University and involve the following two questions:

- On average, how many days per week do you engage in physical activity (such as a brisk walk)?
- On average, how many minutes do you engage in exercise at this level?

By answering these two questions, your patient will give you a snapshot to start discussing how to counsel that individual to gradually increase their physical activity if necessary and ultimately achieve guidelines based on the PAGA 2018 Scientific Report and the CDC as well as the AHA.

2.16.1 Principles of Exercise Prescription

To get a patient started on increased physical activity, it is important to emphasize getting off the couch and taking the first steps to becoming more active (8). This is particularly true for individuals who have been very sedentary. As already indicated, the very sedentary population comprises 30% of all adults, and the intermittently active population comprises an additional 19%.

If an individual wants to then proceed on to a more detailed program of physical activity, the ACSM has developed a framework for exercise prescription, which goes by the acronym FITT. This acronym emphasizes the following four concepts:

- Frequency
- Intensity
- Time
- Type

It should be emphasized that this framework may be particularly appropriate for individuals who are already engaged in physical activity and simply want to increase it further. For the individual who has been completely sedentary, simply getting them to be physically active, even at a low level, and slowly progressing up to eventually meeting the 150 minutes per week of moderate-intensity physical activity is a worthwhile goal. As already indicated, simply getting 30 minutes of physical activity per week is a great start and will enable individuals to reduce their risk of all-cause mortality and heart disease by 20%. For individuals who are looking for a more comprehensive physical activity program, the following recommendations come from ACSM (30):

- *Aerobic Physical Activity*: This type of activity is defined as activities that utilize large muscle groups and require oxygen to produce energy. While there are many possible forms of aerobic physical activity, by far the most commonly prescribed is walking. In fact, when physicians are asked what form of physical activity they would advocate, over 90% recommend walking. There are multiple other possibilities for comparable aerobic activity, which may be found on multiple places on the ACSM website.

- *Muscular Fitness*: Muscular fitness is also an important component of physical activity. Improving muscle mass through resistance strength training can reduce the risk of injuries both in activities of daily living as well as helping maintain balance and the ability to safely perform various types of physical activity. If your patient is new to muscular fitness, it would be a good idea to have them work with a trained exercise specialist either at a health club or a local YMCA. The Physical Activity Guidelines (PGA) 2018 guidelines recommend at least two sessions of muscular strength training per week, separated by at least one day.
- *Flexibility*: Flexibility represents the ability of a joint to move through a whole range of motion. This is an important component of a comprehensive program of physical activity and is particularly important for the aging population. Flexibility training is also recommended in the PAGA 2018 Scientific Report. There are multiple good programs to enhance flexibility, which may be found on various internet websites. Also, a trained professional at the YMCA or a health club can help the individual improve their flexibility.
- *Balance*: Balance is particularly important for individuals over the age of 65. This can be improved either by utilizing specific balance exercises or simply by increasing physical activity and muscular fitness. ACSM has a number of balance exercises which you can refer your patients to in order to improve this aspect of physical activity.
- *Mind/Body Approaches*: Regular physical activity can be very important for stress reduction. In fact, individuals who are involved in regular physical activity report that stress reduction is one of the key benefits that they obtain. Physical activity in outdoor environments has been shown to be particularly beneficial and demonstrated to yield enhanced mind/body benefits. Multiple types of physical activity can yield of mind/body benefits. These include not only walking, but also various forms of yoga and Tai Chi.
- *Duration of Workout*: For many years it was thought that, to attain the most significant benefits, physical activity sessions needed to be 30 minutes per session. Based on additional research, this recommendation was reduced to ten minutes per session in the 1980s in a Position Statement from ACSM and the American Medical Association. As updated in the PAGA 2018, however, it was stated that the duration of physical activity of any duration can yield benefits. Thus, simply making recommendations to take the stairs at work or to walk across the parking lot when shopping can be very beneficial (30). Many people have found that utilizing fitness-tracking devices to determine the number of steps they take each day, with the goal of achieving 10,000 steps per day, can be very motivating.
- *Special Populations*: Some modifications may be needed for physical activity programs for special populations. These would include pregnant individuals, cancer survivors, older individuals, overweight individuals, and many other populations. Recommendations for these should be made using the clinical guidance of the individual physician.

2.17 STEPS FOR PROMOTING REGULAR PHYSICAL ACTIVITY

The most important step for promoting increased physical activity among our patients is to recognize its value and to include it as part of the ongoing regular counseling for every clinical appointment. The PAGA 2018 Scientific Report concludes that "the primary care setting may be an appealing venue for offering physical activity counseling or referral and represents a scalable opportunity to influence population level physical activity." Physical activity counseling has a United States Preventive Services Task Force (USPSTF) "B level" recommendation. Along with nutrition counseling, physical activity must be included in new health plans under the Affordable Care Act Prevention and Health Promotion Activity for Populations at Increased Risk of Cardiovascular Disease. Thus, it is critically important for physicians to become involved and knowledgeable in this area. One good way to get started is to utilize the two questions indicated in the previous section of this chapter. Moreover, seeking further education in this area will help make physicians more effective counselors.

2.18 CHALLENGES TO IMPLEMENTING THE EXERCISE PRESCRIPTION

Despite overwhelming evidence that physical activity is a powerful health-promoting modality, physicians still are not prescribing it enough. We hope that this emphasis in our curriculum will increase the likelihood of physicians not only prescribing physical activity.

Also in many instances, we encourage physicians to collaborate with professionals in the area of physical activity. In one survey for example, only 20% of physicians collaborated with exercise professionals, despite the fact that 75% of physicians expressed interest in such a partnership if it were available to them.

A good step would be for clinicians to become familiar with health clubs and the YMCAs in their area. While there are typically no institutional barriers to consider, the major barrier hindering counseling in the area appears to be at an organizational level, where the absence of staff and resources to support physical activity were cited as the most significant barrier. One good way to overcome these barriers is to become knowledgeable about exercise professionals who can help physicians seamlessly recommend increased physical activity and follow up on it. Various exercise professionals may also assist in implementing exercise prescriptions. There are multiple professionals in the area of physical activity. These include personal trainers, exercise physiologists, physical therapists, and health coaches, among others.

When considering referring one of your patients to a personal trainer look for an individual who has the credential of a certified personal trainer (CPT). There are multiple personal trainer certifying organizations (8). Perhaps the most effective way of determining background and expertise is to look for CPT certification from the ACSM.

The same is true for exercise physiologists. ACSM, for example, offers exams for certified exercise physiologists (ACSM-EP) and certified clinical exercise physiologists (ACSM-CP). One of the most popular areas for exercise physiologists to become involved in the medical profession is through cardiac rehabilitation programs. The Clinical Exercise Physiology Association (CEPA) reports that 45% of exercise physiologists work in cardiac rehabilitation. Despite the demonstrated efficacy of cardiac rehabilitation, the American Heart Association reports that referral rates to cardiac rehabilitation remain suboptimal.

Physical therapists also may be a valuable resource for increasing physical activity. The American Physical Therapy Association (APTA) states that the role of the physical therapist (PT) is to "examine each individual and develop plans using treatment techniques to enhance the ability to move, reduce pain, and restore function and prevent disability." Individual patients who have specific injury issues can particularly benefit from a referral to a physical therapist.

Health coaches have also become more prominent in many areas in the United States. A health coach is a certified clinician trained in patient/client-centered behavior change. While coaches may come from different backgrounds and carry different degrees, perhaps the best way to seek a health coach is through the National Board of Health and Wellness Coaches (NBHWC), which has worked with the National Medical Examining Board to develop accreditation certificates. Coaches are often also self-employed but may work at gyms, fitness or community centers, or corporate wellness programs (31,32). Research on the effectiveness of health coaching for chronic conditions is promising. Research is ongoing to determine the optimal frequency, intensity, and duration of coaching for different conditions.

2.19 RESOURCES

Multiple educational resources are available to help physicians become more knowledgeable in diverse aspects of physical activity. For example, ACSM has developed a program called "Exercise is Medicine" (EIM), which offers useful material. Physicians may also obtain information and even accreditation through ACSM. The American College of Lifestyle Medicine also can provide resources in multiple areas of lifestyle medicine, including physical activity.

2.20 PHYSICAL ACTIVITY IN THE CONTEXT OF OTHER LIFESTYLE MEDICINE MODALITIES

In Part 2 of this book, we place physical activity in the context of other lifestyle medicine modalities and demonstrate their synergistic application to lower the risk factors in developing or treating various chronic diseases. Certainly, other aspects of lifestyle medicine, including proper nutrition, weight management, and avoiding addictive substances such as cigarette smoking and excessive use of alcohol, play critical roles in overall health. Physical activity integrates with all of these other lifestyle medicine modalities.

2.21 BE A ROLE MODEL

We hope that as an additional benefit of adopting this curriculum, physicians will increasingly serve as role models in the area of physical activity for their patients. A number of studies have shown that there is a strong relationship between a physician's own lifestyle and health habits and his or her counseling practices. This is certainly true of many areas, including physical activity. In fact, in one review of 24 studies, there is an 80% correlation between physicians' personal physical activity habits and their likelihood of counseling patients on physical activity (10).

One additional benefit which is often overlooked is that emerging data now suggests that physicians' physical activity helps reduce the likelihood of burnout (33, 34). This may be a function of the potent benefits of reducing anxiety, depression, and stress that can be achieved through regular physical activity.

2.22 CLINICAL APPLICATIONS

Our curriculum will emphasize the fundamental principle articulated in the PAGA 2018 that "some is better than none." Thus, simple counseling, which starts with identifying physical activity as an important health-related modality and asking a few simple questions, can get the conversation started to help patients adopt this strongly health-promoting activity. This will be reiterated throughout every level of the curriculum at various levels of medical education, emphasized in Part 3 of this book.

REFERENCES

1. Physical Activity Guidelines Advisory Committee. 2018 Physical Activity Guidelines Advisory Committee. 2018 Physical Activity Guidelines Advisory Committee Scientific Report. Washington, DC: U.S. Department of Health and Human Services, 2018.
2. Rippe JM. The health benefits of regular physical activity. In Rippe JM (ed.) *Lifestyle Medicine* (4th ed). Boca Raton, FL: CRC Press, 2024.
3. Eckel RH, Jakicic JM, Ard JD, et al. 2013 AHA/ACC guideline on lifestyle management to reduce cardiovascular risk: A report of the American College of Cardiology/American Heart Association Task Force on Practice Guidelines. *J Am Coll Cardiol.* 2014;63(25 Pt B):2960–2984.
4. Lloyd-Jones DM, Hong Y, Labarthe D, et al. Defining and setting national goals for cardiovascular health promotion and disease reduction: the American Heart Association's strategic Impact Goal through 2020 and beyond. *Circulation.* 2010;121(4):586–613.
5. Colberg SR, Sigal RJ, Yardley JE, et al. Physical activity/exercise and diabetes: a position statement of the American Diabetes Association. *Diabetes Care.* 2016;39(11):2065–2079.
6. Healthy People 2020. CDC National Center for Health Statistics. Healthy People – Healthy People 2020. Accessed October 31, 2024.
7. Healthy People 2030. CDC National Center for Health Statistics. Healthy People 2030 | Data & Statistics | DNPAO | CDC. Accessed October 31, 2024.
8. ACSM. American College of Sports Medicine. ACSM | American College of Sports Medicine. Accessed October 31, 2024.

9. ACLM. American College of Lifestyle Medicine. Home – American College of Lifestyle Medicine. Accessed October 31, 2024.
10. Kennedy M. What physicians need to know, do and say to promote physical activity. In Rippe JM (ed.) *Lifestyle Medicine* (3rd ed). Boca Raton, FL: CRC Press, 2019.
11. Rippe JM. Physical activity and fitness in the prevention of cardiovascular disease. In Rippe JM (ed.) *Lifestyle Medicine* (4th ed). Boca Raton, FL: CRC Press, 2023.
12. Centers for Disease Control and Prevention (CDC). Adult participation in aerobic and muscle-strengthening physical activities – United States, 2011. *MMWR Morb Mortal Wkly Rep.* 2013;62(17):326–330.
13. Jamal A, Phillips E, Gentzke AS, et al. Current cigarette smoking among adults – United States, 2016. *MMWR Morb Mortal Wkly Rep.* 2018;67(2):53–59.
14. Blair S, Kohl H, Barlow C. Physical activity, physical fitness, and all-cause mortality in women: do women need to be active? *J Am Coll Nutr.* 1993;12:368–371.
15. American Diabetes Association. Lifestyle management: standards of medical care in diabetes—2019. *Diabetes Care.* 2019;42(Supplement 1):S46–S60.
16. Knowler WC, Barrett-Connor E, Fowler SE et al. Reduction in the incidence of type 2 diabetes with lifestyle intervention or metformin. *N Engl J Med.* 2002;346:393–394.
17. Pan X, Li G, Hu Y. Effects of diet and exercise in preventing NIDDM in people with impaired glucose tolerance: the Da Qing IGT and Diabetes Study. *Diabetes Care.* 1997:20(4):537–544.
18. Lindstrom J, Louheranta A, Mannelin M, et al. The Finnish Diabetes Prevention Study (DPS) lifestyle intervention and 3-year results on diet and physical activity. *Diabetes Care.* 2003;26:3230–3236.
19. 2018 Physical Activity Guidelines Advisory Committee. 2018 Physical Activity Guidelines Advisory Committee Scientific Report. Washington, DC: U.S. Department of Health and Human Services, 2018. Part F. Chapter 10. Individuals With Chronic Conditions. F10–2–F10–101.
20. American College of Obstetricians and Gynecologists. https://www.acog.org/About-ACOG/ACOG-Departments/Deliveries-Before-39-Weeks/ACOG-Clinical-Guidelines. Accessed April 9, 2025.
21. Bassuk SS, Manson JE. Lifestyle and risk of cardiovascular disease and type 2 diabetes in women: a review of the epidemiologic evidence. *Am J Lifestyle Med.* 2008;2:191–213.
22. Manson J, Rich-Edwards J, Colditz A, et al. A prospective study of walking as compared with vigorous exercise in the prevention of coronary heart disease in women. *N Engl J Med.* 1999;341(9):650–658.
23. Lee I, Rexrode K, Cook N, et al. Physical activity and coronary heart disease in women: is "no pain, no gain" passé? *JAMA.* 2001;285(11):1447–1454.
24. Gorelick P, Furie K, Iadecola C, et al. Defining optimal brain health in adults: a presidential advisory from the American Heart Association/American Stroke Association. *Stroke.* 2017;48(10):e284–e303.
25. 2008 Physical Activity Guidelines Advisory Committee. 2008 Physical Activity Guidelines Advisory Committee Scientific Report. Washington, DC: U.S. Department of Health and Human Services, 2008.
26. 2018 Physical Activity Guidelines Advisory Committee. 2018 Physical Activity Guidelines Advisory Committee Scientific Report. Washington, DC: U.S. Department of Health and Human Services, 2018. Part F. Chapter 9. Older Adults. F9-1–F9-42.
27. 2018 Physical Activity Guidelines Advisory Committee. 2018 Physical Activity Guidelines Advisory Committee Scientific Report. Washington, DC: U.S. Department of Health and Human Services, 2018. Part F. Chapter 11. Promoting Physical Activity. F11-1.
28. Abramson S, Stein J, Schaufele M, et al. Personal exercise habits and counseling practices of primary care physicians: a national survey. *Clin J Sport Med.* 2000;10(1):40–48.
29. Exercise is Medicine: A Global Health Initiative. American College of Sports Medicine. https://www.exerciseismedicine.org//. Accessed April 9, 2025.
30. Bushman B. American College of Sports Medicine. Complete Guide to Fitness and Health. Human Kinetics. 2017.
31. Sforzo GA, Kaye MP, Harenberg S, et al. Compendium of health and wellness coaching: 2019 addendum. *Am J Lifestyle Med.* 2019;14(2):155–168.
32. Sforzo GA, Kaye MP, Todorova I, et al. Compendium of the health and wellness coaching literature. *Am J Lifestyle Med.* 2017:19;12(6):436–447.
33. Rippe JM, Ward A. *The Complete Book of Fitness Walking.* New York: Prentice Hall Press, 1990.
34. Merlo G, Rippe J. Physician burnout: a lifestyle medicine perspective. *Am J Lifestyle Med.* 2021; 15(2):148–157.

3 Nutrition

3.1 INTRODUCTION

What individuals consume in their diet profoundly influences their health. Six of the ten leading causes of death worldwide have a nutritional component (1).

Diets that are primarily plant-based, which include increased consumption of fruits and vegetables, more whole grains, etc., yield multiple health benefits. This is why virtually every dietary recommendation from prestigious organizations such as the American Heart Association (AHA) (2–4), the Dietary Guidelines for Americans 2020–2025 (DGA) (5), the World Health Organization (WHO) (6), the American Diabetes Association (ADA) (7), the American Cancer Association (ACA) (8–12), and the Academy of Nutrition and Dietetics (AND) (13) all emphasize this type of diet. The recommendations from these organizations are similar and emphasize primarily a plant-based diet with increased consumption of fruits, vegetables, and whole grains.

Numerous diets have been demonstrated to yield significant health benefits. These include the Mediterranean diet (14), the AHA Prudent Diet (5), the DASH diet, the Nordic diet, various vegetarian diets, the Flexitarian diet, and multiple Asian diets, including those in China, Japan, and Korea, all of which are based on these fundamental principles (5,15).

All of these diets also focus on some restriction of animal products and processed foods and have been shown to yield varying degrees of risk factor reduction, including the prevention, risk factor reduction, and even reversal of some chronic diseases.

For all of these reasons, it is incumbent upon physicians to become knowledgeable about nutrition in general, and plant-based diets in particular. That is the intent of the curriculum and evidence outlined in this book. In this book, we will review the evidence supporting multiple health benefits of plant-based diets and link them to practical strategies for physicians to recommend this approach to their patients. Despite enormous evidence of the multiple benefits of diets that are focused on plants, physicians have typically not advocated nutrition in general or plant-based diets in particular.

Physicians often feel woefully ill-prepared to discuss nutrition with their patients. In fact, less than 40% of physicians routinely counsel their patients on diet at all, and even if they do, they focus on general information such as "follow a balanced diet" (16).

Not surprisingly, several studies have shown that only 21% of patients feel they received adequate nutritional advice from their physicians. This may be due to time constraints. Many physicians, however, also lack specific knowledge about nutrition or how to prescribe healthy diets. This is most likely a consequence of the fact that only 17% of medical schools have specific nutrition courses. Only 14% of individuals who graduate from medical school feel they have adequate nutrition knowledge (17). This is even true in cardiology, where 90% of cardiologists feel they do not have adequate nutritional knowledge (18). The good news in this area is that 95% of cardiologists feel that nutrition counseling is important and try to do it.

Before proceeding with recommendations about plant-based nutrition, it should be noted that not all plant-based diets can be considered "healthy." A recent study divided plant-based diets into "healthy plant-based diets" and "unhealthy plant-based diets" (19). A major difference between the two is that "healthy" plant-based diets emphasize fruits and vegetables, whole grains, and fiber, while reducing tropical oils, sugar, and sodium, as well as red and processed meat. "Unhealthy" plant-based diets, in contrast, do reduce red and processed meat but contain more refined grains, saturated fats, tropical oils, as well as sugar and salt. Studies that have been performed in this area show that "unhealthy" plant-based diets do not lower the risk of heart disease, whereas "healthy" plant-based diets do.

DOI: 10.1201/9781003630043-3

By linking the robust evidence supporting plant-based diets to health and various chronic diseases, and by providing a specific curriculum in this book that guides physicians' steps to efficiently recommend healthy nutrition, we hope to increase the amount of nutrition counseling that occurs in mainstream medicine.

3.2 CURRENT NUTRITIONAL STATUS IN THE UNITED STATES

Unfortunately, the typical eating patterns currently consumed in the United States are not optimal. In fact, they do not align very well with the Dietary Guidelines for Americans. This has been assessed utilizing what is called "The Healthy Eating Index" (HEI) (20). This framework measures current nutritional patterns and compares them with the recommendations from the Dietary Guidelines for Americans. While the average dietary quality, as assessed by the HEI, has improved slightly in the past ten years, it still only has an average score of 59 on a scale of 0–100. This suggests that people have a large opportunity to improve. The HEI scores by age group are found in Figure 3.1. As indicated in this figure, HEI scores across age, sex, race, ethnicity, and income subgroups are all sub-optimum, although they do appear highest in the early ages (2–4) and also ages 60+. When compared to the Healthy US-Style Dietary Pattern aligned in the Dietary Guidelines for Americans 2020–2025 (5), the following issues reflect significant areas where improvement is needed.

- More than 80% of adults in the United States have dietary patterns that are low in vegetables, fruits, and dairy.
- More than half of the population meets the total grain and total protein foods recommendations, but these are based on consuming a considerable amount of refined grains, as well as red meat and processed meat.
- Most Americans exceed the recommendations for added sugars, saturated fats, and sodium.

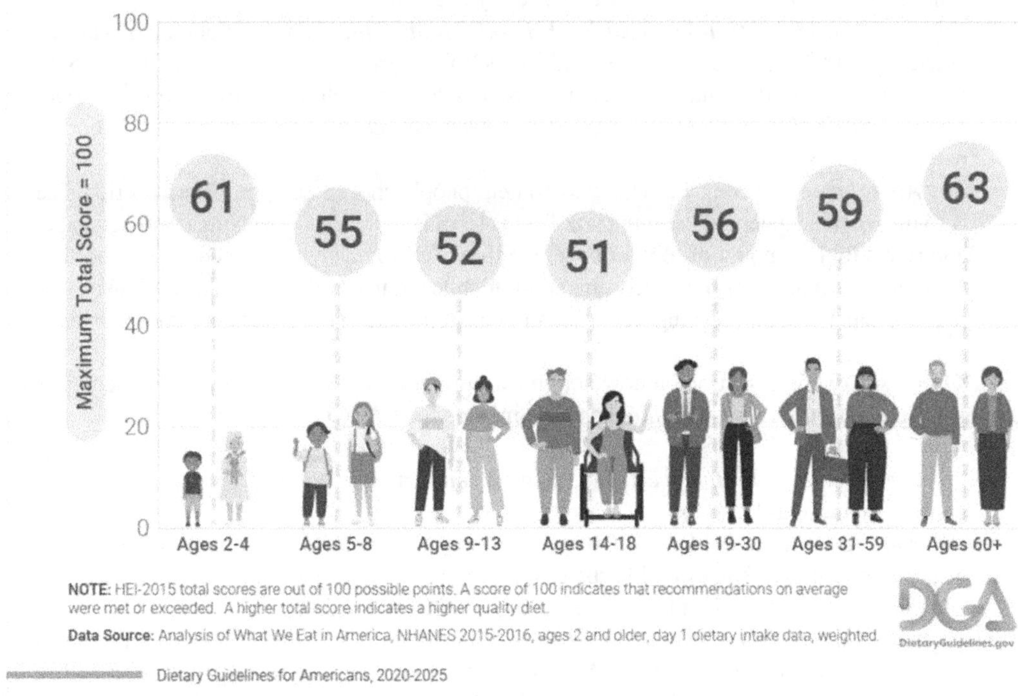

FIGURE 3.1 Adherence of the U.S. population to the *Dietary Guidelines* across life stages, as measured by average Total Healthy Eating Index-2015 scores.

Among nutrients, calcium, potassium, dietary fiber, and vitamin D are considered specific nutrients of public health concern, since intake is associated with health concerns (5). All four of these nutrients are suboptimal in the US population.

All of these findings are of considerable concern because, among the top 17 risk factors identified by the US Burden of Disease Collaborators, poor diet is listed as the leading cause of premature death and disability in the United States. Details about how these suboptimal nutritional patterns impact various chronic diseases can be found in Part 2 of this book.

A key concept in the DGAs is "nutrient density," which, as the name suggests, refers to the amount of nutrients per unit. Units may differ, but it is commonly either nutrients per calorie or nutrients per gram. Nutrient density is relevant to health since nutrient-dense foods are more likely to ensure that both nutrient and energy needs are met. There is good evidence that nutrient density in the usual American diet is much lower than recommended by the DGA 2020–2025 and other frameworks.

3.3 CURRENT NUTRITIONAL RECOMMENDATIONS

The Dietary Guidelines for Americans have listed a number of principles to help both physicians and patients follow the Dietary Guidelines. They have listed the following recommendations:

- *Meet Nutritional Needs Primarily from Foods and Beverages.* The *Dietary Guidelines* 2020–2025 (5) are geared to provide all the essential nutrients within the appropriate range. It is important to recommend that people consume fortified foods and nutrient-containing dietary supplements if they need extra nutrients. It is also important to emphasize to patients to choose nutrient-dense foods, which specifically involves fruits and vegetables, whole grains, etc. In general, dietary patterns are achieved through thoughtful, informed choices. The mantra from the Dietary Guidelines is "one decision, one meal, one day at a time," and to adopt this framework consistently over time.
- *Choose a Variety of Options from Each Food Group.* This allows the choice of various nutrient-dense foods and beverages within each food group and also contributes to both flexibility and cultural and personal preferences. Foods including fresh, canned, dried, frozen, and 100% juices that are in nutrient-dense forms can be included in healthy dietary patterns.
- *Pay Attention to Portion Size.* One way to help people choose an appropriate portion size is to utilize the concept of "serving size." This term is included in the Nutrition Facts label and refers to the amount of food or beverage that is customarily consumed. It is important to emphasize that this is not a recommendation of how much to eat or drink. Obviously, eating less than the stated serving size results in consuming fewer calories and other nutrients.

The DGAs also contain a section on how health care professionals can improve implementation of healthy eating patterns. These recommendations include the following:

- *Start with Personal Preferences*: Once again, healthy dietary patterns involve family preferences in nutrient-dense forms.
- *Incorporate Cultural Traditions*: One specific way that cultural traditions can be emphasized is by utilizing spices and herbs that are common to a particular cultural tradition. This will allow reducing added sugars, saturated fats, and sodium.
- *Consider Budget*: Many people have the misconception that eating healthfully is expensive. As emphasized in the DGAs, a healthy dietary pattern can be affordable and fit within budget constraints. Ways to help individuals achieve this include advanced planning, considering regional and seasonal food availability, and incorporating a variety of fresh, frozen, dried, and canned options.

3.4 HEALTHY DIETS

Multiple different organizations, including the AHA, DGAs 2020–2025, WHO (1), the AHA (3), and many others, recommend healthy dietary patterns. The good news is that these patterns are very consistent with each other. They all basically follow guidelines which are summarized in the following statement from the DGA 2020–2025.

> Within the body of evidence higher intake of vegetables and fruits consistently have been identified as characteristics of healthy eating patterns. Whole grains have been identified as well although with slightly less consistency. Other characteristics of healthy eating patterns have been identified with less consistency including fat free and low fat dairy, seafood, legumes and nuts, lower intakes of meat including processed meats, sugar sweetened foods, particularly beverages, and refined grains have been identified as characteristics of healthy eating patterns.

While there are a variety of plant-based healthy eating patterns, the ones that we focus on in this book are the following:

- *The Healthy US-Style Dietary Pattern* (5): This is the pattern recommended by the DGAs 2020–2025 and is embedded in this document. It focuses on nutrient-dense foods and beverages, including abundant fruits and vegetables, whole grains, low-fat dairy, nuts, seafood, and soy products. This framework allows red meat to be consumed in small quantities, and also poultry and eggs as part of the protein food category.
- *The Mediterranean Diet*: (MedDiet) contains 35%–40% carbohydrates, 12%–20% protein, and fat at a level of 35%–50% (14). The MedDiet emphasizes eating plant-based foods such as fruits, vegetables, whole grains, legumes, nuts, olives, and non-tropical vegetable oils. The MedDiet is relatively high in dietary fat because of the monounsaturated fats in olive oil. The MedDiet allows moderate fish and poultry consumption and is low in red meat. The major trial of the MedDiet that showed it significantly reduced the risk of heart disease was called the PREDIMED Study, which was published in the New England Journal of Medicine (14).
- *The Dietary Approaches to Stop Hypertension (DASH) Diet* (15): This diet contains 60% carbohydrates, protein at 15%–20%, and fat at 20%–30%. This diet also emphasizes eating considerable amounts of fresh fruits and vegetables, low-fat dairy products, whole grains, fish, poultry, beans, seeds, and nuts, and limits consumption of red meat and drinks containing sugar. It is balanced in nutrients, high in fiber, and low in saturated fat. The DASH diet is also a good source of potassium, magnesium, and calcium. It does allow sodium consumption at approximately the average in the US diet of 3,000 mg per day. Subsequent trials of the DASH diet, however, have lowered this to 1,500 mg per day.

This is a diet that is strongly recommended by the AHA. Unfortunately, even though this diet was designed to help control hypertension, only 20% of people with elevated blood pressure follow it.

With regard to specific dietary plans, one survey of physicians reported that 55% recommended the Mediterranean diet, another 40% recommended the low-fat diet, and the DASH diet was recommended by 38%. It is interesting to note that the low-carbohydrate diet was recommended by only 16%. It should be noted that 60% of physicians do not recommend a specific diet for their patients.

3.5 OPPORTUNITIES FOR NUTRITIONAL EDUCATION FOR PHYSICIANS

As already indicated, physician knowledge in the area of healthy nutrition is woefully inadequate. Only 13% of physicians strongly agreed that they were adequately trained to discuss nutrition with their patients. Moreover, a significant majority (78.4%) (21) thought additional training in nutrition would help them provide better clinical care in the prevention of cardiovascular disease and other chronic diseases.

There are multiple opportunities to enhance nutrition education for physicians (22–24). These will be dealt with in detail in the curriculum in Part 3 of this book. There are basically four key opportunities to present nutrition education for physicians. They are the following:

- Medical School
- Residency/Fellowship
- Preparation for STEP and Board Exams
- Continuing Medical Education

Specific opportunities and needs exist at each level of medical education, which will be integrated into the curriculum presented in Part 3 of this book.

The DGA 2020–2025 provides a variety of resources to help educate physicians and also to implement the guidelines in counseling their patients. These resources include MyPlate (5), which is a graphic depiction of key messages about healthy nutrition. This graphic emphasizes the following components of a healthy eating routine:

- Make half your plate fruits and vegetables
- Focus on whole fruits and vary your vegetables
- Make half your grains whole grains
- Vary your protein sources
- Move to low-fat or fat-free dairy milk or yogurt
- Choose fruits and vegetables to consume less added sugars, saturated fat, and sodium

It is important for physicians to emphasize that the benefits of healthy eating add up over time, or as the DGAs summarize, "healthy eating one bite at a time." This mantra emphasizes that small changes matter, and the goal is to start simple with MyPlate. There are also a variety of other resources, including a wide variety of specific educational tools for health professionals, available at *www.dietaryguidelines.gov.*

3.6 NUTRITION AND CHRONIC DISEASE

An enormous body of evidence exists that relates to healthy nutrition and its role in preventing or treating chronic disease. These conditions include the following:

- Cardiovascular disease
- Diabetes, pre-diabetes, and the metabolic syndrome
- Weight gain and obesity
- Cancer
- Brain health and cognition

A separate chapter with detailed references for the background information on the role of nutrition in each of these conditions will be found in Part 2 of this book.

3.7 WOMEN'S HEALTH

Proper nutrition is recommended for all women. Most women currently follow a traditional Western diet, which is an unhealthy diet (5). Women should be counseled to consume more fruits and vegetables and whole grains while avoiding foods high in sugar, fat, and excess sodium. All of these issues apply equally well to women at all life stages, and particularly to women who are pregnant or lactating. These issues are so important that we have devoted a separate chapter in Part 2 to nutritional recommendations for women.

3.8 NUTRITION FOR CHILDREN

It is important to emphasize that healthy nutrition starts in infancy and lasts throughout childhood (5). This emphasis establishes lifelong patterns of healthy nutrition, including increased fruit and vegetable consumption as well as whole grains. All of this is particularly important for children between the ages of 2 and 18. Good nutrition throughout life is a key consideration in lowering the risk of chronic diseases, which are often initiated in childhood but manifest in adulthood. One particular issue that has caused great concern is the increase in childhood obesity in the United States. Establishing healthy nutritional patterns is a highly effective strategy for lowering the risk of obesity and other chronic illnesses, which have their roots in childhood.

All of these issues, with the corresponding background data, will be found in a separate chapter in Part 2 of this book.

3.9 NUTRITION FOR THE ELDERLY

The population of individuals over the age of 65 is the most rapidly growing segment of all age groups. The elderly population is also one in which nutrition plays a particularly important role in lowering the risk or assisting in the treatment of various chronic conditions (25). A number of age-related changes occur that may make healthy eating more challenging for the elderly. Particular nutrients of concern in the elderly are calcium, vitamin D, protein, potassium, and fiber. Malnutrition is also common and not diagnosed frequently enough in the elderly. Screening tools are available to help clinicians make the proper diagnosis. All of these issues will be discussed in more detail in the chapter on Nutrition in the Elderly in Part 2 of this book.

3.10 THE ROLE OF PHYSICIANS IN PRESCRIBING NUTRITION

Substantial evidence supports the efficacy of clinician-initiated nutrition counseling. The recommendation of nutrition should be considered a standard component of clinical care in healthcare settings. This has been strongly recommended by numerous prestigious bodies, including the White House Conference on Hunger, Nutrition and Health, the CDC Foundation, the AHA, the ADA, and the AND, as well as the Physical Activity Guidelines for Americans 2018 (26).

Research strongly shows that nutrition prescription referral to nutritional professionals also effectively helps patients make long-term lifestyle changes. To that end, nutrition counseling has the United States Preventive Services Task Force (USPSTF) level of evidence "B" recommendation. Moreover, nutritional counseling is mandated to be included in new health care plans under the Affordable Care Act Prevention and Health Promotion Activities for Populations at Increased Risk for Cardiovascular Disease.

Multiple resources are available to help physicians prescribe nutrition. Many of them may be obtained by visiting www.dietaryguidelines.gov.

All health care providers should be educated in implementing counseling, prescription, and referral practices. Physicians specifically are beginning to answer the call and successfully include nutrition counseling in their practices. There are still inconsistencies in nutritional counseling and referral practices in the health care setting, but more tools are rapidly becoming available.

3.11 CHALLENGES TO IMPLEMENT THE NUTRITION PRESCRIPTION

Clinicians and health care providers agree that nutrition counseling is essential to evidence-based medicine and that nutrition prescriptions can be an effective strategy to improve nutrition in the clinical population. A robust network of experts exists in this area. However, there still are some perceived barriers to integrating nutrition counseling in clinical practice. Roughly 50% of physicians believe that they play an important role in promoting healthy nutrition to their patients, yet only 20% of patients or fewer are provided with a specific nutrition prescription. We hope to increase that number by offering practical and usable tools in the embedded curriculum in this book.

While barriers are perceived by individual physicians, institutional barriers must also be considered. Lack of structures to support nutrition prescription and the absence of staff resources to facilitate delivery were the most common issues reported when this was surveyed.

3.12 NUTRITIONAL PROFESSIONALS AVAILABLE TO IMPLEMENT PRESCRIPTIONS

Multiple nutrition professionals are available to assist physicians in making an effective nutrition prescription. Most of these can be found through the Academy of Nutrition and Dietetics, which offers certifications for Registered Dietitian Nutritionists (RDNs) (13). Increasingly, both RDNs and nurses have achieved expertise and certification as Diabetes Educators (CDE). If a physician is hoping to refer someone to a nutrition professional, many community health departments and agencies have collected local information to develop resource connections. These referral guides have been shown to be effective and can be helpful in providing patients with specific and evidence-based nutritional counseling.

3.13 EVALUATING PATIENTS FOR HEALTHY NUTRITION

The most important issue for physicians to understand is that ignoring nutrition as a component of counseling sessions with patients suggests that it is not important. Of course, in fact, nothing could be further from the truth!

We have found that one good way to get started is simply to ask the question, "How many servings of fruits and vegetables do you consume in a day?" This is consistent with recommendations from the DGA that individuals should consume four to five servings of fruits and vegetables on a daily basis. This is also consistent with recommendations from the AHA for lowering the risk of heart disease (3). A simple question such as this can often start the discussion about typical nutrition practices and give physicians an opportunity to make some recommendations for ways that it can be easier to consume fruits and vegetables on a daily basis. Unfortunately, only 12% of individuals consume the recommended servings of fruit per day and only 7% consume the recommended number of servings of vegetables.

3.14 SPECIFIC FOODS AND DIETARY PATTERNS

It is important to emphasize to patients that modern nutrition science focuses on overall dietary patterns and not on specific foods. As already indicated, multiple healthy nutritional dietary patterns are available, including the Healthy US-Style Dietary Pattern, the MedDiet, the DASH diet, and the various diets recommended by the AHA, including the Prudent diet. Once this is discussed with your patients, it can lead to a discussion of other healthy components of the diet, including whole grains and dietary fiber, fish, nuts, low-fat dairy products, and soy. Physicians should also emphasize the importance of limiting sugar-sweetened beverages and also limiting red meat and processed meat in the diet. More details on specific foods and dietary patterns will be found in Part 3 of this book.

3.15 HYDRATION

Hydration is an essential part of an overall nutrition plan. Proper hydration is something that physicians should discuss with every patient, but particularly those who are physically active or who live in a warm or high environment (27). Water, of course, is essential to life, and even a small amount of dehydration (as low as 2%–3% of body weight) can result in diminished performance and slight increases in the body's temperature, as well as diminishing the body's ability to control temperature. A good general rule is to consume at least one 8-ounce glass of water more than an individual's thirst indicates. This may vary considerably for patients who are particularly physically active, and is especially important for individuals over the age of 65 and children.

3.16 RESOURCES

Multiple resources are available to help physicians understand healthy nutrition and also how to communicate this to patients. The best source for high-level, credible nutritional information is based on the DGAs 2020–2025. There are a wide variety of both consumer and professional resources available, which can be found at www.dietaryguidelines.gov.

3.17 NUTRITION IN THE CONTEXT OF OTHER LIFESTYLE MEDICINE MODALITIES

We will emphasize throughout this book that the lifestyle medicine modalities act synergistically with each other to promote good health. Thus, while we are focusing on nutrition in this chapter, when it comes to the role of lifestyle medicine modalities in the reduction of risk of chronic diseases, nutrition will be combined with other important lifestyle modalities such as increased physical activity, weight management, avoiding addictive substances, stress reduction, healthy sleep, and positive relationships with other individuals (28,29). All of these contribute to lowering the risk of chronic disease and will be emphasized throughout this book and also in the curriculum found in Part 3 of this book.

3.18 BE A ROLE MODEL

We hope that by utilizing the curriculum and materials found in this book, more physicians will pay closer attention to their own nutritional habits. Numerous research studies have shown that physicians who pay close attention to both nutrition and physical activity are more likely to impart meaningful information in these areas to their patients. Thus, it is very important to be a role model!

3.19 CLINICAL APPLICATIONS

The most important clinical application for physicians in the area of nutrition is simply to inquire in every clinical encounter with patients how they are doing with regard to nutrition. As already indicated, simply asking a few questions about nutrition, such as the level of fruit and vegetable consumption for each patient, can get a positive discussion started.

As we have emphasized throughout this chapter and will emphasize throughout the book, we advocate a plant-forward diet. There are multiple good ones that are evidence-based, including the Healthy US-Style Dietary Pattern, the MedDiet, and the DASH diet, as well as other diets recommended by the AHA. In addition, we have provided a specific seven-day starter program based on an excellent plant-forward nutritional plan called "Full Plate Living." This is found in Appendix A. This would be a great place for physicians to get started on the consumption of plant-forward eating, and it is also something that can be transferred immediately to patients, giving them specific ideas of how to get started with a healthy plant-forward nutritional plan.

REFERENCES

1. World Health Organization. Global Non-Communicable Disease Compact 2020–2030. https://www.who.int/initiatives/global-noncommunicable-diseases-compact-2020-2030. Accessed November 5, 2024.
2. Lichtenstein AH, Appel LJ, Vadiveloo M. 2021 Dietary guidance to improve cardiovascular health: a scientific statement from the American Heart Association. *Circulation*. 2021;114:e72.

3. Lloyd-Jones DM, Hong Y, Labarthe D, et al. American Heart Association Strategic Planning Task Force and Statistics Committee. Defining and setting national goals for cardiovascular health promotion and disease reduction: the American Heart Association's strategic Impact Goal through 2020 and beyond. *Circulation*. 2010; 121(4):586–613.
4. Eckel RH, Jakicic JM, Ard JD, et al. 2013 AHA/ACC guideline on lifestyle management to reduce cardiovascular risk. A report of the American College of Cardiology/American Heart Association Task Force on Practice Guidelines. *Circulation*. 2014;129:S76–S99.
5. U.S. Department of Health and Human Services and U.S. Department of Agriculture. 2020–2025 Dietary Guidelines for Americans. https://health.gov/our-work/ -nutrition-physical activity//-dietary-guidelines2020–2025 Accessed November 4, 2024.
6. World Health Organization on Cardiovascular Disease. https://www.who.int/health-topics/cardiovascular-diseases#tab=tab_1. Accessed November 4, 2024.
7. Colberg SR, Sigal RJ, Yardley JE, et al. Physical activity/exercise and diabetes: a position statement of the American Diabetes Association. *Diabetes Care*. 2016;39(11):2065–79.
8. Wu S, Powers S, Zhu W et al. Substantial contribution of extrinsic risk factors to cancer development. *Nature*. 2016; 201(529):43–47.
9. Doll R, Peto R. The causes of cancer: quantitative estimates of avoidable risks of cancer in the United States today. *J Natl Cancer Inst*. 1981;66(6):1191–308.
10. Campbell TC, The past, present, and future of nutrition and cancer: part 1—was a nutritional association acknowledged a century ago? *Nutr Cancer*. 2017; 69(5):811–817.
11. National Research Council Committee on Diet, N. and Cancer, in Diet, Nutrition, and Cancer. Washington, DC: National Academies Press (US) Copyright © National Academy of Sciences, 1982.
12. World Cancer Research Fund International, A.I.f.C.R., Diet, Nutrition, Physical Activity and Cancer: a Global Perspective: A Summary of the Third Expert Report. London: World Cancer Research Fund International, 2018.
13. Academy of Nutrition and Dietetics. https://www.eatright.org/. Accessed November 5, 2024.
14. Estruch R, Ros E, Salas-Salvado J, et al. Primary prevention of cardiovascular disease with a Mediterranean diet. *N Engl J Med*. 2013;368(14):1279–1290.
15. Mozaffarian D, Appel LJ, Van Horn L. Components of a cardioprotective diet: new insights. *Circulation*. 2011;123(24):2870–2891.
16. Rippe JM. Lifestyle medicine: the health promoting power of daily habits and practices. *Am J Lifestyle Med*. 2018;12(6):499–512.
17. Nestle M, Baron RB. Nutrition in medical education: from counting hours to measuring competence. *JAMA Intern Med*. 2014;174(6):843–844.
18. Devries S, Agatston A, Aggarwal M, et al. A deficiency of nutrition education and practice in cardiology. *Am J Med*. 2017;130(11):1298–1305.
19. Satija A, Bhupathiraju SN, Spiegelman D, et al. Healthful and unhealthful plant-based diets and the risk of coronary heart disease in U.S. adults. *J Am Coll Cardiol*. 2017;25;70(4):411–422.
20. USDA Food and Nutrition Service. U.S. Department of Agriculture. Healthy Eating Index (HEI). Healthy Eating Index (HEI) | Food and Nutrition Service. Accessed November 15, 2024.
21. US Burden of Disease Collaborators, Mokdad AH, Ballestros K, et al. The state of US health, 1990–2016: burden of diseases, injuries, and risk factors among US states. *JAMA*. 2018;10;319(14):1444–1472.
22. Frates B. The evolving state of nutrition education. *Am J Lifestyle Med*. 2023;17(6):759–761.
23. Rippe JM. Physical activity and lifestyle medicine. *Am J Lifestyle Med*. 2021;15(3):212–213.
24. Kushner RF, Van Horn L, Rock CL, et al. Nutrition education in medical school: a time of opportunity. *Am J Clin Nutr*. 2014;99(5 Suppl):1167S–1173S.
25. Lichtenstein A. Optimal nutrition guidance for older adults. In Rippe JM (ed.) *Lifestyle Medicine* (4th ed). Boca Raton, FL: CRC Press, 2023.
26. Physical Activity Guidelines Advisory Committee. 2018 Physical Activity Guidelines Advisory Committee. 2018 Physical Activity Guidelines Advisory Committee Scientific Report. Washington, DC: U.S. Department of Health and Human Services, 2018.
27. Evans G, Maughan J. Effects of an active lifestyle on water balance and water requirements. In Rippe JM (ed.) *Lifestyle Medicine* (4th ed). Boca Raton, FL: CRC Press, 2024.
28. Rippe JM. *Lifestyle Medicine* (4th ed). Boca Raton, FL: CRC Press, 2024.
29. Rippe JM. Lifestyle strategies for risk factor reduction, prevention, and treatment of cardiovascular disease. *Am J Lifestyle Med*. 2018;13(2):204–212.

4 Weight Management and Obesity

4.1 INTRODUCTION

In many ways, overweight and obesity represent quintessential lifestyle diseases. Since overweight and obesity are highly prevalent in the United States, every physician needs to have a sophisticated understanding of how to treat these conditions. Despite the high prevalence of overweight and obesity in the United States and, indeed, around the world (1), physicians are often reluctant to discuss these issues with their patients. Furthermore, they typically do not have the appropriate educational background or understanding of the modern management of these conditions to provide effective counseling.

The purpose of this book and the embedded curriculum is to arm physicians with the appropriate tools to deal with both of these conditions. This is critically important since overweight and obesity underlie multiple other chronic diseases, including cardiovascular disease (CVD), diabetes (T2DM), pre-diabetes, metabolic syndrome (MetS), cancer, arthritis, and many other conditions (2,3). Sadly, the medical profession has not been as active as we should have been in dealing with overweight and obesity. It has been estimated that less than 40% of overweight or obese individuals are counseled concerning these conditions by their physician (4). This represents a wasted opportunity since more than 70% of individuals see their primary care physician on at least an annual basis.

The habits and practices that individuals maintain in their daily lives carry enormous implications for lowering the risk of weight gain and also overweight and obesity. Both physical activity and proper nutrition play crucial roles in weight loss, reducing the likelihood of weight gain, and maintaining a healthy body weight. While proper nutrition and physical activity are dealt with in separate chapters in this book, they will be combined in our curricular approach to preventing weight gain and treating both overweight and obesity.

While it may seem simple that either decreased caloric intake or increased physical activity will contribute to weight maintenance or weight loss, in fact, the process is more complicated, as emphasized in the Consensus Statement on Metabolism from the American Society of Nutrition (5). Multiple factors impact metabolism, including percent body fat and other issues pertaining to metabolism, as well as a host of environmental factors.

At any given time, between 50% and 70% of obese Americans are actively trying to lose weight. Oftentimes, these individuals have misperceptions about how much weight loss is required to yield health benefits. Sustained weight loss of as little as 5%–10% is clinically significant and reduces risk factors for a variety of chronic diseases such as CVD and T2DM (6,7). This was amply demonstrated in the Diabetes Prevention Program (8) and the Look AHEAD Trial (9), both of which showed that a weight loss of 7% of body weight in individuals with obesity resulted in significant improvement in risk factors for both heart disease and diabetes. Thus, clinicians should be aware of these important data and counsel patients about how effective even small amounts of weight loss can be in yielding health benefits. This is particularly important since many patients feel that this amount of weight loss would be a disappointment to them and have misperceptions about how much weight they should lose.

4.2 CURRENT LEVELS OF OVERWEIGHT AND OBESITY IN THE UNITED STATES

Overweight and obesity represent significant public health problems in the United States and, indeed, in other countries around the world. In the United States, the prevalence of overweight as

DOI: 10.1201/9781003630043-4

assessed by body mass index (BMI) has been estimated at approximately 75% of adults (10). This includes overweight, obesity and severe obesity. Obesity itself (BMI $\geq$30 kg/m^2) is estimated at 40% and severe obesity (BMI $\geq$35 kg/m^2) at 16%.

These high levels of overweight and obesity are significant because even small amounts of excess body weight have been associated with multiple chronic diseases. Gaining as little as 10–12 pounds during adulthood is associated with increased risk of multiple chronic diseases, including CVD and T2DM. The cornerstone of obesity treatment relies on lifestyle measures to contribute to balancing energy to prevent weight gain in the first place or creating an energy deficit to achieve weight loss.

A steady increase in the share of people who are overweight or obese has occurred in the past two decades. The rate of obesity, in particular, rose steeply, doubling in adults between 1990 and 2021 to more than 40% and nearly tripling to 29% among girls and women aged 15–24 (10).

Particularly troubling is the increased share of adolescents with obesity. Now, over half of US teens and young adults ages 15–24 are either overweight or obese compared to 29% in 1990 (10). Children who have obesity are more likely to develop high blood pressure and high cholesterol, which can contribute to plaque buildup in their arteries, T2DM, and fat in the liver that causes inflammation. There has been a particularly steep rise in obesity rates among girls and women ages 15–24, reaching 29% in 2021, up from 10% in 1990.

Pharmaceutical therapy and/or bariatric surgery may be needed in addition to these factors in individuals who have obesity. Recently, some new, powerful pharmaceutical agents have significantly increased the ability to lose substantial amounts of weight. These agents, however, need to be prescribed in conjunction with proper nutrition and regular physical activity.

4.3 ASSESSING OVERWEIGHT AND OBESITY IN CLINICAL PRACTICE

On the most fundamental level, obesity refers to an increase in body fat. Unfortunately, the precise measurement of body fat is not easily done in clinical practice. Thus, as a practical matter, most research relies on utilizing BMI. BMI has been demonstrated in multiple studies to correlate with the level of obesity as well as health risk. In order to determine BMI, an accurate measurement of height can be obtained using a wall-mounted stadiometer. Weight should be taken with a regularly calibrated scale. BMI is estimated as the weight in kilograms divided by the height in meters squared. As a practical matter, most clinicians will find it easiest to use charts that are available for various heights and weights, which also yield body mass index. One such chart is found in Figure 4.1.

It should be noted that the distribution of body fat also plays a significant role as a risk factor for CVD and T2DM. It may be more than most clinicians wish to perform measurements of waist circumference, but having a cloth measuring tape can expedite this measurement. Waist circumference is measured with this flexible tape laid horizontally at the level of the superior iliac crest. A waist circumference greater than 40 inches in men (102 cm) or 35 inches in women (89 cm) is considered high and an additional risk for CVD and T2DM (11).

4.4 HEALTH EFFECTS OF OBESITY

The risk factors posed by obesity for multiple chronic diseases will be discussed subsequently in this chapter. The basic underlying health risk appears to relate to the biology of fat cells (adipocytes). It was previously thought that adipocytes were primarily storage sites for excess fat. Research over the last two decades, however, has clarified that adipocytes are, in fact, highly complex inflammatory endocrine and metabolic cells (11–16). Thus, excess adipose tissue essentially serves as a complicated endocrine organ.

Adipocytes function as a potent source of inflammatory molecules such as IL-6, tumor necrosis factor alpha (TNF-α), and many other inflammatory molecules. These complex properties of adipocytes and their role in inflammation appear to underlie the strong relationship between obesity and

Body Mass Index (BMI) based on weight and height

Height		Weight (lb)													
Ft/In	In	120	130	140	150	160	170	180	190	200	210	220	230	240	250
4'10"	58	25	27	29	31	33	36	38	40	42	44	46	48	50	52
4'11"	59	24	26	28	30	32	34	36	38	40	42	44	46	48	50
5'	60	23	25	27	29	31	33	35	37	39	41	43	45	47	49
5'1"	61	23	25	26	28	30	32	34	36	38	40	42	43	45	47
5'2"	62	22	24	26	27	29	31	33	35	37	38	40	42	44	46
5'3"	63	21	23	25	27	28	30	32	34	35	37	39	41	43	44
5'4"	64	21	22	24	26	27	29	31	33	34	36	38	39	41	43
5'5"	65	20	22	23	25	27	28	30	32	33	35	37	38	40	42
5'6"	66	19	21	23	24	26	27	29	31	32	34	36	37	39	40
5'7"	67	19	20	22	23	25	27	28	30	31	33	34	36	38	39
5'8"	68	18	20	21	23	24	26	27	29	30	32	33	35	36	38
5'9"	69	18	19	21	22	24	25	27	28	30	31	32	34	35	37
5'10"	70		19	20	22	23	24	26	27	29	30	32	33	34	36
5'11"	71		18	20	21	22	24	25	26	28	29	31	32	33	35
6'	72		18	19	20	22	23	24	26	27	28	30	31	33	34
6'1"	73			18	20	21	22	24	25	26	28	29	30	32	33
6'2"	74			18	19	21	22	23	24	26	27	28	30	31	32
6'3"	75				19	20	21	22	24	25	26	27	29	30	31
6'4"	76				18	19	21	22	23	24	26	27	28	29	30
6'5"	77				18	19	20	21	23	24	25	26	27	28	30

Body mass index <18 kg/m^2 is not recommended, and therefore these values have not been represented on this table.

From: ACSM Position Stand on Appropriate Intervention Strategies for Weight Loss and Prevention of Weight Regain for Adults

Jakicic JM, Clark, K. Coleman E, et al. American College of Sports Medicine position stand. Appropriate intervention strategies for weight loss and prevention of weight regain for adults. *Med Sci Sports Exerc,* 2001. 33(12): p. 2145-56.

FIGURE 4.1 Body mass index (BMI) based on weight and height. (From: ACSM Position Stand on Appropriate Intervention Strategies for Weight Loss and Prevention of Weight Regain for Adults; Jakicic JM, Clark, K. Coleman E, et al. American College of Sports Medicine position stand. Appropriate intervention strategies for weight loss and prevention of weight regain for adults. *Med Sci Sports Exerc.* 2001;33(12):2145–2156.)

a variety of chronic medical conditions. The metabolic and inflammatory molecules generated by adipocytes are particularly prominent in those located in the abdominal region, which provides the rationale for measuring waist circumference in addition to BMI (11).

4.5 RELATIONSHIP BETWEEN OVERWEIGHT AND OBESITY AND CHRONIC DISEASE

Research has shown that obesity is associated with increased risk of a variety of metabolic diseases. Thus, treatment of obesity mandates an urgent national response articulated by multiple evidence-based documents. For example, the Dietary Guidelines for Americans 2020–2025 characterize obesity as the leading nutritional health problem in the United States (17). The Physical Activity Guidelines for Americans 2018 (PAGA 2018) (18) articulate similar conclusions. The Healthy People 2020 (19) document and the 2030 document set aspirational goals of limiting obesity to no more than 15% of the adult population (20). These goals, however, appear to be wishful thinking since the US population is moving away from these goals rather than toward them. For all of these reasons, it is imperative that physicians play an important role both as individual practitioners and community leaders to help combat the issues of overweight and obesity.

Dramatic increases in obesity among children, adolescents, and young adults are particularly worrisome. In these groups, obesity has tripled over the past 30 years. By the time an individual reaches adolescence and is obese, there is a high likelihood that obesity will continue into adulthood and predispose to a variety of other metabolic abnormalities discussed in this chapter (see next section).

4.6 OVERWEIGHT AND OBESITY AND CHRONIC DISEASE

As already indicated, even a weight gain of 10–12 pounds during adult years significantly increases an individual's likelihood of developing chronic disease (21). This carries great significance, given that the average adult in the United States gains a pound a year after the age of 20. Thus, by the time an individual is 50 years old, the average individual in the United States has gained 30 pounds!

In this section, we will discuss the relationship between overweight and obesity and various chronic diseases. These conditions will be elaborated in more detail when we look at specific chapters on each of these chronic diseases in Part 2 of this book.

- *Cardiovascular Disease (CVD)*: The American Heart Association (AHA) lists obesity as a major risk factor for CVD because of its association with other risk factors (T2DM, dyslipidemias, elevated blood pressure, metabolic syndrome). Obesity and overweight also serve as independent risk factors for CVD (22–24).

  As already indicated, the distribution of body fat also carries additional risk. Abdominal obesity is an independent risk factor for coronary heart disease (CHD) (11–16). This is caused by the accumulation of intra-abdominal fat which can yield insulin resistance, which can further contribute to glucose intolerance, elevated triglycerides, and low HDL, as well as hypertension. These abnormalities, when combined, constitute the MetS.

  The best evidence-based guidelines to help physicians treat obesity were jointly published in 2013 by the AHA, the American College of Cardiology (ACC), and the Obesity Society (TOS) (25). These guidelines include the following five steps:

  1. Use BMI as a first step in establishing criteria to judge potential health risks.
  2. Counsel patients that lifestyle changes can produce modest and sustained weight loss and achieve meaningful health benefits and that greater weight loss produces greater benefits.
  3. Multiple dietary approaches are acceptable for weight loss. However, the diet should be prescribed to achieve reduced caloric intake.
  4. Patients who are overweight or obese should be enrolled in comprehensive lifestyle interventions for weight loss delivered in programs six months or longer.
  5. Advice should be given to patients who might be contemplating bariatric surgery (BMI $\geq$40 kg/m^2) or (BMI $\geq$30 kg/m^2) with obesity comorbid conditions.

  It is important to recognize that when counseling patients, the core therapeutic modalities to treat weight gain and obesity are lifestyle-related, including physical activity and sound nutrition. The large NIH-funded Look AHEAD Trial (Action for Health and Diabetes) showed that individuals who lost 7% of body weight significantly lowered all CVD risk factors, except for LDL cholesterol levels (9).

  The DGA 2020–2025 recommends a variety of healthy anti-inflammatory diets, which, when also combined with caloric control, assist in healthy weight loss. These include the Mediterranean diet (MedDiet) (26), the DASH diet (27), and the Healthy US-Style Dietary Pattern (17).
- *Diabetes, Pre-Diabetes*: Obesity has been clearly linked to increased prevalence of the metabolic syndrome and T2DM as well as CVD. This linkage occurs through dysregulation of multiple endocrine and inflammatory mechanisms, although the specific role of these mechanisms in the pathogenesis of T2DM is incompletely understood (28–30). The mechanisms that link obesity, insulin resistance, and T2DM provide the basis for strategies to prevent and treat insulin resistance.

  Obesity-associated insulin resistance is a major risk factor for T2DM and CVD. Multiple endocrine and inflammatory markers have been demonstrated to be dysregulated in obesity and contribute to insulin resistance.

Fat accumulation, which is the main characteristic of both overweight and obesity, results in adipose tissues storing fats in the form of triglycerides, which increase lipid flow into various blood compartments. This may result in non-adipose tissue such as liver, pancreas, and skeletal muscle accumulating triglycerides (30,31).

Lifestyle interventions, including increased physical activity, healthy nutrition strategies (as already indicated), and behavioral approaches, have been studied and have been demonstrated to lower the risk of developing T2DM. These will be discussed in subsequent sections in this chapter.

These same modalities have been demonstrated in major studies to lower the risk of pre-diabetes turning into diabetes. This was most prominently demonstrated in the Diabetes Prevention Program (DPP) (8) where individuals with glucose intolerance (fasting blood glucose of between 103 and 120 mg/dL) were randomized to lifestyle measures (e.g., increased healthy nutrition, physical activity, and weight loss), metformin, or placebo. Those individuals who were randomized to increase physical activity, consume healthy nutrition, and lose weight lost an average of 7% of their body weight and reduced their risk of developing diabetes by 58%. These lifestyle strategies significantly outperformed both metformin and placebo.

- *Metabolic Syndrome*: Metabolic syndrome (MetS) is a cluster of physiologic variables including hypertension, hyperglycemia, abdominal obesity, and elevated triglycerides. A variety of different definitions for MetS have been proposed. Perhaps the one most commonly used is from the National Cholesterol Education Program Adult Treatment Panel (NCEP-ATP III). NCEP III criteria include the following:
  1. *Abdominal Obesity (Waist Circumference)*: Men >100 cm (>40 inches); women >88 cm (>35 inches).
  2. *HDL Cholesterol*: Men <40 mg/dL; women <50 mg/dL.
  3. *Triglycerides*: >150 mg/dL.
  4. Fasting glucose >100 mg/dL.
  5. *Blood pressure*: (Systolic/diastolic) >130/>85 mm Hg.

  MetS is very common in the adult population in the United States. Estimates have ranged between 27% and 38% of individuals in the United States having MetS (32,33). The AHA recommends that individuals who have MetS be treated as though they already have CHD (30).
- *Cancer*: Physicians often do not recognize the link between obesity and cancer. In fact, obesity is the second leading cause of cancer (only behind cigarette smoking) in the United States (34). The International Agency for Cancer Research (IACR) identified 13 human malignancies related to excess body weight. These include esophageal cancer, colorectal cancer, liver cancer, gallbladder cancer, and pancreatic cancer (35). Obesity is also associated with a variety of endocrine-related cancers, including breast, ovarian, and prostate cancer.

  The leading theory for the relationship between obesity and cancer involves multiple alterations in metabolic parameters resulting from inflammatory markers emitted by adipose tissue. These include IL-6, IL-1, and TNF-α (36,37). Compelling scientific evidence exists to establish the link between inflammatory markers and cancer. In addition, levels of insulin and insulin-like growth factor (IGF-1) also typically increase in obesity and contribute to tumor growth. All of these relationships further underscore the importance of weight loss as a way of reducing the risk of cancer. Utilizing standard lifestyle medicine practices, such as increased physical activity and prioritizing healthy eating patterns while restricting calories, plays essential roles in weight loss and reducing the risk of cancer.
- *Obesity and Arthritis*: Arthritis is common, particularly in individuals over the age of 50 (38). Obesity is the leading cause of osteoarthritis in women and the second leading cause of osteoarthritis in men. This elevated risk is largely due to increased impact

on the bones and joints, particularly of the hip and knee (39,40). In one study 83% of females diagnosed with osteoarthritis of the knee were reported to be obese, compared to 42% in the control group (41). The inflammatory component of obesity, in addition to the mechanical stressors on the bones from excess body weight, also contributes to osteoarthritis. Weight loss is the most significant strategy for assisting in the treatment of osteoarthritis. Dietary interventions, as already indicated in other chronic diseases, are important. Physical activity is also important. It should be noted that patients with osteoarthritis often lead very sedentary lives. Thus, physical activity prescriptions must be geared to start slowly and ramp up gradually in order to accommodate previously sedentary individuals with osteoarthritis.

4.7 PHYSICAL ACTIVITY MANAGEMENT OF OBESITY

Physical activity plays an important role in the prevention of weight gain and, thereby, lowers the risk of developing obesity as an adult (42–45). Thus, physical activity should be stressed in efforts to focus on primary prevention of weight gain and obesity. Physical activity can result in weight loss, even without reduction in energy intake, but the magnitude of weight loss is dependent on the dose of physical activity (46). In contrast, physical activity is a key contributor to long-term weight loss maintenance and prevention of weight regain. Physical activity is, thus, recommended in conjunction with reduced calorie consumption for acute weight loss and ongoing prevention of weight regain. Physical activity is an important lifestyle behavior to include even within medical-based treatments for obesity, such as pharmacologic therapy and bariatric surgery.

Independent of body weight and obesity status, physical activity, as discussed in Chapter 1, yields a variety of health benefits. This justifies the importance of regular physical activity as a key lifestyle behavior not only in patients of optimal body weight, but also in patients with overweight and obesity. Of all the forms of physical activity that may be recommended, most physicians prefer walking as the chief form of moderate physical activity (47). Walking protocols will be provided in Appendix B at the end of this book. While they are not significantly different for overweight or obese individuals, individuals who have been sedentary in the past will need to start any walking program at low levels and slowly ramp up to the levels that are recommended by the CDC and the PAGA 2018.

4.8 BEHAVIORAL MANAGEMENT OF THE PATIENT WITH OBESITY

Modifications of behavior are the foundation of long-term weight control programs for patients with overweight and obesity. The AHA/ACC/TOS Guidelines recommend behavior modification for all patients receiving treatment for obesity (25). Changes in diet and exercise are the ultimate goal, but behavioral strategies are crucial to help patients overcome the challenges to make these needed changes. A wide variety of behavioral strategies are available, and they vary according to individual patients (48–51).

Principles involved in behavior management include setting goals, raising awareness, confronting barriers, and managing stress. In addition, behavioral strategies such as problem-solving are essential for preventing relapse. One strategy that many behavioral specialists utilize is asking the obese patient to sign a behavioral contract. Such contracts typically involve patients agreeing to make one or two healthy changes in their lifestyle between appointments with their health care provider.

In addition, strong support must be available not only from the physician but also from family members and close friends. Currently, guidelines from the AHA, ACC, and TOS for behavioral management of patients' obesity recommend 30–60 minute weekly behavioral counseling sessions with either an individual or a group for the first six months, followed by bi-weekly and then monthly sessions.

4.9 DIETARY MANAGEMENT OF OVERWEIGHT AND OBESITY

The cornerstone for the treatment of overweight and obesity involves effective dietary management. Nutrition assessment may be performed by registered dietitian nutritionists (RDNs) who collect data and analyze it, assisting the patient in making sound choices (52,53).

While numerous dietary interventions are available, the key issue is determining which one will fit best for each patient. Low-fat and low-carbohydrate diets have been compared, and at the end of one year neither resulted in more effective weight loss than the other. The key is to find a healthful diet that will allow an individual to restrict the number of calories that they consume. These healthful diets, according to the DGA 2020–2025, include the Mediterranean diet (26), the DASH diet (27), and the Healthy US-Style Dietary Pattern (17). The key is to find which of these healthy diets works best for an individual patient.

All of these diets have abundant fruits and vegetables and whole grains, and all are, in essence, nutrient-dense, meaning that they deliver high levels of nutrients per calorie. Regular physical activity has been shown to play a significant role in addition to nutritional parameters in helping people achieve long-term weight loss.

Since obesity is a chronic relapsing condition, successful therapy requires long-term strategies and a commitment to shared decision-making and a trusting partnership between the patient and their health care team.

4.10 THE ROLE OF PHARMACOLOGIC THERAPY

For individuals who are obese (BMI≥30 kg/m^2) or severely obese (BMI≥35 kg/m^2), it may be necessary to utilize pharmacologic therapy in addition to lifestyle measures. Currently, eight drugs with good safety profiles are approved by the Federal Drug Administration (FDA) for short- and long-term obesity treatment (semaglutide, liraglutide, naltrexone-bupropion, phentermine-topiramate, orlistat, phentermine, and tirzepatide) (54). If considering prescribing one of these medicines for a patient, the physician must have a clear understanding of the indications and potential side effects.

Recent entries into this area include the GLP-1 medications (55). These medicines, which include Ozempic and Mounjaro, are FDA-approved for diabetes management. GLP-1s work by mimicking a hormone in the body that regulates blood sugar and satiety and help patients lose weight by slowing gastric emptying and causing a feeling of fullness. It should be noted that some physicians are prescribing both Ozempic and Mounjaro off-label for weight loss (56).

The results of the GLP-1 agonists for weight loss have been striking. Many patients lose up to 15% of their initial body weight. Several considerations, however, are important to emphasize. First, it appears that individuals will often regain all of the weight that they lost once they stop taking these medicines. Secondly, they are very expensive. For this reason, many physicians use GLP-1 agents only in the context of also emphasizing healthy nutrition and physical activity.

4.11 BARIATRIC SURGERY

Indications for bariatric surgery include a BMI of >40 kg/m^2, or a BMI of 35–39.9 kg/m^2 with a weight-related condition (57). While most primary care physicians will not have reason to deal with a patient following bariatric surgery, they may be involved with the operative medical management as well as post-operative medical management. These factors will include management of comorbid conditions (e.g., CHD, T2DM, etc.) and also monitoring and prescription of nutritional and physical activity therapies.

4.12 THE ROLE OF THE PHYSICIAN IN OVERWEIGHT AND OBESITY

A key issue for all physicians in the areas of overweight and obesity involves discussions with all patients about weight gain and the risk factors associated with the conditions of overweight and obesity. Unfortunately, only 40% of physicians ever have these discussions with patients who are overweight or obese (58).

In our curriculum, we provide some suggestions on how to initiate this conversation. We also advocate taking a BMI for all patients. If ancillary health care personnel are available, obtaining a waist circumference as outlined in this chapter may also be appropriate.

It is critically important in these discussions not to embarrass or in any way shame a patient who is overweight or obese. Furthermore, these counseling sessions should apply principles of motivational interviewing to help a patient understand in their own terms how to handle issues of weight gain, overweight, and obesity.

4.13 PEDIATRIC OBESITY

Childhood obesity represents a chronic disease epidemic that carries both medical and public health implications. While this book and the enclosed curriculum largely deal with issues in adults, many physicians will end up having discussions with their adult patients about pediatric obesity as well. The prevalence of obesity among children aged 2 to 19 years in the United States is 18.5% (59). The prevalence has continued to rise dramatically in the past three decades in all age groups. The increase in pediatric obesity has resulted in an increase in T2DM and risk factors for CHD in the childhood population (60–65). It is important that physicians focus on supporting the child and the family. Lifestyle changes, including healthy nutrition and, to some degree, caloric reduction, physical activity, sleep, and other behaviors, are important to include in these discussions. While treatment of childhood obesity is beyond the scope of this book, pediatric weight loss programs exist at many hospitals, which can be utilized where pediatric patients and their families can be treated.

4.14 LIFESTYLE MEDICINE, OVERWEIGHT AND OBESITY

As already indicated, obesity in essence represents the quintessential lifestyle medicine condition. Effective treatment of obesity involves both physical activity and healthy nutrition. Lifestyle medicine modalities, which are discussed in detail in various chapters in this book, play significant roles in the short-term and long-term management of obesity. In addition, lifestyle medicine modalities such as regular physical activity and healthy nutrition also lower the risk of a variety of chronic diseases, not only those associated with obesity but those that occur outside of obesity as well. For this reason, utilizing multiple lifestyle medicine modalities can play a critical role in helping patients who are overweight or obese.

In addition, physicians should emphasize lifestyle medicine modalities in individuals who are within the optimal weight range (BMI $\geq$ 19 kg/m^2 and $\leq$ 25 kg/m^2). This is important because lifelong adherence to lifestyle medicine principles and practices will reduce the risk of weight gain in the first place.

4.15 USE OF ANCILLARY PROFESSIONALS AND OBESITY MANAGEMENT PROGRAMS

The key professional group that can assist in helping patients lose weight in the short term is RDNs. They can be found in any large city by accessing the website of the Academy of Nutrition and Dietetics (66). It should be noted, however, that many individuals who advertise themselves as nutrition experts on the internet often do not have the appropriate professional degrees. This can be avoided by going to the Academy of Nutrition and Dietetics website. In addition, most health clubs will have exercise physiologists who can assist in safe physical activity programs that are so important to help people keep weight off in the long term.

4.16 BE A ROLE MODEL

The principles and practices outlined in this chapter can also play an important role in a physician's own health and weight management. It can be very motivating for patients to see that their physician is also following these guidelines. This is particularly true if the physician is either overweight or obese and is working to lower their own risk of chronic disease by adopting these principles.

4.17 CLINICAL APPLICATIONS/CONCLUSIONS

As is emphasized in the embedded curriculum, the key issue is to discuss weight management with all patients.

1. For those who are currently in the "optimal" weight range (BMI $\geq$ 19 kg/m^2 and $\leq$ 25 kg/m^2), the key issue is to emphasize the importance of regular physical activity and healthy nutrition to lower the risk of adult weight gain in the first place.
2. For individuals who have overweight or obesity, a discussion should occur related to the association of overweight or obesity with multiple chronic conditions.
3. For individuals who have overweight or obesity, a good place to start is to obtain a BMI and optimally a waist circumference as outlined in this chapter. This will help initiate the discussion of the links between overweight and obesity and multiple chronic diseases.
4. Discussions about the conditions of overweight and obesity must be done in a professional and non-judgmental fashion, and the techniques of motivational interviewing are appropriate in this setting.

To get your patients started on a walking program, or if you have been sedentary yourself and want to get started with a program, we have provided five walking programs in Appendix B. They start from the least intense to the most intense. They are color-coded. The least intense program is the Blue Walking Program, and the most intense program is the Red Walking Program. Instructions for which program might be best for your patients and/or you are provided along with the program. These walking programs were developed in Dr. Rippe's research laboratory and are based on experience developed from many thousands of patients over many years. The programs are designed so that you can assess your progress and move to the next-level program once you have completed the previous level.

REFERENCES

1. Ng M, Fleming T, Robinson M, et al. Global, regional, and national prevalence of overweight and obesity in children and adults during 1980–2013: a systematic analysis for the Global Burden of Disease Study 2013. *Lancet.* 2014;384(9945):766–781.
2. Anonymous. Clinical guidelines on the identification, evaluation, and treatment of overweight and obesity in adults – the evidence report. National Institutes of Health. *Obes Res.* 1998;6(Suppl 2):51S–209S.
3. Allison DB, Fontaine KR, Manson JE, et al. Annual deaths attributable to obesity in the United States. *JAMA.* 1999;282(16):1530–1538.
4. Rippe JM. Physician education and lifestyle medicine: a key to the future. *Am J Lifestyle Med.* 2024; 18(6):724–726.
5. American Society of Nutrition Statement on Metabolism. https://nutrition.org/publications/fact-sheets-and-position-papers/. Accessed January 29, 2025.
6. Rippe JM, Foreyt JP. *Lifestyle Medicine: Obesity Prevention and Treatment: A Practical Guide.* Boca Raton, FL: CRC Press, 2021.
7. Rippe JM, Angelopoulos T. Obesity and heart disease. In Rippe JM, Angelopoulos TA (eds.) *Obesity: Prevention and Treatment.* Boca Raton, FL: CRC Press, 2012.
8. The Diabetes Prevention Program Research G. The Diabetes Prevention Program (DPP): description of lifestyle intervention. *Diabetes Care.* 2002;25(12):2165–2171.

9. Look Ahead Research Group, Wadden TA, West DS, et al. The Look AHEAD study: a description of the lifestyle intervention and the evidence supporting it. *Obesity*. 2006;14(5):737–752.
10. Collaborators GUOF. National-level and state-level prevalence of overweight and obesity among children, adolescents, and adults in the USA, 1990–2021, and forecasts up to 2050. *Lancet*. 2024;404 (10469):2278–2298.
11. Despres JP. Excess visceral adipose tissue/ectopic fat: the missing link in the obesity paradox? *J Am Coll Cardiol*. 2011;57(19):1887–1889.
12. Zamboni M, Armellini F, Sheiban I, et al. Relation of body fat distribution in men and degree of coronary narrowings in coronary artery disease. *Am J Cardiol*. 1992;70(13):1135–1138.
13. Bjorntorp P. Abdominal obesity and the development of noninsulin-dependent diabetes mellitus. *Diabetes/Metab Rev*. 1988;4(6):615–622.
14. Folsom AR, Kaye SA, Sellers TA, et al. Body fat distribution and 5-year risk of death in older women. *JAMA*. 1993;269(4):483–487.
15. Folsom AR, Prineas RJ, Kaye SA, et al. Incidence of hypertension and stroke in relation to body fat distribution and other risk factors in older women. *Stroke*. 1990;21(5):701–706.
16. Price GM, Uauy R, Breeze E, et al. Weight, shape, and mortality risk in older persons: Elevated waist-hip ratio, not high body mass index, is associated with a greater risk of death. *Am J Clin Nutr*. 2006;84(2):449–460.
17. U.S. Department of Agriculture, U.S. Department of Health and Human Services. Dietary guidelines for Americans, 2020–2025 (9th ed). December 2020. Available at DietaryGuidelines.gov. https://www.dietaryguidelines.gov/resources/2020-2025-dietary-guidelines-online-materials. Accessed December 23, 2024.
18. Physical Activity Guidelines Advisory Committee. 2018 Physical Activity Guidelines Advisory Committee. 2018 Physical Activity Guidelines Advisory Committee Scientific Report. Washington, DC: U.S. Department of Health and Human Services, 2018.
19. CDC National Center for Health Statistics. Healthy People 2020. Healthy People – Healthy People 2020. Accessed December 23, 2024.
20. CDC National Center for Health Statistics. Healthy People 2030. Healthy People – HP2030. Accessed December 23, 2024.
21. Bassuk SS, Manson JE. Lifestyle and risk of cardiovascular disease and type 2 diabetes in women: a review of the epidemiologic evidence. *Am J Lifestyle Med*. 2008;2(3):191–213.
22. Lloyd-Jones DM, Hong Y, Labarthe D, et al. Defining and setting national goals for cardiovascular health promotion and disease reduction: the American Heart Association's strategic Impact Goal through 2020 and beyond. *Circulation*. 2010; 121(4):586–613.
23. American Heart Association. Council on Lifestyle and Cardiometabolic Health. Council on Lifestyle and Cardiometabolic Health – Professional Heart Daily | American Heart Association. Accessed December 23, 2024.
24. Eckel RH, Jakicic JM, Ard JD, et al. 2013 AHA/ACC guideline on lifestyle management to reduce cardiovascular risk. *Circulation*. 2014;129(25_suppl_2):S76–S99.
25. Jensen MD, Ryan DH, Apovian CM, et al. 2013 AHA/ACC/TOS guideline for the management of overweight and obesity in adults: a report of the American College of Cardiology/American Heart Association Task Force on Practice Guidelines and The Obesity Society. *J Am Coll Cardiol*. 2014;63 (25 Pt B):2985–3023.
26. Estruch R, Ros E, Salas-Salvado J, et al. Primary prevention of cardiovascular disease with a Mediterranean diet. *N Engl J Med*. 2013;368(14):1279–1290.
27. Appel LJ, Moore TJ, Obarzanek E, et al. A clinical trial of the effects of dietary patterns on blood pressure. DASH Collaborative Research Group. *N Engl J Med*. 1997;336(16):1117–1124.
28. The Emerging Risk Factor Collaboration. Separate and combined associations of body-mass index and abdominal adiposity with cardiovascular disease: collaborative analysis of 58 prospective studies. *Lancet* 2011:377:1085–1095.
29. Montague C, O'Rahilly S. The perils of portliness: causes and consequences of visceral adiposity. *Diabetes*. 2000; 49:883–893.
30. National Cholesterol Education Program. Executive summary of the third report of the National Cholesterol Education Program (NCEP) expert panel on detection, evaluation and treatment of high blood cholesterol in adults (adult treatment panel III). *JAMA*. 2001;285:2486–2497.
31. Mitrakou A, Kelley D, Veneman T., et al. Contribution of abnormal muscle and liver glucose metabolism to postprandial hyperglycemia in non-insulin dependent diabetes mellitus. *Diabetes*. 1990;39: 1381–1390.

32. Ford E. Increasing prevalence of the metabolic syndrome among U.S. adults. *Diabetes Care*. 2004; 27:2444–2449.
33. Ford E, Giles W, Dietz W. Prevalence of the metabolic syndrome among U.S. adults. Findings from the third National Health and Nutrition Examination Survey. *JAMA*. 2002;287:356–359.
34. Lauby-Secretan B, Scoccianti C, Loomis D, et al. Body fatness and cancer—viewpoint of the IARC working group. *N Engl J Med.* 2016;375(8):794–798.
35. Berger N. Obesity and cancer pathogenesis. *Ann N Y Acad Sci.* 2014;1311:57–76.
36. Hotamisligil G. Inflammation and metabolic disorders. *Nature.* 2006; 444 (7121): 860–867.
37. Reilly S, Saltiel A. Adapting to obesity with adipose tissue inflammation. *Nat Rev Endocrin.* 2017;13(11):633–643.
38. Arthritis Related Statistics 2006. Accessed January 17, 2025.
39. Leach R, Baumgard S, Broom J. Obesity: its relationship to osteoarthritis of the knee. *Clin Orthop Relat Res.* 1973;(93):271–273.
40. Coggon D, Reading I, Croft P, et al. Knee osteoarthritis and obesity. *Int J Obes Relat Metab Disord.* 2001;25:622–627.
41. Liu B, Balkwill A, Banks E, et al. Relationship of height, weight and body mass index to the risk of hip and knee replacements in middle-aged women. *Rheumatology.* 2007;46:861–867.
42. Williamson D, Madans J, Anda R, et al. Recreational physical activity and ten-year weight change in a US national cohort. *Int J Obes.* 1993;17:279–286.
43. DiPietro L, Dziura J, Blair S. Estimated change in physical activity level (PAL) and prediction of 5-year weight change in men: the Aerobics Center Longitudinal Study. *Int J Obes.* 2004;28:1541–1547.
44. Lee I, Djousse L, Sesso H, et al. Physical activity and weight gain prevention. *JAMA.* 2010;303: 1173–1179.
45. Shiroma E, Sesso H, Lee I. Physical activity and weight gain prevention in older men. *Int J Obes.* 2012;36:1165–1169.
46. Jakicic J, Otto A, Semler L, et al. Effect of physical activity on 18-month weight change in overweight adults. *Obesity.* 2011;19:100–109.
47. Rippe JM, Ward A. *The Complete Book of Fitness Walking.* New York: Prentice Hall Press, 1990.
48. Foreyt JP. Need for lifestyle intervention: how to begin. *Am J Cardiol.* 2005;96(4A):11E–14E.
49. Renjilian DA, Perri MG, Nezu AM, et al. Individual versus group therapy for obesity: effects of matching participants to their treatment preferences. *J Consult Clin Psychol.* 2001;69(4):717–721.
50. Johnston CA, Moreno JP, Foreyt JP. Cardiovascular effects of intensive lifestyle intervention in type 2 diabetes. *Curr Atheroscler Rep.* 2014;16(12):457.
51. Kramer FM, Jeffery RW, Forster JL, et al. Long-term follow-up of behavioral treatment for obesity: patterns of weight regain among men and women. *Int J Obes.* 1989;13(2):123–136.
52. Academy of Nutrition and Dietetics Evidence Analysis Library. Adult weight management: executive summary of recommendations 2014 academy of nutrition and dietetics. https://www.eatrightpro.org/. Accessed April 18, 2025.
53. Esper DH. Utilization of nutrition-focused physical assessment in identifying micronutrient deficiencies. *Nutr Clin Pract.* 2015;30(2):194–202.
54. Pasarica M., Dhurandar NV. A clinical approach to pharmacological management of the patient with obesity. In Rippe JM, Foreyt JP (eds.) *Lifestyle Medicine: Obesity Prevention and Treatment: A Practical Guide.* Boca Raton, FL: CRC Press, 2021.
55. Jastreboff AM, Aronne LJ, Ahmad NN, et al. Tirzepatide once weekly for the treatment of obesity. *N Engl J Med.* 2022;387(3):205–216.
56. Wilding JPH, Batterham RL, Calanna S, et al. Once-weekly semaglutide in adults with overweight or obesity. *N Engl J Med.* 2021;384(11):989–1002.
57. American Society for Metabolic and Bariatric Surgery. Estimate of Bariatric Surgery Numbers, 2011–2018 Estimate of Bariatric Surgery Numbers, 2011–2022 – American Society for Metabolic and Bariatric Surgery. Accessed January 17, 2025.
58. Rippe JM. Lifestyle medicine: the health promoting power of daily habits and practices. *Am J Lifestyle Med.* 2018;12(6):499–512.
59. Skinner AC, Skelton JA. Prevalence and trends in obesity and severe obesity among children in the United States, 1999–2012. *JAMA Pediatr.* 2014;168(6):561–566.
60. Katzmarzy PT. Cardiovascular risk and physical activity in children. In Rippe JM (ed.) *Lifestyle Medicine* (4th ed). Boca Raton, FL: CRC Press, 2024.
61. Faulkner C, Couch SC, Hemingway J. Cardiovascular risk and diet in children. In Rippe JM (ed.) *Lifestyle Medicine* (4th ed). Boca Raton, FL: CRC Press, 2024.

62. Landsbaugh Kaar J, Simon SL. Sleep and obesity prevention in children and adolescents. In Rippe JM (ed.) *Lifestyle Medicine* (4th ed). Boca Raton, FL: CRC Press, 2024.
63. Moore J, Haemer M. Childhood obesity. In Rippe JM (ed.) *Lifestyle Medicine* (4th ed). Boca Raton, FL: CRC Press, 2024.
64. Shustak RJ, Brothers JA, Daniels SR. Identification and management of children with dyslipidemia. In Rippe JM (ed.) *Lifestyle Medicine* (4th ed). Boca Raton, FL: CRC Press, 2024.
65. Baker-Smith C, Gidding S. Diagnosis, management and treatment of systemic hypertension in youth. In Rippe JM (ed.) *Lifestyle Medicine* (4th ed). Boca Raton, FL: CRC Press, 2024.
66. Academy of Nutrition and Dietetics. Academy of Nutrition and Dietetics. eatright.org. Accessed January 17, 2025.

5 Substance Abuse and Addiction

5.1 INTRODUCTION

All primary care physicians and lifestyle medicine physicians need to have a good grasp of the diagnosis and treatment of addiction and substance abuse. Avoiding addictive substances is one of the pillars of lifestyle medicine. There is good reason for this. Individuals who are suffering from addiction and substance abuse disorders typically do not get the help they require to tackle their medical problems.

Substance abuse and addiction problems should be regarded as similar to hypertension and diabetes since they require specialized care and diagnosis as a critical first step. They may also require long-term or lifelong treatment for risk reduction. For all these reasons, it is important to become knowledgeable about the signs, symptoms, diagnosis, and treatment options available for individuals suffering from substance abuse and addiction disorders.

A good example of this issue is cigarette smoking, which is a major cause of disease and a leading risk factor for heart disease and multiple types of cancer (1). Cigarette smoking is often first discussed and treated by primary care physicians or physicians practicing lifestyle medicine. In addition, primary care practitioners will also treat patients who drink alcohol (sometimes in excess), use cannabis, or may use opioids. For this reason, knowing how to recognize and diagnose when these issues become a problem and what the available treatment options are is critically important for all primary care physicians. This is particularly true for those who focus on the area of lifestyle medicine.

Oftentimes, individuals who suffer from significant problems with these substances may be reluctant to discuss this with their physician. Because substance abuse disorders can either be missed or ignored, it is essential for lifestyle medicine practitioners and, indeed, all primary care physicians to be knowledgeable about these issues.

The naming of the field of addiction medicine has been somewhat controversial. Currently, the preferred term and one used by the DSM-5 (Diagnostic and Statistical Manual of Mental Disorders) is "substance use disorder" (SUD) (2). SUD refers to a group of disorders that involve compulsive and repeated use of substances that are associated with negative physical and psychological health consequences. The field has become particularly important for primary care physicians in the context of the opioid health crisis. The concept of SUDs has expanded to the imperative for primary care physicians and lifestyle medicine practitioners to become knowledgeable about other SUDs in addition to opioids. Many of these SUDs are seen with some frequency in primary care practices. These include cigarette smoking, alcohol use, opioid use, and cannabis use disorders.

Overall, SUD is a major public health problem in the United States. Over 19 million Americans aged 19 or older (7.8%) suffer from some form of SUD (3). For example, the National Epidemiologic Surveys of Alcohol and Related Conditions estimate that the lifetime prevalence of alcohol and related disorders is 23% and drug use disorders is 10.3%. Males experience SUDs at a much higher rate than females (10.7% of US males compared to 5.7% of US females) (4).

Typically, individuals begin to meet criteria for SUDs during young adulthood (ages 18–25). This corresponds to a period of life when there is insufficient development of the frontal lobes of the brain, which makes individuals more susceptible to engaging in risky behaviors.

Tobacco is the most commonly abused substance. Currently, it is estimated that 12% of Americans continue to regularly use tobacco products (5). This results in more than 480,000 deaths

DOI: 10.1201/9781003630043-5

attributable to tobacco use each year in the United States, which is more than deaths from all other SUDs combined.

Alcohol is also frequently used in the United States. Over 86% of the population has consumed alcohol at least occasionally at some point in their lifetime (6). It should be noted that almost 27% of the US population has reported binge drinking (defined as drinking more than five drinks in one setting for men or four for women) (6), and 7% of the population (16.3 million) reported heavy drinking on five or more days within the past month. The use of opioids and synthetically produced opioids such as fentanyl has dramatically increased in the United States over the past two decades, although there has been some decrease in this in the past five years (7). Nonetheless, overdoses from opioids remain alarmingly high, with over 100,000 annual deaths. This problem appears to be particularly focused on the African American population, where it has continued to rise, whereas it has diminished somewhat in the Caucasian population (8).

A number of issues have added to the problem of physicians not adequately diagnosing SUDs. For example, a typical primary care physician has been well trained to handle the most common illnesses such as diabetes, obesity, hypertension, and coronary artery disease, but the background and education in SUDs have been largely lacking. This omission may be somewhat a result of the misperception that SUDs are a result of moral failure or criminal behavior. We hope that by including avoidance of addictive substances as one of the key pillars in lifestyle medicine and providing background in this area in this book and embedded curriculum, we can begin to correct the problem of suboptimal education among physicians in this area.

In this chapter, we will focus specifically on cigarette smoking, alcohol use disorders, opioid use disorders, and cannabis use disorder (CUD).

5.2 CIGARETTE SMOKING

Cigarette smoking in the United States remains the leading cause of preventable disease, disability, and death. More than 16 million Americans are currently living with a disease caused by smoking (9,10). There is some evidence that technology-based interventions utilizing the prevalence of mobile phone apps may help some individuals to quit. There is also some evidence that exercise may help with short-term abstinence. Perhaps the most efficacious approach involves targeted behavioral interventions built on the current and unique skills and beliefs of those who smoke. The goal is to ultimately give smokers the best chance to achieve long-term abstinence. Obviously, this is an area where lifestyle medicine practitioners and primary care physicians need specific and detailed knowledge.

A. *The Health Consequences of Smoking*: The adverse health consequences of cigarette smoking are well known. Smoking harms virtually every organ in the body and is strongly associated with cardiovascular disease (CVD), stroke, pneumonia, and erectile dysfunction (10). Cigarette smoking is also associated with cancer of the lung, bladder, cervix, oral cavity, and many others. In addition, smoking harms reproductive health.
B. *Epidemiology*: In the United States, about 12.5% of the adult population (over the age of 18) and 1.5% of youths (middle and high school students) currently smoke cigarettes (11). Cigarette smoking is more common in persons of color, those not currently married, those who have not completed a high school education, and/or those who live below the Federal poverty line, experience anxiety, or have a disability.
C. *Health Consequences of Excessive Alcohol Consumption*: Multiple severe health problems result from excessive alcohol consumption. These include increased risk of pancreatitis and liver disease, as well as increased risk of a variety of cancers (breast, mouth, esophagus, and colon). In addition, increased risk of cardiovascular issues such as heart disease and stroke occurs with excessive alcohol consumption.

   Excessive alcohol consumption may also contribute to mental health conditions such as depression and anxiety and may lead to cerebral damage, including memory problems and dementia. Furthermore, excessive alcohol consumption can lead to a variety of digestive problems and weakened immunity.

It is well known that excessive alcohol use increases the risk of injuries from falls, violence, and accidents and is also linked to social issues such as family problems.

Recent data have suggested that any amount of alcohol consumption may be hazardous to an individual's health and may contribute to increased risk of multiple different cancers. Excessive alcohol consumption is also associated with increased risk of acute respiratory distress syndrome, bacterial pneumonia, and respiratory interstitial virus infection. People who drink excessively and frequently are more liable to contract diseases such as pneumonia and tuberculosis than people who do not drink excessively. In short, excessive alcohol consumption has adverse effects on virtually every bodily system.

D. *Rates of Smoking Cessation*: The risk and severity of diseases caused by smoking are directly related to how long an individual has smoked and the number of cigarettes smoked per day. It is beneficial to quit smoking at any age. For example, after cigarette smoking cessation, the risk of heart attack drops sharply after one year. After quitting, the risk of stroke is approximately the same as that of non-smokers after two to five years. The risk of various cancers of the mouth and larynx declines by 50% after five years (12). The risk of dying of lung cancer drops by half in ten years. Current estimates indicate that 68% of current smokers would like to stop smoking, and 7.4% were able to quit for more than six months in the past year.

E. *Pharmacologic Aides for Smoking Cessation*: The combination of behavioral counseling and medication has been more effective than either treatment alone for smoking cessation. Thus, this should be the preferred recommendation (13,14). A variety of medications have been approved by the FDA, including over-the-counter products (e.g., nicotine gum, lozenges, and patches) and prescription-only medications (e.g., nicotine inhaler, sustained-release bupropion, and varenicline) (15,16). These may help increase the likelihood of smoking cessation, particularly when used in combination with counseling.

F. *Behavioral Smoking Cessation Strategies*: A variety of strategies are available. These include individual counseling, group therapy, telephone counseling, and motivational interviewing. All have shown some efficacy in helping individuals with smoking cessation. Perhaps the most efficacious of these is individual counseling, which has been shown to increase the likelihood of quitting smoking by 40%–60% (17).

G. *Primary Care Visits*: As indicated elsewhere in this book, over 70% of people see their primary care provider (PCP) each year (18). This number includes individuals who are currently smoking. Thus, primary care–based cessation interventions are a highly effective way to reach most cigarette users (19). It may be difficult for many PCPs to spend time assisting an individual with smoking cessation. Many large primary care practices also have behavioral health providers who can assist in this area or can be trained to help with smoking cessation.

H. *Community-based Approaches*: A variety of community-based approaches may also be successful (20). These include mass media campaigns and worksite programs, both of which have been shown to be efficacious.

I. *Technology*: Technology-driven approaches with the wide dissemination of handheld devices and the prevalence of the population using Internet-based approaches may also be efficacious for helping individuals with smoking cessation (21–24).

J. *Other Lifestyle/Behavioral Approaches*: Exercise has been promoted by a variety of sources, including the US Department of Health and Human Services, to help at least with short-term abstinence (25). Of course, this is a key consideration for lifestyle practitioners and is discussed in considerable detail elsewhere in this book and in the embedded curriculum.

K. *Electronic Cigarettes*: Electronic cigarettes have been advertised as a way to help with cigarette smoking cessation (26). The research in this area, however, is controversial.

Although moderate evidence of efficacy exists when comparing e-cigarettes to nicotine replacement therapy (27).

L. *Abrupt Quitting versus Tapering*: One traditional behavioral method is to advocate either abrupt quitting (using a predetermined quit day) or gradual reduction of cigarettes, which has also shown some efficacy (28,29).

All of these approaches to helping individuals with the very important health consideration of cigarette smoking cessation should be familiar to all primary care physicians and lifestyle medicine practitioners. This will allow these physicians to choose the most efficacious recommendation or group of recommendations for current smokers.

5.3 ALCOHOL USE DISORDERS

Alcohol consumption is very common in the United States and around the world. As a result, alcohol use disorder (AUD) also has a high prevalence in the United States. The criteria for AUD will be discussed subsequently in this chapter.

A. *Screening*: Effective screening tools exist that can be implemented in clinical practice for primary care physicians and lifestyle medicine physicians (30). In addition, evidence-based treatments are available, which will also be discussed in this chapter. It should be noted that during the coronavirus disease 2019 (COVID-19) pandemic, alcohol use substantially increased. This further emphasizes why it is important for physicians at all levels of clinical practice to be aware of when alcohol consumption verges into AUD.
B. *Epidemiology*: The prevalence of AUD in one study was 13.9%, with a lifetime prevalence of 29.1% (31). These estimates are based on the National Epidemiologic Survey on Alcohol and Related Conditions, which involved interviewing 36,390 individuals. In this study, AUD had increased by almost 50% compared to a prior estimate in 2001–2002 (31). Increases were particularly noted in women, African Americans, individuals over the age of 65, and participants aged 45–64. The mean age of onset for AUD was 26.2 years. A family history of AUD increases the likelihood of developing this disorder, making family history a relevant part of screening.
C. *Stages of Addiction*: Most public health publications and websites characterize the stages of addiction using either a three-stage or a four-stage model. The three-stage model utilizes a framework of early, middle, and late stages. The early stage is defined by increasing tolerance to alcohol (32). The middle stage is when individuals crave alcohol and have symptoms of withdrawal and may suffer consequences in their personal or professional lives. The late stage is characterized by loss of control, when serious personal and physical consequences occur from alcohol use.

   Stages in the four-stage model are "adaptive," "dependence," "progression," and "conclusion" (33). The first stage also involves the development of tolerance. In the next stage, the individual's amount of alcohol consumption increases, and the individual may start to plan his or her life around drinking. In the progression stage, a sense of loss of control is experienced. The concluding stage is defined by physical symptoms and serious personal and professional consequences. All physicians should be familiar with these stages of addiction since they can be employed in questions related to individual patients and their use of alcohol.
D. *Diagnosis*: The *Diagnostic and Statistical Manual of Mental Disorders*, 5th edition (DSM-5) has a list of diagnostic criteria (34). These are found in Figure 5.1.
E. *Screening Tools*: The diagnostic criteria in DSM-5 lend themselves to screening tools. The most commonly used extensive screen is called the AUD Identification Test (AUDIT), shown in Figure 5.2, and may be useful for individual patient use (35).

F. *Special Populations*: Three populations are at particular risk for alcohol use disorder. These include the elderly (individuals over the age of 65), college students, and physicians. With regard to the elderly, the exact prevalence of AUD is controversial. It may be as low as 1%–3% or as high as 33% (36). With regard to college students, it should be noted that alcohol consumption among college students is common (37). One study reported that binge drinking (e.g., five or more consecutive drinks in one sitting in the past two weeks) is at a level of 40% among college students. There is good information about binge drinking on the National Institute for Alcohol Abuse and Alcoholism website. There is also a website called collegedrinkingprevention.gov, which contains excellent educational material.

It may surprise physicians to know that AUD is prevalent among physicians. Some estimates indicate that 10%–12% of doctors develop some type of SUD (about 50% of this begin AUD) (38). Specialties most at risk are anesthesia, emergency medicine, and psychiatry. AUD may be difficult to diagnose in this population due to high professional stigma and underreporting by colleagues.

A problematic pattern of alcohol use leading to clinically significant impairment or distress, as manifested by at least two of the following, occurring within a 12-month period:

Impaired Control

1. Alcohol is often taken in larger amounts or over a longer period than was intended.
2. There is a persistent desire or unsuccessful efforts to cut down or control alcohol use.
3. A great deal of time is spent in activities necessary to obtain alcohol, use alcohol, or recover from its effects.
4. Craving, or a strong desire or urge to use alcohol.

Social Impairment

5. Recurrent alcohol use resulting in a failure to fulfill major role obligations at work, school, or home.
6. Continued alcohol use despite having persistent or recurrent social or interpersonal problems caused or exacerbated by the effects of alcohol.
7. Important social, occupational, or recreational activities are given up or reduced because of alcohol use.

Risky Use

8. Recurrent alcohol use in situations in which it is physically hazardous.
9. Alcohol use is continued despite knowledge of having a persistent or recurrent physical or psychological problem that is likely to have been caused or exacerbated by alcohol.

Physiological Indicators

10. Tolerance, as defined by either of the following:
    a. A need for markedly increased amounts of alcohol to achieve intoxication or desired effect.
    b. A markedly diminished effect with continued use of the same amount of alcohol.
11. Withdrawal, as manifested by either of the following:
    a. The characteristic withdrawal syndrome for alcohol
    b. Alcohol (or a closely related substance, such as a benzodiazepine) is taken to relieve or avoid withdrawal symptoms.

FIGURE 5.1 DSM-5 diagnostic criteria. (From: Chen A. Alcohol use and disorders: diagnosis and treatment. *Substance-related and Addictive Disorders. Diagnostic and Statical Manual of Mental Disorders.* American Psychiatric Association, 2013. In Rippe JM (ed.) Lifestyle Medicine (4th ed). Boca Raton, FL: CRC Press, 2024. Used with Permission from Dr. James Rippe.)

Questions	0	1	2	3	4	
1. How often do you have a drink containing alcohol?	Never	Monthly or less	2 to 4 times a month	2 to 3 times a week	4 or more times a week	
2. How many drinks containing alcohol do you have on a typical day when you are drinking?	1 or 2	3 or 4	5 or 6	7 to 9	10 or more	
3. How often do you have 5 or more drinks on one occasion?	Never	Less than monthly	Monthly	Weekly	Daily or almost daily	
4. How often during the last year have you found that you were not able to stop drinking once you had started?	Never	Less than monthly	Monthly	Weekly	Daily or almost daily	
5. How often during the last year have you failed to do what was normally expected of you because of drinking?	Never	Less than monthly	Monthly	Weekly	Daily or almost daily	
6. How often during the last year have you needed a first drink in the morning to get yourself going after a heavy drinking session?	Never	Less than monthly	Monthly	Weekly	Daily or almost daily	
7. How often during the last year have you had a feeling of guilt or remorse after drinking?	Never	Less than monthly	Monthly	Weekly	Daily or almost daily	
8. How often during the last year have you been unable to remember what happened the night before because of your drinking?	Never	Less than monthly	Monthly	Weekly	Daily or almost daily	
9. Have you or someone else been injured because of your drinking?	No		Yes, but not in the last year		Yes, during the last year	
10. Has a relative, friend, doctor, or other health care worker been concerned about your drinking or suggested you cut down?	No		Yes, but not in the last year		Yes, during the last year	

FIGURE 5.2 Alcohol use disorders identification test (AUDIT).

G. *Treatment*: A variety of treatments are available for AUD. The first step involves managing withdrawal symptoms. The mainstay for this stage is benzodiazepines, which have been shown to be highly effective. The preferred benzodiazepines to be used include long-acting ones, including chlordiazepoxide and diazepam (39,40). The second stage is maintenance of sobriety and relapse prevention. The highest risks of relapse are in the three months and one year after the date of sobriety. A variety of behavioral treatments are also available, which include motivational interviewing and mutual-help groups such as Alcoholics Anonymous (AA).

H. *When to Refer*: It may be appropriate to involve an addiction medicine specialist to help clarify issues related to the diagnosis, as well as assist in the process of detoxification.

I. *AUD and COVID-19*: The COVID-19 pandemic led to a dramatic increase in AUD, including a 25% increase in alcohol-related deaths between 2019 and 2020. This was far above the 16.6% increase in all-cause mortality typically observed before COVID-19. In one survey study, 75% of adults reported alcohol use on one additional day per month during the COVID-19 pandemic (30). This has led to the recommendation from the World

Health Organization (WHO) and other experts to encourage annual screening for AUD and comorbid psychiatric diagnoses.

With the high prevalence of alcohol consumption in the United States and elsewhere, knowledge of the way that alcohol can lead to addiction is particularly relevant to primary care and lifestyle medicine–practicing physicians.

5.4 OPIOID USE DISORDERS

Diagnosis and treatment of opioid use disorders (OUDs) is very important for all clinicians, but particularly primary care clinicians and individuals practicing with an emphasis on lifestyle medicine. The opioid epidemic in the United States has gotten somewhat better over the past few years. As late as 2023–2024, however, there were still over 100,000 annual deaths from drug overdoses (8). This has been a particular problem with synthetic opioids such as fentanyl. Of note, deaths from overdoses among Caucasians have decreased by 20% while increasing by 40% in the African American population. In addition, it appears that the COVID-19 pandemic worsened limited access to treatment among rural, poor, and minority populations (41). For all these reasons, it is essential that all primary care physicians, and particularly those practicing in the area of lifestyle medicine, be aware of risk factors, how to diagnose, and how to treat OUDs.

A. *Risk Factors*: Opioids play an important role in treating patients with severe pain that is not well controlled with other therapies. Risk factors for the use of opioids, however, are important to understand. Physician prescribing practices have changed dramatically since the 1990s and early 2000s (41). In the 1990s and early 2000s, liberal use of opioids peaked because physicians were urged to be more aggressive in treating pain. Moreover, with longer-acting opioids, it was thought that there was a reduced risk of addiction. In addition, this concept was aggressively promoted by a number of pharmaceutical companies. This led to the overprescribing of opioid pills without sufficient follow-up visits. The pendulum has now swung in the opposite direction. In the period between 2012 and 2015, prescriptions for opioids fell by about 50% (42).

   Since opioids are useful in treating intractable pain, it is important that clinicians understand the risk factors for the overuse of opioids. Risk factors exist that predict misuse of opioids when prescribed for chronic pain. A screening tool has now been developed to assist physicians in evaluating risk. This screening instrument is the Screener and Opioid Assessment for Patients and Pain (SOAPP) (43). This screening tool is found in Table 5.1.

   Anyone who scores 18 or higher on this screening tool is rated as being at risk for opioid misuse.

B. *Diagnosis*: The DSM-5 has developed criteria for OUDs (44). These are found in Table 5.2. There are three clusters of symptoms that are centered around this diagnosis:
   1. Impaired control and drug cravings
   2. Psychosocial impairment
   3. Pharmacologic adaptation

   To meet the criteria for opioid use disorder, an individual needs to have at least two of the specified 11 criteria outlined in Table 5.2.

C. *Treatment Options*: The average primary care physician or individual focusing on lifestyle medicine will rarely be called upon to treat someone with OUD. These cases require specialized expertise, and a referral will usually be required. Possible treatment options from a pharmacological standpoint include methadone maintenance treatment and buprenorphine office-based treatment. Use of buprenorphine requires a special DEA waiver for

TABLE 5.1
Screening Tool to Assess Risk for Opioid Misuse in Pain Patients

Screener and Opioid Assessment for Patients with Pain (SOAPP)® Version 1.0 - 14Q

Name: ____ ____ ____ ____ ____ ____ ____ ____ __ Date: ____________

The following are some questions given to all patients at the Pain Management Center who are on or being considered for opioids for their pain. Please answer each question as honestly as possible. This information is for our records and will remain confidential. Your answers alone will not determine your treatment. Thank you.

Please answer the questions below using the following scale:

0 = Never, 1 = Seldom, 2 = Sometimes, 3 = Often, 4 = Very Often

1. How often do you have mood swings?
2. How often do you smoke a cigarette within an hour after you wake up?
3. How often have any of your family members, including parents problem with alcohol or drugs?
4. How often have any of your close friends had a problem with alcohol or drugs?
5. How often have others suggested that you have a drug or alcohol problem?
6. How often have you attended an AA or NA meeting?
7. How often have you taken medication other than the way that it was prescribed?
8. How often have you been treated for an alcohol or drug problem?
9. How often have your medications been lost or stolen?
10. How often have others expressed concern over your use?
11. How often have you felt a craving for medication?
12. How often have you been asked to give a urine screen for substance abuse?
13. How often have you used illegal drugs (for example, marijuana, cocaine, etc.) in the past five years?
14. How often, in your lifetime, have you had legal problems or been arrested?

Please include any additional information you wish about the above answers. Thank you.

Tool for Assessing Risk of Developing Opioid Use Disorders

TABLE 5.2
DSM-5 Diagnostic Criteria

A problematic pattern of alcohol use leading to clinically significant impairment or distress, as manifested by *at least two of the following, occurring within a 12-month period*:

Impaired Control

1. Alcohol is often *taken in larger amounts* or over a longer period than was intended.
2. There is a *persistent desire or unsuccessful efforts to cut down* or control alcohol use.
3. A *great deal of time is spent in activities necessary to obtain alcohol*, use alcohol, or recover from its effects.
4. *Craving*, or a strong desire or urge to use alcohol.

Social Impairment

5, Recurrent alcohol use resulting in a *failure to fulfill major role obligations* at work, school, or home.
6. Continued alcohol use despite having *persistent or recurrent social or interpersonal problems* caused or exacerbated by the effects of alcohol.
7. Important social, occupational, or recreational *activities are given up or reduced* because of alcohol use.

Risky Use

8. Recurrent alcohol *use in situations in which it is physically hazardous*.
9. Alcohol use is continued despite *knowledge of having a persistent or recurrent physical or psychological problem* that is likely to have been caused or exacerbated by alcohol.

(*Continued*)

TABLE 5.2 (*Continued*)
DSM-5 Diagnostic Criteria

Physiological Indicators

10. *Tolerance*, as defined by either of the following:
    a. A need for markedly increased amounts of alcohol to achieve intoxication or the desired effect.
    b. A markedly diminished effect with continued use of the same amount of alcohol.
11. *Withdrawal*, as manifested by either of the following:
    a) The characteristic withdrawal syndrome for alcohol
    b) Alcohol (or a closely related substance, such as a benzodiazepine) is taken to relieve or avoid withdrawal symptoms.

qualified physicians (45). The third option is naltrexone, which is an opioid antagonist used to prevent relapse to opioids in patients who have completed opioid detoxification (46,47).

D. *Psychosocial Treatment*: Pharmacotherapy is typically not sufficient when used alone for opioid addiction. Therefore, clinicians have the added responsibility for patients with OUD problems to go beyond prescribing medicine. This typically involves psychosocial treatment modalities. The classic treatment modality is cognitive behavioral therapy (CBT) to help patients develop appropriate coping skills (48,49). There are also self-help groups, such as 12-step group offerings, including Alcoholics Anonymous or Narcotics Anonymous (NA). In addition, alternatives to 12-step meetings include Self-Management and Recovery Training (SMART) therapy, rational recovery (RR), or Secular Organizations for Sobriety (SOS) (30). It should be noted that individuals who are on medication as part of their recovery for OUD may not be allowed to join some of the 12-step groups.

5.5 CANNABIS USE DISORDER

A. *Introduction*: Cannabis is the most commonly used psychoactive drug in the United States (48). Approximately 12% of the population aged 12 or over have reported cannabis use in the past month (49). Changes in state laws legalizing cannabis for medical and recreational use have coincided with changes in public perception of cannabis use (50–52). While many people increasingly view cannabis as harmless, significant risks are associated with its use (53). There is also evidence suggesting national increases in cannabis use, with higher levels of potency and increases in adult use leading to increased prevalence of cannabis use disorder (CUD) diagnoses (54,55). Between 20% and 30% of cannabis users now meet criteria for CUD (56).

B. *Harms and Risk Associated with Cannabis Use*: Cannabis is a commonly used drug during pregnancy (57,58). Many women see cannabis as a natural, safe substance to use throughout pregnancy. There are, however, some risks to the fetus. Therefore, the American College of Obstetrics and Gynecologists recommends that women who are pregnant, contemplating pregnancy, or breastfeeding not use marijuana (59).

Childhood exposure to cannabis often involves unintended ingestion of high-potency edible cannabis products (60). This can lead to a variety of untoward symptoms such as dizziness, respiratory depression, and vomiting (61). Primary care physicians have increasingly reported severe or intractable vomiting (hyperemesis) in some heavy users of cannabis.

In the adolescent population, cannabis use can potentially result in negative impacts on brain development, educational outcomes, cognition, and IQ (62,63). This is an area of active current study.

There are also potential adverse effects of adult exposure, including adverse impacts on driving safety. The major psychoactive compound in cannabis can impair motor and cognitive functions. It has been demonstrated that driving under the influence of cannabis increases the risk of fatal and nonfatal motor vehicle accidents (64,65). Legislation prohibits driving while under the influence of cannabis. There are no reliable tests, however, to determine cannabis levels in drivers.

C. *Cannabis Use Disorder*: The DSM-5 provides specific criteria for making a CUD diagnoses (66). These are found in Table 5.3. Cannabis withdrawal can also be significant. The DSM-5 criteria for cannabis withdrawal are found in Table 5.4.

   Psychiatric comorbidities also constitute a risk factor for CUD and are also associated with other substance and psychiatric disorders, including alcohol or nicotine use disorders (67).

D. *Screening for CUD*: Primary care physicians should screen all patients for cannabis use (68). Utilization of the DSM-5 (Table 5.2) criteria may be helpful in determining whether or not CUD is present.

   Treatment for CUD: The US Preventive Services Task Force recommends screening for health risk factors for CUD utilizing the screening, brief intervention, and referral to treatment (SBIRT) model (69). This has been developed for risky alcohol use. Its effectiveness for other substances remains unclear.

   The mainstay of treatment involves psychosocial interventions to increase patient awareness of the negative consequences of cannabis use in combination with enhancing motivation to reduce use (70). The most efficacious strategy involves the use of CBT and/or motivational interviewing/motivational enhancement therapy (MI/MET), or their combination. CUD treatment involves the management of external triggers, thoughts, and behaviors that encourage substance use and promote better coping skills. There are currently no pharmacological interventions for CUD.

E. *Use of Cannabis for Pain*: Chronic pain is a common indication for cannabis use (71). This has become particularly prevalent as people have attempted to use marijuana as a replacement for opioids. Many medical marijuana patients use cannabis for pain relief and may achieve relief as a partial or complete substitute for opioids.

TABLE 5.3
DSM-IV and DSM-5 Criteria for Cannabis Use Disorder (CUD)

	DSM-IV Abuse[a]	DSM-IV Dependence[b]	DSM-5 CUD[c]
Hazardous use (e.g., driving under the influence)	X		X
Social/interpersonal problems related to use	X		X
Neglected major roles to use	X		X
Legal problems	X		
Withdrawal			X
Tolerance		X	X
Used large amounts/longer than intended		X	X
Repeated attempts to quit/control use		X	X
Much time spent using		X	X
Physical/psychological problems related to use		X	X
Activities given up for use		X	X
Craving[d]			X

[a] One or more criteria within a 12-month period.
[b] Three or more criteria within a 12-month period.
[c] Two or more criteria within a 12-month period.
[d] New criterion added in DSM-5.

TABLE 5.4
DSM-5 Cannabis Withdrawal

A. Cessation of heavy, prolonged cannabis use (i.e., daily or almost daily use over at least a few months).

B. Three or more of these symptoms within a week after cessation of heavy, prolonged use:
  - Irritability, anger, or aggression
  - Nervousness or anxiety
  - Sleep difficulty (e.g., insomnia, disturbing dreams)
  - Decreased appetite or weight loss
  - Restlessness
  - Depressed mood
  - At least one of these physical symptoms causing significant discomfort: abdominal pain, shakiness/tremors, sweating, fever, chills, headache

C. The symptoms cause clinically significant distress or impairment in social, occupational, or other important areas of functioning.

D. The symptoms are not due to another medical condition or another mental disorder, including intoxication or withdrawal from another substance.

F. *Use of Cannabis for Psychiatric Conditions*: No compelling evidence exists for the use or efficacy of cannabis in the treatment of depression or anxiety disorders (72,73). Anecdotal testimonies exist, however, from some individuals stating that cannabis relieves depression or anxiety.

5.6 USE OF LIFESTYLE MEDICINE MODALITIES FOR SUBSTANCE ABUSE OR ADDICTION

As will be emphasized in multiple chapters throughout this book, a combination of other lifestyle modalities, such as regular exercise and stress reduction, can play very important roles in lowering the risk of addiction to various substances such as cigarettes, alcohol, opioids, or cannabis. For this reason, it is important that physicians have a basic understanding of the presence of these substances and their potential use among their patients. Knowledge and avoidance of addictive substances is one of the pillars of lifestyle medicine.

5.7 CONCLUSIONS/CLINICAL APPLICATIONS

It is important for primary care physicians and lifestyle medicine physicians to have a good grasp of the diagnosis and treatment options for various substance use disorders and addictions. Primary care physicians, and particularly those practicing in the area of lifestyle medicine, are often the first individuals who encounter a patient who has a substance use disorder. In this chapter, we have highlighted some of the most common substance use disorders and offered some suggestions about how to screen and treat them. On the most fundamental level, it is vital for primary care or lifestyle medicine physicians simply to inquire whether individuals are having any problems with cigarette smoking (if they currently smoke), the amount of alcohol consumed, and whether there is any potential for opioid use disorder or cannabis use disorder. This chapter has provided details, and the embedded curriculum will provide further details on how to initiate conversations in this area and the possible treatment options available.

REFERENCES

1. Mokdad AH, James S. Marks M, et al. Actual causes of death in the United States, 2000. *JAMA*. 2004;291(10):1238–1245.
2. American Psychiatric Association. American Psychiatric Association's Diagnostic and Statistical Manual of Mental Disorders (DSM-5). American Psychiatric Publishing, April, 2013. 947p.

3. Park-Lee E, Lipari RN, Hedden SL, et al. Receipt of services for substance use and mental health issues among adults: results from the 2016 National Survey on Drug Use and Health 2017. NSDUH Data Review.
4. Center for Behavioral Health Statistics and Quality. Behavioral health trends in the United States: results from the 2014 National Survey on Drug Use and Health 2015. HHS Publication No. SMA 15–4927, NSDUH Series H-50.
5. U.S. Department of Health and Human Services. The health consequences of smoking—50 years of progress: a report of the surgeon general. Atlanta, GA: U.S. Department of Health and Human Services, 2014.
6. National Institute of Alcohol Abuse and Alcoholism. Alcohol use in the United States. Alcohol facts and statistics. June 2017. www.niaaa.nih.gov/alcohols-effects-healthy/alcohol-topics/alcohol-facts-and-statistics. Accessed November 15, 2024.
7. Volkow ND. America's addiction to opioids: heroin and prescription drug abuse (testimony to congress). National Institute on Drug Abuse. 2014. https://www.drugabuse.gov/about-nida/legislative-activities/testimony-to-congress/2016/americas-addiction-to-opioids-heroin-prescription-drug-abuse. Accessed November 15, 2024.
8. Volpicelli JR. Diagnosis and treatment of opioid use disorder. In Rippe JM (ed.) *Lifestyle Medicine* (4th ed). Boca Raton, FL: CRC Press, 2024.
9. Ciccolo JT, Santa Barbara NJ. Behavioral approaches to enhancing cigarette smoking cessation. In Rippe JM (ed.) *Lifestyle Medicine* (4th ed). Boca Raton, FL: CRC Press, 2024.
10. U.S. Department of Health and Human Services. *The Health Consequences of Smoking—50 Years of Progress: A Report of the Surgeon General.* Atlanta, GA: U.S. Department of Health and Human Services, Centers for Disease Control and Prevention, National Center for Chronic Disease Prevention and Health Promotion, Office on Smoking and Health, 2014.
11. U.S. Department of Health and Human Services. The Health Consequences of Smoking—50 Years of Progress: A Report of the Surgeon General. Atlanta, GA: U.S. Department of Health and Human Services, Centers for Disease Control and Prevention, National Center for Chronic Disease Prevention and Health Promotion, Office on Smoking and Health, 2014.
12. Babb S, Malarcher A, Schauer G, Asman K, Jamal A. Quitting smoking among adults – United States 2000–2015. *MMWR Morb Mort Wkly Rep.* 2017;65(52):1457–1464.
13. Patnode CD, Henderson JT, Coppola EL, Melnikow J, Durbin S, Thomas RG. Interventions for tobacco cessation in adults, including pregnant persons: updated evidence report and systematic review for the US Preventive Services Task Force. *JAMA.* 2021;325(3):280–298.
14. Hartmann-Boyce J, Hong B, Livingstone-Banks J, Wheat H, Fanshawe TR. Additional behavioural support as an adjunct to pharmacotherapy for smoking cessation. *Cochrane Database Syst Rev.* 2019;6:CD009670.
15. Stead LF, Lancaster T. Combined pharmacotherapy and behavioural interventions for smoking cessation. *Cochrane Database Syst Rev.* 2012;(10):CD008286.
16. Shahab L, McEwen A. Online support for smoking cessation: a systematic review of the literature. *Addiction.* 2009;104(11):1792–804.
17. Lancaster T, Stead LF. Individual behavioural counselling for smoking cessation. *Cochrane Database Syst Rev.* 2005;(2):CD001292.
18. Jamal A, Dube SR, Babb SD, et al. Tobacco use screening and cessation assistance during physician office visits among persons aged 11–21 years—National Ambulatory Medical Care Survey, United States, 2004–2010. *MMWR Morb Mort Wkly Rep Surveill Summ.* 2014;63(Suppl 2):71–79.
19. Bartsch AL, Härter M, Niedrich J. et al. A systematic literature review of self-reported smoking cessation counseling by primary care physicians. *PloS One.* 2016;11(12):e0168482.
20. Leeks KD, Hopkins DP, Soler RE, et al. Task force on community preventive services. Worksite-based incentives and competitions to reduce tobacco use. A systematic review. *Am J Prev Med.* 2010;38(2): S263–S274.
21. Shahab L, McEwen A. Online support for smoking cessation: a systematic review of the literature. *Addiction.* 2009;104(11):1792–1804.
22. Bock B, Graham A, Sciamanna C, et al. Smoking cessation treatment on the Internet: content, quality, and usability. *Nicotine Tob Res.* 2004;6(2):207–219.
23. Walters ST, Wright JA, Shegog R. A review of computer and Internet-based interventions for smoking behavior. *Addict Behav.* 2006;31(2):264–277.
24. Hall AK, Cole-Lewis H, Bernhardt JM. Mobile text messaging for health: a systematic review of reviews. *Annu Rev Public Health.* 2015;36:393–415.

25. Ussher MH, Faulkner GEJ, Angus K, et al. Exercise interventions for smoking cessation. *Cochrane Database Syst Rev.* 2019(10):CD002295.
26. Hartmann-Boyce J, McRobbie H, Butler AR, et al. Electronic cigarettes for smoking cessation. *Cochrane Database Syst Rev.* 2021(9):CD010216.
27. Wagener TL, Siegel M, Borrelli B. Electronic cigarettes: achieving a balanced perspective. *Addiction.* 2012;107(9):1545–1548.
28. Carpenter MJ, Hughes JR, Solomon LJ, et al. Both smoking reduction with nicotine replacement therapy and motivational advice increase future cessation among smokers unmotivated to quit. *J Consult Clin Psychol.* 2004;72(3):371–381.
29. Hughes JR, Callas PW. Is delaying a quit attempt associated with less success? *Nicotine Tob Res.* 2011;13(12):1228–1232.
30. Chen C-Y, Slatkin S. Alcohol use disorders: diagnosis and treatment. In Rippe JM (ed.) *Lifestyle Medicine* (4th ed). Boca Raton, FL: CRC Press, 2024.
31. Grant BF, Goldstein RB, Saha TD, et al. Epidemiology of DSM-5 alcohol use disorder: results from the national epidemiologic survey on alcohol and related conditions III. *JAMA Psychiatry.* 2015;72(8):757–766.
32. Top Treatment Centers. Early, Mid, Late Stages of Alcoholism – The 3 or 4 Stage Paradigm [Internet]. 2017. https://www.projectknow.com/research/stages-of-alcoholism/. Accessed November 26, 2024.
33. Ashwood Recovery. The Stages of Alcoholism Explained. https://www.ashwoodrecovery.com/blog/stages-alcoholism-explained/. Accessed November 26, 2024.
34. Substance-Related and Addictive Disorders. Diagnostic and Statistical Manual of Mental Disorders. American Psychiatric Association, 2013.
35. Fleming MF. Screening and brief intervention in primary care settings. *Alcohol Res Health.* 2004;28:57–62.
36. Caputo F, Vignoli T, Leggio L, et al. Alcohol use disorders in the elderly: a brief overview from epidemiology to treatment options. *Exp Gerontol.* 2012;47(6):411–416.
37. O'Malley PM, Johnston LD. Epidemiology of alcohol and other drug use among American college students. *J Stud Alcohol Suppl.* 2002;(14):23–39.
38. Berge KH, Seppala MD, Schipper AM. Chemical dependency and the physician. *Mayo Clin Proc.* 2009;84(7):625–631.
39. Kattimani S, Bharadwaj B. Clinical management of alcohol withdrawal: a systematic review. *Ind Psychiatry J.* 2013;22(2):100–108.
40. McHugh, R. Kathryn, et al. Benzodiazepine misuse in adults with alcohol use disorder: prevalence, motives and patterns of use. *J Subst Abuse* Treat. 2020;117:108061.
41. Vandergrift JL, Weng W, Gray BM. The association between physician knowledge and inappropriate medications for older populations. *J Am Geriatr Soc.* 2021;69(12):3584–3594.
42. Zhu W, Chernew ME, Sherry TB, et al. Initial opioid prescriptions among US commercially insured patients, 2012–2017. *N Engl J Med.* 2019;380(11):1043–1052.
43. Butler SF, Budman SH, Fernandez K, et al. Validation of a screener and opioid assessment measure for patients with chronic pain. *Pain.* 2004;112(1–2):65–75.
44. O'Brien C. Addiction and dependence in DSM-V. *Addiction.* 2011;106(5):866–867.
45. Andorn AC, Haight BR, Shinde S, et al. Treating opioid use disorder with a monthly subcutaneous buprenorphine depot injection: 12-month safety, tolerability, and efficacy analysis. *J Clin Psychopharmacol.* 2020;40(3):231–239.
46. Ockert DM, Volpicelli JR, Baier AR, et al. A nonopioid procedure for outpatient opioid detoxification. *J Addict Med.* 2011;5(2):110–114.
47. Sigmon SC, Bisaga A, Nunes E, et al. Opioid detoxification and naltrexone induction strategies: recommendations for clinical practice. *Am J Drug Alcohol Abuse.* 2012;38(3):187–199.
48. Fiellin DA, Barry DT, Sullivan LE, et al. A randomized trial of cognitive behavioral therapy in primary care-based buprenorphine. *Am J Med.* 2013;126(1):74.e11–74.e17.
49. Pan S, Jiang H, Du J, et al. Efficacy of cognitive behavioral therapy on opiate use and retention in methadone maintenance treatment in China: a randomised trial. *PLoS One.* 2015;10(6):127598.
50. Compton WM, Han B, Jones CM, et al. Marijuana use and use disorders in adults in the USA, 2002–14: analysis of annual cross-sectional surveys. *Lancet Psychiatry.* 2016;3(10):954–964.
51. Azofeifa A, Mattson ME, Schauer G, et al. National estimates of marijuana use and related indicators – national survey on drug use and health, United States, 2002–2014. *MMWR Surveill Summ.* 2016; 65(11):1–28.

52. Levy NS, Mauro PM, Mauro CM, et al. Joint perceptions of the risk and availability of Cannabis in the United States, 2002–2018. *Drug Alcohol Depend.* 2021;226:108873.
53. Fischer B, Russel C, Sabioni P, et al. Lower-risk cannabis use guidelines: a comprehensive update of evidence and recommendations. *Am J Public Health.* 2017;107(8):1277.
54. El-Sohly MA, Mehmedic Z, Foster S, et al. Changes in Cannabis potency over the last 2 decades (1995–2014): analysis of current data in the United States. *Biol Psychiatry.* 2016;79(7):613–619.
55. Carliner H, Mauro PM, Brown QL, et al. The widening gender gap in marijuana use prevalence in the U.S. during a period of economic change, 2002–2014. *Drug Alcohol Depend.* 2017;170:51–58.
56. Hasin DS, Saha TD, Kerridge BT, et al. Prevalence of marijuana use disorders in the United States between 2001–2002 and 2012–2013. *JAMA Psychiatry.* 2015;72(12):1235–1242.
57. Volkow ND, Compton WM, Wargo EM. The risks of marijuana use during pregnancy. *JAMA.* 2017;317(2):129–130.
58. Brown QL, Sarvet AL, Shmulewitz D, et al. Trends in marijuana use among pregnant and nonpregnant reproductive-aged women, 2002–2014. *JAMA.* 2017;317(2):207–209.
59. The American College of Obstetricians and Gynecologists. Marijuana and Pregnancy. https://www.acog.org/womens-health/infographics/marijuana-and-pregnancy. Published 2018. Accessed April 18, 2025.
60. National Academies of Sciences and Medicine. The health effects of cannabis and cannabinoids: the current state of evidence and recommendations for research. Washington, DC: National Academies of Sciences and Medicine, 2017.
61. Emoto J, Weeks K, Kallail KJ. Accidental acute Cannabis intoxication presenting as seizure in pediatrics patients. *Kans J Med.* 2020;13:129–130.
62. Fergusson DM, Boden JM, Horwood LJ. Psychosocial sequelae of cannabis use and implications for policy: findings from the Christchurch Health and Development Study. *Social Psychiatry Psychiatric Epidemiol.* 2015;50(9):1317–1326.
63. Dhein S. Different effects of Cannabis abuse on adolescent and adult brain. *Pharmacology.* 2020;105(11–12):609–617.
64. Asbridge M, Hayden JA, Cartwright JL. Acute cannabis consumption and motor vehicle collision risk: systematic review of observational studies and meta-analysis. *BMJ.* 2012;344:e536.
65. Brady JE, Li G. Trends in alcohol and other drugs detected in fatally injured drivers in the United States, 1999–2010. *Am J Epidemiol.* 2014;179(6):692–699.
66. Hasin DS, O'Brien CP, Auriacombe M, et al. DSM-5 criteria for substance use disorders: recommendations and rationale. *Am J Psychiatry.* 2013;170(8):834–851.
67. Hasin DS, Kerridge BT, Saha TD, et al. Prevalence and correlates of DSM-5 Cannabis use disorder, 2012–2013: findings from the national epidemiologic survey on alcohol and related conditions-III. *Am J Psychiatry.* 2016;173(6):588–599.
68. Turner S, Spithoff S, Kahan M. Approach to cannabis use disorder in primary care: focus on youth and other high-risk users. *Can Fam Physician.* 2014;60(9):801–808.
69. Moyer VA, Force PST. Screening and behavioral counseling interventions in primary care to reduce alcohol misuse: U.S. preventive services task force recommendation statement. *Ann Intern Med.* 2013;159(3):210–218.
70. Jonas DE, Garbutt JC, Amick HR, et al. Behavioral counseling after screening for alcohol misuse in primary care: a systematic review and meta-analysis for the US preventive services task force. *Ann Intern Med.* 2012;157(9):645–654.
71. Hardt J, Jacobsen C, Goldberg J, et al. Prevalence of chronic pain in a representative sample in the United States. *Pain Med.* 2008;9(7):803–812.
72. Walsh Z, Gonzalez R, Crosby K, et al. Medical cannabis and mental health: a guided systematic review. *Clin Psychol Rev.* 2017;51:15–29.
73. Lowe DJE, Sasiadek JD, Coles AS, et al. Cannabis and mental illness: a review. *Eur Arch Psychiatry Clin Neurosci.* 2019;269(1):107–120.

6 Sleep

6.1 INTRODUCTION

Healthy sleep is essential for virtually every organ system, indeed, for life itself and optimal health (1–4). Sleep plays a significant role in metabolism, cardiovascular function, brain function, systemic physiology, appetite regulation, etc. It also plays a very significant role in the function of the immune system and hormonal systems (5–7). Healthy sleep is one of the pillars of lifestyle medicine since lifestyle factors play important roles in maintaining healthy sleep and, in turn, sleep plays a crucial role in other lifestyle factors.

Normal healthy sleep is characterized by good quality, adequate duration, appropriate timing and regularity, as well as the absence of sleep disorders (8). We emphasize sleep as part of this book and the embedded curriculum since it is a critical and often neglected component of clinical interactions with patients.

Up to 70 million people in the United States have a chronic sleep disorder that impacts their daily functioning and health (9). There are over 100 sleep disorders. Sleep disorders are typically manifested in one of the following ways: failure to obtain the necessary amount or quantity of sleep (sleep deprivation), inability to maintain sleep continuity (disrupted sleep), difficulty maintaining sleep (insomnia), and events that occur during sleep (e.g., sleep apnea, restless leg syndrome) (10). In this chapter, we will focus on normal sleep as well as problems that can disrupt sleep and their health implications. The chapter will also include ways that clinicians can assess sleep in patients, as well as the importance of addressing sleep in every clinical encounter. We conclude this chapter with information on what has been called "sleep hygiene," which includes tips on healthy sleeping.

6.2 CHARACTERISTICS OF NORMAL SLEEP

Stages of sleep have typically been divided into two components. The first is rapid eye movement (REM) sleep, and then four stages of non-rapid eye movement (NREM) sleep characterized by increased sleep depth (11). Stages 3 and 4 are typically considered the most restorative types of sleep and typically occur in the first one-third of the night. REM sleep, in contrast, increases as the night progresses and is longest in the last third of sleep. A number of physiologic changes occur in both REM and NREM sleep. These include changes in brain activity, heart rate, blood pressure, sympathetic nervous system activity, and muscle tone, as well as blood flow to the brain, respiration, airway resistance, renal and endocrine function, body temperature, and sexual arousal. It is important to understand that the sleep/wake cycle is controlled by daily rhythms called circadian rhythms. These are regulated by the hypothalamus. Circadian rhythms synchronize sleep to external day/night cycles (6).

6.3 SLEEP DISRUPTION

Various kinds of sleep disruption are very common (12). The National Sleep Foundation in a 2014 survey, reported that 35% of American adults rated their sleep quality as "poor" or "only fair." In this same survey, prolonged sleep at least one night per week was reported by only 45% of respondents (13). In contrast, 53% of respondents had trouble staying asleep at least one night in the previous week, and 23% of respondents had trouble staying asleep for five or more nights. Snoring was also common, as reported in this survey. Unfortunately, only 17% of respondents had been told by a physician that they had a sleep disorder. Most of these (68%) were told that they had sleep apnea (12).

DOI: 10.1201/9781003630043-6

Multiple risk factors contribute to sleep disruption. They include a variety of lifestyle, biological, psychological, genetic, and social factors (14). The lifestyle factors that play a role include consuming excessive amounts of caffeine or drinking alcohol. Individuals who work the night shift are also at risk for sleep disruption, as is being a college student. Excessive nighttime light pollution may also disrupt circadian rhythm and create sleep disruptions. Stressful life circumstances may also disrupt sleep, as can a terminal illness or being a parent of a young infant.

Sleep disruption is a broad category and may include a sleep disorder such as obstructive sleep apnea (OSA) or restless leg syndrome. Major medical conditions may also be associated with sleep disruption, particularly those that require nighttime medical monitoring.

Sleep deprivation studies have shown that various types of sleep disruption can result in both short- and long-term adverse health effects. These effects are thought to be related to increased levels of catecholamines, as well as decreased oxygen consumption and carbon dioxide production. These findings suggest that the sympathetic nervous system is activated in sleep disruption (15–17).

In addition, hormonal changes may accompany sleep disruption. For example, increased insulin resistance may occur with sleep disruption in individuals with type 2 diabetes (T2DM) (18,19). It has also been shown that decreased leptin or increased ghrelin are metabolic changes that may be associated with sleep disruption. These may lead to increased appetite and weight gain.

Inflammatory cytokines such as tumor necrosis factor (TNFα), interleukin one (IL-1) and six (IL-6), and C-reactive protein (CRP) may also be associated with sleep disruption (20,21). In addition, insufficient sleep may contribute to adverse alterations in the neuroendocrine stress response, which can ultimately lead to stress, mood disorders, and depression (22).

6.4 SHORT-TERM HEALTH CONSEQUENCES OF SLEEP DISRUPTION

Short-term sleep disruption can result in a variety of adverse health consequences. These include sympathetic activation, which is associated with an increased risk of cardiovascular disease (CVD), and psychiatric conditions may also ensue (23,24). Short-term sleep disruption can directly influence both cognition and mood, which may increase the likelihood of depression. Short-term sleep disruption may also alter cognition and cognitive performance. One study of primary care physicians reported that disturbed sleep was associated with levels of high burnout.

6.5 COMMON SLEEP DISORDERS

Sleep disorders are very common. There are over 100 different types of sleep disorders, which may range from difficulty sleeping at night to problems of excessive daytime sleepiness. Some of the most common lifestyle-responsive sleep disorders are listed here:

- *Obstrutive Sleep Apnea*: Obstructive Sleep Apnea (OSA) is found in 15%–30% of males and 10%–15% of females in North America (25). There are two types of sleep apnea—obstructive and central. The most common (greater than 85%) is obstructive sleep apnea (OSA). OSA is associated with complete or partial collapse of the upper airway for ten seconds or longer, repeated throughout the night. Upper airway tissues may create a blockage of the airway sufficient to limit airflow and disrupt sleep-related breathing. This, in turn, may result in a drop in oxygen levels in the blood, which leads to arousal and awakenings, although the awakenings may be so brief that the individual is not aware that they occur during sleep. Even though these awakenings are very short, they can create adverse effects on health. Central sleep apnea (CSA) is responsible for prolonged breathing pauses, which can lead to hypoventilation and hypoxia syndrome. This condition also adversely affects sleep quantity and quality, similar to OSA, even though the mechanisms are different.
- *Periodic Limb Movement Disorder (PLMD)*: This condition has been commonly called "restless leg syndrome." It is characterized by sensorimotor discord when resting or lying

down, which results in discomfort, aching, jerking, twitching, tingling, or crawling sensations in the legs, causing the urge to move or shift the legs (26,27). A wide variety of different etiologies are responsible for this condition, including third-trimester pregnancy, endocrine disorders, and Parkinson's disease (27,28).

- *Insomnia*: This is the most common of all sleep complaints (29). This sleep disorder is characterized by difficulty falling asleep, staying asleep, or experiencing disordered sleep for at least one month and may lead to daytime dysfunction or disturbance. A wide variety of etiologies are potentially responsible for insomnia, including late-night eating, stress, medical comorbidities, or psychiatric comorbidities, including anxiety and depression. Other causes may include side effects from medication, excessive caffeine, nicotine, or another sleep disorder (30).
- *Long-term Health Consequences of Sleep Deprivation*: There are multiple long-term consequences of sleep disruption, which may have particularly significant effects on the cardiovascular system, including hypertension, dyslipidemia, and weight-related issues, as well as metabolic syndrome and T2DM. The adverse effects on the cardiovascular system are thought to be due to increased activity of the central nervous system, which contributes to elevated blood pressure. The ARIC Study (the Atherosclerosis Risk in Communities study) showed a 50% increase in CVD in individuals who have difficulty falling asleep or non-restorative sleep compared to individuals with healthy sleep. Studies of long-term adverse consequences of sleep disruption have suggested that disruption of sympathetic activity, glucose metabolism, and possibly inflammation may contribute to the increased likelihood of adverse CVD effects.

6.6 SLEEP DISORDERED BREATHING (SDB) AND CHRONIC DISEASE

Sleep-disordered breathing consists of a spectrum of disease-related breathing disorders, which includes OSA, CSA, Cheyne-Stokes respiration, and sleep-related hypoventilation. All of these are tied together by being associated with impaired ventilation during sleep and sleep disruption. One of the key chronic diseases that SDB is associated with is CVD since it can exacerbate cardiac ischemia and reduce systolic and diastolic function, as well as create an increased risk of cardiac arrhythmias and sudden death. Unfortunately, SDB often goes unrecognized even in cardiology practice (31).

The most common SDB is OSA, which is characterized by either periods of complete cessation of breathing (apnea) or partial cessation (hypopnea), upper airway occlusion, and lower airway occlusion. OSA affects 34% of middle-aged males and 17% of middle-aged females. OSA and SDB have multiple shared risk factors, including central obesity. OSA has been shown to be present in 40%–80% of individuals with hypertension, heart failure, CHD, or cerebrovascular disease. Individuals with OSA typically experience loud snoring and impaired quality of life. Sleep studies are typically utilized to diagnose the degree of apnea or hypopnea.

> *The Pathophysiology of Obstructive Sleep Apnea*: Multiple different factors increase the risk of OSA (32). These include an anatomically small airway and lying in the supine position. In addition, reduced lung volume in individuals with obesity can increase the risk of OSA. Pregnancy or allergies associated with nasal swelling can increase the risk of OSA. OSA can worsen following acute ingestion of alcohol, particularly when a person is in the supine position. Typically, blood CO_2 mildly increases during sleep, which helps activate respiratory muscles and protect the upper airway. Depressed sensitivity to CO_2, however, is common in obesity, hypoventilation, and sleep hypoventilation syndromes.

A variety of risk factors increase the risk of OSA. In addition to male sex, older age and obesity are recognized as OSA risk factors. Central obesity is more commonly found in men than in women and predisposes to OSA.

Having the diagnosis of overweight or obesity accounts for 40%–60% of cases of OSA. Middle-aged obese individuals are four times as likely to have OSA compared with normal-weight individuals. A 1% increase in body mass based on BMI increases the episodes of apnea by 3% (33). It should be noted, however, that approximately 20% of OSA patients are not obese, so normal weight does not eliminate the possibility of OSA. It has been estimated that 80% of individuals with moderate or severe OSA are undiagnosed (34,35). The role of screening for OSA, however, is not established. The US Preventive Services Task Force in 2017 concluded that insufficient evidence exists to recommend routine screening for sleep apnea in primary care settings (36). Individuals with elevated BMI or whose partner reports loud snoring, as well as older age, should also be considered as risk factors for OSA.

Linkages Between Sleep-Disordered Breathing and Cardiovascular Disease: Sleep disordered breathing has been shown to increase sympathetic nervous system activity (37). This may result in acute blood pressure elevations and intermittent hypoxia, which, in turn, may augment inflammatory and hypercoagulable states as well as exacerbate insulin resistance and hypopnea. Oxygen desaturation may also compromise oxygenation of myocardial tissue.

Sleep-Disordered Breathing and Hypertension: It has been estimated that up to 30% of individuals with essential hypertension and 80% of individuals with resistant hypertension have OSA (38). The Joint National Commission on Prevention, Detection, Evaluation, and Treatment of High Blood Pressure (JNC 7) identified OSA as a treatable cause of hypertension (39). Treatment of OSA typically involves continuous positive airway pressure (CPAP), which has been shown to reduce both systolic and diastolic pressure by 1.5–3 mm Hg.

CPAP combined with medication and weight loss or increased physical activity may generate greater effects than single therapy (40). This underscores the importance of lifestyle measures as key components in the treatment of OSA.

Sleep-Disordered Breathing and Coronary Heart Disease: SDB contributes to atherosclerosis by a variety of mechanisms. These mechanisms include triggering the sympathetic nervous system and augmenting the release of pro-inflammatory proteins. In addition, SDB may contribute to other metabolic abnormalities such as dyslipidemia, insulin resistance, and endothelial dysfunction. OSA may contribute to acute ischemia due to decreased oxygen delivery. More than 75% of patients presenting with acute coronary syndromes have been reported to have SDB (41). SDB is an independent risk factor for CHD. Multiple studies have shown that SDB is associated with a 35% increase in the risk of acute coronary syndromes. CHD in younger individuals and by the age of 70 increases by 70% with SDB (41,42). Individuals with OSA using CPAP have significantly reduced rates of both fatal and non-fatal CVD compared to untreated patients (25).

Sleep-Disordered Breathing and Cardiac Arrhythmias: Patients with SDB are predisposed to both ventricular and atrial arrhythmias largely as a result of underlying cardiac risk factors and CVD (43–45). In one study, a 17-fold increase in arrhythmias was reported during an episode of apnea compared to a period of normal breathing (46). CPAP use in patients with OSA reduces atrial fibrillation risk by 44%, as shown in one study.

Other chronic conditions associated with sleep-disordered breathing include adverse effects on the endocrine system and also adverse impacts on the neurochemistry of hunger, as well as hormonal health.

Obesity and Sleep: Adults with shorter sleep duration and sleep loss are at increased risk of becoming obese (47–49). This association may be due to disruptions in neuroendocrine function, including increased levels of ghrelin and decreased levels of leptin, as well as increased appetite, increased glucose intolerance, and insulin sensitivity, which, in turn, may result in increased fat accumulation.

Autoimmune Disorders and Sleep: Sleep disorders are associated with autoimmune disorders such as systemic lupus erythematosus (SLE), rheumatoid arthritis, and systemic sclerosis (50).

Neurologic Disorders and Sleep: Poor sleep accelerates the progression of major neurodegenerative disorders such as Parkinson's disease and Alzheimer's disease (51). A variety of potential etiologies associated with poor sleep may contribute to these diseases. In addition, stroke is associated with SDB. For example, patients with insomnia have a 54% increase in stroke risk, and conversely, half of stroke patients suffer from insomnia.

Psychiatric Disorders and Sleep: Many psychiatric conditions are linked to sleep disturbances, including depression, anxiety, and Attention Deficit Hyperactivity Disorder (ADHD) (52,53). There is a bidirectional relationship that exists particularly between sleep disturbance and depression. Patients with depression have an increased likelihood of comorbid insomnia and vice versa. In addition, sleep disturbances are a cardinal symptom of anxiety disorders.

6.7 SLEEP AND NORMAL AGING

Both the quality and duration of sleep change as people grow older. As many as 50% of individuals over the age of 65 complain about sleep problems, including "disturbed" or "light" sleep, frequent awakenings, early morning awakenings, and undesired daytime sleepiness (54–56). These changes make it all the more important for primary care physicians and individuals practicing in the area of lifestyle medicine to inquire about sleep in patients of all ages, but particularly those over the age of 65. The most significant change that older individuals experience is repeated and frequent interruption of sleep and long periods of wakefulness. It is speculated that this results from age-dependent decreases in sleep-related homeostatic processes.

It should be emphasized that even if older individuals are carefully screened and do not complain of sleep disturbance, they may still show these changes as described when compared to younger adults. This suggests that sleep disturbances may be a part of the aging process per se and independent of any primary sleep disorder. Thus, they are often referred to as "age-related sleep changes." For all of these reasons, it is important to discuss lifestyle practices and sleep during every consultation and clinic visit, particularly for individuals over the age of 65. Issues related to how to counsel individuals concerning sleep and chronic illnesses, with a particular emphasis on lifestyle factors, are discussed in subsequent sections of this chapter and are also discussed in detail in the embedded curriculum.

6.8 INTERVENTIONS AND TREATMENTS FOR DISRUPTED AND DISORDERED SLEEP

Treatment of Sleep-Related Breathing Disorders: Sleep apnea or hypoxia are complicated issues when it comes to both causes and treatments. If an individual is complaining of or apparently experiencing sleep apnea, a thorough clinical evaluation is warranted, and an interdisciplinary team should be involved. Sleep testing is recommended so that the patient receives an appropriate diagnosis and treatment options (57).

Non-surgical approaches to OSA begin by treating underlying medical conditions, including nutritional therapy and lifestyle modifications (58,59). Both nutrition and exercise should be emphasized. If there is underlying allergic rhinitis or hypothyroidism, pharmacotherapy may be instituted to treat these conditions. In central sleep apnea, it is particularly important to assess medications in general, particularly narcotic medications, and propose alternative recommendations. Nasal dilators and mandibular advancement devices may be required. Positive airway pressure (PAP) is the most common recommendation. CPAP is often the treatment of choice.

Treatment of Insomnia: Over 50% of primary care patients may experience insomnia; however, less than one-third of these individuals will report this problem to their physicians (60). The majority of individuals with insomnia have a poor understanding of treatment options and may turn to alcohol (28%) or untested over-the-counter remedies (23%). Benzodiazepines may also be used by some patients but carry significant issues related to cognitive behavioral changes. Cognitive behavioral therapy (CBT) has been shown to be helpful and is well established as an efficacious treatment for insomnia (61–63). CBT focuses on healthful sleep habits and unhealthful sleep behaviors and environments. These will be discussed in more detail at the end of this chapter under the framework of "Sleep Hygiene."

Lifestyle Factors and Sleep: Given the high value of healthy sleep and the relationship between disturbed sleep and increased risk of various chronic diseases, it is important to find strategies to help individuals minimize disruptions in their sleeping patterns. This starts with inquiring of patients about both the quality and duration of their sleep. This is frequently neglected in clinical visits but represents a very important part of lifestyle medicine and, in fact, is one of the major pillars of lifestyle medicine.

Lifestyle factors that can impact sleep include the following:

- *Weight*: As already discussed, individuals who are obese are significantly more susceptible to sleep disturbances than individuals in the healthy weight range (64). Obesity significantly increases the risk of OSA and, of course, is associated with multiple other risk factors (see Chapter 20).

  The good news is that weight loss in individuals who are obese can reduce the likelihood of OSA by 50%. This is particularly important to address since over 70% of the adult population in the United States is either overweight or obese.
- *Physical Activity*: As discussed in multiple chapters in this book and incorporated throughout the embedded curriculum, physical activity is beneficial for many reasons, including lowering the risk of CVD. Research studies have also shown that physical activity helps people sleep better (65). Regular moderate physical activity can help extend sleep duration and improve sleep quality, as well as decrease time to sleep onset.
- *Nutrition*: Both diet and nutrition, as well as meal timing, can influence the quality of sleep. Eating a large amount of food before bed can make it difficult to fall asleep and maintain sleep. In addition, certain foods and drinks may make it either easier or harder to get to sleep. The important role of nutrition in multiple chronic conditions has been emphasized in multiple chapters in this book. Of note, dietary patterns that follow the healthy principles of consuming ample fruits and vegetables, whole grains, and fiber, such as the Mediterranean diet (66) and the DASH diet (67), have both been shown to have a positive impact on sleep.

  Of note, a body of information exists that suggests that people who do not get enough sleep have a tendency to select high-calorie foods. This may be due to hormonal changes that relate to appetite and hunger, which are disrupted by inadequate sleep. This, of course, can contribute to weight gain, overweight, and obesity. There is a bidirectional relationship between weight management and sleep.

  The timing of food consumption may also impact sleep. During the coronavirus disease 2019 (COVID-19) epidemic, many aspects of individuals' daily routines were interrupted, causing people not only to consume more alcohol but also to consume more food and increase the likelihood of overweight or obesity.
- *Sleep and Tobacco*: As emphasized in multiple sections of this book, tobacco use has multiple adverse effects on health. In addition to its addictive potential, tobacco adversely affects the quality and quantity of sleep (68–70). Nicotine adversely impacts circadian rhythm. Individuals who smoke tobacco are more than twice as likely to have OSA. In addition, tobacco leads to difficulty initiating sleep due to its stimulant and withdrawal

effects. For all of these reasons, it is important to emphasize that tobacco cessation is not only vital for general health considerations but also for restorative sleep.

- *Sleep and Caffeine*: Caffeine is a standard part of many of our lives. Caffeine may also adversely affect sleep. Caffeine has a half-life of three to seven hours, depending on the individual's cytochrome P450 and genotype. Unfortunately, almost half of Americans are "very likely" to use caffeinated beverages to combat daytime sleepiness (71). This can create a vicious cycle, with poor sleep leading to daytime sleepiness and increased caffeine consumption. This, of course, is an important issue to discuss with patients.
- *Sleep and Alcohol*: Alcohol is often used as a sleep aid. In the short term, alcohol may induce sleep, but research has demonstrated a reduction in sleep quality in the second half of the night (72). Thus, just like with caffeine consumption, alcohol should be part of sleep discussions with patients.

6.9 INTEGRATED AND PREVENTIVE APPROACHES

As already indicated, numerous lifestyle approaches may be employed, which could make a big difference in helping combat various sleep disorders. These include regular physical activity, healthy nutrition, weight management, avoiding addictive substances such as cigarette smoking and alcohol, and modifying caffeine consumption. These factors, along with creating a proper environment to emphasize and support healthy sleep, are all important. We will focus on the environment in the next section.

6.10 SLEEP HYGIENE

Sleep hygiene is the phrase used for the creation of an optimum environment for healthy sleep (73). This is a broad concept that includes not only having the proper bedroom environment but also the daily routines that promote consistent, uninterrupted sleep. A key part of sleep hygiene is maintaining a stable sleep schedule and making the bedroom comfortable and free of disruptions. It is also important to maintain a relaxing pre-bed routine and to build healthy habits throughout the day, which can contribute to ideal sleep hygiene. This is an area where the multiple components of lifestyle medicine come into play. Here are some specific recommendations to establish good sleep hygiene:

- *Setting a Consistent Sleep Schedule*: This includes practices to establish a fixed wake-up time regardless of whether it is a weekday or weekend, making sleep a priority, and making gradual adjustments if sleep has become disordered. Napping is acceptable as long as the naps are relatively short and take place in the early afternoon.
- *Follow a Nightly Routine*: Most people find it helpful to budget 30 minutes for winding down, as well as dimming the lights and keeping away from bright lights, which can hinder the production of melatonin. It is particularly important not to use handheld devices immediately prior to going to bed since the blue light in these devices can hinder melatonin production.
- *Cultivate Healthy Daily Habits*: This involves getting daylight exposure, being physically active, not smoking cigarettes, reducing alcohol consumption, and cutting down on caffeine, particularly in the afternoon and evening. In bed activities should be restricted to sleep, with the only exception being sexual relations.
- *Optimizing the Bedroom*: The bedroom should be configured to be an environment that invites healthy sleep. This includes a comfortable mattress and pillow, setting a slightly cooler, although comfortable, temperature (74) and blocking out as much light and noise as possible (75).

All of these components of sleep hygiene are essential lifestyle habits to promote healthy sleep, although people frequently neglect them. Healthy sleep is very important for lowering the risk of chronic disease and should be emphasized in all clinical encounters.

6.11 CONCLUSIONS/CLINICAL APPLICATIONS

The most important clinical application is to inquire about sleep in all clinical encounters. This can stimulate a discussion of the key components of healthy sleep and why it is so important for lowering the risk of chronic disease. The factors outlined in this chapter can play a very important role in promoting healthy sleep and should be included in discussions of this very important lifestyle habit. These components are also included in the embedded curriculum.

REFERENCES

1. Ramar K, Malhotra RK, Carden KA, et al. Sleep is essential to health: an American Academy of Sleep Medicine position statement. *J Clin Sleep Med.* 2021;17(10):2115–2119.
2. Matricciani L, Paquet C, Galland B, et al. Children's sleep and health: a meta-review. *Sleep Med Rev.* 2019;46:136–150.
3. Bruce ES, Lunt L, McDonagh JE. Sleep in adolescents and young adults. *Clin Med.* 2017;17(5):424–428.
4. Foster RG. Sleep, circadian rhythms and health. *Interface Focus.* 2020;10(3):20190098.
5. Consensus Conference Panel, Watson NF, Badr MS, et al. Joint consensus statement of the American academy of sleep medicine and sleep research society on the recommended amount of sleep for a healthy adult: methodology and discussion. *Sleep.* 2015;38(8):1161–1183. Epub 2015 Jul 22.
6. Institute of Medicine, Committee on Sleep Medicine and Research, Board of Health Sciences Policy. Sleep Disorders and Sleep Deprivation: An Unmet Public Health Problem. Washington, DC: National Academic Press, 2006.
7. Watson NF, Badr MS, Belenky G, et al. Recommended amount of sleep for a healthy adult: a joint consensus statement of the American Academy of Sleep Medicine and Sleep Research Society. *Sleep.* 2015;38(6):843–844. Epub 2015 Jun 4.
8. Office of Disease Prevention and Health Promotion. Sleep Health. U.S. Department of Health and Human Services, Washington, DC. https://odphp.health.gov/healthypeople/objectives-and-data/browse-objectives/sleep. Accessed February 27, 2025.
9. Rippe JM. Sleep and cardiovascular disease. In Rippe JM (ed.) *Integrating Lifestyle Medicine in Cardiovascular Health and Disease Prevention.* Boca Raton, FL: CRC Press, 2022.
10. Moser D, Anderer P, Gruber G, et al. Sleep classification according to AASM and Rechtschaffen & Kales: effects on sleep scoring parameters. *Sleep.* 2009;32(2):139–149.
11. Rechtschaffen A, Kales A. *A Manual of Standardized Terminology, Techniques and Scoring System for Sleep Stages of Human Subjects.* Bethesda, MD: National Institutes of Health, National Institute of Neurological Diseases and Blindness, Neurological Information Network, 1968.
12. National Sleep Foundation. 2014 Sleep Health Index. Arlington, VA: National Sleep Foundation, 2014.
13. Younes M, Hanly PJ. Immediate post-arousal sleep dynamics: an important determinant of sleep stability in obstructive sleep apnea. *J Appl Physiol.* 2016;120(7):801–808.
14. Chen X, Wang R, Zee P, et al. Racial/ethnic differences in sleep disturbances: the multi-ethnic study of atherosclerosis (MESA). *Sleep.* 2014;125:162–167.
15. Bailey TS, Grunberger G, Bode BW, et al. American Association of Clinical Endocrinologists and American College of Endocrinology 2016 outpatient glucose monitoring consensus statement. *Endocr Pract.* 2016;22(2):231–261.
16. Pulak LM, Jensen L. Sleep in the intensive care unit: a review. *J Intensive Care Med.* 2016;31(1):14–23.
17. Elliott R, Rai T, McKinley S. Factors affecting sleep in the critically ill: an observational study. *J Crit Care.* 2014;29(5):859–863.
18. Vgontzas AN, Bixler EO, Lin HM, et al. Chronic insomnia is associated with nyctohemeral activation of the hypothalamic-pituitary-adrenal axis: clinical implications. *J Clin Endocrinol Metab.* 2001;86(8):3787–3794.
19. Bonnet MH, Berry RB, Arand DL. Metabolism during normal, fragmented, and recovery sleep. *J Appl Physiol.* 1991;71(3):1112–1118.
20. Ali T, Choe J, Awab A, et al. Sleep, immunity and inflammation in gastrointestinal disorders. *World J Gastroenterol.* 2013;19(48):9231–9239.
21. Hurtado-Alvarado G, Dominguez-Salazar E, Pavon L, et al. Blood-brain barrier disruption induced by chronic sleep loss: low-grade inflammation may be the link. *J Immunol Res.* 2016;2016:4576012.
22. Tiemeier H, Pelzer E, Jonck L, et al. Plasma catecholamines and selective slow wave sleep deprivation. *Neuropsychobiology.* 2002;45(2):81–86.

23. Irwin M, Thompson J, Miller C, et al. Effects of sleep and sleep deprivation on catecholamine and interleukin-2 levels in humans: clinical implications. *J Clin Endocrinol Metab.* 1999;84(6):1979–1985.
24. Ekstedt M, Akerstedt T, Soderstrom M. Microarousals during sleep are associated with increased levels of lipids, cortisol, and blood pressure. *Psychosom Med.* 2004;66(6):925–931.
25. Javaheri S, Barbe F, Campos-Rodriguez F, et al. Sleep apnea: types, mechanisms, and clinical cardiovascular consequences. *J Am Coll Cardiol.* 2017;69(7):841–858.
26. Eckert DJ, Jordan AS, Merchia P, Malhotra A. Central sleep apnea: pathophysiology and treatment. *Chest.* 2007;131(2):595.
27. Klingelhoefer L, Bhattacharya K, Reichmann H. Restless legs syndrome. *Clin Med.* 2016;16(4):379.
28. Natarajan R. Review of periodic limb movement and restless leg syndrome. *J Postgrad Med.* 2010; 56(2):157–162.
29. Roth T. Insomnia: definition, prevalence, etiology, and consequences. *J Clin Sleep Med.* 2007;3(5 Suppl):S7.
30. Singareddy R, Vgontzas AN, Fernandez-Mendoza J, et al. Risk factors for incident chronic insomnia: a general population prospective study. *Sleep Med.* 2012;13(4):346.
31. Meisinger C, Heier M, Löwel H, et al. Sleep duration and sleep complaints and risk of myocardial infarction in middle-aged men and women from the general population: the MONICA/KORA Augsburg cohort study. *Sleep.* 2007;30(9):1121–1127.
32. Jordan AS, Wellman A, Edwards JK, et al. Respiratory control stability and upper airway collapsibility in men and women with obstructive sleep apnea. *J Appl Physiol.* 2005;99(5):2020–2027.
33. Peppard PE, Young T, Barnet JH, et al. Increased prevalence of sleep-disordered breathing in adults. *Am J Epidemiol.* 2013;177(9):1006–1014.
34. Redline S, Sotres-Alvarez D, Loredo J, et al. Sleep-disordered breathing in Hispanic/Latino individuals of diverse backgrounds. The Hispanic Community Health Study/Study of Latinos. *Am J Respir Crit Care Med.* 2014;189(3):335–344.
35. Physical Activity Guidelines Advisory Committee. 2018 Physical Activity Guidelines Advisory Committee. 2018 Physical Activity Guidelines Advisory Committee Scientific Report. Washington, DC: U.S. Department of Health and Human Services, 2018.
36. Jonas DE, Amick HR, Feltner C, et al. Screening for obstructive sleep apnea in adults: evidence report and systematic review for the US preventive services task force. *JAMA.* 2017;317(4):415–433.
37. Baltzis D, Bakker JP, Patel SR, et al. Obstructive sleep apnea and vascular diseases. *Compr Physiol.* 2016;6(3):1519–1528.
38. Pedrosa RP, Drager LF, Gonzaga CC, et al. Obstructive sleep apnea: the most common secondary cause of hypertension associated with resistant hypertension. *Hypertension.* 2011;58(5):811–817.
39. Chobanian AV, Bakris GL, Black HR, et al. Seventh report of the joint national committee on prevention, detection, evaluation, and treatment of high blood pressure. *Hypertension.* 2003;42(6):1206–1252.
40. Liu L, Cao Q, Guo Z, et al. Continuous positive airway pressure in patients with obstructive sleep apnea and resistant hypertension: a meta-analysis of randomized controlled trials. *J Clin Hypertens.* 2016;18(2):153–158.
41. Fox H, Purucker HC, Holzhacker I, et al. Prevalence of sleep-disordered breathing and patient characteristics in a coronary artery disease cohort undergoing cardiovascular rehabilitation. *J Cardiopulm Rehabil Prev.* 2016;36(6):421–429.
42. Yeboah J, Redline S, Johnson C, et al. Association between sleep apnea, snoring, incident cardiovascular events and all-cause mortality in an adult population: MESA. *Atherosclerosis.* 2011;219(2):963–968.
43. Mehra R, Stone KL, Varosy PD, et al. Nocturnal arrhythmias across a spectrum of obstructive and central sleep-disordered breathing in older men: outcomes of sleep disorders in older men (MrOS sleep) study. *Arch Intern Med.* 2009;169(12):1147–1155.
44. Hohl M, Linz B, Bohm M, et al. Obstructive sleep apnea and atrial arrhythmogenesis. *Curr Cardiol Rev.* 2014;10(4):362–368.
45. Ayas NT, Taylor CM, Laher I. Cardiovascular consequences of obstructive sleep apnea. *Curr Opin Cardiol.* 2016;31(6):599–605.
46. Qureshi WT, Nasir UB, Alqalyoobi S, et al. Meta-analysis of continuous positive airway pressure as a therapy of atrial fibrillation in obstructive sleep apnea. *Am J Cardiol.* 2015;116(11):1767–1773.
47. Potter GDM, Cade JE, Hardie LJ. Longer sleep is associated with lower BMI and favorable metabolic profiles in UK adults: findings from the national diet and nutrition survey. *PLoS One.* 2017;12(7):e0182195.
48. Beccuti G, Pannain S. Sleep and obesity. *Curr Opin Clin Nutr Metab Care.* 2011;14(4):402.
49. Kim HO, Kang I, Choe W, Yoon KS. Sleep duration and risk of obesity: a genome and epidemiological study. *World Acad Sci J.* 2021;3(2):1.

50. Hsiao YH, Chen YT, Tseng CM, et al. Sleep disorders and increased risk of autoimmune diseases in individuals without sleep apnea. *Sleep.* 2015;38(4):581.
51. Bishir M, Bhat A, Essa MM, et al. Sleep deprivation and neurological disorders. *Biomed Res Int.* 2020;2020:5764017.
52. Franzen PL, Buysse DJ. Sleep disturbances and depression: risk relationships for subsequent depression and therapeutic implications. *Dialogues Clin Neurosci.* 2008;10(4):473–481.
53. Fang H, Tu S, Sheng J, Shao A. Depression in sleep disturbance: a review on a bidirectional relationship, mechanisms and treatment. *J Cell Mol Med.* 2019;23(4):2324.
54. Foley DJ, Monjan AA, Brown SL, et al. Sleep complaints among elderly persons: an epidemiologic study of three communities. *Sleep.* 1995;18(6):425–432.
55. Foley DJ, Monjan A, Simonsick EM, et al. Incidence and remission of insomnia among elderly adults: an epidemiologic study of 6,800 persons over three years. *Sleep.* 1999;22 Suppl 2:S366–S372.
56. Vitiello M, Foley DJ, Stratton K, et al. Prevalence of sleep complaints and insomnia in the vitamins and lifestyle (VITAL) study cohort of 77,000 older men and women. *Sleep*; 2004;27:120.
57. Virk JS, Kotecha B. When continuous positive airway pressure (CPAP) fails. *J Thorac Dis.* 2016;8(10):E1112–E1121.
58. Stepanski EJ, Rybarczyk B. Emerging research on the treatment and etiology of secondary or comorbid insomnia. *Sleep Med Rev.* 2006;10(1):7–18.
59. Joosten SA, Edwards BA, Wellman A, et al. The effect of body position on physiological factors that contribute to obstructive sleep apnea. *Sleep.* 2015;38(9):1469–1478.
60. Spielman AJ, Caruso LS, Glovinsky PB. A behavioral perspective on insomnia treatment. *Psychiatr Clin North Am.* 1987;10(4):541–553.
61. Siebern AT, Manber R. New developments in cognitive behavioral therapy as the first-line treatment of insomnia. *Psychol Res Behav Manag.* 2011;4:21.
62. Espie CA. “Stepped care”: a health technology solution for delivering cognitive behavioral therapy as a first line insomnia treatment. *Sleep.* 2009;32(12):1549–1558.
63. McCurry SM, Logsdon RG, Teri L, et al. Evidence-based psychological treatments for insomnia in older adults. *Psychol Aging.* 2007;22(1):18–27.
64. Lauderdale DS, Knutson KL, Rathouz PJ, et al. Cross-sectional and longitudinal associations between objectively measured sleep duration and body mass index: the CARDIA Sleep Study. *Am J Epidemiol.* 2009;170(7):805–813.
65. Dolezal BA, Neufeld EV, Boland DM, et al. Interrelationship between sleep and exercise: a systematic review. *Adv Prev Med.* 2017;2017:1364387.
66. Medline Plus. National Library of Medicine. Review date 2020 Jul 13. A.D.A.M. Medical Encyclopedia. Mediterranean Diet. Mediterranean Diet: MedlinePlus Medical Encyclopedia. Accessed February 27, 2025.
67. Medline Plus. National Library of Medicine. Review date 2020 Aug 13. A.D.A.M. Medical Encyclopedia. Understanding the DASH Diet. Understanding the DASH diet: MedlinePlus Medical Encyclopedia. Accessed February 27, 2025.
68. Hwang JW, Sundar IK, Yao H, et al. Circadian clock function is disrupted by environmental tobacco/cigarette smoke, leading to lung inflammation and injury via a SIRT1-BMAL1 pathway. *FASEB J.* 2014;28(1):176–194.
69. Kashyap R, Hock LM, Bowman TJ. Higher prevalence of smoking in patients diagnosed as having obstructive sleep apnea. *Sleep Breath* 2001 54. 2001;5(4):167–172.
70. McNamara JPH, Wang J, Holiday DB, et al. Sleep disturbances associated with cigarette smoking. *Psychol Health Med.* 2014;19(4):410–419.
71. Clark I, Landolt HP. Coffee, Caffeine, and sleep: a systematic review of epidemiological studies and randomized controlled trials. *Sleep Med Rev.* 2017;31:70–78.
72. Angarita GA, Emadi N, Hodges S, et al. Sleep abnormalities associated with alcohol, cannabis, cocaine, and opiate use: a comprehensive review. *Addict Sci Clin Pract.* 2016;11(1):9.
73. National Institute of Health (NIH) 2012 January. NIH News in Health: Breaking Bad Habits. Breaking Bad Habits | NIH News in Health. Accessed February 27, 2025.
74. Harding EC, Franks NP, Wisden W. The temperature dependence of sleep. *Front Neurosci.* 2019;13:336.
75. Hume KI, Brink M, Basner M. Effects of environmental noise on sleep. *Noise Health.* 2012;14(61):297–302.

7 Positive Connections with Others

7.1 INTRODUCTION

Recently, numerous books and articles have documented the decline of social connectedness both in the United States and in a variety of other countries. In fact, this topic has formed the centerpiece of an important Surgeon General's Advisory from the former US Surgeon General, Dr. Vivek Murthy, entitled "Our Epidemic of Loneliness and Isolation" (1). The exact title of the Advisory is "The Healing Effects of Social Connection and Community." Dr. Murthy expands on this Surgeon General's Advisory with a wonderful book entitled *Together: The Healing Power of Human Connections in a Sometimes Lonely World* (2).

The issue of declining connectedness and the accompanying feelings of loneliness and social isolation have prompted articles from the American Medical Association (AMA) about what physicians need to know about this emerging health problem (3). In addition, the American College of Lifestyle Medicine (ACLM) was one of the first medical organizations to clearly acknowledge that social connections are a key component of overall health and well-being. ACLM did this by including "positive social connections" as one of the six pillars of lifestyle medicine (4).

The purpose of this chapter is to underscore the interactions between social connectedness and health. We will also provide some specific recommendations for physicians and other healthcare workers to assess the issues of social connectedness and/or loneliness in their patients. In addition, we will provide specific recommendations based on those made by Dr. Murthy in his Surgeon General's Advisory on what healthcare providers need to know and how physicians can help both assess and potentially ameliorate issues of loneliness in their patients by encouraging increased social connection.

The issue of social connection carries profound health implications. The inverse of this, loneliness, can carry multiple adverse health consequences. In addition, loneliness is sometimes hidden in plain sight since individuals may feel ashamed of acknowledging their feelings of loneliness.

Thus, it is very important that physicians have the tools to inquire about and counsel individuals in the areas of social connection. Many of the recommendations made in this chapter are drawn directly from the Surgeon General's Advisory on Social Connection and Community. We strongly urge individuals to access this important, evidence-based document.

7.2 WHY SOCIAL CONNECTIONS MATTER

Multiple levels of social connections exist, and all of them matter. Some of our connections are with family, friends, and colleagues (5–10). Others involve neighbors, colleagues at work, schools, and even the internet. Unfortunately, many individuals lack a variety of social connections, and this can lead to poor health and other negative outcomes. One way that the lack of social connection is measured is by measuring loneliness and social isolation.

It is important to understand that social isolation and loneliness are related but they are not synonymous. Social isolation means having few social relationships (11). On the other hand, loneliness is a subjective internal state resulting from the unmet need between an individual's preferred and actual experience (12). Loneliness and social isolation increase the risk of premature death by 26% and 29%, respectively.

Dr. Murthy writes that poor or insufficient social connections are associated with an increased risk of disease, including a 29% increased risk of heart disease (CVD) and a 32% increased risk

DOI: 10.1201/9781003630043-7

of stroke. Lack of social connection can also have multiple other health impacts, as will be considered later in this chapter. In addition to the health consequences of a lack of social connections, there are also significant economic impacts. For example, excess Medicare spending and increased hospital and nursing facility expenditures are estimated at 6.7 million dollars annually (13), and stress-related absenteeism, often based on loneliness, costs employers an estimated 154 billion dollars annually (14–16).

It is important to understand that social connection is a fundamental human need and is as essential to survival as food, water, and shelter. Human beings are biologically wired for social connections. Living alone means having to fulfill many of the basic demands for survival on one's own. Social isolation and loneliness are also critical public health concerns. For example, in 2022, a study showed that when people were asked how close they felt to others emotionally, only 39% of adults said they felt very connected to others (17). In addition, the experience of loneliness has dramatically increased in the United States, particularly among young adults.

Loneliness is more widespread than any other major health issue, including smoking, diabetes, and even obesity (18–20). However, even though loneliness is very prevalent, fewer than 20% of individuals who always feel lonely recognize it as a health consideration (21). For all of these reasons, social connection is both an important social and societal imperative.

7.3 WHAT IS SOCIAL CONNECTION?

Social connections involve a variety of different components. It is not just the number of close relationships that a person has. Rather, it involves, as Dr. Murthy writes, three separate but inter-related domains: namely, structure, function, and quality (1,22,23).

Structure encompasses the number and variety of relationships and frequent interactions that people have. These may include marital and partnership status, family size, and the number of friends that an individual has. *Function* denotes the degree to which relationships serve needs, such as emotional support, mentorship, or support in a crisis. Finally, *quality* consists of how positive or negative relationships and interactions are. This involves satisfaction, strain, and inclusion or exclusion.

Social connection is a continuum. For example, we tend to think of people as either being lonely or not, but in fact, there is a continuum (24,25). Everyone feels lonely at times. This underscores the fact that social connection is dynamic, that social connections change over time and can be either enhanced or compromised for a variety of reasons such as life events, illnesses, moves, or job transitions. The third component of social connection encompasses a variety of factors that can either serve as deficits or strengths. For example, individuals may have a very strong and supportive family that provides a connection or multiple connections at work, which provide such a strength. These factors may not be adequately assessed when thinking about a deficit such as loneliness.

7.4 IS SOCIAL CONNECTION DECLINING?

As Dr. Murthy points out in the Surgeon General's Advisory, it appears that in the United States, individuals have felt less connected over time. It is hard to put a precise number on this, but the components that have declined include social connections, connections with family, companionship, social engagement with friends, and a variety of other social engagements. All of these appear to have been in decline in the United States (26,27).

7.5 FACTORS THAT CAN SHAPE SOCIAL CONNECTIONS

A wide variety of factors can shape social connections. These are articulated by Dr. Murthy as occurring in four major domains: individual, relationship, community, and society. *Individual* factors such as chronic disease, physical and mental health, personality, race, gender, socioeconomic status, and life changes are all important. In the *relationship* category, household size as well as the components of structure, function, and quality, already outlined in the previous section, all matter. *Community* can also play a significant role in social connection (28,29). This factor involves the quality of outdoor space, the type of housing available, the impact of schools and workplace, as well as a variety of issues that have to do with local government and community organizations. Finally, on a macro level, *society* can also impact social connectedness. This factor involves the norms and values of society, public policies, and historical inequities.

Technology can also impact social connections (30–32). This was first identified in the classic book *Bowling Alone* by Robert Putnam (26). This book, while published over 20 years ago, was the first to articulate that use of the internet could have a significantly negative effect on social connection. This will be discussed in more detail later in this chapter.

It is also essential to understand that social connections can lead to better health for an individual (33). This was first illustrated many years ago in a study in California, where individuals who were laid off from work either served as volunteers in organizations or remained isolated. This study showed that the individuals who remained active in volunteerism significantly improved their health and their chances of gaining employment again. This underscored a profound message, particularly in the area of volunteerism, since it suggested that doing good for others often resulted in personal health benefits.

7.6 IMPACT FROM THE COVID-19 PANDEMIC

The coronavirus disease 2019 (COVID-19) pandemic exacerbated the already present trends in declining social connection (34). Lockdowns and stay-at-home orders underscored the value of social connection and how fragile it is. Many people experienced isolation or loneliness in a way that they had not experienced before. For example, major life events such as celebrations of birthdays, weddings, etc., were either postponed or shifted to online. In addition, individuals experienced anxiety, stress, fear, sadness, and grief to some degree because of the loss of these relationships with other individuals. The COVID-19 pandemic affected different populations in different ways. Individuals who worked on the front lines in either transportation or health care experienced the COVID-19 pandemic differently than those who were forced to stay at home (35).

Older individuals and those living in managed care environments were particularly at risk for the loss of social connections. Perhaps one surprising effect of the COVID-19 pandemic was that half of the adult population in the United States reported informally helping others, which allowed them to find or create connections with others during this public health crisis (33). Certainly, the COVID-19 pandemic brought to the forefront the value of social connections and the impact of their loss.

7.7 INDIVIDUAL HEALTH OUTCOMES

Perhaps the most relevant portion of the Surgeon General's Advisory written by Dr. Murthy relates to the impact of social connection on a variety of health outcomes. Dr. Murthy has put together an extensive, evidence-based report on multiple health outcomes related to connectedness.

A. *Survival and Mortality*: Over four decades of research have produced robust evidence that lacking social connection—and in particular, scoring high on measures of social isolation—is associated with a significantly increased risk of early death from all causes (36–41).

   Abundant evidence exists from multiple medical and scientific disciplines that socially connected people live longer. The linkage between social connection and mortality risk dates back as early as 1979 in epidemiologic studies. This research showed that individuals who lacked social connection were more than twice as likely as individuals with greater social connection to die within a 7.5-year follow-up period, even accounting for age, health status, socioeconomic status, and health practices.

Since that time, more recent estimates looking across data from 148 studies show that social connection increases odds of survival by 50% (39). In these studies, social connection was more powerful than smoking, alcohol consumption, or physical inactivity and risk factors such as high blood pressure, body mass index, or cholesterol levels on survival (41). This underscores the importance of social connections for good health. Multiple studies have now shown that lack of social connection independently predicts death from all causes, including deaths caused by diseases.

B. *Cardiovascular Disease*: Heart disease and stroke are the entities where the strongest evidence linking social connection to health exists (24,42). Multiple studies taken together have shown that there is an increased risk of 29% for heart disease and a 32% risk of stroke in individuals who lack social connections (43). In addition, childhood isolation is also associated with increased risk factors for cardiovascular disease.

In patients who suffer from heart failure, high levels of loneliness were associated with a 68% increase in hospitalization, a 57% higher risk of emergency department visits, and a 26% increased risk of outpatient visits (44, 45). In addition, for those individuals who have suffered a heart attack, those who have poor social connections are more likely to die from the heart attack.

C. *Hypertension*: Several studies have shown that the more social support one has, the greater the reduction in the likelihood of developing high blood pressure (46). This holds true in a variety of populations. In Black Americans, those with positive social connections have a greater than 36% lower risk of high blood pressure (47). In older individuals, the effects of social isolation on hypertension are greater than any other risk factor, including diabetes (25).

Other research studies have shown that strong social connections are helpful in high blood pressure control. The National Social Life, Health and Aging Project (NSHAP) has reported a "causal role of social connections in reducing hypertension (25)." This is true particularly for individuals over the age of 50.

D. *Diabetes*: Social connections have been clearly shown in multiple studies to have an impact on the development and management of diabetes (48–50). Low social connections have been linked to the development of type 2 diabetes (T2DM) in both men and women, particularly women over the age of 70. In addition, social connection is associated with better self-rated health and disease management among individuals with T2DM. Individuals with pre-diabetes have fewer complications and are less likely to advance to T2DM if they have strong social connections (48–50). The National Health and Nutrition Examination Survey (NHANES) showed that older individuals with T2DM who have a large social network had a significantly reduced risk of all-cause mortality (51).

E. *Infectious Diseases*: Socially connected individuals appear to have stronger immune responses when they are exposed to infectious diseases. In contrast, individuals who experience loneliness and poor social support have an increased risk of developing and severity of infectious diseases. Studies in even relatively minor infectious diseases, such as the common cold, have shown that individuals with strong social ties are at fourfold lower risk of developing colds when exposed to people with a virus (52). This is also true with immune responses to the COVID-19 vaccine, where lack of social connections resulting in loneliness was associated with weaker antibody responses to vaccines (53).

F. *Cognitive Function*: Multiple studies have shown that social isolation and loneliness result in accelerated cognitive decline and increased risk of dementia, including Alzheimer's disease in older adults (54). One study showed that the risk of developing dementia increased by 50% in older adults, and cognitive abilities declined 20% faster than those who did not have strong social connections and reported loneliness (55).

G. *Depression and Anxiety*: Social isolation and loneliness predict the risk of developing depression and anxiety and can exacerbate these conditions over time. This is particularly true of older adults, although it is also true of younger people (56). In a review of 63 studies, loneliness and social isolation among children and adolescents increased the risk of anxiety and depression (57).

H. *Suicidality and Self-Harm*: According to a 2010 study, "The Interpersonal Theory of Suicide," socialization is arguably the strongest and most reliable predictor for reducing suicidal ideation, attempts, and suicidal behavior among samples varying in age, nationality, and clinical severity. This finding has been supported by multiple studies over many years (58). The findings have clearly shown that social connection protects against suicide as a cause of death, especially for men. In one study of over 500,000 middle-aged adults, the probability of dying by suicide more than doubled among men who lived alone (59).

Loneliness and low social support are also associated with increased risk of self-harm. In one review of 40 studies involving more than 60,000 older adults, increases in loneliness were reported to be the primary motivation for self-harm (59).

Often, the relationship between social connection and various chronic illnesses may be influenced by both biological and psychological processes, as well as behaviors. These will be discussed in the next few sections.

7.8 BIOLOGICAL PROCESSES AND SOCIAL CONNECTION

Multiple connections to biology exist that involve social connections. These involve risk and protection from disease and many other issues. Since biological processes work in concert with each other, the previous section on health consequences for social connection is highly relevant (60–63).

An emerging biological pathway of considerable interest in all branches of medicine is inflammation. Inflammation is now thought to be a major underlying cause of many chronic illnesses. Being isolated can increase inflammation to the same degree as physical inactivity (64). Inflammation is thought to be an underlying component of CVD, T2DM, hypertension, cancer, and cognitive decline. Thus, the underlying link between social connection and inflammation is an important one that relates to numerous metabolic diseases.

7.9 PSYCHOLOGICAL IMPACTS OF SOCIAL CONNECTION

Physical health and mental health are inextricably intertwined. Social connection can also impact multiple psychological processes, including the likelihood of anxiety and depression (as outlined in the previous section), as well as issues such as sense of meaning and purpose (65). In addition, individuals who have high levels of social connections are more likely to engage in health-promoting behaviors and use preventive health care services (66,67).

The way stress is perceived may also be impacted by social connections (68–71). Individuals who have high levels of social connection are likely to seek support to minimize stress. As indicated in other chapters in this book, stress reduction is a key health consideration, and it is strongly linked to social connection (72).

7.10 SOCIAL CONNECTION AND BEHAVIORS

Health-related behaviors are also linked to social connection (73–75). These include adhering to treatments such as taking medication, engaging in preventive measures, etc. Social connections can also encourage individuals to get more sleep (76) and may impact other behaviors such as getting vaccinated, ceasing cigarette smoking, and engaging in regular physical activity.

7.11 EDUCATIONAL AND ECONOMIC BENEFITS OF SOCIAL CONNECTION

Multiple educational and economic benefits are also associated with social connections.

For example, positive social connections are associated with a higher likelihood of graduating from college and obtaining a four-year college degree (77,78). Among medical students, feeling socially isolated is associated with dropping out. This represents an important issue for why levels of burnout are so prevalent among medical students and house officers and should be noted carefully by attending physicians (79).

Better job performance is also associated with social connection. Social connections help prevent work stress and burnout (80). In addition, social connection is associated with shorter recovery time from injury and illness.

In addition, social connection in the workplace plays an important role in individuals' employment situations. Social connections with individuals of varying social and economic backgrounds influence where individuals can find employment opportunities (81,82). Social connections can also help individuals acquire appropriate skills from their peers.

7.12 SOCIAL CONNECTIONS AND COMMUNITY

Social connections and population health have been studied for many years and are strongly associated with each other (83). Cities with higher levels of social connectedness have better outcomes, including population health for the community, safety, resilience, and prosperity (84,85).

7.13 THE ROLE OF PHYSICIANS AND OTHER HEALTH CARE PROFESSIONALS AND SOCIAL CONNECTIONS

Dr. Murthy advocated adopting a national strategy for improving connectedness to improve health. In this area, physicians and other health care workers can play critical roles.

Physicians and other health care organizations, such as hospitals and public health organizations, play an important role in preventing the loss of social connection (39). This applies not only to individual patients who express loneliness but also plays an important role in helping others achieve greater connectedness.

Physicians can also play an important role in multiple ways, such as including social connections as a key health consideration for individuals and engaging their patients about this. This is true at primary, secondary, and tertiary levels, where it is important that physicians actively assess patients' social connections to help identify those individuals at increased risk or already experiencing social disconnection and loneliness, and help evaluate and provide support. Educating patients about the benefits of social connections is also an important role that physicians can play, both in primary and secondary prevention. In addition, physicians can help with interventions to provide social support for patients, particularly those at risk for loneliness and isolation.

The American Medical Association has also provided information in a series of articles and podcasts entitled "What Doctors Wish Patients Knew about Loneliness and Health" (3). By using the tools provided by the AMA, physicians can become more knowledgeable about the effects of loneliness and isolation and provide specific counseling to help ameliorate these conditions.

7.14 THE ROLE OF TECHNOLOGY

Technology has advanced rapidly over the last ten years. There is no question that technology has impacted how we live and work and on social connectivity.

The benefits of technology, however, may come at a cost. While technology may enhance social connectivity, it can also distract people and occupy a great deal of mental bandwidth while making individuals of all ages feel worse about their relationships and diminishing their ability to connect deeply with each other.

These potential downsides of technology were first identified in the seminal publication in the year 2000 in the book *Bowling Alone: Collapse and Revival of the American Community* (26).

In this book, Dr. Putnam identified that there was a deterioration in aspects of communities in the United States. Even though the book was published 25 years ago, the evidence was already present. For example, in the late 1990s, many investigators thought that the advent of the internet would yield more connections. Actually, what happened was exactly the opposite. What occurred was a serious decline in interpersonal connections. Dr. Putnam documented that there was a 50% decrease in individuals who had at least one friend with whom they could share deep thoughts and secrets. There were often more connections, but much less presence of a real social community.

While the internet has brought many wonderful advantages, it can also create hazards. A study published by the University of Pittsburgh several years ago involving 1,787 individuals compared people who spent two hours or more on a daily basis on the internet with those who spent one hour or less (2). Those who spent more than two hours on the internet each day were twice as likely to report being lonely as those who spent less time.

Recently, Dr. Putnam has taken a more measured view of the impact of modern technology, in general, and on the internet, in particular, on social connections. In the afterword to the 20th anniversary edition of Bowling Alone, which was published in 2020 in the midst of the COVID-19 pandemic, Dr. Putnam wrote that while the internet did allow connections between people who were forced to isolate because of the pandemic, he still raised issues about whether or not the level of social connection (in his words, "social capital") had really advanced because of this technology (84). In this afterword, he indicated that the response of the internet to the COVID-19 pandemic needed to be further evaluated, although he did raise a number of cautions, including hyperpolarization and balkanization that do not lead to truly satisfying social connections.

7.15 EXPERIENCING "THE GOOD LIFE"

A book published in 2023 by Waldinger and Shultz, entitled *The Good Life,* documents the surprising finding from a long scientific study conducted among Harvard students and lower-income students in downtown Boston on happiness (85). After studying these participants for over 80 years, the investigators concluded, much to their surprise, that the most important component to establishing a "good life" was relationships with other people. Thus, they provided a ringing endorsement for the positive value of social connections. This is worth emphasizing for physicians as they discuss social connections with their patients. Connectedness is not just an antidote to loneliness; it is also a key, and perhaps the most crucial component of having a happy life.

7.16 HOW TO ENHANCE SOCIAL CONNECTIONS AND OVERCOME LONELINESS

As an antidote to loneliness, Dr. Murthy outlined four potential strategies in his book entitled *The Healing Power of Human Connection in a Sometimes Lonely World.* Here are his four potential strategies (2).

- *Spend Time Each Day with Those You Love*: Dr. Murthy emphasizes that this is not limited to people in your immediate household. His recommendation is to devote at least a few minutes each day to connecting with those you care most about.
- *Focus on Each Other*: This recommendation focuses on trying to eliminate distractions while interacting with each other. Forget multitasking. It is important to give the other person the gift of your full attention. It is important as well to make eye contact and listen respectfully, and give the other person full attention.
- *Embrace Solitude*: As we have already indicated, and as Dr. Murthy also describes, there is a clear distinction between solitude and loneliness. Embracing solitude is the first step in building stronger connections with yourself, which is a vital underpinning of building connections to other people. Thus, as physicians counsel individuals on loneliness, it is

important to recognize that solitude is an important consideration for developing a connection with yourself and that loneliness and solitude are not the same concept.

- *Help and Be Helped*: As indicated in the study that we have quoted from California, service is a very important form of human connection which underscores the value of purpose in life, as well as creating a stronger social response.

7.17 CONCLUSIONS/CLINICAL APPLICATIONS

There is no longer any question that social connections carry profound physical and mental benefits. Conversely, loneliness can create adverse health consequences and increase the likelihood of developing multiple chronic diseases. With this in mind, it is important that physicians become knowledgeable and embrace the concept of social connections and their interactions with health.

The process of connecting with others is a highly appropriate pillar in lifestyle medicine and one that physicians should embrace. This is why we have focused on ways not only to counsel people, but to consider social connections as an important health consideration. We also hope that physicians themselves will recognize and embrace this concept.

Perhaps the easiest way to start the conversation with individuals and obtain information is to inquire from patients about the other people that they interact with. "Tell me about the people you interact with?" "Do you feel you have satisfying relationships?" "Have you ever felt lonely?" All of these questions may seem difficult to start with, but they will allow patients to understand that the physician cares about this topic and that it is not shameful to experience loneliness. It should also be emphasized to make the distinction between solitude and loneliness. Solitude can be a very powerful way to make connections with oneself, whereas loneliness may layer negative psychological aspects on solitude that are not necessarily present.

REFERENCES

1. Murthy V, Office of the Surgeon General (OSG). Our Epidemic of Loneliness and Isolation: The U.S. Surgeon General's Advisory on the Healing Effects of Social Connection and Community. Washington, DC: US Department of Health and Human Services, 2023.
2. Murthy VH. *Together: The Healing Power of Human Connection in a Sometimes Lonely World*. New York: Wellcome Collection, 2021.
3. Berg S. What doctors wish patients knew about loneliness and health. AMA. 2023. What doctors wish patients knew about loneliness and health | American Medical Association. Accessed February 21, 2025.
4. American College of Lifestyle Medicine. Home – American College of Lifestyle Medicine. Accessed February 21, 2025.
5. Hu T, Zheng X, Huang M. Absence and presence of human interaction: the relationship between loneliness and empathy. *Front Psychol.* 2020;11:768.
6. Ehsan A, Klaas HS, Bastianen A, Spini D. Social capital and health: a systematic review of systematic reviews. *SSM – Popul Health.* 2019;8:100425.
7. Holt-Lunstad J. Social connection as a public health issue: the evidence and a systemic framework for prioritizing the "social" in social determinants of health. *Annu Rev Public Health.* 2022;43(1):193–213.
8. John S, James L. Knight Foundation, Gallup Inc. Knight Soul of the Community 2010. 2010.
9. 34. Aldrich DP, Meyer MA. Social capital and community resilience. *Am Behav Sci.* 2015;59(2):254–269.
10. Aldrich D. (2012). *Building Resilience: Social Capital in Post-Disaster Recovery.* Chicago, IL: The University of Chicago Press, 2012. doi:10.7208/chicago/9780226012896.001.0001.
11. Badcock JC, Holt-Lunstad J, Bombaci P, et al. Position statement: addressing social isolation and loneliness and the power of human connection. Global Initiative on Loneliness and Connection (GILC), 2022.
12. Holt-Lunstad J, Steptoe A. Social isolation: an underappreciated determinant of physical health. *Curr Opin Psychol.* 2021;43:232–237.
13. Flowers L, Houser A, Noel-Miller C, et al. *Medicare Spends More on Socially Isolated Older Americans.* Washington, DC: AARP Public Policy Institute, 2017.

14. Bowers A, Wu J, Lustig S, Nemecek D. Loneliness influences avoidable absenteeism and turnover intention reported by adult workers in the United States. *J Organ Eff People Perform*. 2022;9(2): 312–335.
15. Ozcelik H, Barsade SG. No employee an Island: workplace loneliness and job performance. *Acad Manag J*. 2018;61(6):2343–2366.
16. United States Department of Health and Human Services. The U.S. Surgeon General's Framework for Workplace Mental Health and Well-being. Washington, DC: U.S. Department of Health and Human Services, Office of the U.S. Surgeon General, 2022.
17. Gallup Inc., Meta. *The State of Social Connections*. Washington DC: Gallup Inc., 2022.
18. Office on Smoking and Health National Center for Chronic Disease Prevention and Health Promotion. Current Cigarette Smoking Among Adults in the United States. Current Cigarette Smoking Among Adults in the United States | Smoking and Tobacco Use | CDC. Accessed February 21, 2025.
19. Centers for Disease Control and Prevention. Prevalence of Both Diagnosed and Undiagnosed Diabetes. Centers for Disease Control and Prevention. Prevalence of Total, Diagnosed, and Undiagnosed Diabetes Among Adults: United States, 2013–2016 | Blogs | CDC. Accessed February 21, 2025.
20. Division of Nutrition Physical Activity and Obesity, National Center for Chronic Disease Prevention and Health Promotion. Adult Obesity Facts. Centers for Disease Control and Prevention. Adult Obesity Facts | Obesity | CDC. Accessed February 21, 2025.
21. DiJulio B, Hamel L, Muñana C, Brodie M. Loneliness and Social Isolation in the United States, the United Kingdom, and Japan: An International Survey, 2018.
22. Holt-Lunstad J, Robles TF, Sbarra DA. Advancing social connection as a public health priority in the United States. *Am Psychol*. 2017;72(6):517–530.
23. Holt-Lunstad J. Why social relationships are important for physical health: a systems approach to understanding and modifying risk and protection. *Annu Rev Psychol*. 2018;69:437–458.
24. Holt-Lunstad J. The major health implications of social connection. *Curr Dir Psychol Sci*. 2021;30(3): 251–259.
25. Yang YC, Boen C, Gerken K, et al. Social relationships and physiological determinants of longevity across the human life span. *Proc Natl Acad Sci USA*. 2016;113(3):578–583.
26. Putnam RD. Bowling alone: America's declining social capital. In Crothers L, Lockhart C (eds.) *Culture and Politics: A Reader*. New York: Palgrave Macmillan US; 2000:223–234.
27. Kannan V, Veazie P. US trends in social isolation, social engagement, and companionship—nationally and by age, sex, race/ethnicity, family income, and work hours, 2003–2020. *SSM Popul Health*. 2022; 25;21:1013312023.
28. Atwell M, Stillerman B, Bridgeland JM. Health Index 2021: Citizenship During Crisis. Civic, National Conference on Citizenship, University of Virginia's Miller Center, Democracy Initiative and the Partnership for American Democracy, 2021.
29. Parker K, Horowitz J, Brown A, et al. What Unites and Divides Urban, Suburban and Rural Communities. Pew Research Center, 2018.
30. Perrin M, Atske S. About three-in-ten U.S. adults say they are 'almost constantly' online. Pew Research Center, 2021.
31. Vogels E, Gelles-Watnick R, Massarat N. Teens, Social Media and Technology 2022. Pew Research Center, 2022.
32. Ortiz-Ospina E. The rise of social media. Our World in Data, 2019.
33. Brown KM, Hoye R, Nicholson M. Self-esteem, self-efficacy, and social connectedness as mediators of the relationship between volunteering and well-being. *J Soc Serv Res*. 2012;38(4):468–483.
34. McClain C, Vogels E, Perrin A, et al. The Internet and the Pandemic. Pew Research Center, 2021.
35. Leigh-Hunt N, Bagguley D, Bash K, et al. An overview of systematic reviews on the public health consequences of social isolation and loneliness. *Public Health*. 2017;152:157–171.
36. Shor E, Roelfs DJ. Social contact frequency and all-cause mortality: a meta-analysis and meta-regression. *Soc Sci Med*. 2015;128:76–86.
37. Pinquart M, Duberstein PR. Associations of social networks with cancer mortality: a meta-analysis. *Crit Rev Oncol Hematol*. 2010;75(2):122–137.
38. Rico-Uribe LA, Caballero FF, Martin-Maria N, et al. Association of loneliness with all-cause mortality: a meta-analysis. *PLoS One*. 2018;13(1):e0190033.
39. Holt-Lunstad J, Smith TB, Layton JB. Social relationships and mortality risk: a meta-analytic review. *PLoS Med*. 2010;7(7):e1000316.
40. Berkman LF, Syme SL. Social networks, host resistance, and mortality: a nine-year follow-up study of Alameda County residents. *Am J Epidemiol*. 1979;109(2):186–204.

41. Pantell M, Rehkopf D, Jutte D, et al. Social isolation: a predictor of mortality comparable to traditional clinical risk factors. *Am J Public Health.* 2013;103(11):2056–2062.
42. National Academies of Sciences Engineering and Medicine (NASEM). *Social Isolation and Loneliness in Older Adults: Opportunities for the Health Care System.* Washington, DC: The National Academies Press, 2020.
43. Valtorta NK, Kanaan M, Gilbody S, et al. Loneliness and social isolation as risk factors for coronary heart disease and stroke: systematic review and meta-analysis of longitudinal observational studies. *Heart.* 2016;102(13):1009–1016.
44. Heidari Gorji MA, Fatahian A, Farsavian A. The impact of perceived and objective social isolation on hospital readmission in patients with heart failure: a systematic review and meta-analysis of observational studies. *Gen Hosp Psychiatry.* 2019;60:27–36.
45. Manemann SM, Chamberlain AM, Roger VL, et al. Perceived social isolation and outcomes in patients with heart failure. *J Am Heart Assoc.* 2018;7(11).
46. National Center for Chronic Disease Prevention and Health Promotion. Heart Disease and Stroke. Centers for Disease Control and Prevention. About the Division for Heart Disease and Stroke Prevention | National Center for Chronic Disease Prevention and Health Promotion (NCCDPHP) | CDC. Accessed February 26, 2025.
47. Harding BN, Hawley CN, Kalinowski J, et al. Relationship between social support and incident hypertension in the Jackson heart study: a cohort study. *BMJ Open.* 2022;12(3):e054812.
48. de Wit M, Trief PM, Huber JW, Willaing I. State of the art: understanding and integration of the social context in diabetes care. *Diabet Med.* 2020;37(3):473–482.
49. Brinkhues S, Dukers-Muijrers N, Hoebe C, et al. Socially isolated individuals are more prone to have newly diagnosed and prevalent type 2 diabetes mellitus – the Maastricht study. *BMC Public Health.* 2017;17(1):955.
50. Brinkhues S, Dukers-Muijrers N, Hoebe C, et al. Social network characteristics are associated with type 2 diabetes complications: the Maastricht study. *Diabetes Care.* 2018;41(8):1654–1662.
51. Loprinzi PD, Ford MA. Effects of social support network size on mortality risk: considerations by diabetes status. *Diabetes Spectr.* 2018;31(2):189–192.
52. LeRoy AS, Murdock KW, Jaremka LM, et al. Loneliness predicts self-reported cold symptoms after a viral challenge. *Health Psychol.* 2017;36(5):512–520.
53. Stephen G, Siobhán H, Muldoon OT, et al. Social cohesion and loneliness are associated with the antibody response to COVID-19 vaccination. *Brain Behav Immun.* 2022;103:179–185.
54. Akhter-Khan SC, Tao Q, Ang TFA, et al. Associations of loneliness with risk of Alzheimer's disease dementia in the Framingham heart study. *Alzheimer's Dement.* 2021;17(10):1619–1627.
55. Donovan NJ, Wu Q, Rentz DM, et al. Loneliness, depression and cognitive function in older U.S. adults. *Int J Geriatr Psychiatry.* 2017;32(5):564–573.
56. Domènech-Abella J, Mundó J, Haro JM, et al. Anxiety, depression, loneliness and social network in the elderly: longitudinal associations from The Irish Longitudinal Study on Ageing (TILDA). *J Affect Disord.* 2019;246:82–88.
57. Loades ME, Chatburn E, Higson-Sweeney N, et al. Rapid systematic review: the impact of social isolation and loneliness on the mental health of children and adolescents in the context of COVID-19. *J Am Acad Child Adolesc Psychiatry.* 2020;59(11):1218–1239.e1213.
58. Shaw RJ, Cullen B, Graham N, et al. Living alone, loneliness and lack of emotional support as predictors of suicide and self harm: a nine-year follow up of the UK Biobank cohort. *J Affect Disord.* 2021;279:316–323.
59. Troya MI, Babatunde O, Polidano K, et al. Self-harm in older adults: systematic review. *Br J Psychiatry.* 2019;214(4):186–200.
60. Cacioppo JT, Cacioppo S, Capitanio JP, Cole SW. The neuroendocrinology of social isolation. *Annu Rev Psychol.* 2015;66:733–767.
61. Mattos Dos Santos R. Isolation, social stress, low socioeconomic status and its relationship to immune response in COVID-19 pandemic context. *Brain Behav Immun Health.* 2020;7:100103.
62. Muscatell KA. Social psychoneuroimmunology: understanding bidirectional links between social experiences and the immune system. *Brain Behav Immun.* 2021;93:1–3.
63. Robles TF. Annual research review: social relationships and the immune system during development. *J Child Psychol Psychiatry.* 2021;62(5):539–559.
64. Furman D, Campisi J, Verdin E, et al. Chronic inflammation in the etiology of disease across the life span. *Nat Med.* 2019;25(12):1822–1832.

65. Silver L, Van Kessel P, Huang C et al. What Makes Life Meaningful? Views From 17 Advanced Economies. Pew Research Center, 2021.
66. Petrova D, Garcia-Retamero R, Catena A. Lonely hearts don't get checked: on the role of social support in screening for cardiovascular risk. *Prev Med.* 2015;81:202–208.
67. Kim ES, Strecher VJ, Ryff CD. Purpose in life and use of preventive health care services. *Proc Natl Acad Sci USA.* 2014;111(46):16331–16336.
68. Southwick SM, Sippel L, Krystal J, et al. Why are some individuals more resilient than others: the role of social support. *World Psychiatry.* 2016;15(1):77–79.
69. Kivimäki M, Steptoe A. Effects of stress on the development and progression of cardiovascular disease. *Nat Rev Cardiol.* 2018;15(4):215–229.
70. Chandola T, Brunner E, Marmot M. Chronic stress at work and the metabolic syndrome: prospective study. *BMJ.* 2006;332(7540):521–525.
71. McEwen BS. Neurobiological and systemic effects of chronic stress. *Chronic Stress.* 2017;1:2470547017692328.
72. Birmingham WC, Holt-Lunstad J. Social aggravation: understanding the complex role of social relationships on stress and health-relevant physiology. *Int J Psychophysiol.* 2018;131:13–23.
73. Kobayashi LC, Steptoe A. Social isolation, loneliness, and health behaviors at older ages: longitudinal cohort study. *Ann Behav Med.* 2018;52(7):582–593.
74. Schrempft S, Jackowska M, Hamer M, et al. Associations between social isolation, loneliness, and objective physical activity in older men and women. *BMC Public Health.* 2019;19(1):74.
75. Christakis NA, Fowler JH. Social contagion theory: examining dynamic social networks and human behavior. *Stat Med.* 2013;32(4):556–577.
76. Kent de Grey RG, Uchino BN, Trettevik R, et al. Social support and sleep: a meta-analysis. *Health Psychol.* 2018;37(8):787–798.
77. DuBois DL, Portillo N, Rhodes JE, et al. How effective are mentoring programs for youth? A systematic assessment of the evidence. *Psychol Sci Public Interest.* 2011;12(2):57–91.
78. Steiner RJ, Sheremenko G, Lesesne C, et al. Adolescent connectedness and adult health outcomes. *Pediatrics.* 2019;144(1):e20183766.
79. Maher BM, Hynes H, Sweeney C, et al. Medical school attrition-beyond the statistics a ten year retrospective study. *BMC Med Educ.* 2013;13(1):13.
80. Velando-Soriano A, Ortega-Campos E, Gómez-Urquiza JL, et al. Impact of social support in preventing burnout syndrome in nurses: a systematic review. *Jpn J Nurs Sci.* 2020;17(1):e12269.
81. Chetty R, Jackson MO, Kuchler T, et al. Social capital I: measurement and associations with economic mobility. *Nature.* 2022;608(7921):108–121.
82. Chetty R, Jackson MO, Kuchler T, et al. Social capital II: determinants of economic connectedness. *Nature.* 2022;608(7921):122–134.
83. Patel A, Plowman S. The Increasing Importance of a Best Friend at Work. Workplace. Gallup Inc., 2022.
84. Putnam R. *Bowling Alone Revised and Updated: The Collapse and Revival of American Community.* New York: Simon & Schuster, 2020.
85. Waldinger R, Schulz M. *The Good Life.* New York: Simon & Schuster, 2023.

8 The Combined Power of Lifestyle Medicine Modalities to Lower Risk Factors and Assist in Treatment of Chronic Disease

8.1 INTRODUCTION

In Part 1, we focused on the robust evidence supporting the health benefits for each of the seven major components of lifestyle medicine. In Part 2, we now move on from these individual lifestyle factors to show how a combination of these components can make a significant difference in either lowering the risk or assisting in the treatment of various chronic diseases. The combination of these key components of lifestyle medicine has been demonstrated in multiple studies to enhance their power. Moreover, there are synergies among the seven components, which show that a number of these modalities strongly interact with each other, thereby further enhancing the benefits of each.

8.2 THE SEVEN COMPONENTS OF LIFESTYLE MEDICINE

In Part 1, we outlined seven chapters, each of which was devoted to the robust scientific evidence behind each of the seven components of lifestyle medicine. These seven components are:

- Physical activity
- Healthy nutrition
- Weight management
- Stress reduction
- Avoidance of addictive substances
- Sleep
- Positive relations with others

While each of these components individually yields significant health benefits, many of them interact strongly with each other. They also act synergistically to further enhance the health benefits of each other. That synergistic factor will be the focus of each of the nine chapters found in Part 2 of this book. This synergy will also be a key consideration in the embedded curriculum found in Part 3.

8.3 THE POWER OF COMBINING COMPONENTS OF LIFESTYLE MEDICINE

Robust evidence exists demonstrating that the combination of the modalities that we have outlined for lifestyle medicine acts synergistically to lower the risk of developing chronic disease and/or assist in its treatment. The research that supports this is multifaceted and found across a variety of fields.

DOI: 10.1201/9781003630043-8

Perhaps the most compelling early evidence of how the components of lifestyle medicine interact with each other comes from two studies from the Harvard School of Public Health. The first of these studies, the Nurses' Health Trial, was conducted on over 110,000 nurses (largely female), who have now been followed for more than 20 years. This study showed that individuals who follow five simple lifestyle factors substantially improve their health and lower their risk of chronic disease. The five factors are:

- Regular physical activity (30 minutes at least five days per week)
- Healthy nutrition (more fruits, vegetables, and whole grains)
- Health weight management (BMI $\geq$ 19 and $\leq$ 25 Kg/m^2)
- Avoiding cigarettes
- And perhaps the most controversial, consuming one alcoholic beverage per day.

Nurses who followed these five lifestyle habits reduced their risk of diabetes by 91% and lowered their risk of coronary heart disease (CHD) by 83%.

Similar findings occurred in the Physicians' Health Study, which consisted largely of male physicians. This latter study showed the same robust decrease in the likelihood of developing diabetes and heart disease for individuals who followed these five lifestyle habits and practices. Of note, adopting even one of these lifestyle practices or habits lowered an individual's risk of developing diabetes or heart disease by 50%. This powerful finding is employed as we move forward into the curriculum found in Part 3 of this book.

Of note, and unfortunately, when these health care professionals were surveyed concerning their lifestyle habits, only 5% adopted all five of these powerful lifestyle habits and actions. This finding, in a sense, is not surprising since the Behavioral Risk Factor Study had shown similar very low adherence to simple lifestyle factors. We simply need to do better! We hope that physicians who use this book and follow the embedded curriculum can move the needle not only to more healthy habits for their patients but also in their own lives.

Multiple other organizations have utilized combinations of components of lifestyle medicine to make recommendations on how to enhance health. These include the Dietary Guidelines for Americans 2020–2025, multiple documents from the American Heart Association (AHA), including their 2021 nutritional recommendations, as well as their document for Defining and Setting National Goals for Cardiovascular Health Promotion and Disease Reduction, and the 2013 lifestyle practice guidelines.

In addition, a strong research base exists for utilizing multiple lifestyle modalities to lower the risk of both heart disease (CVD) and type 2 diabetes (T2DM). This research base was provided in the Diabetes Prevention Program (DPP), where healthy nutrition and regular physical activity combined with weight loss were the most effective treatment for people with glucose intolerance to prevent progression to T2DM. Similar results were obtained in the Look AHEAD Trial, where, once again, sound nutrition, weight loss, and regular physical activity were recommended. Multiple components of lifestyle change were also present in the weight loss guidance produced by the AHA/ACC/The Obesity Society (TOS). The Presidential Advisory from the AHA and the American Stroke Association (ASA) also recommended a similar multi-component approach to lower the risk of both CVD and cognitive decline.

Of note, the AHA initially published a framework called "Life's Simple Seven," which contains multiple lifestyle recommendations in a simple framework to reduce the risk of CVD. Several years ago, the AHA added an eighth component and turned it into "Life's Essential Eight." The eighth component that was added was healthy sleep.

Thus, multiple different organizations have utilized the power of combining multiple components of lifestyle medicine in their recommendations to lower the risk and assist in the treatment of chronic disease.

8.4 THE SEVEN COMPONENTS OF LIFESTYLE MEDICINE ARE SYNERGISTIC WITH EACH OTHER

Even though we divided the seven components of lifestyle medicine into individual chapters in Part 1, it is important to recognize that these components are synergistic with each other. For example, both physical activity and healthy nutrition are essential for healthy weight management. In addition, regular physical activity is central to one of the recommendations to avoid addictive substances and also enhances sleep and provides stress reduction. Positive relations with other people have also been shown to improve sleep and result in stress reduction and increase the likelihood of following healthy nutrition and obtaining regular physical activity while lowering the risk of CVD, stroke, and cognitive decline. Thus, these seven components of lifestyle medicine have been shown to be effective in combination for both lowering the risk of chronic disease and also in its treatment. The main underlying reason for this is that the components act synergistically with each other.

8.5 CONCLUSIONS/CLINICAL APPLICATIONS

In Part 2, we now look at the robust literature from multiple sources for how the seven components of lifestyle medicine may be used in combination with each other to provide maximum benefit for lowering the risk of chronic disease or assist in its treatment if already present. We do not mean to suggest that utilizing all of these components is essential to get benefits. In fact, as is shown in the embedded curriculum, we recommend starting with one or two of the components and then building from the success of that into more components until people have achieved multiple health benefits from combining a grouping of the seven components in lifestyle medicine.

9 Cardiovascular Disease

9.1 INTRODUCTION

Profound linkages exist between daily habits and practices in the area of lifestyle medicine for both lowering the risk of cardiovascular disease (CVD) and playing a significant role in its treatment (1–10). For this reason, primary care physicians and those particularly interested in lifestyle medicine should focus considerable attention on this area. This is all the more important given that CVD remains the leading killer of both men and women in the United States, resulting in over 37% of annual mortality (11).

Literally thousands of studies support the concept that regular physical activity, maintenance of proper weight, sound nutritional practices, avoiding tobacco products, obtaining proper sleep, lowering stress, and engaging in positive relationships with other people all significantly lower the risk of CVD (1–10,12). While these principles have been incorporated in virtually every evidence-based clinical guideline addressing the prevention and treatment of metabolically related diseases, they are particularly prominent in a newly developed literature supporting the concept of "cardiovascular health" (2). Guidelines from both the American Heart Association (AHA) and the American College of Cardiology (ACC) strongly support the prominent role of positive lifestyle measures in reducing the risk and, oftentimes, assisting in the treatment of cardiovascular disease (1–10, 13,14). The AHA and ACC have also been leaders in promoting the new concept of "cardiovascular health" (CVH), which is defined as reducing or eliminating cardiovascular risk factors in the first place (2).

Despite the overwhelming evidence supporting the health benefits of these positive lifestyle measures, it remains a challenge to help individuals incorporate the major lifestyle principles into their daily habits and actions. A good example of this is that in the past twenty years, there has been a significant reduction in cardiovascular disease. For example, coronary heart disease (CHD) in the United States fell by more than 40% during this period of time. This suggests that there has been some benefit from lifestyle measures since approximately half of the reduction of CVD between 1980 and 2018 came from improved lifestyle risk factors such as smoking cessation, increased physical activity, and better control of cholesterol and blood pressure (15). Nonetheless, unfortunately, several lifestyle factors rose strongly in the opposite direction. It has been estimated that increases in obesity and diabetes, which both substantially increased during this period of time, could potentially obliterate all the gains achieved by other lifestyle-related risk factors unless these trends can be reversed (15).

When the AHA released its Strategic Management Plan in 2020, it concluded that less than 1% of individuals achieved "ideal cardiovascular health," which is focused on a series of lifestyle factors such as regular physical activity, sound nutrition, weight management, and avoidance of tobacco, as well as lifestyle-related factors such as control of cholesterol, blood pressure, and glucose (1).

Clearly, significant challenges remain. In the last twenty years, both the AHA and ACC have been leaders in promoting the power of lifestyle habits and practices as key factors promoting cardiovascular health. In the Strategic Plan from the AHA in 2020, for example, the concept of "primordial" prevention (prevention of risk factors from occurring in the first place) was introduced into the cardiovascular lexicon, in addition to the construct of "ideal" cardiovascular health (1). This concept was updated and expanded in another Scientific Statement in 2022 (2). Moreover, in 2013, the AHA and ACC issued "Guidelines for Lifestyle Management to Reduce Cardiovascular Risk" (13). In addition, the council within the AHA, which previously was called the "Council on Nutrition, Physical Activity and Metabolism" in 2013, changed its name to the "Council on Lifestyle and Cardiometabolic Health" (16).

DOI: 10.1201/9781003630043-9

Other factors point to the fact that daily habits and actions are key parameters in reducing the risk of and oftentimes treating cardiovascular disease. For example, the Physical Activity Guidelines for Americans 2018 (PAGA 2018) focused considerable emphasis on regular physical activity as a key component of lowering the risk of CVD (17). The American College of Lifestyle Medicine (ACLM) has also focused attention on employing lifestyle habits and actions for lowering the risk of CVD (18). Thus, while there are many areas where the synergistic benefits of multiple lifestyle factors play an important role in lowering the risk of various metabolic diseases, it is important to start a discussion of these diseases with a focus on CVD. CVD remains the dominant metabolic condition where lifestyle practices play an important role in reducing risk and oftentimes assisting in treatment (1–10,19).

In this chapter, we will focus on how the synergistic effects of lifestyle factors play an important role in lowering the risk of CVD, which remains the leading killer of both men and women in the United States.

9.2 DEFINING CARDIOVASCULAR HEALTH

The Strategic Plan from the AHA in 2020 articulated the goal, which was "by 2020 to improve the cardiovascular health of all Americans by 20%, while reducing death from CVD and stroke by 20%" (1). To achieve these goals, the AHA made an effort to define a fundamentally new concept and emphasis on cardiovascular health. The AHA outlined a series of steps to accomplish this goal, many of which depend on lifestyle modalities. The overall strategy was based on three central concepts:

- Primordial prevention
- Evidence that risk factors for CVD develop early in life
- Balancing individual risk approaches with population-level approaches

The AHA Strategic Plan also introduced the concept of "primordial prevention" as a key component of cardiovascular health. Primordial prevention incorporates strategies to avoid developing adverse levels of cardiovascular risk factors in the first place rather than treating the risk factors (1,20). The AHA also introduced the concept of "ideal" cardiovascular health. This was initially defined as a series of seven health behaviors and health factors, including not smoking, maintaining a healthy body mass index, achieving the appropriate levels of physical activity, achieving a healthy diet, maintaining a total cholesterol of <200 mg/dL, maintaining a blood pressure of <120/<80 mm Hg, and maintaining a fasting glucose of <100 mg/dL. The cholesterol, blood pressure, and glucose parameters were all defined as "untreated" values (1).

Several years later, the AHA added an eighth factor related to healthy sleep. This has now become the overall framework that the AHA recommends for individuals who wish to achieve ideal cardiovascular health. It is called "Life's Essential 8." It is clear that lifestyle factors provide the core strategies that the AHA uses to define cardiovascular health.

9.3 EPIDEMIOLOGY OF CARDIOVASCULAR DISEASE

CVD remains the leading cause of death worldwide. It is also the leading cause of non-communicable diseases (NCDs) and is a major component of the World Health Organization (WHO) initiative to combat NCDs around the world. The WHO has stated that 74% of all deaths each year are the result of NCDs (21). The WHO has also stated that CVD is largely preventable through the reduction of behavioral risk factors, namely tobacco use, physical inactivity, harmful use of alcohol, and an unhealthy diet. Thus, lifestyle measures form the core of the WHO initiative to combat NCDs.

Some decreases in CVD have occurred in high-income countries. However, the prevalence of CVD in low- and middle-income countries has risen from 26% to 32% of deaths (22). Thus, it is important to understand that CVD represents a worldwide pandemic and that lifestyle medicine interventions can play a critically important role not only in lowering the risk of CVD in the United States but also around the world. Lifestyle medicine modalities can also serve as an important component of its treatment when CVD is already present.

9.4 LIFESTYLE MEDICINE FOCUSED HISTORY AND PHYSICAL EXAMINATION

Obtaining an accurate history and performing a comprehensive physical examination are cornerstones of good medical practice. When it comes to CVD, some nuances exist that can make a big difference in helping an individual adopt those habits and actions that have been shown to significantly reduce the risk of cardiovascular disease.

As already indicated, multiple lifestyle modalities, including proper nutrition, regular physical activity, weight management, stress management, avoiding addictive substances, healthful sleep, and positive relations with other individuals, all have been shown to lower the risk of CVD. Thus, these modalities should be emphasized, particularly in a lifestyle medicine-focused history.

In the area of nutrition, some sample questions emphasized by the AHA Guidelines (23), which can emphasize healthy nutrition, include the following:

- How many fruits and vegetables do you eat on a daily basis?
- How often do you eat fish (preferably oily fish)?
- How often do you eat fiber-rich whole grains?
- Do you take steps to reduce the amount of sodium (salt) in your diet?
- How often do you consume sugar-sweetened beverages?

These questions highlight key considerations that form the basis of virtually every heart-healthy nutritional diet recommended either by the AHA or the Dietary Guidelines for Americans 2025 (DGAs 2020–2025) (24). In the 2022 update on "Life's Essential Eight," the AHA broadened the recommendations to include the following: "A plant-forward nutritional plan such (25) as the Mediterranean Diet or DASH diet" (26).

In the area of physical activity, a good and simple way to start the dialogue would be to employ the two-item questionnaire developed at Stanford University. Simply ask your patient:

- How often do you engage in regular physical activity on a weekly basis?
- How much time do you spend each time you engage in physical activity?

These two questions can lead to a discussion of the role of physical activity in reducing the risk of CVD (27).

With regard to *weight*, some sample questions to get the dialogue started would be:

- Has your weight been stable over the past five years, or "How much did you weigh when you graduated from high school?" (28). These questions can open the door to discussing both weight gain and overweight and obesity.

In the area of *stress*, a good opening question is:

- How much stress do you experience in your daily life at work or at home?

In the area of *sleep*:

- How well do you sleep? How often do you get at least seven hours of sleep per night?

With regard to avoiding *addictive substances*, questions related to how much alcohol you consume include:

- How often do you consume five alcoholic drinks or more in a short period of time (binge drinking)?
- How many alcoholic drinks do you consume in an average day? In an average week?

In the area of *cigarette smoking*:

- Do you smoke?
- Have you ever smoked? If so, when did you quit?
- Are you exposed to secondhand smoke?

All are relevant.

With regard to *positive relationships* with others, a good place to start is:

- How supportive is your significant other and/or family?
- Do you have a wide circle of friends?
- Do you sometimes or often feel isolated or lonely?

In the area of *lifestyle-focused physical examination,* the following factors should be included:

- In addition to the normal parameters that every physician is trained to evaluate, we also recommend that weight and height should be measured and body mass index (BMI) computed and discussed with every patient.
- In addition, additional beneficial information will be obtained if the waist circumference is measured, so that you can discuss with an individual the issue of abdominal obesity as an additional risk factor for CVD.
- Blood pressure should be measured utilizing standard criteria and techniques that every physician learns. The American College of Cardiology also has published recommendations related to arm position and pausing for at least 5–10 minutes with the patient in a comfortable seated position, etc., before taking blood pressure (29).
- Some specialized tests may also provide valuable information. For example, a 3-day food record, which is typically administered by a nutritionist, can give a detailed analysis of current nutritional habits (30). An exercise tolerance test may be appropriate for individuals who have been quite sedentary or who have a history of cardiovascular disease. Dual-energy X-ray absorptiometry (DEXA) may also be helpful if you are fortunate to have a DEXA machine or access to one. This is an accurate test to determine the amount of body fat and muscle tissue.

9.5 LIFESTYLE MEDICINE, PHYSICAL ACTIVITY, AND CARDIOVASCULAR DISEASE

Regular physical activity has been repeatedly shown to lower the risk of CVD in general, as well as CHD, hypertension, heart failure, and Type 2 Diabetes Mellitus (T2DM) (18,31). Assessment of the levels of physical activity and recommendations for appropriate increases should be part of every patient encounter with physicians.

The key recommendation for physical activity is to help every patient avoid an inactive lifestyle. In fact, the PAGA 2018 has adopted the simple mantra "some is better than none." To illustrate this recommendation, they published a figure that contains information shown in Figure 9.1 (18).

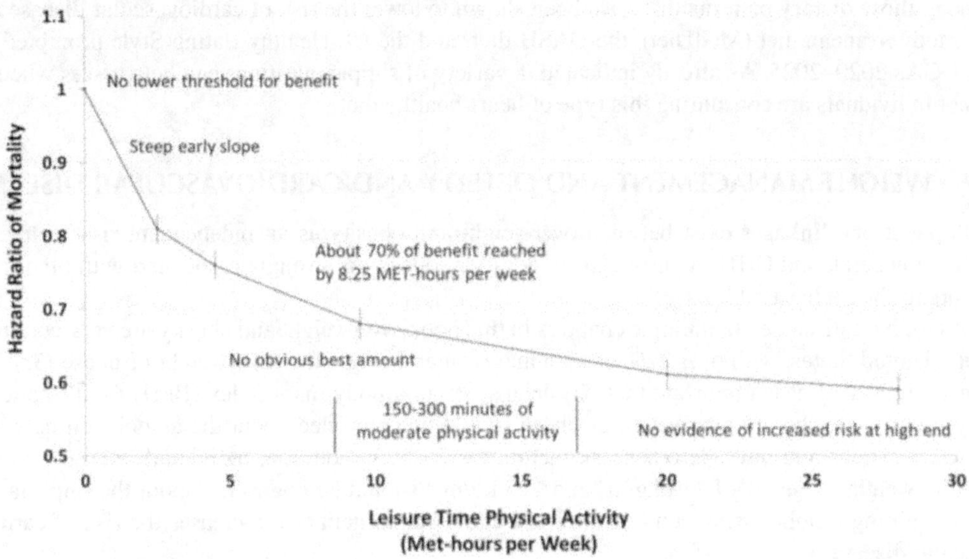

FIGURE 9.1 Relationships of moderate-to-vigorous physical activity to all-cause mortality, with highlighted characteristics common to studies of this type.

This figure illustrates that the most benefit comes from individuals who accumulate 150 minutes of moderate-intensity physical activity per week (typically in five sessions of 30 minutes each). As depicted in this graph, however, there is no lower threshold for benefit. Indeed, if individuals only obtain 30 minutes of physical activity per week, they receive a 20% reduction in all-cause and CVD mortality.

It should be emphasized that initial recommendations from the American Heart Association suggested physical activity should be conducted in 30-minute sessions. This recommendation subsequently was changed, however, to 10-minute sessions and then recently to the accumulation of any time spent with physical activity that adds up to the equivalent of 30 minutes in a day, which was shown to lower the risk of cardiovascular disease (18).

The key issue is to discuss physical activity with every patient. As we discuss in this chapter, there are synergies between physical activity and weight management, as well as stress reduction and sleep. Thus, physical activity is a cornerstone to the synergistic benefits of multiple lifestyle medicine modalities, which interact with each other and all contribute to lowering the risk of CVD.

9.6 NUTRITION AND CARDIOVASCULAR DISEASE

Proper nutrition plays a critically important role in reducing the risk of cardiovascular disease. Healthy dietary pattern recommendations are consistent across various prestigious organizations and guidelines, including the AHA (24), DGAs 2020–2025 (25), as well as recommendations from the Academy of Nutrition and Dietetics (AND) (32).

All of these organizations recommend dietary patterns that emphasize increased fruit and vegetable consumption, whole grains, seafood (oily fish), legumes and nuts, and low- or non-fat dairy products. The recommendations also emphasize lowering consumption of red meats and processed meats, lowering sugar-sweetened beverages, and refined grains. These healthy, plant-based patterns have been repeatedly shown to lower the risk of CVD.

Implementation of plant-forward diets such as those recommended by these organizations represents a key mandate for clinicians to employ to help their patients develop healthier eating habits. Modern nutrition science focuses on dietary patterns rather than individual foods or nutrients.

Among those dietary patterns that have been shown to lower the risk of cardiovascular disease are the Mediterranean diet (MedDiet), the DASH diet, and the US Healthy Eating Style promoted by the DGAs 2020–2025. As already indicated, a variety of simple questions can help assess whether or not individuals are consuming this type of heart-healthy diet.

9.7 WEIGHT MANAGEMENT AND OBESITY AND CARDIOVASCULAR DISEASE

Multiple strong linkages exist between overweight and obesity as an independent risk factor for CVD in general, and CHD in particular. In addition, obesity is strongly associated with other risk factors for heart disease (29).

As we have discussed in multiple chapters in this book, overweight and obesity are very common in the United States, with over 72% of men and women being either overweight or obese (33). As already indicated, it is important that physicians obtain a body mass index (BMI) for all patients they see. Those who are overweight or obese should be counseled about the association between those conditions and multiple other risk factors for CVD. In addition, individuals who are in the healthy weight range (BMI ≥19 kg/m^2 and ≤25 kg/m^2) should be counseled about the importance of not gaining weight during adult years, since adult weight gain also increases the risk of cardiovascular disease.

9.8 TOBACCO CESSATION AND CARDIOVASCULAR DISEASE

Cigarette smoking is a significant risk factor for CHD. While cigarette smoking prevalence has decreased in the last forty years in the United States, over 12% of individuals in the United States still smoke cigarettes (34,35). A variety of counseling programs and strategies are available to help people quit smoking. The good news is that individuals who are able to stop cigarette smoking rapidly decrease their risk factors for both CVD and a variety of cancers that are associated with this deadly habit (see Chapter 5 on avoiding addictive substances) (36).

A variety of pharmaceutical therapies are available to help with smoking cessation. A combination of pharmaceutical therapy and counseling has been shown to be the most effective way of stimulating cigarette smoking cessation. Other lifestyle interventions, such as regular physical activity, may also play important roles as adjunct therapy, particularly in the initial stages of smoking cessation. For all of these reasons, it is important that physicians discuss smoking with their patients who are still smoking and recommend a variety of lifestyle medicine strategies to help them discontinue this very dangerous and difficult habit to stop.

9.9 STRESS REDUCTION AND CARDIOVASCULAR DISEASE

Acute and chronic stress are associated with increased risk of CVD (37–39). Multiple stress-reduction mind/body techniques are available and can be effective in helping people reduce stress in their daily lives. More detail about available stress reduction techniques is found in Chapter 9. Lifestyle medicine physicians should initiate a discussion about stress in every patient counseling session.

9.10 SLEEP AND CARDIOVASCULAR DISEASE

Healthy sleep is very important to all bodily systems and, indeed, life itself. While healthy sleep interacts with multiple organ systems, it exerts a particularly profound effect on the cardiovascular system (40–43). Up to 70 million people in the United States have chronic sleep disorders (44,45). Disordered sleep is a significant risk factor for hypertension and is particularly common in individuals who are overweight or obese. Disrupted sleep can create an increased risk for obstructive sleep apnea, which can lead to cardiac ischemia (46,47). A variety of other lifestyle factors, such as weight loss (for overweight or obese individuals), increased physical activity, and nutrition are all lifestyle factors that can positively impact sleep and improve quality of life while reducing the risk of cardiovascular disease.

Sleep disorders are particularly prevalent in individuals over the age of 65 (48,49). Because of this, it is particularly important to inquire about sleep in older individuals, although all patients should have at least a brief discussion with their physician about the quality and quantity of sleep. Much more detail about sleep is found in Chapter 6 of this book. It is important, however, to specifically emphasize the interaction between sleep and other lifestyle medicine modalities, particularly when it comes to lowering the risk of cardiovascular disease.

9.11 POSITIVE RELATIONS WITH OTHERS AND CARDIOVASCULAR DISEASE

Multiple strong connections exist between social connections and physical health in general, and particularly in CVD and stroke outcomes (50). Many studies have shown that social isolation and loneliness may increase the risk of morbidity from these conditions (51). In fact, a number of studies have shown that social isolation and loneliness increase the risk of CVD by 29% and the risk of stroke by 32% (51). The AHA concluded in a 2022 statement that "social isolation and loneliness are common, yet under-recognized determinants of cardiovascular health and brain health." Thus, for all these reasons, it is important to inquire of individuals about their level of social connections and whether or not they are experiencing loneliness. Social connections also interact with multiple other lifestyle issues, including physical activity, nutrition, stress, and avoidance of addictive substances (52). Conversely, good social connections can synergistically interact with other lifestyle medicine modalities to further reduce the risk of CVD (50).

9.12 CARDIOVASCULAR RISK FACTORS/UNIFYING THEMES

Some unifying themes have begun to emerge that show why various positive lifestyle factors strongly interact with multiple types of CVD to lower their risk. Many research studies now point to underlying inflammation as a cause of multiple CVD problems. It used to be thought, for example, that atherosclerosis was largely a function of LDL cholesterol. New research has shown that the initial inciting event for atherosclerosis is typically inflammation of the inner lining of the arteries, which ultimately leads to accumulation of cholesterol and inflammatory cells (53,54). Moreover, other conditions such as obesity, T2DM, and metabolic syndrome all appear to share a major underlying etiology of increased inflammation (53,54). To further exacerbate the issue of inflammation, the standard American diet is, in and of itself, inflammatory (55). This is one of the reasons why less inflammatory diets such as the MedDiet and DASH diet seem to be so effective in lowering the risk and manifestations of CVD (26,27). In addition, cigarette smoking has been clearly shown to exert multiple inflammatory effects.

The good news is that multiple lifestyle medicine modalities, such as regular physical activity, healthy nutrition, weight management, avoiding cigarette smoking, and stress reduction, all interact synergistically with each other and exert anti-inflammatory effects. This may be the underlying reason why the combination of lifestyle medicine modalities is so powerful in lowering the risk of CVD.

9.13 OTHER MANIFESTATIONS OF CARDIOVASCULAR DISEASE

It is important to understand that atherosclerosis, which is the underlying cause of most CVD, has manifestations throughout the body. Thus, peripheral artery disease (56), carotid artery disease (57), chronic kidney disease, and erectile dysfunction may all be manifestations of the same process of atherosclerosis that causes narrowing of the coronary arteries.

Thus, when an individual is being counseled for lowering the risk factors of CHD, it should also be mentioned that some of these other manifestations of this systemic problem may also be present. It has even been suggested that erectile dysfunction, which is a common condition, particularly in men over the age of 50 who have multiple risk factors for CVD, may be an early manifestation of systemic atherosclerosis, which will ultimately cause CHD. In addition, individuals who have peripheral artery disease are three to four times as likely to have CHD as individuals who do not (56).

It is also important to emphasize that many of the same processes that can create adverse conditions within the coronary arteries can also create adverse conditions in the arteries in the brain. A Presidential Advisory from the AHA and the American Stroke Association entitled "Optimal Brain Health" advised that the same strategies utilized for lowering the risk of heart disease should also be employed to lower the risk of deterioration of brain function and cognitive decline (58). Thus, it is important to emphasize to patients, but particularly to those over the age of 65, that cognitive decline may also be a manifestation of underlying CVD. The good news is that the same lifestyle medicine modalities that are utilized to lower the risk of CVD are also effective in lowering the risk of cognitive decline (58).

9.14 SPECIALIZED TOPICS

- *Women and Cardiovascular Disease*: It is important to understand that CVD is the leading cause of morbidity and mortality in both men and women (59). In women, the symptomatology of CHD may be somewhat different than in men (60), so physicians need to be particularly cognizant of these differences (61). Unfortunately, in one survey, fewer than one in five physicians knew that more women than men die each year of heart disease. Furthermore, once women develop CHD, they have a worse prognosis than men. Among women over the age of 40, 42% die within five years after the first myocardial infarction, but only 32% of men suffer this (61). Perhaps one reason why there is less understanding and emphasis on heart disease in women than in men is that women tend to develop symptomatic CHD ten years later than men. (See also Chapter 16 for more detail.)

  The risk factors for cardiovascular disease in women are very similar to those in men. They include age, presence of hypertension, dyslipidemia, T2DM, obesity, cigarette smoking, inactivity, and metabolic syndrome. The good news is that in one major study (the Nurses' Heart Trial), women who followed five simple lifestyle practices, such as regular physical activity, proper nutrition, weight management, and not smoking, reduced their risk of heart disease by 83% (62). This good news message should be communicated to women. The most important issue for physicians is to recognize that, for female patients, heart disease remains the leading killer and to have detailed discussions with them about lowering risk factors for CVD, just like the discussions that occur with men about the very positive effects of lifestyle factors.
- *Genetics, Epigenetics, and Precision Medicine*: Significant progress has been made over the last decade in identifying lifestyle-related risk factors for CVD. These advances have typically come from applying data across large population groups (63,64). There is an emerging field of genetics, epigenetics, and precision medicine, which may offer an opportunity to apply these lifestyle medicine techniques with more precision in the future to lower the risk of CVD (65). While most of the information from these new techniques is not currently available for clinical application, it carries great potential for the future (66). It appears that lifestyle medicine techniques have a particular impact on the area of epigenetics, which is the field of how external processes influence gene transcription. These factors can result in altered levels of methylation of RNA, which impacts the way DNA is transcribed, and this can, in turn, alter levels of protein.

  The most common epigenetic modification is methylation of cysteine bases in DNA, which may result in reduced transcription or "silencing" of the gene. It has been postulated that most lifestyle practices may alter the methylation of DNA. Thus, epigenetics is destined to become an important and widely studied area related to the impact of lifestyle habits and practices on CVD risk. This area may even yield dramatic advances in what the AHA has called "primordial" prevention, which has the potential to lower risk factors even before they develop. Lifestyle medicine is likely to play a very important role in fulfilling this vision.

- *Reversing Heart Disease*: A number of studies generated over the past two decades have shown that intensive therapeutic lifestyle change measures (ITLC) can result in dramatic reversal of CHD (67–69). The area of ITLC typically involves very low-fat nutrition, regular physical activity, and stress reduction as key components that may contribute to reversing heart disease. A number of studies have led to the emergence of ITLC as an important and emerging component of the practice of lifestyle medicine. Many individuals are not willing to make these dramatic changes. For those who do, however, there is a significant opportunity to potentially even reverse CVD.
- *Children and Adolescents*: While this book and the embedded curriculum focus on adults, it is important to remember that many aspects of CVD, which are manifested in adults, have their roots in childhood. Recently, risk factors for heart disease in children and adolescents have increased significantly (70–74). The prevalence of dyslipidemia and hypertension has also risen sharply, as well as dramatic increases in the prevalence of overweight and obesity (Chapter 17).

  While a detailed review of these increasingly prevalent risk factors for CVD in children is beyond the scope of this book and the embedded curriculum, the same types of lifestyle measures that are applicable for the prevention and treatment of CVD in adults are highly relevant to children (see also Chapter 17). Good information on physical activity for children has recently been presented in the PAGA 2018 Scientific Report (18), and abundant evidence may also be found in the DGAs 2020–2025 (75). Since many of the lifestyle measures employed in adults are highly relevant to children, issues related to lifestyle medicine modalities are highly appropriate to be recommended for entire families.
- *Future of Lifestyle Medicine and Cardiovascular Disease: Research and Applications*: Great progress has been made in understanding the etiology of CVD and how lifestyle modalities lower its risk and assist in its treatment. In the future, technologies such as advanced computational techniques and genomic sequencing can potentially offer important information for advancing our understanding of how to lower the risk of CVD (76–80). These technologies may also offer potential for identifying patients at birth who are highly susceptible to CVD. This overall approach has been articulated by the American Heart Association as "primordial" prevention (1,2). While most of these technologies are not currently available in clinical practice, they have great potential for the future.

9.15 CONCLUSIONS/CLINICAL APPLICATIONS

The area of reducing risk for CVD is one where there has been enormous progress, particularly related to lifestyle medicine modalities. In this chapter, we have focused on ways to utilize some of this information as components of counseling for every patient. In particular, questions about physical activity, nutrition, tobacco use, sleep, stress, and positive relationships with others are all highly relevant for discussion with individual patients, since all of these show significant linkages between lifestyle modalities and risk of CVD. This is very important since CVD remains the leading cause of morbidity and mortality in the United States and around the world.

REFERENCES

1. Lloyd-Jones DM, Hong Y, Labarthe D, et al. Defining and setting national goals for cardiovascular health promotion and disease reduction: the American Heart Association's strategic impact goal through 2020 and beyond. *Circulation*. 2010; 121(4):586–613.

2. Lloyd-Jones DM, Allen NB, Anderson CAM, Life's essential 8: updating and enhancing the American Heart Association's construct of cardiovascular health: a presidential advisory from the American Heart Association. *Circulation.* 2022; 146(5):e18–e43.
3. Rippe JM. Lifestyle strategies for risk factor reduction, prevention, and treatment of cardiovascular disease. *Am J Lifestyle Med.* 2019;13(2):204–212.
4. Huffman MD, Capewell S, Ning H, et al. Cardiovascular health behavior and health factor changes (1988–2008) and projections to 2020: results from the National Health and Nutrition Examination Surveys. *Circulation.* 2012;125:2595–2602.
5. Pilkerton CS, Singh SS, Bias TK, et al. Changes in cardiovascular health in the United States, 2003–2011. *J Am Heart Assoc.* 2015;4:e001650.
6. Fang N, Jiang M, Fan Y. Ideal cardiovascular health metrics and risk of cardiovascular disease or mortality: a meta-analysis. *Int J Cardiol.* 2016;214:279–283.
7. Folsom AR, Yatsuya H, Nettleton JA, et al. ARIC Study Investigators. Community prevalence of ideal cardiovascular health, by the American Heart Association definition, and relationship with cardiovascular disease incidence. *J Am Coll Cardiol.* 2011;57:1690–1696.
8. Polonsky TS, Ning H, Daviglus ML, et al. Association of cardiovascular health with subclinical disease and incident events: the multi-ethnic study of atherosclerosis. *J Am Heart Assoc.* 2017;6: e004894.
9. Allen NB, Krefman AE, Labarthe D, et al. Cardiovascular health trajectories from childhood through middle age and their association with subclinical atherosclerosis. *JAMA Cardiol.* 2020;5:557–566.
10. Khera AV, Emdin CA, Drake I, et al. Genetic risk, adherence to a healthy lifestyle, and coronary disease. *N Engl J Med.* 2016;375:2349–2358.
11. Virani SS, Alonso A, Benjamin EJ, et al. On behalf of the American Heart Association Council on Epidemiology and Prevention Statistics Committee and Stroke Statistics Subcommittee. Heart disease and stroke statistics—2020 update: a report from the American Heart Association. *Circulation.* 2020;141:e139–e596.
12. Rippe JM. *Lifestyle Medicine* (4th ed). Boca Raton, FL: CRC Press, 2024.
13. Eckel RH, Jakicic JM, Ard JD, et al. 2013 AHA/ACC guideline on lifestyle management to reduce cardiovascular risk. *Circulation.* 2014;129(25_suppl_2):S76–S99.
14. Grundy SM, Stone NJ, Bailey AL, et al. 2018 AHA/ACC/AACVPR/AAPA/ABC/ACPM/ADA/AGS/APhA/ASPC/NLA/PCNA guideline on the management of blood cholesterol: executive summary: a report of the American College of Cardiology/American Heart Association Task Force on clinical practice guidelines. *Circulation.* 2019;139(25):e1046–e1081.
15. Ford ES, Ajani UA, Croft JB, et al. Explaining the decrease in U.S. deaths from coronary disease, 1980–2000. *N Engl J Med.* 2007;356(23):2388–2398.
16. American Heart Association. American Heart Association | To be a relentless force for a world of longer, healthier lives. Accessed January 30, 2025.
17. Physical Activity Guidelines Advisory Committee. 2018 Physical Activity Guidelines Advisory Committee. 2018 Physical Activity Guidelines Advisory Committee Scientific Report. Washington, DC: U.S. Department of Health and Human Services, 2018.
18. American College of Lifestyle Medicine. Home – American College of Lifestyle Medicine. Accessed January 30, 2025.
19. Rippe JM. *Integrating Lifestyle Medicine in Cardiovascular Health and Disease Prevention.* Boca Raton, FL: CRC Press, 2022.
20. Strasser T. Reflections on cardiovascular disease. National Heart Lung and Blood Institute. Clinical guidelines on the identification, evaluation, and treatment of overweight and obesity in adults. Bethesda, MD, 1998. *Interdiscip Sci Rev.* 1978:225–230.
21. World Health Organization. Global Non Communicable Disease Compact 2020–2030. https://www.who.int/initiatives/global-noncommunicable-diseases-compact-2020-2030. Accessed January 30, 2025.
22. The Global Burden of Disease 2013. https://ghdx.healthdata.org/gbd-data-tool. Accessed January 30, 2025.
23. Lichtenstein AH, Appel LJ, Vadiveloo M, et al. 2021 Dietary guidance to improve cardiovascular health: a scientific statement from the American Heart Association. *Circulation.* 2021;144(23):e472–e487.
24. U.S. Department of Health and Human Services and U.S. Department of Agriculture. 2020–2025 Dietary Guidelines for Americans (9th ed). 2020:164.
25. Estruch R, Ros E, Salas-Salvado J, et al. Primary prevention of cardiovascular disease with a Mediterranean diet. *N Engl J Med.* 2013;368(14):1279–1290.

26. Sacks FM, Svetkey LP, Vollmer WM, et al. Effects on blood pressure of reduced dietary sodium and the Dietary Approaches to Stop Hypertension (DASH) diet. DASH-Sodium Collaborative Research Group. *N Engl J Med.* 2001;344(1):3–10.
27. Exercise is Medicine. Home – Exercise is Medicine Home – Exercise is Medicine. Accessed January 30, 2025.
28. Jensen MD, Ryan DH, Apovian CM, et al. 2013 AHA/ACC/TOS guideline for the management of overweight and obesity in adults: a report of the American College of Cardiology/American Heart Association Task Force on Practice Guidelines and The Obesity Society. *J Am Coll Cardiol.* 2014;63(25 Pt B):2985–3023.
29. Appel LJ, Brands MW, Daniels SR, et al. Dietary approaches to prevent and treat hypertension: a scientific statement from the American Heart Association. *Hypertension.* 2006;47(2):296–308.
30. Rippe JM. *Lifestyle Nutrition: Eating for Good Health to Lower the Risk of Chronic Diseases.* Boca Raton, FL: CRC Press, 2024.
31. Rippe JM. *Lifestyle Medicine: Increasing Physical Activity: A Practical Guide.* Boca Raton, FL: CRC Press, 2020.
32. Nutrition and Physical Activity: General Population (NPA-GP) Guideline (2022–2023). EAL. Accessed January 31, 2025.
33. National Center for Health Statistics. United States, 2016: With Chartbook on Long-Term Trends in Health. Hyattsville, MD: National Center for Health Statistics, 2017.
34. US Centers for Disease Control and Prevention. The Health Consequences of Smoking: 50 Years of Progress: A Report of the Surgeon General. Atlanta, GA, 2014.
35. Jamal A, Phillips E, Gentzke AS, et al. Current cigarette smoking among adults: United States, 2016. *MMWR Morb Mortal Wkly Rep.* 2018;67:53–59.
36. Creamer MR, Wang TW, Babb S, et al. Tobacco product use and cessation indicators among adults: United States, 2018. *MMWR Morb Mortal Wkly Rep.* 2019;68:1013–1019.
37. Holman EA, Silver RC, Poulin M, et al. Terrorism, acute stress, and cardiovascular health: a 3-year national study following the September 11th attacks. *Arch Gen Psychiatry.* 2008;65(1):73–80.
38. Ming EE, Adler GK, Kessler RC, et al. Cardiovascular reactivity to work stress predicts subsequent onset of hypertension: the air traffic controller health change study. *Psychosom Med.* 2004;66(4):459–465.
39. Nielsen NR, Kristensen TS, Schnohr P, et al. Perceived stress and cause-specific mortality among men and women: results from a prospective cohort study. *Am J Epidemiol.* 2008;168(5):481–491.
40. Grandner MA, Fernandez FX. The translational neuroscience of sleep: a contextual framework. *Science.* 2021;374:568–573.
41. Kryger MH, Roth T, Goldstein CA. *Principles and Practice of Sleep Medicine.* Amsterdam: Elsevier Health Sciences, 2021.
42. Pienaar PR, Kolbe-Alexander TL, van Mechelen W, et al. Associations between self-reported sleep duration and mortality in employed individuals: systematic review and meta-analysis. *Am J Health Promot.* 2021;35:853–865.
43. Yin J, Jin X, Shan Z, et al. Relationship of sleep duration with all-cause mortality and cardiovascular events: a systematic review and dose-response meta-analysis of prospective cohort studies. *J Am Heart Assoc.* 2017;6:e005947.
44. National Sleep Foundation. 2014 Sleep Health Index. Arlington, VA: National Sleep Foundation, 2014.
45. Moser D, Anderer P, Gruber G, et al. Sleep classification according to AASM and Rechtschaffen & Kales: effects on sleep scoring parameters. *Sleep.* 2009;32(2):139–149.
46. Peppard PE, Young T, Barnet JH, et al. Increased prevalence of sleep-disordered breathing in adults. *Am J Epidemiol.* 2013;177(9):1006–1014.
47. Jordan AS, McSharry DG, Malhotra A. Adult obstructive sleep apnea. *Lancet.* 2014;383(9918):736–747.
48. Foley DJ, Monjan AA, Brown SL, et al. Sleep complaints among elderly persons: an epidemiologic study of three communities. *Sleep.* 1995;18(6):425–432.
49. Foley DJ, Monjan A, Simonsick EM, et al. Incidence and remission of insomnia among elderly adults: an epidemiologic study of 6,800 persons over three years. *Sleep.* 1999;22 Suppl 2:S366–S372.
50. Levine GN, Cohen BE, Commodore-Mensah Y, et al. Psychological health, well-being, and the mind-heart-body connection: a scientific statement from the American Heart Association. *Circulation.* 2021;143(10):e763–e83.
51. Vivek M. Office of the Surgeon General (OSG). Our Epidemic of Loneliness and Isolation: The U.S. Surgeon General's Advisory on the Healing Effects of Social Connection and Community. Washington, DC: US Department of Health and Human Services, 2023.

52. Unger E, Diez-Roux AV, Lloyd-Jones DM, et al. Association of neighborhood characteristics with cardiovascular health in the multi-ethnic study of atherosclerosis. *Circ Cardiovasc Qual Outcomes.* 2014;7:524–531.
53. Libby P, Bornfeldt KE, Tall AR. Atherosclerosis: successes, surprises, and future challenges. *Circ Res.* 2016;118(4):531–534.
54. Shapiro MD, Fazio S. From lipids to inflammation: new approaches to reducing atherosclerotic risk. *Circ Res.* 2016;118(4):732–749.
55. Christ A, Lauterbach M, Latz E. Western diet and the immune system: an inflammatory connection. *Immunity.* 2019;51(5):794–811.
56. Gerhard-Herman MD, Gornik HL, Barrett C, et al. 2016 AHA/ACC guideline on the management of patients with lower extremity peripheral artery disease: a report of the American College of Cardiology/American Heart Association Task Force on clinical practice guidelines. *Circulation.* 2017;135(12):e726–e779.
57. Meschia JF, Bushnell C, Boden-Albala B, et al. Guidelines for the primary prevention of stroke: a statement for healthcare professionals from the American Heart Association/American Stroke Association. *Stroke.* 2014;45(12):3754–3832.
58. Gorelick PB, Furie KL, Iadecola C, et al. Defining optimal brain health in adults: a presidential advisory from the American Heart Association/American Stroke Association. *Stroke.* 2017;48(10):e284–e303.
59. Mosca L, Benjamin EJ, Berra K, et al. Effectiveness-based guidelines for the prevention of cardiovascular disease in women – 2011 update: a guideline from the American Heart Association. *Circulation.* 2011;123(11):1243–1262.
60. Canto JG, Goldberg RJ, Hand MM, et al. Symptom presentation of women with acute coronary syndromes: myth vs reality. *Arch Intern Med.* 2007;167(22):2405–2413.
61. McSweeney JC, Rosenfeld AG, Abel WM, et al. Preventing and experiencing ischemic heart disease as a woman: state of the science: a scientific statement from the American Heart Association. *Circulation.* 2016;133(13):1302–1331.
62. Liu S, Stampfer MJ, Hu FB, et al. Whole-grain consumption and risk of coronary heart disease: results from the nurses' health study. *Am J Clin Nutr.* 1999;70(3):412–419.
63. Musunuru K, Kathiresan S. Principles of cardiovascular genetics. In Zipes DP, Libby P, Bonow RO, Mann DL, Tomaselli GF (eds.) *Braunwald's Heart Disease* (11th ed). Philadelphia, PA: Elsevier, 2019.
64. Shah SH, Arnett D, Houser SR, et al. Opportunities for the cardiovascular community in the precision medicine initiative. *Circulation.* 2016;133(2):226–231.
65. O'Donnell CJ, Nabel EG. Genomics of cardiovascular disease. *N Engl J Med.* 2011;365(22):2098–2109.
66. Rippe JM. The future of lifestyle medicine. In Rippe JM (ed.) *Manual of Lifestyle Medicine.* Boca Raton, FL: CRC Press, 2021.
67. Ornish D, et al. Intensive lifestyle changes for reversal of coronary heart disease. *JAMA.* 1998;280: 2001–2007.
68. Ornish D, et al. Can lifestyle changes reverse coronary atherosclerosis? The lifestyle heart trial. *Lancet.* 1990;336:129–133.
69. Kelly J. High intensity therapeutic lifestyle change. In Rippe JM (ed.) *Lifestyle Medicine* (3rd ed). Boca Raton, FL: CRC Press, 2019.
70. Berenson GS, Srinivasan SR, Bao W, et al. Association between multiple cardiovascular risk factors and atherosclerosis in children and young adults. The Bogalusa Heart Study. *N Engl J Med.* 1998; 338(23):1650–1656.
71. McMahan CA, Gidding SS, Malcom GT, et al. Pathobiological determinants of atherosclerosis in youth risk scores are associated with early and advanced atherosclerosis. *Pediatrics.* 2006;118(4):1447–1455.
72. Newman WP 3rd, Freedman DS, Voors AW, et al. Relation of serum lipoprotein levels and systolic blood pressure to early atherosclerosis. The Bogalusa Heart Study. *N Engl J Med.*1986;314(3):138–144.
73. Raitakari OT, Juonala M, Kahonen M, et al. Cardiovascular risk factors in childhood and carotid artery intima-media thickness in adulthood: the cardiovascular risk in young Finns study. *JAMA.* 2003;290(17):2277–2283.
74. Shustak RJ, Brothers JA, Daniels SR. Identification and management of children with dyslipidemia. In Rippe JM (ed.) *Lifestyle Medicine* (4th ed). Boca Raton, FL: CRC Press, 2024.
75. Schunkert H, König IR, Kathiresan S, et al. Large-scale association analysis identifies 13 new susceptibility loci for coronary artery disease. *Nat Genet.* 2011;6;43(4):333–338.
76. Hernandez-Saavedra D, Moody L, Xu GB, et al. Epigenetic regulation of metabolism and inflammation by calorie restriction. *Adv Nutr.* 2019;10(3):520–536.

77. Ellsworth DL, Croft DT, Weyandt J, et al. Intensive cardiovascular risk reduction induces sustainable changes in expression of genes and pathways important to vascular function. *Circ Cardiovasc Genet.* 2014;7(2):151–160.
78. Samani NJ, Erdmann J, Hall AS, et al. Genome wide association analysis of coronary artery disease. *N Engl J Med.* 2007;357(5):443–453.
79. Tada H, Melander O, Louie JZ, et al. Risk prediction by genetic risk scores for coronary heart disease is independent of self-reported family history. *Eur Heart J.* 2016;37(6):561–567.
80. Antman EM, Loscalzo J. Precision medicine in cardiology. *Nat Rev Cardiol.* 2016;13(10):591–602.

10 Diabetes, Pre-Diabetes, and the Metabolic Syndrome

10.1 INTRODUCTION

The prevalence of diabetes, pre-diabetes, and the metabolic syndrome (MetS) has grown substantially over the past 30 years in the United States and in other affluent countries around the world. According to the Centers for Disease Control (CDC) in 2021, the last year for which reliable data was available, 11.6% of the United States population, or 38.4 million people, had diabetes (1). This includes:

- *Diagnosed Diabetes*: 29.7 million adults with diagnosed diabetes.
- *Undiagnosed Diabetes*: 8.7 million adults with undiagnosed diabetes, which represents 22% of all patients with diabetes.

In 2015, the CDC recorded that more than 110 million US adults were living with diabetes and pre-diabetes (2). As already indicated, 29.7 million adults were diagnosed with diabetes and another 84.1 million had pre-diabetes (33.9% of adults). Nearly one fourth of all adults (87 million adults) do not know they have diabetes and are included in the 110 million figure (3). In children and adolescents, approximately 193,000 have either type 1 diabetes (T1DM) or type 2 diabetes (T2DM).

Lifestyle therapies, including medical nutrition therapy (MNT), physical activity, and/or education and counseling support, all play a critically important role in both the prevention and management of T2DM (4,5). Multiple large studies have shown that lifestyle interventions implemented in individuals with pre-diabetes can effectively prevent T2DM in some instances for up to 15–20 years (6). Lifestyle interventions continue to be effective throughout the disease process and have shown their greatest impact early in the course of the disease (7).

10.2 EPIDEMIOLOGY

The prevalence of diabetes varies by age, sex, weight status, race/ethnicity, and education level (1).

- *Age*: The prevalence of diabetes increases with age, reaching 29.2% for those aged 65 or older
- *Sex*: Men are more likely to have diabetes than women
- *Weight Status*: The prevalence of diabetes increases with increasing weight status
- *Race and Ethnicity*: The prevalence of diabetes varies by race and ethnicity
- *Education Level*: The prevalence of diabetes decreases with increasing educational attainment

Between 90% and 95% of people with diabetes have T2DM. T2DM most often develops in people 45 years or older (7). Unfortunately, more children, teens, and young adults are also developing this condition. The increase in prevalence seems to coincide with the significant increase in overweight and obesity among children and adolescents (8).

10.3 LIFESTYLE MEDICINE THERAPIES IN THE MANAGEMENT OF DIABETES

Lifestyle medicine modalities play crucially important roles at all stages in both the development and management of insulin resistance, pre-diabetes, T2DM, and MetS. Among the lifestyle

DOI: 10.1201/9781003630043-10

interventions, preventing obesity, increasing physical activity, and following healthy nutrition are all priorities in the prevention of pre-diabetes and T2DM (8).

The goal of MNT in diabetes is to support healthy eating patterns and achieve individualized glycemia, blood pressure, and lipid goals. As diabetes progresses, the goal of MNT changes to delay, prevent, or help manage any potential complications. Many registered dietitian nutritionists (RDNs) have an additional degree as certified diabetes educators (CDE), which allows them to deliver MNT in an evidence-based mode (5). MNT must address the individual needs of literacy and access to healthy food choices, as well as the willingness of the person to make behavior changes.

Multiple other lifestyle medicine modalities play central roles in both the prevention of T2DM, pre-diabetes, and MetS, as well as the management of these conditions. These will be discussed throughout this chapter.

10.4 TYPE 1 DIABETES AND LIFESTYLE MEDICINE

T1DM accounts for only 5% of diagnosed diabetes. T1DM is thought to be due to a disruption of insulin-producing pancreatic beta cells by an autoimmune process, which leads to an absolute insulin deficiency. This beta cell destruction varies considerably among individuals. T1DM commonly occurs in childhood and adolescence, but it can occur at any age, even into the eighth or ninth decade of life. Children and adolescents may present with ketoacidosis as the first symptom of this disease (9). Adults may retain enough beta cell function to prevent ketoacidosis, but many of these individuals ultimately become dependent on insulin for survival and are at risk for ketoacidosis.

- Treatment of T1DM
    - *Insulin and Blood Glucose Monitoring*: An individual with T1DM must be treated with daily subcutaneous injections (or basal insulin and rapid-acting insulin after meals or continuous subcutaneous insulin (CSI) infusion). The Diabetes Control Complications Trial (DCCT) showed that intensive therapy with MDI or CSI delivered by multidisciplinary teams of physicians, registered dietitian nutritionists (RDNs), nurses, and behavioral scientists, among others, resulted in improved glycemia, reduced total complication risk, and improved long-term outcomes.

  Recommended levels for blood glucose are found in Table 10.1.
- Lifestyle Interventions for T1DM
    - *Medical and Nutrition Therapy*: Enormous evidence exists that MNT, which employs carbohydrate counting and insulin-to-carbohydrate ratios, contributes to significant decreases in HBA1C and significant improvements in quality of life (10). MNT is optimally delivered through frequent encounters with RDNs and patient use of carbohydrate counting to guide mealtime insulin dosage. Half of insulin needs are for basal glucose control, and the other half is for prandial requirements. Carbohydrate intake is a primary determinant of bolus insulin needs, but if a meal contains more protein and fat than usual, bolus insulin doses may be needed to compensate for delayed postprandial glucose rises.
    - *Physical Activity/Exercise*: The Physical Activity Guidelines for Americans (PAGA 2018) Scientific Report advocates that youth with T1DM should engage in 60 minutes or more of daily moderate or vigorous activity and muscle-strengthening exercise for at least two days per week (11). These are similar to the recommendations made for all children. Adults with T1DM are recommended by PAGA 2018 to engage in 150 minutes or more of moderate physical activity per week. Most individuals typically divide physical activity into five 30-minute sessions. Prevention of hypoglycemia with exercise is a significant concern (12). Individuals may have to adjust by increasing carbohydrates if pre-exercise glucose levels are less than 100 mg/dL.

TABLE 10.1
Recommended Levels for Blood Glucose

A1C	Preprandial Capillary PG[a]	Peak Postprandial Capillary PG	Bedtime/Overnight
Adults			
ADA; <7.0% (53 mmol/mol)[b] AACE/ACE: ≤6.5%[c]	80–130 mg/dL (4.4–7.2 mmol/L)[b]	<180 mg/dL (10.0 mmol/L)[b,d]	
Children and adolescents with type 1 diabetes[b,e]			
<7.5% (58 mmol/mol)	90–130 mg/dL (5.0–7.2 mmol/L)		90–150 mg/dL (5.0–8.3 mmol/L)

Sources: See Refs. [8,12]. From Franz M. Lifestyle therapies for the management of diabetes. In Rippe JM (ed.) *Lifestyle Medicine*, 3rd ed, CRC Press, Boca Raton, FL, 2019. Used with permission of the editor Dr. James Rippe.

[a] Plasma glucose.

[b] More or less stringent glycemic goals may be appropriate for individual persons. Blood glucose goals should be modified in children with frequent hypoglycemia or hypoglycemia unawareness.

[c] Goal if it can be achieved safely.

[d] Postprandial PG may be used if A1C goals are not met despite reaching preprandial PG goals.

[e] In children and adolescents, postprandial PG values should be measured when there is a discrepancy between pre-prandial PG values and A1C levels and to assess pre-prandial insulin doses in those on basal-bolus or CSII regimens.

- *Education/Counselling*: It is important that individuals with diabetes and their families receive diabetes self-management education and support (DSMES). This provides support for individuals to take self-control of T1DM (7).
- *Social Care*: Clinically significant emotional disorders such as anxiety, depression, and disordered eating behaviors are common in people with T1DM and may require screening and referrals for treatment. Overutilizing insulin, causing hypoglycemia in an attempt to lose weight, is the most common eating disorder in individuals with T1DM (13,14).

10.5 TYPE 2 DIABETES

T2DM is responsible for 90%–95% of all diabetes (7). Many of the people who have T2DM are obese. Obesity itself causes some degree of insulin resistance. Individuals who are not obese by BMI criteria may still have T2DM. They may also have an increased percentage of body fat disproportionately distributed in the abdominal region, which also causes insulin resistance.

T2DM is the result of a combination of insulin resistance and beta-cell failure. Insulin resistance may be present in a variety of target tissues, namely muscle, liver, and adipose cells (15,16). Insulin levels may be normal but are not able to overcome this insulin resistance. Hyperglycemia results and may be first exhibited as elevations in postprandial blood glucose. Ultimately, increases in fasting glucose concentration also occur.

T2DM is a progressive disease and may ultimately require increased dosages of either oral hypoglycemic agents or, eventually, insulin. T2DM is a risk factor for cardiovascular disease. Three-quarters of individuals with T2DM die of CVD. In addition to its intrinsic risk of CVD, T2DM is also associated with hypertension and dyslipidemia, which must be managed aggressively in individuals with T2DM (see the subsequent section in this chapter).

- *Medical Nutrition Therapy*: MNT is a vital component of the medical management of diabetes (5). Diabetes educators such as RDNs or nurses with diabetes education credentials (DECs) are most effective in delivering MNT, which includes carbohydrate counting, particularly within meals. Reduced energy intake should also be established. A summary of MNT interventions for adults with diabetes is found in Table 10.2.

- *Physical Activity*: Physical activity plays an important role in every stage of T2DM (11,12). Regular physical activity reduces the risk of developing T2DM and can also play an important role in its management for people who already have the condition. These facts are recognized in the Position Statement from the American Diabetes Association on Physical Activity/Exercise (17) and Diabetes, the PAGA 2018 (11) Scientific Report, as well as the ADA Lifestyle Management Standards for Medical Care in Diabetes (10). Regular physical activity can lower the risk and prevent or delay T2DM. Aerobic activity such as walking,

TABLE 10.2
Academy of Nutrition and Dietetics Evidence-Based Nutrition Therapy Intervention Recommendations for Type 1 and Type 2 Diabetes in Adults

Topic	Recommendations	Rating
Nutrition prescription	Individualize in collaboration with the adult; a variety of eating patterns are acceptable based on the individual's preferences.	Fair
Energy intake	- For overweight or obese adults: a reduced-energy, healthful eating plan with the goal of weight loss, weight maintenance, and/or prevention of weight gain. - For appropriate-weight adults: a healthful eating plan with the goal of weight maintenance and/or prevention of weight gain.	Strong Consensus
Macronutrient composition	An individualized, healthful eating plan within appropriate energy intake. Differing amounts of carbohydrate (39%–57%) and fat (27%–40%) report no significant effects on A1C or insulin levels, independent of weight loss.	Fair
Carbohydrate management strategies	- Adults on MDI or CSII: educate on carbohydrate counting using insulin-to-carbohydrate ratios. - Adults on fixed insulin doses or on insulin secretagogues: educate on carbohydrate consistency (timing and amount). - Adults on MNT alone or on diabetes medication (other than insulin secretagogues): educate on carbohydrate management strategy. - All recommendations are based on the individual's abilities, preferences, and management goals. Monitoring carbohydrate intake is a key strategy for achieving glycemic goals.	Strong Fair Fair Fair
Fiber intake	Encourage consumption of dietary fiber from foods, such as fruits, vegetables, whole grains, and legumes at the levels recommended by the Dietary Reference Intakes of the US Department of Agriculture due to the overall health benefits of dietary fiber.	Fait
Glycemic index (GI) and glycemic load (GL)	Lowering GI or GL may or may not have a significant effect on glycemic control. Studies longer than 12 weeks report no significant influence of GI or GL, independent of weight loss, on A1C levels.	Fair
Nutritive sweeteners	- Nutritive sweeteners, when substituted isocalorically for other carbohydrates, will not have a significant effect on A1C or insulin levels. - Advise against excessive intake of nutritive sweeteners to avoid excessive calorie and carbohydrate intake.	Fair Fair
Nonnutritive sweeteners (NNS)	- Intake of FDA-approved NNS within the recommended daily intake levels established by the FDA does not have a significant influence on glycemic control. - Substituting foods and beverages containing FDA-approved NNS within the recommended daily intake can reduce overall calorie and carbohydrate intake; however, the other sources of calories and carbohydrates in these foods and beverages need to be considered.	Weak Fair

(continued)

TABLE 10.2 (*Continued*)
Academy of Nutrition and Dietetics Evidence-Based Nutrition Therapy Intervention Recommendations for Type 1 and Type Diabetes in Adults

Topic	Recommendations	Rating
Protein intake	- Adding protein to meals and/or snacks does not prevent or assist in the treatment of hypoglycemia. Ingested protein appears to increase the insulin response without increasing plasma glucose concentrations; therefore, protein should not be used to treat or prevent hypoglycemia. - Adults with diabetes and diabetic kidney disease do not need protein restriction; there is no significant influence of protein intake. - Type of protein (vegetable-based vs. animal-based) does not have a significant effect on glomerular filtration rate.	Fair Strong Weak
Cardioprotective eating patterns	- Encourage consumption of a cardioprotective eating pattern within the recommended energy intake. - Encourage an individualized reduction in sodium intake. Less than 2,000 mg of sodium per day is appropriate; for adults with both diabetes and hypertension, further reduction in sodium should be individualized.	Strong Fair
Nutrient adequacy: vitamin, mineral, and/or herbal supplements	If proposed as a diabetes management strategy, advise that there is no clear benefit from supplementation in people who do not have deficiencies.	Fair
Alcohol	When adults choose to drink alcohol, they should do so in moderation (up to one drink/day for women and up to two drinks/day for men). Alcohol consumption may place adults using insulin or insulin secretagogues at increased risk for delayed hypoglycemia.	Weak
Physical activity	Encourage an individualized physical activity plan, unless medically contraindicated, to gradually achieve the following: • Accumulating 150 minutes or more of physical activity per week; • Moderate-intensity aerobic exercise spread over at least three days/week with no more than two consecutive days without exercise; • Resistance training at least twice per week; and • Reduce sedentary time by breaking up extended periods (more than 90 minutes) spent sitting.	Strong
Glucose monitoring	Ensure that adults are educated about glucose monitoring and using data to adjust therapy.	Fair

Source: MacLeod J, Franz MJ, Handu D, et al. Academy of nutrition and dietetics nutrition practice guideline for type 1 and type 2 diabetes in adults: nutrition intervention evidence reviews and recommendations. *J Acad Nutr Diet.* 2017;117:1637–1658. Reprinted from *Lifestyle Medicine*, 3rd ed, CRC Press, Boca Raton, FL, 2019. With permission of the Editor, James M. Rippe, MD.

cycling, jogging, or swimming has been shown in particular to lower the risk of diabetes and/or assist in its treatment. Recommendations from the American College of Sports Medicine (ACSM) (18) and PAGA 2018 all recommend 150 minutes of moderate-intensity physical activity per week, as well as two episodes of strength training per week, for people with T2DM.

- *Education/Counseling Support*: Every person with diabetes should be managed with education, self-management, and management planning along with their health care team (7,8). A particular emphasis on healthy eating in this area involves consuming nutrient-dense foods and reduced energy intake. Both the Mediterranean diet (MedDiet) (19) and the DASH diet (20) are plant-forward diets that are examples of healthy eating patterns.

- *Psychosocial Care*: Individuals with T2DM can also benefit from psychosocial care, particularly in the area of stress reduction. This will help improve adherence to diabetes care recommendations. This is particularly true of individuals who have obesity. Unfortunately, some health care providers have negative attitudes or stereotypes about people with obesity.

10.6 THE RELATIONSHIP BETWEEN DIABETES AND CARDIOVASCULAR DISEASE

There is a strong association between T2DM and multiple aspects of CVD. Individuals with T2DM have a two- to four-fold increased risk of mortality from coronary heart disease (CHD) compared to those without T2DM (21). T2DM is also associated with increased risk of myocardial infarction (MI) and multiple other aspects of acute coronary syndrome (ACS) events. T2DM is also associated with risk of other manifestations of atherosclerotic vascular disease, including stroke, cerebral vascular disease, and peripheral artery disease (22). T2DM is also associated with a two- to four-fold increase in heart failure (HF) (22). HF is a key driver of CVD morbidity and mortality (23,24). In addition, T2DM increases the risk of atrial fibrillation (AF). It also increases the stroke rate by 2%–5% per year (7). For this reason, the American Heart Association (AHA) guidelines recommend anticoagulation for all patients with T2DM who have a history of atrial fibrillation due to increased stroke risk (see the subsequent section in this chapter).

10.6.1 Pathophysiologic Link between Coronary Heart Disease and Diabetes

As already indicated, risk factors for CHD include hypertension, dyslipidemia, and adiposity. These risk factors tend to cluster in individuals with T2DM (25). The underlying pathophysiology is not completely understood. Hyperglycemia associated with T2DM is associated with endothelial basal cell dysfunction and an increased risk of systemic inflammation (26) (see also Chapter 9). Abnormalities in coagulation and fibrogenic pathways, and also changes in platelet biology, further contribute to increased risk of thrombotic conditions in individuals with T2DM (27).

10.7 THE ROLE OF LIFESTYLE MANAGEMENT IN PREVENTION OF CORONARY HEART DISEASE AND ITS COMPLICATIONS IN DIABETES

Multiple different lifestyle medicine modalities play very important roles in reducing the risk and manifestations of CHD in individuals with T2DM. Here are some of the key lifestyle medicine modalities associated with lowering the risk of CVD in the T2DM population.

- *Therapeutic Lifestyle Counseling*: This is the essence of behavioral management. Therapeutic lifestyle counseling (TLC) is central to including multiple other lifestyle medicine behavioral strategies, including regular physical activity, healthy nutrition, smoking cessation, and weight management (7).
- *Lipids*: Lipids should be routinely and regularly measured in all patients with T2DM (7). The major pharmacologic treatment in dyslipidemia is statin therapy. The goal with statin therapy is to maintain LDL-C levels less than 70 mg/dL. Modalities such as regular physical activity may serve to raise HDL, which can further lower the risk of CHD.
- *Blood Pressure*: Maintaining a healthy blood pressure is particularly important in individuals with T2DM (7). Blood pressure should be measured during every clinical visit in these patients. The ADA recommends a blood pressure target of no higher than 140/85 mm Hg

and optimally below 130/80 mm Hg if possible. Multiple lifestyle interventions have been demonstrated to help with weight management, including regular physical activity, dietary sodium restriction, and weight loss. Angiotensin-converting enzyme (ACE) inhibitors are the preferred medication for blood pressure control in individuals with T2DM in addition to these lifestyle modalities (7).

- *Physical Activity*: Major organizations, including the AHA, PAGA 2018 (11), the ACSM, and Practice Guidelines from the American Diabetes Association (ADA) (12,17), all recommend 150 minutes of moderate-intensity aerobic physical activity on a weekly basis or 75 minutes of vigorous aerobic activity.
- *Tobacco*: Individuals with T2DM should refrain from tobacco use or be advised to quit (see also Chapter 5 on Substance Abuse) (7).
- *Antiplatelet Agents*: Both the ADA and AHA recommend aspirin therapy (75–162 mg dL) for primary prevention in patients with diabetes who are at increased risk for CVD (7). Individuals allergic to aspirin, however, should be treated with other antiplatelet agents.
- *Glycemic Control*: The HbA1C goal for most patients with T2DM is less than 7% in the absence of CVD. The ADA recognizes that higher targets, such as 8%, may be appropriate for individuals with moderate or severe risk of CVD (7).
- *Sleep Hygiene*: Healthy sleep is also an important consideration for individuals with T2DM (27). Disruptive sleep promotes insulin resistance and impairs pancreatic β-cell function. In addition, cross-sectional studies demonstrate a close association between reduced sleep time and weight gain (28). Food preferences may also be affected by sleep for reasons that are not completely understood (29,30). In addition, interventional treatment for obstructive sleep apnea (OSA) is important. It is also important for people with T2DM since OSA is associated with increased risk of hypertension and increased risk of heart disease (30). Thus, healthy sleep is a key consideration for all individuals with T2DM (see also Chapter 6). The recommendation for modalities to increase sleep hygiene is, therefore, very important for people with T2DM.
- *Environmental Lighting*: Disturbed circadian clocks are influenced by environmental lighting (31). One of these is the pancreatic clock, which influences glucose tolerance. Several studies in healthy individuals have demonstrated that increased postprandial insulin and glucose levels occur with exposure to bright light at night. The quality of light also affects insulin resistance (32). For example, the light produced by screen devices (e.g., smartphones, tablets, and computers) has been demonstrated to be associated with insulin resistance in healthy individuals (33). This is an area of ongoing research in people with T2DM.
- *Stress Reduction*: Chronic stress impacts multiple system functions (34). Chronic stress activates the hypothalamic-pituitary-adrenal axis and the sympathetic nervous system, thereby increasing cortisol and catecholamine levels and worsening insulin resistance (35). This, in turn, can increase cardiovascular complications associated with T2DM.
- *Alcohol Intake*: While there are multiple controversial research trials in the area of alcohol intake, there is no clear association between moderate alcohol intake and T2DM (36,37).
- *Endocrine Disruptors*: A number of chemicals that have various industrial uses may disrupt hormone signaling (38–40). These endocrine-disrupting compounds may be associated with the development of T2DM.
- *Positive Interaction with Others*: Given the multiple social components of a chronic illness such as T2DM, it is particularly important to have a supportive group of individuals around the person who has this condition (7,8). This includes not only his or her physician but also family members, significant others, friends, etc. These positive connections have been shown to help with the management of not only the physical but also the psychological manifestations of chronic diseases such as T2DM.

10.8 LIFESTYLE MEDICINE AND THE MANAGEMENT OF PRE-DIABETES

Pre-diabetes is a condition where hyperglycemia is present but blood glucose levels are below the T2DM thresholds (7). Pre-diabetes is very common in the United States. It has been estimated to occur in over 33% of adults (41,42).

The lifestyle medicine goals for pre-diabetes should focus on achieving and maintaining a healthy body weight, improving dietary patterns, and increasing physical activity to prevent pre-diabetes from evolving into diabetes or perhaps even reversing pre-diabetes (43,44).

The diagnosis of pre-diabetes occurs when there is a fasting blood sugar (FBG) between 100 and 125 mg/dL (7). This typically reflects hepatic insulin resistance, which is an early phase of insulin secretion. In addition, high FBG may also reflect muscle insulin resistance. In addition to the 33% of adults aged 18–64 who have pre-diabetes, there are 48% of individuals 65 or older who have pre-diabetes, according to data from the American Diabetes Association 2015. Pre-diabetes prevalence is higher in men (36.6%) than in women (29.3%) (7).

10.9 THE ROLE OF LIFESTYLE FACTORS IN THE DEVELOPMENT OF PRE-DIABETES

Pre-diabetes typically represents impaired insulin secretion, insulin resistance, and disproportionate body fat distribution or a combination of these factors (7). Excessive calorie intake and physical inactivity increase insulin resistance and, therefore, pre-diabetes risk. Insulin resistance is also shown to increase with age. Smoking has also been found to result in a 78% increased risk of impaired glucose tolerance (IGT) (41,42). Reducing body weight and increasing exercise are key lifestyle factors, particularly given the effects of obesity on hyperglycemia. It is especially important to emphasize these lifestyle changes to restore normal glycemia early in the history of pre-diabetes, since these lifestyle changes alone are less likely to restore normal glycemia later in the natural history of glucose intolerance (44).

10.10 THE DIABETES PREVENTION PROGRAM (DPP)

The DPP showed that overweight participants who had elevated IGT and/or FBG who were randomized to intensive lifestyle interventions experienced 58% decrease in the likelihood of progressing to diabetes (45). This was a much stronger performance than either metformin or placebo. Lifestyle modification included 16 weeks of educational sessions and eight monthly sessions, all focusing on reducing body weight by 7% and increasing physical activity to greater than or equal to 150 minutes per week. Lifestyle modification lowered the risk of diabetes by 58%. Other studies have also shown similar results (46). For all these reasons, it is very important to identify pre-diabetes in adult patients who are already overweight or obese. A fasting blood sugar should be obtained in all patients and followed on a yearly basis to assist in this diagnosis, so that lifestyle medicine modalities can be implemented at the earliest possible time.

- *Components of Effective Lifestyle Intervention and Pre-Diabetes*: Weight loss programs have been routinely shown to improve glucose regulation and help re-establish normal glycemia. In addition to the DPP, the Finnish Diet Diabetes Prevention Study (FDDPS) showed that weight loss of 7% improved insulin sensitivity and beta-cell function (46). The most successful lifestyle modification programs implement multiple strategies promoting weight loss, improving diet, and increasing physical activity (47,48). All of these are critically important for physicians to advocate for individuals who have pre-diabetes.
- *Pre-Diabetes and the Metabolic Syndrome*: A significant overlap exists between pre-diabetes, diabetes, and the MetS. MetS involves multiple components of disordered metabolism

(49,50). Various criteria have been promulgated by different organizations concerning what constitutes MetS. The most commonly used criteria are contained in the National Cholesterol Education Program III (NCEP III), which include the following:

- Blood pressure > 140/85 mm Hg
- Fasting blood glucose > 100 mg/dL
- Triglycerides > 150 mg/dL
- Waist circumference in men >40 inches and in women >35 inches
- HDL < 40 mg/dL

Utilizing these criteria, between 36% and 38% of individuals in the United States have MetS (49). There is significant overlap between metabolic syndrome, diabetes, and pre-diabetes. The AHA recommends that individuals with MetS should be treated with lifestyle measures similar to those used to reduce the risk of CVD, specifically, physical activity, weight loss (if necessary), and control of lipids and high blood pressure (50).

10.11 HEART FAILURE IN PATIENTS WITH DIABETES

T2DM is associated with a significant heart failure risk. T2DM is associated with a two- to five-fold increase in individuals for heart failure (22). Pharmacologic treatment for heart failure in patients with T2DM focuses largely on ACE inhibitors (7). Blood pressure and blood glucose control are also critically important in the treatment of heart failure in patients with T2DM. Lifestyle measures, including weight loss (if necessary), decreased sodium in the diet, and regular physical activity as tolerated, also play important roles in the treatment of heart failure in individuals who have T2DM.

10.12 SECONDARY PREVENTION

Individuals who have already established CVD should be managed with secondary prevention measures similar to those for patients without T2DM. Some studies have suggested that individuals with diabetes who require coronary revascularization may do better with angioplasty or coronary artery bypass grafting. This debate is not yet resolved.

10.13 DYSGLYCEMIA

Doctors Jeffrey Mechanic and Michael Via from Mount Sinai Hospital have proposed a novel framework for approaching individuals who typically have been diagnosed as either having pre-diabetes, T2DM, or metabolic syndrome (51,52). They argue that abnormalities in glucose management encompass the major pathophysiologic events that yield all of these conditions. They argue that by utilizing a different framework that focuses on dysglycemia, individuals can be treated earlier and complications diminished. Their model basically involves four stages. They are as follows:

Stage 1: Insulin Resistance – Insulin resistance is extremely common. In fact, in the United States, it is estimated that 74.5% of individuals have insulin resistance. The formal diagnosis of insulin resistance is made by obtaining insulin levels. Insulin resistance, however, is so prominent and unhealthy lifestyles and normal adiposity are so common that these investigators argue that it is reasonable to approach individuals who are overweight or obese or are very inactive as though they already have insulin resistance. This allows treatment at the earliest stages and can avoid individuals progressing on to pre-diabetes, diabetes, or complications from diabetes.

In their framework, *Stage 2 is pre-diabetes.* Criteria for this, as already discussed, are impaired fasting glucose with glucose levels between 100 and 125 mg/dL. As already indicated, pre-diabetes occurs in 28–35% of individuals in the US and 30–45% of individuals worldwide.

In their framework, *Stage 3 represents T2DM,* which should be subject to all of the lifestyle and other treatments already discussed in this chapter.

Stage 4 involves type 2 diabetes with vascular complications. This condition involves 6.0% of individuals in the United States and 1–2% of individuals worldwide (25).

The benefit of utilizing this novel framework is that it emphasizes many lifestyle targets to be performed at the very earliest stages before any significant sequelae, even at the level of pre-diabetes, occur. This approach is very similar to that adopted by the American Heart Association when it recommends focusing on "primordial" factors in heart health, namely identifying and treating issues before they even turn into risk factors (53,54).

10.14 PREVENTING AND MANAGING DIABETES IN THE REAL WORLD

The research studies already discussed in this chapter are labor-intensive and may be difficult to achieve outside of a research environment. Nonetheless, T2DM prevention programs may be launched utilizing a variety of delivery formats, including individual and group sessions (47,48). They also may be administered by health care professionals or community members in diverse settings such as clinics, churches, or fitness centers. In all of these settings, individuals with pre-diabetes are likely to receive benefits.

10.15 CONCLUSIONS/CLINICAL APPLICATIONS

Pre-diabetes, T2DM, and MetS are interrelated. As outlined in this chapter, lifestyle medicine modalities are critically important for all of these conditions. Thus, it is particularly important for clinicians to have an understanding of how various lifestyle medicine modalities such as increased physical activity, healthy nutrition, weight management or weight loss (if necessary), avoidance of cigarette smoking, stress reduction, and positive relations with others all play very important roles in both lowering the risk of pre-diabetes turning into T2DM or assisting in the management of these conditions. It has also been argued that the initial inciting event in these conditions is insulin resistance. Thus, adopting positive lifestyle measures for all individuals, but particularly those who are overweight or obese, can significantly reduce the burden of pre-diabetes, diabetes, and metabolic syndrome.

REFERENCES

1. Centers for Disease Control and Prevention. https://www.cdc.gov/. Accessed March 26, 2025.
2. Centers for Disease Control and Prevention. National Diabetes Statistics Report, 2017. Centers for Disease Control and Prevention. Atlanta, GA: US Department of Health and Human Services, 2017.
3. Gregg EW, Williams DE, Geiss L. Changes in diabetes-related complications in the United States. *N Engl J Med.* 2014;371(3):286–287.
4. Diabetes Prevention Program Research Group; Knowler WC, Fowler SE, et al. 10-year follow-up of diabetes incidence and weight loss in the Diabetes Prevention Program Outcomes Study. *Lancet.* 2009;374(9702):1677–1686.
5. Franz MJ, MacLeod J, Evert A, et al. Academy of nutrition and dietetics nutrition practice guideline for type 1 and type 2 diabetes in adults: systematic review of evidence for medical nutrition therapy effectiveness and recommendations for integration into the nutrition care process. *J Acad Nutr Diet.* 2017;117(10):1659–1679.
6. Holman RR, Paul SK, Bethel MA, et al. 10-year follow-up of intensive glucose control in type 2 diabetes. *N Engl J Med.* 2008;359(15):1577–1589. Epub 2008 Sep 12.
7. American Diabetes Association. Standards of medical care in diabetes 2017. *Diabetes Care.* 2017;40 (Suppl 1):S1–S127.
8. Handelsman Y, Bloomgarden ZT, Grunberger G, et al. American association of clinical endocrinologists and American College of Endocrinology – clinical practice guidelines for developing a diabetes mellitus comprehensive care plan – 2015. *Endocr Pract.* 2015;21(Suppl 1):1–87.
9. Diabetes Control and Complications Trial (DCCT)/Epidemiology of Diabetes Interventions and Complications (EDIC) Study Research Group. Mortality in type 1 diabetes in the DCCT/EDIC versus the general population. *Diabetes Care.* 2016;39:1378–1383.

10. Chamberlain JJ, Kalyani RR, Leal S, et al. Treatment of type 1 diabetes: synopsis of the 2017 American Diabetes Association standards of medical care in diabetes. *Ann Intern Med.* 2017;167(7):493–498.
11. Physical Activity Guidelines Advisory Committee 2018 Physical Activity Guidelines Advisory Committee. 2018 Physical Activity Guidelines Advisory Committee Scientific Report. Washington, DC: US Department of Health and Human Services, 2018.
12. Keshel TE, Coker RH. Exercise training and insulin resistance: a current review. *J Obes Weight Loss Ther.* 2015;5(Suppl 5):S5-003.
13. Phelan SM, Burgess DJ, Yeazel MW, et al. Impact of weight bias and stigma on quality of care and outcomes for patients with obesity. *Obes Rev.* 2015;16(4):319–326.
14. Ochner CN, Tsai AG, Kushner RF, et al. Treating obesity seriously: when recommendations for lifestyle change confront biological adaptations. *Lancet Diabetes Endocrinol.* 2015;3(4):232–234.
15. Inzucchi SE, Bergenstal RM, Buse JB, et al. Management of hyperglycemia in type 2 diabetes, 2015: a patient-centered approach: update to a position statement of the American Diabetes Association and the European Association for the Study of Diabetes. *Diabetes Care.* 2015;8(1):140–149.
16. Garber AJ, Abrahamson MJ, Barzilay JI, et al. Consensus statement by the American Association of Clinical Endocrinologists and American College of Endocrinology on the comprehensive type 2 diabetes management algorithm – 2020 executive summary. *Endocr Pract.* 2020;26(1):107–139.
17. Colberg SR, Sigal RJ, Yardley JE, et al. Physical activity/exercise and diabetes: a position statement of the American Diabetes Association. *Diabetes Care.* 2016;39(11):2065–2079.
18. ACSM Physical Activity Guidelines. https://acsm.org/education-resources/trending-topics-resources/physical-activity-guidelines/. Accessed March 26, 2025.
19. Estruch R, Ros E, Salas-Salvado J, et al. Primary prevention of cardiovascular disease with a Mediterranean diet. *N Engl J Med.* 2013;368(14):1279–1290.
20. Sacks FM, Svetkey LP, Vollmer WM, et al. Effects on blood pressure of reduced dietary sodium and the Dietary Approaches to Stop Hypertension (DASH) diet. DASH-sodium collaborative research group. *N Engl J Med.* 2001;344(1):3–10.
21. Bassuk SS, Manson JE. Lifestyle and risk of cardiovascular disease and type 2 diabetes in women: a review of the epidemiologic evidence. *Am J Lifestyle Med.* 2008;2(3):191–213.
22. Nanayakkara N, Ranasinha S, Gadowski A, et al. Age, age at diagnosis and diabetes duration are all associated with vascular complications in type 2 diabetes. *J Diabetes Complic.* 2018;32(3):279–290.
23. Malick W, Mechanick J. Context: impact of dysglycemia and lifestyle medicine on cardiometabolic-based chronic disease. In Rippe JM (ed.) *Lifestyle Medicine* (4th ed). Boca Raton, FL: CRC Press, 2024.
24. Srinath R. Rosa T, Shah L, et al. Management: lifestyle medicine approaches to insulin resistance, prediabetes, type 2 diabetes, and diabetes complications. In Rippe JM (ed.) *Lifestyle Medicine* (4th ed). Boca Raton, FL: CRC Press, 2024.
25. Dal Canto E, Ceriello A, Rydén L, et al. Diabetes as a cardiovascular risk factor: an overview of global trends of macro and micro vascular complications. *Eur J Prev Cardiol.* 2019;26(2_suppl):25–32.
26. Wu H, Ballantyne CM. Metabolic inflammation and insulin resistance in obesity. *Circ Res.* 2020;126(11):1549–1564.
27. Katsiki N. Mikhailidis D, Banach M. Cardiovascular diseases and type 2 diabetes mellitus. *Acta Pharmacol Sin.* 2018;39(7):1176–1188.
28. Keith SW, Redden DT, Katzmarzyk PT, et al. Putative contributors to the secular increase in obesity: exploring the roads less traveled. *Int J Obes.* 2006;30(11):1585–1594.
29. Simon SL, Field J, Miller LE, et al. Sweet/dessert foods are more appealing to adolescents after sleep restriction. *PLoS One.* 2015;10(2):e0115434.
30. Matricciani L, Olds T, Petkov J. In search of lost sleep: secular trends in the sleep time of school-aged children and adolescents. *Sleep Med Rev.* 2012;16(3):203–11.
31. Saper CB, Scammell TE, Lu J. Hypothalamic regulation of sleep and circadian rhythms. *Nature.* 2005;437(7063):1257–1263.
32. Stenvers DJ, Scheer F, Schrauwen P, et al. Circadian clocks and insulin resistance. *Nat Rev Endocrinol.* 2019;15(2):75–89.
33. Albreiki MS, Middleton B, Hampton SM. A single night light exposure acutely alters hormonal and metabolic responses in healthy participants. *Endocr Connect.* 2017;6(2):100–110.
34. Sharma VK, Singh TG. Chronic stress and diabetes mellitus: interwoven pathologies. *Curr Diabetes Rev.* 2020;16(6):546–556.
35. Osborne MT, Shin LM, Mehta NN, et al. Disentangling the links between psychosocial stress and cardiovascular disease. *Circ Cardiovasc Imaging.* 2020;13(8):e010931.

36. Brien SE, Ronksley PE, Turner BJ, et al. Effect of alcohol consumption on biological markers associated with risk of coronary heart disease: systematic review and meta-analysis of interventional studies. *BMJ.* 2011;342:d636.
37. Suliga E, Koziel D, Ciesla E, et al. Consumption of alcoholic beverages and the prevalence of metabolic syndrome and its components. *Nutrients.* 2019;11(11):2764.
38. Nadal A, Quesada I, Tuduri E, et al. Endocrine-disrupting chemicals and the regulation of energy balance. *Nat Rev Endocrinol.* 2017;13(9):536–546.
39. Vafeiadi M, Roumeliotaki T, Myridakis A, et al. Association of early life exposure to bisphenol A with obesity and cardiometabolic traits in childhood. *Environ Res.* 2016;146:379–387.
40. Heindel JJ, Blumberg B, Cave M, et al. Metabolism disrupting chemicals and metabolic disorders. *Reprod Toxicol.* 2017;68:3–33.
41. World Health Organization. About Diabetes. Intermediate States of Hyperglycemia. https://www.who.int/news-room/fact-sheets/detail/diabetes. Accessed March 26, 2025.
42. Nathan D, Davidson M, DeFronzo R, et al. American Diabetes Association. Impaired fasting glucose and impaired glucose tolerance: implications for care. *Diabetes Care.* 2007;30(3):753–759.
43. Garber A, Abrahamson M, Barzilay J, et al. Consensus statement by the American Association of Clinical Endocrinologists and American College of Endocrinology on the comprehensive type 2 diabetes management algorithm – 2017 executive summary. *Endocrine Practice.* 2017;23(2):207–238.
44. Berger S, Huggins G, McCaffery J, et al. Comparison among criteria to define successful weight-loss maintainers and regainers in the action for health in diabetes (Look AHEAD) and diabetes prevention program trials. *Am J Clin Nutr.* 2017;106:1337–1346.
45. Diabetes Prevention Program (DPP). National Institute of Diabetes, Digestive and Kidney Diseases. https://www.niddk.nih.gov/about-niddk/research-areas/diabetes/diabetes-prevention-program-dpp. Accessed March 26, 2025.
46. Lindström J, Louheranta A, Mannelin M, et al., The Finnish Diabetes Prevention Study (DPS). Lifestyle intervention and 3-year results on diet and physical activity. *Diabetes Care.* 2003;26:3230–3236.
47. Flay B. Efficacy and effectiveness trials (and other phases of research) in the development of health promotion programs. *Prev Med.* 1986;15(5):451–474.
48. Ackermann R, Finch E, Brizendine E, et al. Translating the diabetes prevention program into the community: the DEPLOY pilot study. *Am J Prev Med.* 2008;35(4):357–363.
49. Dietz WH, Robinson TN. Clinical practice. Overweight children and adolescents. *N Engl J Med.* 2005;352(20):2100–2109.
50. Rezaianzadeh A, Namayandeh SM, Sadr SM. National cholesterol education program adult treatment panel III versus international diabetic federation definition of metabolic syndrome, which one is associated with diabetes mellitus and coronary artery disease? *Int J Prev Med.* 2012:3(8):552–558.
51. Via M, Mechanic J. Lifestyle medicine and diabetes, pre-diabetes and the metabolic syndrome. In Rippe JM (ed.) *Lifestyle Medicine* (4th ed). Boca Raton, FL: CRC Press, 2024.
52. Via M, Mechanick J. Overview: dysglycemia-based chronic disease – exposing lifestyle medicine targets. In Rippe JM (ed.) *Lifestyle Medicine* (4th ed). Boca Raton, FL: CRC Press, 2024.
53. Lloyd-Jones DM, Hong Y, Labarthe D, et al. Defining and setting national goals for cardiovascular health promotion and disease reduction: the American Heart Association's strategic impact goal through 2020 and beyond. *Circulation.* 2010;121(4):586–613.
54. Lloyd-Jones DM, Allen NB, Anderson CAM, et al. American Heart Association. Life's essential 8: updating and enhancing the American Heart Association's construct of cardiovascular health: a presidential advisory from the American Heart Association. *Circulation.* 2022;146(5):e18–e43.

11 Cancer

11.1 INTRODUCTION

Cancer is the second leading cause of mortality worldwide (1). There were 19.3 million new diagnoses of cancer and approximately 10 million deaths from cancer in 2020 in the United States. By the year 2040, this is expected to rise to 28.4 million diagnoses of cancer. It is anticipated that cancer will become the leading cause of death by 2060 (2). Cancers of the liver, lung, and colorectal area are the most common causes of cancer death.

There are multiple ways that lifestyle medicine modalities can interact with cancer. Regular physical activity, healthy nutrition, weight management, avoidance of addictive substances such as tobacco, and excessive consumption of alcohol all potentially contribute in significant ways to reducing the cancer burden (3,4). There are also a variety of environmental exposures that represent a significant area where lifestyle medicine can have an impact.

11.2 THE GLOBAL BURDEN OF CANCER

Cancer is a disease of aging. As shown in Figure 11.1, the prevalence of cancer starts to significantly increase after the age of 50 and peaks after the age of 80 (5). While this book and the embedded curriculum are largely focused on adults, it is important to remember that cancer is a leading cause of death in children, adolescents, and young adults. Each year, approximately 10,500 children receive a diagnosis of cancer, while 77,000 adolescent and young adult patients are newly diagnosed each year (6) in the United States. The good news is that survival rates for cancer in children have significantly improved in the past 20 years. Today, almost 85% of children, adolescents, and young adults are living at least five years following a diagnosis of cancer (7).

For all of these reasons, it is essential that primary care physicians and those focusing on lifestyle medicine have a comprehensive understanding of how lifestyle measures can impact both the likelihood of developing cancer and also assist in its treatment.

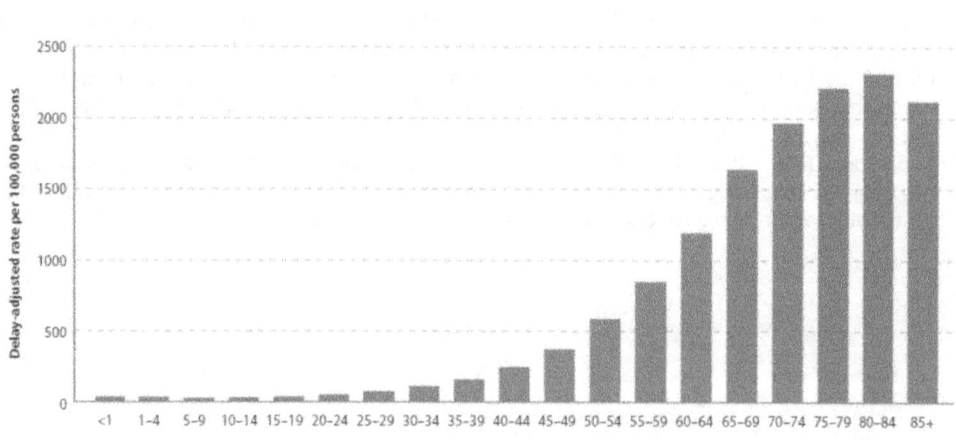

Incidence rates by age at diagnosis, all cancer types. (From National Cancer Institute 2021. *Age and Cancer Risk*. Reproduced by permission of NCI.)

FIGURE 11.1 The likelihood of being diagnosed with cancer increases with age

DOI: 10.1201/9781003630043-11

11.3 PHYSICAL ACTIVITY AND CANCER PREVENTION

Physical activity plays an important role in the regulation of multiple physiologic systems (8,9). Abundant evidence exists for the multiple health benefits of regular physical activity, which has been accumulated in the Physical Activity Guidelines for Americans 2018 (PAGA 2018), discussing the role of physical activity in reducing the risk of various chronic diseases, including cancer (10). As indicated in multiple chapters in this book, the PAGA 2018 Scientific Report recommends that people should engage in at least 150 minutes of moderate-intensity physical activity and two days of muscular strength training on a weekly basis. This includes individuals who are over the age of 65. These individuals also have the recommendation to add activities to improve their balance. The PAGA 2018 report also concludes that inactivity is a major health problem and should be avoided (10).

Most patients with cancer who do not engage in regular physical activity expose themselves to a higher risk of a variety of chronic diseases, including cancer, as well as other causes of premature death. For this reason, the American Cancer Society (ACS) has issued guidelines for both nutrition and physical activity in cancer prevention (11). In addition, the American College of Sports Medicine (ACSM) has endorsed the updated consensus statement and guidelines for exercise for adult patients with cancer (11). For all of these reasons, clinicians should counsel patients and support physical activity as a key strategy across the cancer prevention continuum, regardless of the age of their patients.

11.4 PHYSICAL ACTIVITY IN PRIMARY PREVENTION

Primary prevention is, of course, preventing a chronic disease such as cancer before it occurs. Healthy lifestyle behaviors in this area are essential to lower risk factors for multiple chronic diseases. The World Health Organization (WHO) has reported that 30%–50% of cancers can be prevented by avoiding risk factors and also by engaging in regular physical activity (12). Of course, a variety of other lifestyle-related behaviors, such as tobacco use, poor diet, physical inactivity, and alcohol consumption, are also important and are estimated to represent the underlying cause of half of all deaths in the United States, including increased risk of death from cancer (13,14).

The relationship between regular physical activity and lower risk of cancer has been established in a number of studies (15,16). In one study, women who engaged in athletic training had a lower risk of breast cancer and cancers of the uterus, ovaries, cervix, and vagina compared to non-athletic counterparts (17). A systematic review and meta-analysis showed that running was associated with a reduction of 23% in cancer mortality (18). Researchers from the American Cancer Society and the American Cancer Institute pooled data from 12 US and European cohort studies which included 1,440,000 adults, and showed that leisure time physical activity was associated with a lower risk of developing 13 cancers including esophageal, liver, lung, kidney, gastric, cardiac, endometrial, leukemia, myeloma, colon, head and neck, rectal, bladder, and breast cancers (19).

Emerging data suggest that physical activity may exert all of these positive effects by enhancing patients' anti-inflammatory and immune functions (20). In addition, physical activity has the potential to reduce the amount of adipose tissue and the production of sex hormones, insulin, leptin, and inflammatory markers (21,22).

Physical activity interacts with patients' age, gender, and body composition. It may also impact a variety of underlying mechanisms (23). The mechanisms by which physical activity exerts its positive benefits are still not completely understood and are an area of significant ongoing research.

- *Physical Activity and Secondary Prevention*: Physical activity in secondary prevention is designed to reduce the impact of cancer on patients' health, psychosocial, and physical function. Cancer can adversely impact many areas of individuals' lives. Patients with cancer may experience more anxiety, pain, depressive symptoms, fatigue, and physical function impairment compared to individuals who do not have cancer (24,25).

Strong evidence exists in favor of regular physical activity in patients with cancer to improve reported outcomes, including diminishing fatigue and anxiety, reducing depressive symptoms, and improving quality of life and physical function.

These symptoms may vary depending on the type of cancer. One meta-analysis showed that regular physical activity is more effective in reducing cancer-related fatigue than available pharmaceutical options (26,27). One major longitudinal study of 4,643 women diagnosed with invasive breast cancer showed that women who engaged in regular physical activity before their diagnosis had lower all-cause mortality than non-exercisers (28). Multiple potential mechanisms exist for why physical activity may be valuable in secondary prevention. This is an area of significant ongoing research.

- *Physical Activity in Tertiary Prevention*: Physical activity is also very helpful in managing the long-term impact of the complex conditions that are often related to cancer. Physical activity can help prevent long-term problems not only in cancer recovery but also in improving physical function. Pooled data from the National Cancer Institute consortium of six prospective cohort studies involving a total of 654,827 adults showed that leisure-time physical activity was associated with a longer life expectancy of up to four to five years (29).

  In patients with colorectal cancer, individuals who participated in regular lifestyle medicine activities such as regular physical activity, avoiding tobacco use, lowering alcohol consumption, and maintaining an ideal body weight, as well as healthy nutrition, have been shown to reduce cancer-specific and overall mortality by up to 40% (30). These factors also improve health-related quality of life. Physical activity in multiple cancers, including breast cancer and colon cancer, has been shown to significantly reduce the rate of recurrence. Multiple hypotheses exist about why physical activity in tertiary prevention is so effective. This is an area of ongoing research. For all these reasons, it is important for physicians to continue to emphasize to patients how valuable regular physical activity is, even in tertiary prevention.
- *Physical Activity Guidelines and Practice Before and After the Diagnosis of Cancer*: During the pre-treatment timeframe, once the diagnosis of cancer has been made, regular physical activity can lower anxiety while increasing or maintaining muscle mass and physical function (31). Once active treatment has begun, physical activity can help with coping with or reducing symptoms and also help maintain healthy body composition and physical function.
- *Physical Activity Guidelines and Practice During and After Cancer Treatment*: A number of organizations have reviewed the evidence and concluded that regular exercise can be recommended during cancer treatment. This includes the National Comprehensive Cancer Network (32), the American Cancer Society, the Clinical Oncology Society of Australia (33), the American College of Sports Medicine (34), and the American College of Clinical Oncology (35). These organizations have agreed that regular physical activity reduces anxiety, depression, and fatigue, and improves health-related quality of life, including sleep and physical function. Recommendations from these organizations include that patients should be advised to perform moderate-intensity aerobic exercise for 30 minutes three times per week, as well as two times weekly progressive resistance training. The ACSM has also offered guidelines that are even more specific than these.

  A summary of this evidence is found in Figure 11.2.
- *The Role of Physicians in Recommending Physical Activity*: One difficulty in making physical activity standard for cancer patients at all stages involves convincing physicians to focus on exercise recommendations during and after cancer treatment. In fact, only 14.7% of patients receive discussions of exercise from their oncology care team (36). A validated triage tool is available that can be included in the process to ease this challenge. It is called

Effects of Exercise on Health-Related Outcomes in Those with Cancer

What can exercise do?

- **Prevention of 7 common cancers***
  Dose: 2018 Physical Activity Guidelines for Americans: 150-300 min/week moderate or 75-150 min/week vigorous aerobic exercise
- **Survival of 3 common cancers****
  Dose: Exact dose of physical activity needed to reduce cancer-specific or all-cause mortality is not yet known; Overall more activity appears to lead to better risk reduction

*bladder, breast, colon, endometrial, esophageal, kidney and stomach cancers
**breast, colon and prostate cancers

Overall, avoid inactivity, and to improve general health, aim to achieve the current physical activity guidelines for health (150 min/week aerobic exercise and 2x/week strength training).

Outcome	Aerobic Only	Resistance Only	Combination (Aerobic + Resistance)
Strong Evidence	Dose	Dose	Dose
Cancer-related fatigue	**3x**/week for **30** min per session of moderate intensity	**2x**/week of **2** sets of **12-15** reps for major muscle groups at moderate intensity	**3x**/week for **30** min per session of moderate aerobic exercise, plus **2x**/week of resistance training **2** sets of **12-15** reps for major muscle groups at moderate intensity
Health-related quality of life	**2-3x**/week for **30-60** min per session of moderate to vigorous	**2x**/week of **2** sets of **8-15** reps for major muscle groups at a moderate to vigorous intensity	**2-3x**/week for **20-30** min per session of moderate aerobic exercise plus **2x**/week of resistance training **2** sets of **8-15** reps for major muscle groups at moderate to vigorous intensity
Physical Function	**3x**/week for **30-60** min per session of moderate to vigorous	**2-3x**/week of **2** sets of **8-12** reps for major muscle groups at moderate to vigorous intensity	**3x**/week for **20-40** min per session of moderate to vigorous aerobic exercise, plus **2-3x**/week of resistance training **2** sets of **8-12** reps for major muscle group at moderate to vigorous intensity
Anxiety	**3x**/week for **30-60** min per session of moderate to vigorous	Insufficient evidence	**2-3x**/week for **20-40** min of moderate to vigorous aerobic exercise plus **2x**/week of resistance training of **2** sets, **8-12** reps for major muscle groups at moderate to vigorous intensity
Depression	**3x**/week for **30-60** min per session of moderate to vigorous	Insufficient evidence	**2-3x**/week for **20-40** min of moderate to vigorous aerobic exercise plus **2x**/week of resistance training of **2** sets, **8-12** reps for major muscle groups at moderate to vigorous intensity
Lymphedema	Insufficient evidence	**2-3x**/week of progressive, supervised, program for major muscle groups does not exacerbate lymphedema	Insufficient evidence
Moderate Evidence			
Bone health	Insufficient evidence	**2-3x**/week of moderate to vigorous resistance training plus high impact training (sufficient to generate ground reaction force of **3-4** time body weight) for at least **12** months	Insufficient evidence
Sleep	**3-4x**/week for **30-40** min per session of moderate intensity	Insufficient evidence	Insufficient evidence

Citation: bit.ly/cancer_exercise_guidelines

Moderate intensity (40%-59% heart rate reserve or VO_2R) to vigorous intensity (60%-89% heart rate reserve or VO_2R) is recommended

Exercise is Medicine | AMERICAN COLLEGE of SPORTS MEDICINE

FIGURE 11.2 Physical activity and cancer

EXCEEDS-S (37). This tool is found in Figure 11.3. It is hoped that this validated instrument may further encourage physicians to recognize the value of regular physical activity in all stages of cancer diagnosis and treatment.

Another source of useful information on physical activity and cancer comes from the program developed by the ACSM entitled Exercise is Medicine. This program provides tools for many chronic conditions concerning how physical activity can be very valuable.

- *Barriers to Physical Activity*: In adult cancer survivors, the most common barriers to physical activity are getting motivated, a lack of self-discipline, health issues, and adverse effects from treatment such as fatigue or pain (37,38). Fatigue is extremely common in cancer patients undergoing treatment and also in cancer survivors. Regular physical activity has been demonstrated to yield the benefit of reducing cancer-related fatigue.

  Another barrier is cancer-related pain, which is also extremely common (39,40). Physical activity, in addition to pain medicine, has been demonstrated to reduce patients' pain. Potential barriers need to be recognized and addressed by all physicians.
- *Health Equity and Physical Activity*: Health equity represents an issue related to levels of physical activity in all populations in the United States. It is not surprising that these issues also exist in patients with cancer (41–43). Physicians need to be attuned to health equity issues in all patients they see. Regular physical activity is shown to be an excellent predictor of cardiac health in patients with cancer. Therefore, efforts are important to make physical activity equally accessible to all patients regardless of their socioeconomic status, gender, or sexual orientation (43).

The Exercise in Cancer Evaluation and Decision Support - Survivor (EXCEEDS-S) Tool

Directions: Answer "yes" or "no" to the questions below. When you answer "yes", review the corresponding recommendation. Use the ACSM Exercise is Medicine, Moving Through Cancer registry[2] to locate a program near you.

Note: Always discuss with your doctor before starting a new exercise program.

Question	Answer	Recommendation
1. Do any of the following limit your ability to complete daily activities including work, hobbies, home care, socializing, and caring for yourself or loved ones? ☐ Difficulty with any of the following activities: • getting in or out of a vehicle, or using public transportation • walking one block without using a mobility aid like a cane or a walker • moving or reaching with your arms ☐ Difficulty being without a caregiver or another person who can assist you with activities ☐ New or worsening of any of the following conditions: • muscle weaknesses or coordination • difficulty with eating or drinking • difficulty with memory, multitasking, or thinking • numbness or loss of sensation in feet or hands • dizziness or blurred vision, or feeling lightheaded or disoriented ☐ Moderate to high pain that you rate as 7 out of 10 (0 = no pain, 10 = highest pain) ☐ Moderate to high fatigue that you rate as 7 out of 10 (0 = no fatigue, 10 = highest fatigue)	Yes No	**Outpatient cancer rehabilitation**
Continue to the next section if you answered "no" above or if there are no recommended programs in your area		
2. Have you fallen in the past 6 months?	Yes No	**Clinically supervised exercise program**
3. In the past 3 months, have you had any of the following cancer treatments? ☐ Surgery ☐ Stem cell transplant ☐ Chemotherapy ☐ Targeted therapy or immunotherapy ☐ Radiation therapy or brachytherapy	Yes No	
4. In the past week, have you experienced any of the following conditions? ☐ Mild daily fatigue that you rate as 3 to 6 out of 10 (0 = no fatigue, 10 = highest fatigue) ☐ Tingling sensation or loss of feeling in your feet or hands ☐ Difficulty with memory, multitasking, or thinking ☐ Dizziness after you stand up from either sitting in a chair or from lying down ☐ Nausea or frequent vomiting/diarrhea that interferes with daily activities ☐ Frequent feelings of dehydration ☐ Loss or gain of more than 5% body weight ☐ Lack of voluntary control over urination or defecation (incontinence) ☐ Persistent heaviness or swelling in your arm(s), leg(s), or trunk (lymphedema) ☐ Immunosuppression due to anemia, neutropenia, or thrombocytopenia	Yes No	
Continue to the next section if you answered "no" above or if there are no recommended programs in your area		
5. Do you currently have or are you planning to receive a catheter? *Including but not limited to: peripherally Inserted Central Cather (PICC), port, intraperitoneal catheter, or ostomy*	Yes No	**Cancer-specific community-based exercise program**
6. Confidence for independent exercise *Would you describe yourself as "highly confident" that you will exercise at moderate or vigorous intensity for 30 minutes, at least 3 times a week, for the next 12 weeks without receiving support from an exercise professional?*	Yes No	
Continue to the next section if you answered "no" above or if there are no recommended programs in your area		
Independent exercise *Try to do at least 150 minutes of moderate-intensity physical activity every week* *Examples: brisk walk, water aerobics, casual biking, doubles tennis*		

[1] https://www.exerciseismedicine.org/eim-in-action/moving-through-cancer/exercise-program-registry/

Version 1.2022 | ©Kelley C. Wood PhD, ACSM-CEP, CET

Validated triage tool "The Exercise in Cancer Evaluation and Decision Support - Survivor (EXCEEDS-S) Tool." (From Covington, K. R., Marshall, T., Campbell, G., Williams, G. R., Fu, J. B., Kendig, T. D., ... & Pergolotti, M. (2021). Development of the exercise in cancer evaluation and decision support (EXCEEDS) algorithm. *Supportive Care in Cancer*, 29(11), 6469–6480. Reproduced by permission of Springer Nature.)

FIGURE 11.3 Evaluating Exercise in Cancer

11.5 NUTRITION IN CANCER PREVENTION

Environmental and lifestyle factors account for up to 90% of the lifetime risk of developing cancer (3). This high level of non-hereditary influence on risk indicates that primary risk factors associated with carcinogenesis are important and potentially modifiable. Nutrition is certainly one of these modifiable lifestyle factors. In 1981, Doll and Peto published a seminal article entitled "The Causes of Cancer," which focused on modifiable environmental lifestyle factors (4). They estimated that at least 35% of cancer burden (10%–70%) was attributable to dietary factors. They also highlighted dietary factors that were hypothesized to be protective against cancer, as well as multiple dietary factors, including excessive caloric consumption and alcohol, that increased risk.

The National Academy of Sciences (NAS) published the first major institutional report on diet, nutrition, and cancer in 1982 (44). This report provided evidence-based dietary guidelines for the prevention of cancer and included the recommendation to decrease dietary fat intake, increase plant-based foods, and not consume nutrients through supplements. These recommendations are consistent with modern nutritional science, which concludes that focus should be maintained on dietary patterns rather than individual foods or nutrients.

Multiple national and international tools for exploring dietary recommendations and making guidelines for cancer prevention are now available. Perhaps the most important are the Dietary Guidelines for Americans (DGAs) 2020–2025, which outline multiple factors related to nutrition and cancer risk (45). The Healthy Eating Index (HEI 2015) is also very useful in this area (46). Important information on nutrition and cancer prevention was established by the World Cancer Research Fund International (WCRF) and the American Institute for Cancer Research (AICR). The WCRF/AICR issued cancer prevention recommendations, including increased consumption of plant-based foods and limits on alcohol consumption. The recommendations are found graphically in Figure 11.4.

- *Supplements*: The 2018 WCRF/AICR cancer prevention guidelines specifically recommended that patients not use supplements for cancer prevention (47,48). This is consistent with the messaging recommended by the National Academy of Sciences in 1982. In the United States, supplement use is common. According to NHANES data, over 57% of adults and 80% of women aged 60 and over use dietary supplements (49). Most often these are multivitamins/mineral supplements, as well as vitamin D and omega-3 fatty acid supplements.

  There has been considerable interest in antioxidant supplements, including beta-carotene, vitamin E, vitamin C, and vitamin A. Data from a variety of studies have shown that these supplements, or combinations of these supplements, do not protect against the incidence of the particular cancer being investigated (50). Several of the studies actually reported increased cancer risk with supplementation. Some short-term, randomized controlled trials using vitamin D or calcium supplements have shown mixed results regarding cancer outcomes. The scientific consensus has concluded that the use of whole foods and, in particular, plant-based diets offers the best nutritional advice for lowering the risk of cancer.
- *Plant-based Dietary Patterns*: As recommended throughout multiple chapters in this book, a wide variety of prestigious medical organizations, including the AHA (51), ACS, and the DGAs 2020–2025, all recommend dietary patterns that emphasize plant-based foods. These diets include a variety of fruits and vegetables, whole grains, nuts, legumes, herbs, and spices. They also uniformly recommend that the vitamins, minerals, and polyphenols found in these types of foods are most beneficial when consumed as whole foods, such as whole grains, fruits, and vegetables. These diets also include significant fiber, which further lowers the risk of cancer. In addition, soybeans and other legumes such as beans, nuts, peas, and lentils are major protein sources in plant-based diets and also contribute to lowering the risk of cancer.

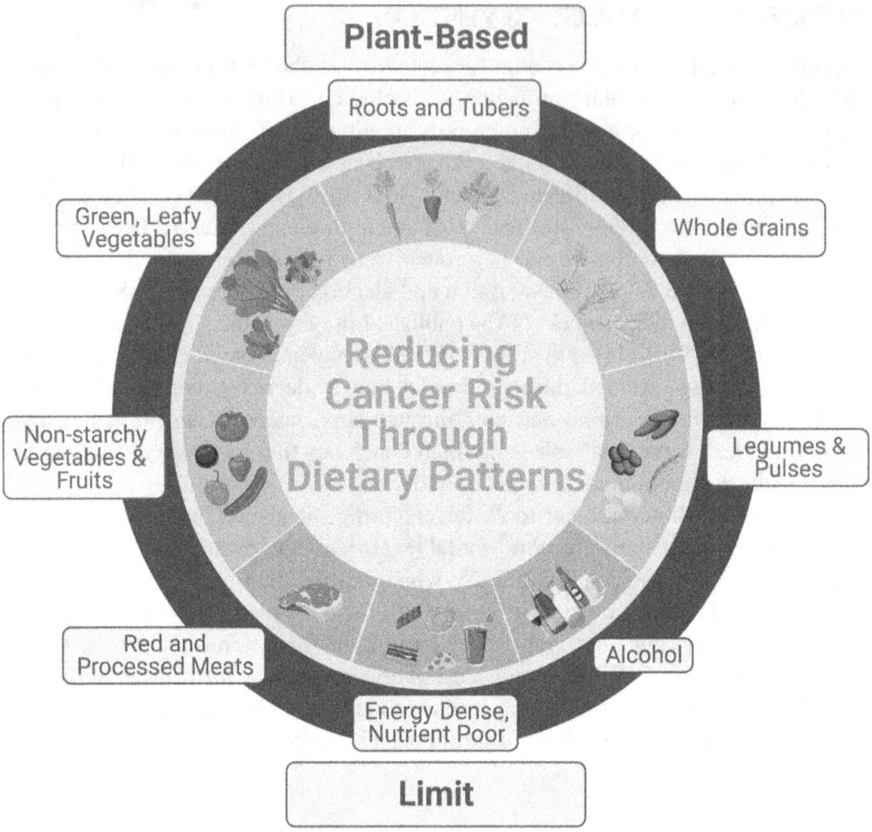

FIGURE 11.4 Dietary patterns and cancer risk

Plant-based diets have been recommended by multiple organizations, including the Continuous Update Project, to lower the risk of cancer (47). Dietary pattern recommendations issued by the WCRF/AICR include the Mediterranean diet (MedDiet) (52), DASH diet (53), the US Healthy Eating Style, and the DGAs 2020–2025 (45). No scientific evidence exists that suggests that one specific plant-based diet over another is more efficacious for lowering cancer risk. Individuals should be encouraged to follow the plant-based dietary pattern that best fits their lifestyle and personal preferences.

- *Energy Balance/Healthy Weight*: Plant-based diets, in addition to providing nutrients, may also assist in the reduction of cancer risk by helping to maintain a healthy body weight. In the 2018 WCRF/AICR Cancer Prevention Recommendations, one of the recommendations was to maintain a healthy body weight (54). The other recommendations include being physically active, eating a plant-based diet, limiting fast foods, limiting bread and processed meat, cutting down on sugary treats, and limiting alcohol consumption. All of these recommendations contribute to influencing energy balance and the healthy weight recommendations.

As already indicated in numerous chapters of this book, obesity contributes to chronic inflammation and insulin resistance (55). This, in turn, leads to increased levels of cytokines and growth hormones, which promote cancer initiation and progression. Obesity and the metabolic syndrome are associated with an increased incidence of at least 13 cancers.

The standard American dietary pattern is typically energy-dense and contains a high percentage of processed foods, bread, and processed meat. This type of dietary pattern is associated with increased body fat and increased risk of cancer, including colorectal cancer and hormone-sensitive postmenopausal breast cancer.

- *Processed Foods*: Food processing represents a double-edged sword. The US Department of Agriculture defines processed food as one that has undergone changes from its natural state (56). This includes multiple different processing techniques such as milling, cutting, pasteurizing, cooking, and canning. By this definition, most foods within the food supply are processed to some degree, and not all foods with some processing are unhealthy.

  A variety of food processing classification systems have been developed. Most do not include nutrient profiling parameters. The European Prospective Investigation into Cancer and Nutrition (EPIC) makes an attempt to rationalize the balance between nutrient benefits and the level of processing (57).

  A category entitled "Ultra Processed Foods" consists of highly processed foods that are processed in a way that nutrient density decreases and energy density increases with the addition of sugars and fats. These foods are ready to eat and consist of foods such as sugar-sweetened beverages, cookies and packaged baked goods, salty snacks, fast food, and frozen dinners. Americans consume more than half of their calories from these ultra-processed foods, which contribute to increased energy consumption (58,59). For this reason, ultra-processed food intake is associated with higher overall cancer risk and breast cancer risk (60).
- *Red and Processed Meat*: In 2015, the AICR classified processed meat as carcinogenic (61). Epidemiologic studies have long supported the association between red and processed meat and colorectal cancer (62,63). The association between red meat and cancer risk is complicated (64). There may be an association between consumption of red meat and colorectal cancer. The WCRF/AICR acknowledges that there are methodological limitations to the epidemiologic studies that have supported this. At the current time, the scientific consensus concludes that more evidence from rigorously designed studies is needed to fully understand the relationship between red meat consumption and cancer risk. It should also be noted that red meat is an excellent source of protein, vitamin B12 (almost exclusively found in animal products), niacin, vitamin B6, zinc, and phosphorus (65). The WCRF/AICR guidelines attempt to weigh the risk versus benefit by recommending limiting intake of red meat to 12–18 ounces (approximately three portions) per week in conjunction with a plant-based diet.
- *Alcohol*: Alcohol is consumed widely around the world. On average, adults worldwide consume one alcoholic drink per day. There is considerable variation among populations. Ethanol increases reactive oxygen species production in cells, and it is metabolized to formaldehyde, which can damage DNA and proteins. There is strong evidence supporting a positive association between alcohol intake and risk of cancer of the larynx, esophagus, liver, colorectum, and postmenopausal breast cancer (66–68). Most cancer-related dietary recommendations endorse limiting or complete avoidance of alcohol. More details about the health risks of overconsumption of alcohol and the diagnosis of alcohol use disorder (AUD) may be found in Chapter 5.
- *Clinical Applications*: A good summary of clinical nutritional recommendations for cancer prevention and control has been issued by the WCRF/AICR in a summary table from their 3rd Annual Expert Report in 2018 (69). These data are found in Table 11.1.
- *Tobacco Use and Addiction*: Tobacco smoking is highly addictive and harmful to every organ in the body. Continued smoking causes a loss of an average of 10 years of life (70). Clinical practice guidelines recommend implementation of the "five As" for every smoker. The five A's are: ask, advise, assess, assist, and arrange (follow-up). A number of analyses have demonstrated the efficacy of numerous pharmacotherapies in the context of behavioral support or counseling. Even brief interventions with smokers remain among the most cost-effective health care interventions.

TABLE 11.1
Recommendations Concerning Nutrition and Cancer Risk

Recommendation	Strategies for Implementation
Use a patient-centered treatment approach	• Use SMART (Specific, Measurable, Achievable, Relevant, and Time-Bound) goals; set personalized goals for each individual • Consider and address socio-economic barriers • Treat emotional or disordered eating behaviors • Consider consultation with or referral to other healthcare providers or agencies that can assist in treating or managing nutrition-related problems
Achieve and maintain a healthy weight throughout the lifecycle	• Consume a nutrient-dense, balanced diet • Participate in physical activity or exercise most days of the week • Follow obesity treatment guidelines considering lifestyle, pharmacological, and surgical treatment options as appropriate (78–80)

Eat a plant-based diet	• Balance meals and snacks according to The New American Plate with at least two-thirds of the plate being vegetables, fruits, whole grains, and beans and one-third or less animal protein
	• Follow a vegan, vegetarian, or Mediterranean dietary pattern
	• Consume 30 g/d of fiber from food sources
	• Eat a variety of:
	  • fruits (e.g., berries, oranges, apples, avocado)
	  • non-starchy vegetables (e.g., broccoli, okra, asparagus, peppers, cabbage)
	  • green, leafy vegetables (e.g., spinach, lettuce, kale)
	  • roots and tubers (e.g., carrots, sweet potatoes, turnips, beets)
	  • whole grains (e.g., brown rice, wheat, oats, barley, and rye)
	  • legumes and pulses (e.g., beans and lentils)

Limit consumption of red and processed meat	• Limit intake of red meat (e.g., beef, pork, lamb) to 12–18 ounces (or three portions) per week • Eat little, if any, processed meat (e.g., bacon, hot dog, sausage, pepperoni, deli meats)
Limit consumption of sugar-sweetened beverages (e.g., soda, sweet tea, juices)	• Enjoy mostly low-calorie beverages such as water, sparkling water, and unsweet tea
Limit or avoid alcohol consumption	• It is best not to drink alcohol
Limit consumption of processed foods high in fat, starches, or sugars	• Limit consumption of "fast foods," many pre- prepared or packaged foods, baked goods, desserts, and candy • Consume fresh, frozen, or no salt added vegetable options • Prepare more meals at home and avoid adding fat, sugar, and salt during and after cooking • When eating out, choose foods lower in fat and sugar • Eat fruit or yogurt as a sweet food option
Do not use supplements for cancer prevention	• Aim to meet nutritional needs through diet alone • Use macro- and micro-nutrient supplementation to correct known deficiencies • Do not mega-dose or use high dose dietary supplements

Source: Data from World Cancer Research Fund International and American Institute for Cancer Research. *Diet, Nutrition, Physical Activity and Cancer: A Global Perspective: A Summary of the Third Expert Report*. London: World Cancer Research Fund International, 2018 and Shams-White, MM et al., Operationlizing the 2008 World Cancer Research Fund/American Institute for cancer prevention recommendations: A standardized scoring system. *Nutrients* 2019; 11(7).

Zunica E, Gilmore A. The importance of nutrition in cancer prevention. From Rippe JM. *Lifestyle Medicine*, 4th ed. CRC Press, Boca Raton, FL, 2018. Used with permission from the editor, James Rippe, M.D.

- *Cigarette Smoking and Health*: Cigarette smoking in the United States has declined precipitously since the 1964 US Surgeon General's Report, when over 50% of males and 30% of females were cigarette smokers (71). By 2020, 14% of men and 11% of women in the United States still smoked cigarettes "every day" or "some days" (72). In addition, 3.7% used electronic cigarettes, 3.5% smoked cigars, and 2.3% used smokeless tobacco products (72).

  Even though cigarette smoking has declined rapidly in the United States, it is still far too high. It is estimated that tobacco smoking causes over 400,000 premature deaths per year in the United States and over six million premature deaths worldwide (73,74). In addition to the number of deaths from cigarette smoking, it is estimated that there are over 20 types of non-fatal serious smoking conditions that cause illness in people who do not die in that year (75). The vast majority of these illnesses are chronic respiratory diseases such as chronic obstructive pulmonary disease (COPD).

  Organ-related diseases in people who continue to smoke create an average loss of ten years of life compared to never smokers. By the age of 70, 42% of smokers have died versus 19% of never smokers. It is estimated that over 90% of smokers are aware that smoking cigarettes causes lung cancer, but fewer individuals know that cigarette smoking also increases cancer risk at nine other sites, including the mouth, esophagus, stomach, pancreas, larynx, cervix, bladder, kidney, and acute leukemia (74). The age-adjusted risk of death from COPD is tenfold higher for smokers than for never smokers. In addition, smokers triple their risk of dying of coronary heart disease (CHD), stroke, and other manifestations of atherosclerosis between the ages of 35 and 64 (74).
- *The Benefits of Smoking Cessation*: The benefits of smoking cessation are very strong. Smokers who quit smoking by age 50 cut their risk of dying in half over the next 15 years compared to those who continue smoking (74). For example, the excess risk of death from CHD is cut in half within one year of stopping smoking. The same level of risk reduction, however, may take 10–15 years for lung cancer (75,76).

  Detailed issues related to counseling and screening for tobacco use and tobacco use disorder may be found in Chapter 5 and will not be repeated here.

  The "Five As" model for approaching cigarette smokers includes the following: "Ask," which mandates screening for the use of tobacco or nicotine products. "Advice," which represents a brief motivational intervention. "Assess," which involves assessing the frequency of use and potential for addiction/dependence. "Assist," which focuses on helping individuals understand ways to quit smoking. The last A is "Arrange," which means following up with the individual to determine whether or not they have been able to cease cigarette smoking (77). These are all discussed in detail in Chapter 20.

11.6 LIFESTYLE APPROACHES TO OBESITY MANAGEMENT FOR CANCER CONTROL

Overweight and obesity promote, accelerate, and worsen the prognosis of multiple malignancies. Overweight and obesity currently account for 14% of all cancer deaths in men and 20% in women (78–82). Obesity control can prevent and/or reduce the incidence of many cancers. In 1962, only 14.3% of the United States adult population was estimated to be obese. Recent data indicate that in the United States, the prevalence of obesity is 42.5% in adults and 19.7% in those under 20, with equal prevalence in both men and women.

The public is well aware of the impact of obesity on CVD, stroke, and diabetes. According to a 2017 report from the AICR, however, only 50% of Americans were aware that obesity stimulates cancer growth (83). The ACS issued a series of landmark reports, as well as a prospective observational study of more than one million US adults, which clearly demonstrated that overweight and obesity are associated with increased cancer incidence and deaths (78–80). As already indicated in Chapter 4, the etiology of the link between overweight and obesity and multiple chronic diseases appears to

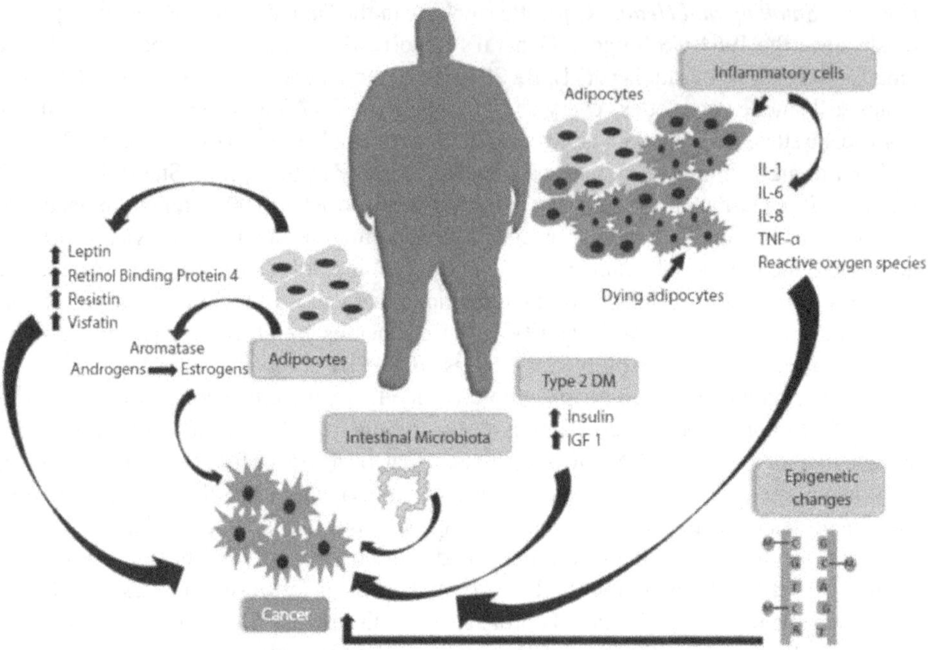

FIGURE 11.5 There are multiple mechanisms which link obesity to cancer

stem from the role of adipocytes (fat cells). Adipocytes stimulate intensive metabolic functions, most prominently inflammation and modulation of insulin sensitivity, nutrient uptake, and storage.

- *Mechanism of Obesity's Impact on Cancer*: Multiple mechanisms are hypothesized by which obesity affects cancer. These are indicated in Figure 11.5. It is important to understand that obesity does not initiate the carcinogenic process but rather promotes and accelerates cancer progression (84,85).

  The linkages between obesity and cancer appear to be largely related to the inflammatory response generated by substances secreted by adipocytes (86). In addition, insulin-like growth factor (IGF-1) is typically increased in obesity and can contribute to tumor growth (87,88).

  Also, in obesity, epigenetic changes are thought to shift cellular metabolism to fatty acid synthesis and oxidation (89,90). These metabolic changes have been shown to occur in as little as three days of high-fat diet consumption. It is important to note that epigenetic changes can become heritable through multiple generations of cell division and may be transgenerationally passed from parent to offspring.

  In addition to obesity itself being associated with increased risk of cancer, different dietary fats may also have different effects on cancer development. For example, saturated tropical oils such as coconut oil and palm oil promote tumor growth, while equal amounts of olive oil promote obesity but not tumor growth (91). It should also be noted that monounsaturated fat, such as that found in olive oil, has actually been shown to be associated with decreased risk of various cancers, including those of the digestive tract and breast (92), as have polyunsaturated fatty acids (PUFAs). High-carbohydrate diets, which may result in hyperglycemia and insulin resistance, particularly in obese or diabetic individuals, have been shown to contribute to cancer progression and its adverse effects.
- *Strategies to Disrupt the Obesity/Cancer Linkage*: The most effective way to prevent increased cancer risk associated with obesity is by maintaining a lean body mass

throughout life, utilizing multiple lifestyle strategies that are indicated throughout this book. In addition, weight loss in individuals who are obese or overweight by using lifestyle medicine modifications can significantly reduce circulating cancer risk factors (93–95). It is important to emphasize, however, that these effects require sustained weight loss.

A large pooling project, involving prospective studies on diet and cancer from the United States, Australia, and Japan, concluded that weight loss of 20 pounds in obese individuals resulted in a 32% lower incidence of breast cancer.

The beneficial consequences of intentional weight loss have been clearly demonstrated in bariatric surgery (96). For example, the Swedish Obesity Study (SOS), which compared over 2,000 individuals following metabolic bariatric surgery (MBS) versus control subjects, was associated with a 40% reduction in cancer incidence after 10.9 years (97,98). The SPLENDID study of surgical procedures and long-term effectiveness in neoplastic disease incidence and death showed that the prevalence of cancer was highly correlated with the degree of weight loss (97).

- *Lifestyle Recommendations to Disrupt The Obesity/Cancer Linkage*: The vast majority of recommendations for primary prevention of cancer involve maintaining a lean body weight and avoiding obesity throughout life (98,99). These involve the modalities already discussed in this book, including healthy nutrition and regular physical activity.

  Also, specifically, these recommendations involve avoiding high-calorie foods and sugary drinks (100) and prioritizing healthy eating patterns such as those recommended in multiple chapters in this book, including the MedDiet and the DASH diet.

  Maintaining good sleep hygiene is also very important for weight management. Lack of adequate sleep specifically has been associated with many diseases, including obesity. Recently, it has been shown that sleep restriction can modify appetite and food intake, leading to an increase in BMI (101). Sleep deprivation also worsens insulin sensitivity, which is a risk factor for T2DM. There has been some success in approaching chronic insomnia with cognitive behavioral therapy, which typically involves healthy sleep practices and relaxation techniques (see also Chapter 6).

  In addition, a strategy for primary cancer prevention by following cancer screening guidelines is very important (102–108). Regular screening is particularly important for overweight or obese individuals who have a tendency to avoid cancer screening. It is important to emphasize to individuals that overweight and obesity result in increased cancer occurrence and that early detection increases the chance of a cure.

11.7 SECONDARY PREVENTION IN CANCER SURVIVORS

Over 18 million cancer survivors currently reside in the United States, two-thirds of whom are over the age of 65 (109,110). Obesity remains a risk factor for cancer recurrence after initial diagnosis. Cancer survivors are more likely to develop complications following cancer treatment; therefore, it is important to avoid weight gain after cancer diagnosis. For all these reasons, the strategies of regular physical activity, healthy nutritional patterns, and good sleep hygiene are all important.

11.8 TYPE 2 DIABETES (T2DM) AND CANCER RISK

Obesity is also a major risk factor for the development of T2DM (see also Chapter 10). Insulin resistance found in T2DM results in hyperinsulinemia and hyperglycemia, which have been associated with increased risk of multiple different types of malignancies. The hypothesized mechanism for the increased risk of cancer in T2DM is the tumor-promoting effect of insulin and IGF-1, which are particularly elevated in the obese population with T2DM (111–113).

11.9 CANCER PREVENTION VACCINES

Each year, more than two million cases of cancer are attributable to infectious agents that occur around the globe (114). Vaccines that target viral surface proteins are available to protect against infection and prevent viral-mediated malignant transformation. The hepatitis B virus vaccine is typically administered to newborn children and prevents the development of hepatitis B virus-mediated hepatocellular cancer (115).

The Human Papillomavirus (HPV) vaccine is also safe and is typically given to adolescents before initiation of sexual activity. The HPV vaccine prevents high-risk infection of the cervix, vulva, vagina, penis, and oral pharynx and thereby prevents cancer development in these tissues (116,117).

Since many tumor cells have unique antigens, there has been significant focus on developing vaccines to prevent, destroy, and block tumor cell progression. This is an area of ongoing research. Information about cancer prevention vaccines is very important for parents of young children and also parents of newborns. Thus, these vaccines should be discussed with these patients during regular counseling sessions.

11.10 CONCLUSION/CLINICAL APPLICATION

Multiple interactions between lifestyle medicine principles and practices and both the prevention and treatment of cancer exist. Unfortunately, the public at large and even the medical community often do not appreciate the importance of these lifestyle modalities when it comes to the prevention and treatment of cancer. Regular physical activity, healthy nutrition, avoiding tobacco products, and avoiding or treating obesity all play essential roles in all phases of the prevention and treatment of cancer. All of these issues should be discussed in routine counseling sessions for all patients.

REFERENCES

1. Sung H, Ferlay J, Siegel RL, et al. Global cancer statistics 2020: GLOBOCAN estimates of incidence and mortality worldwide for 36 cancers in 185 countries. *CA Cancer J Clin.* 2021;71(3):209–249.
2. Mattiuzzi C, Lippi G. Current cancer epidemiology. *J Epidemiol Glob Health.* 2019;9(4):217–222.
3. Wu S, Powers S, Zhu W, et al. Substantial contribution of extrinsic risk factors to cancer development. *Nature.* 2016;529(7584):43–47.
4. Doll R, Peto R. The causes of cancer: quantitative estimates of avoidable risks of cancer in the United States today. *JNCI.* 1981;66(6):1192–1308.
5. National Cancer Institute. Age and Cancer. Risk Factors: Age – NCI. https://www.cancer.gov/about-cancer/causes-prevention/risk/age. Accessed March 20, 2025.
6. Ries L, Eisner M, Kosary C, et al. Surveillance, Epidemiology, and End Results (SEER) Program SEER* Stat Database: Incidence—SEER 9 Regs Public-Use, Nov 2004 Sub (1973–2002). National Cancer Institute, Division of Cancer Control and Population Sciences, Surveillance Research Program, Cancer Statistics Branch. Released April 2005, based on the November 2004 submission. National Cancer Institute, Division of Cancer Control and Population Sciences, Surveillance Research Program, Cancer Statistics Branch Released April. 2005.
7. National Cancer Institute. Childhood Cancer Survivor Study: An Overview. Bethesda, MD: U.S. Department of Health and Human Services, 2021. https://www.cancer.gov/types/childhood-cancers/ccss.
8. Phillips SM, Padgett LS, Leisenring WM, et al. Survivors of childhood cancer in the United States: prevalence and burden of morbidity. *Cancer Epidemiol Biomarkers Prev.* 2015;24(4):653–663.
9. Wogksch MD, Goodenough CG, Finch ER, et al. Physical activity and fitness in childhood cancer survivors: a scoping review. *Aging Cancer.* 2021;2(4):112–128.
10. Physical Activity Guidelines Advisory Committee. 2018 Physical Activity Guidelines Advisory Committee. 2018 Physical Activity Guidelines Advisory Committee Scientific Report. Washington, DC: U.S. Department of Health and Human Services, 2018.
11. Rock CL, Thomson C, Gansler T, et al. American Cancer Society guideline for diet and physical activity for cancer prevention. *CA Cancer J Clin.* 2020;70(4):245–71.

12. World Health Organization. Cancer. Geneva: World Health Organisation, 2022. https://www.who.int/cancer/en/. Accessed March 20, 2025.
13. Mokdad AH, Marks JS, Stroup DF, et al. Actual causes of death in the United States, 2000. *JAMA*. 2004;291(10):1238–1245.
14. Mokdad AH, Marks JS, Stroup DF, et al. Correction: actual causes of death in the United States, 2000. *JAMA*. 2005;293(3):293–294.
15. Mok A, Khaw KT, Luben R, et al. Physical activity trajectories and mortality: population based cohort study. *BMJ*. 2019;365:l2323.
16. Blond K, Brinkløv CF, Ried-Larsen M, Crippa A, Grøntved A. Association of high amounts of physical activity with mortality risk: a systematic review and meta-analysis. *Br J Sports Med*. 2020;54(20):1195.
17. Frisch RE, Wyshak G, Albright NL, et al. Lower prevalence of breast cancer and cancers of the reproductive system among former college athletes compared to non-athletes. *Br J Cancer*. 1985;52(6): 885–891.
18. Pedisic Z, Shrestha N, Kovalchik S, et al. Is running associated with a lower risk of all-cause, cardiovascular and cancer mortality, and is the more the better? A systematic review and meta-analysis. *Br J Sports Med*. 2020;54(15):898–905.
19. Moore SC, Lee IM, Weiderpass E, et al. Association of leisure-time physical activity with risk of 26 types of cancer in 1.44 million adults. *JAMA Intern Med*. 2016;176(6):816–825.
20. Gustafson MP, Wheatley-Guy CM, Rosenthal AC, et al. Exercise and the immune system: taking steps to improve responses to cancer immunotherapy. *J Immunother Cancer*. 2021;9(7):e001872.
21. McTiernan A. Mechanisms linking physical activity with cancer. *Nat Rev Cancer*. 2008;8(3):205–211.
22. Friedenreich CM, Orenstein MR. Physical activity and cancer prevention: etiologic evidence and biological mechanisms. *J Nutr*. 2002;132(11 Suppl):3456s–364s.
23. Zhang X, Ashcraft KA, Betof Warner A, et al. Can exercise-induced modulation of the tumor physiologic microenvironment improve antitumor immunity? *Cancer Res*. 2019;79(10):2447–2456.
24. Hammermüller C, Hinz A, Dietz A, et al. Depression, anxiety, fatigue, and quality of life in a large sample of patients suffering from head and neck cancer in comparison with the general population. *BMC Cancer*. 2021;21(1):94.
25. Kokkonen K, Tasmuth T, Lehto JT, et al. Cancer patients' symptom burden and health-related quality of life (HRQoL) at tertiary cancer center from 2006 to 2013: a cross-sectional Study. *Anticancer Res*. 2019;39(1):271.
26. Weis J. Cancer-related fatigue: prevalence, assessment and treatment strategies. *Expert Rev Pharmacoecon Outcomes Res*. 2011;11(4):441–446.
27. Mustian KM, Alfano CM, Heckler C, et al. Comparison of pharmaceutical, psychological, and exercise treatments for cancer-related fatigue: a meta-analysis. *JAMA Oncol*. 2017;3(7):961–968.
28. Irwin ML, McTiernan A, Manson JE, et al. Physical activity and survival in postmenopausal women with breast cancer: results from the women's health initiative. *Cancer Prev Res*. 2011;4(4):522–529.
29. Moore SC, Patel AV, Matthews CE, et al. Leisure time physical activity of moderate to vigorous intensity and mortality: a large pooled cohort analysis. *PLoS Med*. 2012;9(11):e1001335.
30. Scott JM, Li N, Liu Q, et al. Association of exercise with mortality in adult survivors of childhood cancer. *JAMA Oncol*. 2018;4(10):1352–1358.
31. Courneya KS, Friedenreich CM. Physical activity and cancer control. *Semin Oncol Nurs*. 2007; 23(4):242–252.
32. Rock CL, Thomson CA, Sullivan KR, et al. American Cancer Society nutrition and physical activity guideline for cancer survivors. *CA Cancer J Clin*. 2022;72(3):230–262.
33. Cormie P, Atkinson M, Bucci L, et al. Clinical Oncology Society of Australia position statement on exercise in cancer care. *Med J Aust*. 2018;209(4):184–187.
34. Patel AV, Friedenreich CM, Moore SC, et al. American College of Sports medicine roundtable report on physical activity, sedentary behavior, and cancer prevention and control. *Med Sci Sports Exerc*. 2019;51(11):2391–2402.
35. Ligibel JA, Bohlke K, May AM, et al. Exercise, diet, and weight management during cancer treatment: ASCO guideline. *J Clin Oncol*. 2022:JCO2200687.
36. Ligibel JA, Pierce LJ, Bender CM, et al. Attention to diet, exercise, and weight in oncology care: results of an American Society of Clinical Oncology National Patient Survey. *Cancer*. 2022;15;128(14):2817–2825.
37. Covington KR, Marshall T, Campbell G, et al. Development of the exercise in cancer evaluation and decision support (EXCEEDS) algorithm. *Support Care Cancer*. 2021;29(11):6469–6480.
38. Kuhnt S, Ernst J, Singer S, et al. Fatigue in cancer survivors – prevalence and correlates. *Onkologie*. 2009;32(6):312–317.

39. Huang IC, Brinkman TM, Kenzik K, et al. Association between the prevalence of symptoms and health-related quality of life in adult survivors of childhood cancer: a report from the St Jude lifetime cohort study. *J Clin Oncol.* 2013;31(33):4242–4251.
40. Sluka KA, Frey-Law L, Hoeger Bement M. Exercise-induced pain and analgesia? Underlying mechanisms and clinical translation. *Pain.* 2018;159(Suppl 1):S91–s97.
41. National Center for Chronic Disease Prevention and Health Promotion. Adult Physical Inactivity Prevalence Maps by Race/Ethnicity. Atlanta, GA: Centers for Disease Control and Prevention, 2022 Adult Physical Inactivity Outside of Work I Physical Activity I CDC.
42. Saffer H, Dave D, Grossman M, et al. Racial, ethnic, and gender differences in physical activity. *J Hum Cap.* 2013;7(4):378–410.
43. Clarke M, Lewin J, Lazarakis S, et al. Overlooked minorities: the intersection of cancer in lesbian, gay, bisexual, transgender, and/or intersex adolescents and young adults. *J Adolesc Young Adult Oncol.* 2019;8(5):525–528.
44. National Research Council Committee on Diet, Nutrition and Cancer. Diet Nutrition Cancer. Washington, DC: National Academies Press. US Copyright @ National Academy of Sciences, 1982.
45. U.S. Department of Agriculture and U.S. Department of Health and Human Services. U.S. Department of Agriculture and U.S. Department of Health and Human Services. Dietary Guidelines for Americans, 2020–2025. 9th edition. December 2020. Available at DietaryGuidelines.gov. 2020. https://www.dietaryguidelines.gov/resources/2020-2025-dietary-guidelines-online-materials.
46. Krebs-Smith SM, Pannucci TE, Subar AF, et al. Update of the healthy eating index: HEI-2015. *J Acad Nutr Diet.* 2018;118(9):1591–1602.
47. World Cancer Research Fund/American Institute for Cancer Research, Diet, Nutrition, Physical Activity and Cancer: A Global Perspective: A Summary of the Third Expert Report. London, UK: World Cancer Research Fund International, 2018.
48. Kaluza J, Harris HR, Hakansson N, et al. Adherence to the WCRF/AICR 2018 recommendations for cancer prevention and risk of cancer: prospective cohort studies of men and women. *Br J Cancer.* 2020;122(10):1562–1570.
49. Dietary Supplement use among Adults: United States, 2017–2018. In NCHS Data Briefs, S. National Center for Health Editor. Hyattsville, MD, 2021. doi: 10.15620/cdc:101131. Accessed April 30, 2025.
50. Yang CS, Chen JX, Wang H, et al. Lessons learned from cancer prevention studies with nutrients and non-nutritive dietary constituents. *Mol Nutr Food Res.* 2016;60(6):1239–1250.
51. Lichtenstein AH, Appel LJ, Vadiveloo M, et al. 2021 Dietary guidance to improve cardiovascular health: a scientific statement from the American Heart Association. *Circulation.* 2021;144(23):e472–e487.
52. Schwingshackl L, Schwedhelm C, Galbete C, et al. Adherence to mediterranean diet and risk of cancer: an updated systematic review and meta-analysis. *Nutrients.* 2017;9(10):1063.
53. Sacks FM, Svetkey LP, Vollmer WM, et al. Effects on blood pressure of reduced dietary sodium and the Dietary Approaches to Stop Hypertension (DASH) diet. *N Engl J Med.* 2001;344(1):3–10.
54. World Cancer Research Fund/American Institute for Cancer Research. Body fatness and weight gain and the risk of cancer. Continuous Update Project Expert Report. World Cancer Research, 2018.
55. Lauby-Secretan B, Scoccianti C, Loomis D, et al., Body fatness and cancer – viewpoint of the IARC Working Group. *N Engl J Med.* 2016;375(8):794–798.
56. Jones JM. Food processing: criteria for dietary guidance and public health? *Proc Nutr Soc.* 2019;78(1):4–18.
57. Slimani N, Deharveng G, Southgate DA, et al., Contribution of highly industrially processed foods to the nutrient intakes and patterns of middle-aged populations in the European Prospective Investigation into Cancer and Nutrition study. *Eur J Clin Nutr.* 2009;63(4):S206–S225.
58. Lian M. Salted fish and processed foods intake and nasopharyngeal carcinoma risk: a dose-response meta-analysis of observational studies. *Eur Arch Otorhinolaryngol.* 2022;279(5):2501–2509.
59. Martínez Steele E, Popkin BM, Swinburn B, et al. The share of ultra-processed foods and the overall nutritional quality of diets in the US: evidence from a nationally representative cross-sectional study. *Popul Health Metr.* 2017;15(1):6.
60. Fiolet T, Srour B, Sellem L, et al. Consumption of ultra-processed foods and cancer risk: results from NutriNet-Santé prospective Cohort. *BMJ.* 2018;360:k322.
61. Bouvard V, Loomis D, Guyton KZ, et al. Carcinogenicity of consumption of red and processed meat. *Lancet Oncol.* 2015;16(16):1599–600.
62. Cross AJ, Leitzmann MF, Gail MH, et al. A prospective study of red and processed meat intake in relation to cancer risk. *PLoS Med.* 2007;4(12):e325.
63. Huang Y, Cao D, Chen Z, et al. Red and processed meat consumption and cancer outcomes: umbrella review. *Food Chem.* 2021;356:129697.

64. Hur SJ, Jo C, Yoon Y, et al. Controversy on the correlation of red and processed meat consumption with colorectal cancer risk: an Asian perspective. *Crit Rev Food Sci Nutr.* 2019;59(21):3526–3537.
65. U.S. Department of Agriculture. Agricultural Research. FoodData Central, Editor. USDA FoodData Central, 2019. Accessed March 20, 2025.
66. Report on Carcinogens. National Toxicology Program: Research Triangle Park, North Carolina. National Toxicology Program, 2021. 15th Report on Carcinogens. Accessed March 20, 2025.
67. Maasland DH, van den Brandt PA, Kremer B, et al. Alcohol consumption, cigarette smoking and the risk of subtypes of head-neck cancer: results from the Netherlands Cohort Study. *BMC Cancer.* 2014;14:187.
68. McNabb S, Harrison TA, Albanes D, et al. Meta-analysis of 16 studies of the association of alcohol with colorectal cancer. *Int J Cancer.* 2020;146(3):861–873.
69. Wiseman M, Cannon G, Butrum R. et al. Policy and Action for Cancer Prevention. Food, Nutrition and Physical Activity: A Global Perspective. 2009. COVER.pdf. Accessed April 17, 2025.
70. Doll R, Peto R, Boreham J, et al. Mortality in relation to smoking: 50 years' observations on male British doctors. *BMJ.* 2004;328(7455):1519.
71. Center for Disease Control and Prevention (CDC). Achievements in public health, 1900–1999: Tobacco Use – United States, 1900–1999. *MMWR.* 1999;48(43):986–993.
72. Cornelius ME, Loretan CG, Wang TW, et al. Tobacco product use among adults – United States, 2020. *MMWR Morb Mortal Wkly Rep.* 2022;71(11):397–405.
73. Thun, MJ, Apicalla LF, Henley S.J. Smoking vs. other risk factors as the cause smoking-attributable deaths: confounding in the Courtroom. *JAMA.* 2020;284:706–712.
74. U.S. Department of Health and Human Services. The Health Consequences of Smoking: 50 Years of Progress. A Report of the Surgeon General. Atlanta, GA: U.S. Department of Health and Human Services, Centers for Disease Control and Prevention, National Center for Chronic Disease Prevention and Health Promotion, Office on Smoking and Health, 2014.
75. Center for Disease Control and Prevention (CDC). Cigarette smoking-attributable morbidity—United States, 2000. *MMWR Morb Mortal Wkly Rep.* 2003;52(35):842–844.
76. U.S. Department of Health and Human Services. The Health Benefits of Smoking Cessation. Washington, DC: CDC Office on Smoking and Health, 1990.
77. Fiore M for the 2008 Clinical Practice Update Panel. A clinical practice guideline for treating tobacco use and dependence: 2008 update. A US public health service report. *Am J Prev Med.* 2008;35(2):158–176.
78. Calle EE, Kaaks R. Overweight, obesity and cancer: epidemiological evidence and proposed mechanisms. *Nat Rev Cancer.* 2004;4(8):579–91.
79. Calle EE, Rodriguez C, Walker-Thurmond K, et al. Overweight, obesity, and mortality from cancer in a prospectively studied cohort of U.S. adults. *N Engl J Med.* 2003;348(17):1625–1638.
80. Calle EE, Thun MJ, Petrelli JM, et al. Body-mass index and mortality in a prospective cohort of U.S. adults. *N Engl J Med.* 1999;341(15):1097–1105.
81. Fryar CD, Carroll MD, Afful J. Prevalence of Overweight, Obesity, and Severe Obesity Among Adults Aged 20 and over: United States, 1960–1962 through 2017–2018.2020 11-29-22. NCHS Health E-Stats. https://www.cdc.gov/nchs/data/hestat/obesity-adult-17-18/obesity-adult.htm#Citation.
82. Stierman B, Afful J, Carroll M. National Health and Nutrition Examination Survey 2017–March 2020 prepandemic data files development of files and prevalence estimates for selected health outcomes. *Natl Health Stat Rep.* 2021;(158):106273.
83. American Institute for Cancer Research. Cancer Risk Awareness Survey Report Cancer Awareness Infographic, 2017. https://www.aicr.org/assets/docs/pdf/reports/AICR%20Cancer%20Awareness%20Report%202017_jan17%202017.pdf. Accessed March 25, 2025.
84. Berger NA. Obesity and cancer pathogenesis. *Ann NY Acad Sci.* 2014;1311:57–76.
85. Berger NA. Young adult cancer: influence of the obesity pandemic. *Obesity.* 2018;26(4):641–650.
86. Park EJ, Lee JH, Yu GY, et al. Dietary and genetic obesity promote liver inflammation and tumorigenesis by enhancing IL-6 and TNF expression. *Cell.* 2010;140(2):197–208.
87. Reilly SM, Saltiel AR. Adapting to obesity with adipose tissue inflammation. *Nat Rev Endocrinol.* 2017;13(11):633–643.
88. Ouchi N, Parker JL, Lugus JJ, et al. Adipokines in inflammation and metabolic disease. *Nat Rev Immunol.* 2011;11(2):85–97.
89. Jang H, Serra C. Nutrition, epigenetics, and diseases. *Clin Nutr Res.* 2014;3(1):1–8.
90. Choi SW, Friso S. Epigenetics: a new bridge between nutrition and health. *Adv Nutr.* 2010;1(1):8–16.
91. Doerner SK, Reis ES, Leung ES, et al. High-fat diet-induced complement activation mediates intestinal inflammation and neoplasia, independent of obesity. *Mol Cancer Res.* 2016;14(10):953–965.

92. Pelucchi C, Bosetti C, Negri E, et al. Olive oil and cancer risk: an update of epidemiological findings through 2010. *Curr Pharm Des.* 2011;17(8):805–812.
93. Linkov F, Maxwell GL, Felix AS, et al. Longitudinal evaluation of cancer-associated biomarkers before and after weight loss in RENEW study participants: implications for cancer risk reduction. *Gynecol Oncol.* 2012;125(1):114–119.
94. Parker ED, Folsom AR. Intentional weight loss and incidence of obesity-related cancers: the Iowa Women's Health Study. *Int J Obes Relat Metab Disord.* 2003;27(12):1447–1452.
95. Byers T, Sedjo RL. Does intentional weight loss reduce cancer risk? *Diabetes Obes Metab.* 2011; 13(12):1063–1072.
96. Teras LR, Patel AV, Wang M, et al. Sustained weight loss and risk of breast cancer in women 50 years and older: a pooled analysis of prospective data. *J Natl Cancer Inst.* 2020;112(9):929–937.
97. Sjostrom L, Gummesson A, Sjostrom CD, et al. Effects of bariatric surgery on cancer incidence in obese patients in Sweden (Swedish Obese Subjects Study): a prospective, controlled intervention trial. *Lancet Oncol.* 2009;10(7):653–662.
98. Sjostrom L. Review of the key results from the Swedish Obese Subjects (SOS) trial – a prospective controlled intervention study of bariatric surgery. *J Intern Med.* 2013;273(3):219–234.
99. Massetti GM, Dietz WH, Richardson LC. Excessive Weight Gain, Obesity, and cancer: opportunities for clinical intervention. *JAMA.* 2017:1975–1976.
100. Rolls BJ. Dietary energy density: applying behavioural science to weight management. *Nutr Bull.* 2017;42(3):246–253.
101. Hanlon EC, Tasali E, Leproult R, et al. Sleep restriction enhances the daily rhythm of circulating levels of endocannabinoid 2-arachidonoylglycerol. *Sleep.* 2016;39(3):653–664.
102. Oeffinger KC, Fontham ET, Etzioni R, et al. Breast cancer screening for women at average risk: 2015 guideline update from the American Cancer Society. *JAMA.* 2015;314(15):1599–1614.
103. Siu AL, U.S. Preventive Services Task Force. Screening for breast cancer: U.S. preventive services task force recommendation statement. *Ann Intern Med.* 2016;164(4):279–296.
104. Aberle DR, Adams AM, Berg CD, et al. Reduced lung-cancer mortality with low-dose computed tomographic screening. *N Engl J Med.* 2011;365(5):395–409.
105. Winawer SJ, Zauber AG, Ho MN, et al. Prevention of colorectal cancer by colonoscopic polypectomy. The National Polyp Study Workgroup. *N Engl J Med.* 1993;329(27):1977–1981.
106. Imperiale TF, Ransohoff DF, Itzkowitz SH, et al. Fecal DNA versus fecal occult blood for colorectal-cancer screening in an average-risk population. *N Engl J Med.* 2004;351(26):2704–2714.
107. Lin JS, Piper MA, Perdue LA, et al. Screening for colorectal cancer: updated evidence report and systematic review for the US preventive services task force. *JAMA.* 2016;315(23):2576–2594.
108. Saslow D, Solomon D, Lawson HW, et al. American Cancer Society, American Society for Colposcopy and Cervical Pathology, and American Society for Clinical Pathology screening guidelines for the prevention and early detection of cervical cancer. *CA Cancer J Clin.* 2012;62(3):147–172.
109. National Cancer Institute. Statistics and Graphs. Sciences CCP, editors. Cancer.gov. National Cancer Institute, 2022.
110. Miller KD, Nogueira L, Devasia T, et al. Cancer treatment and survivorship statistics, 2022. *CA Cancer J Clin.* 2022;72(5):409–436.
111. Shlomai G, Neel B, LeRoith D, et al. Type 2 diabetes mellitus and cancer: the role of pharmacotherapy. *J Clin Oncol.* 2016;34(35):4261–4269.
112. Barone BB, Yeh HC, Snyder CF, et al. Long-term all-cause mortality in cancer patients with preexisting diabetes mellitus: a systematic review and meta-analysis. *JAMA.* 2008;300(23):2754–2764.
113. Hu FB, Manson JE, Liu S, et al. Prospective study of adult onset diabetes mellitus (type 2) and risk of colorectal cancer in women. *J Natl Cancer Inst.* 1999;91(6):542–547.
114. De Martel C, Georges D, Bray F, et al. Global burden of cancer attributable to infections in 2018: a worldwide incidence analysis. *Lancet Glob Health.* 2019;8(2):e180–e190.
115. Poland GA, Jacobson RM. Clinical practice: prevention of hepatitis B with the hepatitis B vaccine. *N Engl J Med.* 2004;351(27):2832–2838.
116. Meites E, Szilagyi PG, Chesson HW, et al. Human papillomavirus vaccination for adults: updated recommendations of the advisory committee on immunization practices. *MMWR Morb Mortal Wkly Rep.* 2019;68:698–702.
117. McQuillan G, Kruszon-Moran D, Markowitz LE, et al. Prevalence of HPV in adults aged 18–69: United States, 2011–2014. NCHS data brief, no 280. Hyattsville, MD: National Center for Health Statistics, 2017.

12 Lifestyle Modalities and Weight Management/Obesity

12.1 INTRODUCTION

In Chapter 4, we focused on the conditions of weight gain, weight management, and obesity. As indicated in that chapter, these conditions represent quintessential lifestyle diseases. They are, unfortunately, extremely prevalent in the United States. For example, over 72% of the adult population in the United States is either overweight or obese (1,2). The average adult in the United States gains 2.2 pounds a year after the age of 20. Thus, by the age of 50, the average adult in the United States has gained between 30 and 45 pounds over their weight at age 20.

While Chapter 4 focused largely on the treatment of obesity per se, this chapter will focus on how various lifestyle medicine modalities play important and synergistic roles in lowering the likelihood of weight gain and obesity. We will also focus some attention on the established linkages between obesity and multiple other chronic diseases such as cardiovascular disease (CVD), type 2 diabetes (T2DM), metabolic syndrome (MetS), cancer, cognitive decline, and even Alzheimer's disease.

Given the prevalence of overweight and obesity in the United States, it is incumbent upon all physicians, but particularly those who practice in the area of lifestyle medicine, to have a sophisticated understanding of the modern science of obesity and, of equal importance, to be able to counsel all patients about the importance of maintaining a healthy body weight.

Sadly, despite the fact that over 70% of individuals see their primary care physician on an annual basis, less than 40% of physicians counsel overweight or obese patients about the significant health risks that are associated with these conditions (3).

In the curriculum that is embedded in this book, our goal is to provide appropriate tools for physicians to address weight gain, overweight, and obesity. Some specific ideas will also be provided about how to start counseling sessions to emphasize the significant relationship between weight gain, overweight, obesity, and numerous chronic conditions.

Multiple studies have now shown that what individuals do in their daily lives carries enormous implications for all of these conditions. Physical activity and proper nutrition are critically important in the area of weight loss, but also have been demonstrated to reduce the likelihood of weight gain in the first place and to help maintain a healthy body weight. Proper nutrition and physical activity have been discussed in detail in separate chapters on each of these lifestyle factors. This chapter will focus attention on how to combine these modalities to help individuals either control weight or lose weight.

Multiple factors contribute to weight gain, overweight, and obesity. It would seem to make sense that reducing calories and increasing physical activity would be all that is required for both weight loss and maintaining a healthy body weight. The issue of maintaining a healthy body weight, however, is much more complex than that. The American Society of Nutrition, in its consensus statement on metabolism, emphasized multiple other important factors (4). The environment, genetic background, interaction with other individuals, level of stress, as well as national and international food and agricultural policies, all play roles in the likelihood that people will gain weight and become overweight or obese.

For individuals who are overweight or obese, further complications come from prospective studies that have shown that when individuals are asked how much weight they would like to lose, they typically respond that they would like to lose 15%–20% of their body weight to get back to their high

DOI: 10.1201/9781003630043-12

school or college weight (5). In fact, weight loss of 5%–10% is all that is required to substantially lower the risk of multiple chronic diseases, including CVD, T2DM, MetS, and even cancer (6–11).

When this current level of recommended weight loss is discussed with individuals, a number of studies have shown that patients describe this amount of weight loss as either "disappointing" or "extremely disappointing." It will require good counseling skills on the part of physicians to emphasize that an achievable weight loss of 5%–10% of body weight makes a huge difference in terms of the reduction of risk of chronic disease. There is solid a evidence base for these assumptions, which comes from large NIH-funded studies, including the Diabetes Prevention Program (DPP) (12) and the Look AHEAD trial (13).

12.2 EPIDEMIOLOGY

The current levels of overweight and obesity in the United States have been discussed in detail in Chapter 4. The data supporting the high prevalence of overweight and obesity in the United States are drawn largely from body mass index (BMI) determinations (this is the weight in kilograms divided by the height in meters squared). As a practical matter, most physicians will find it more expeditious to refer to readily available charts that provide BMI based on various heights and weights. One of the charts is found in Table 12.1.

TABLE 12.1
Body Mass Index (BMI) Body Weight (lbs)

HT (inches)	120	130	140	150	160	170	180	190	200	210	220	230	240	250
58	25	27	29	31	33	36	38	40	42	44	46	48	50	52
59	24	26	28	30	32	34	36	38	40	42	44	46	48	50
60	23	25	27	29	31	33	35	37	39	41	43	45	47	49
61	23	25	26	28	30	32	34	36	38	40	42	43	45	47
62	22	24	26	27	29	31	33	35	37	38	40	42	44	46
63	21	23	25	27	28	30	32	34	35	37	39	41	43	44
64	21	22	24	26	27	29	31	33	34	36	38	39	41	43
65	20	22	23	25	27	28	30	32	33	35	37	38	40	42
66	19	21	23	24	26	27	29	31	32	34	36	37	39	40
67	19	20	22	23	25	27	28	30	31	33	34	36	38	39
68	18	20	21	23	24	26	27	29	30	32	33	35	36	38
69	18	19	21	22	24	25	27	28	30	31	32	34	35	37
70		19	20	22	23	24	26	27	29	30	32	33	34	36
71		18	20	21	22	24	25	26	28	29	31	32	33	35
72		18	19	20	22	23	24	26	27	28	30	31	33	34
73			18	20	21	22	24	25	26	28	29	30	32	33
74			18	19	21	22	23	24	26	27	28	30	31	32
75				19	20	21	22	24	25	26	27	29	30	31
76				18	19	21	22	23	24	26	27	28	29	30
77				18	19	20	21	23	24	25	26	27	28	30

Source: From ACSM Position Stand on Appropriate Intervention Strategies for Weight Loss and Prevention of Weight Regain for Adults. Jakicic JM, Clark, K. Coleman E, et al. American College of Sports Medicine position stand. Appropriate intervention strategies for weight loss and prevention of weight regain for adults. *Med Sci Sports Exerc*, 2001;33(12):2145–2156.

Note: Body mass index <18 is not recommended, and therefore these values are not represented in this table. Body mass index based on weight and height.

It should be noted that while BMI provides a reasonable correlation between weight and risk of developing chronic diseases (14), it does not provide a highly accurate estimate of body fat. A variety of other methodologies are available to obtain more accurate measurements of body fat. These include dual energy X-ray absorptiometry (DEXA), magnetic resonance imaging (MRI), and computerized tomography (CT). Unless the physician is fortunate enough to have access to DEXA scanning, MRI or CT scanning are options. These methodologies, however, are typically not necessary and may be prohibitively expensive in any setting other than research studies.

Overweight and obesity represent significant public health problems in the United States and also in other countries around the world. It is estimated that over 2.1 billion people around the world are currently obese, and this number is projected to grow to over 3 billion by 2050 (15). As already indicated, in the United States, the prevalence of overweight and obesity as assessed by BMI has now been estimated at over 72% of adults. Obesity itself has grown rapidly, and it is now estimated at 40% and severe obesity at 16% (16). The rate of obesity has risen steeply and doubled in adults between 1990 and 2021 to more than 40% and has nearly tripled to 29% among girls and women ages 15–24 (2,17).

Particularly troubling is that there has been an increased proportion of adolescents with obesity. Over half of US teens and young adults ages 15–24 are now overweight or obese compared to 29% in 1990 (17). These are particularly worrisome numbers since obesity in younger age groups tends to strongly predict obesity as adults and creates an increased risk for all the adverse events associated with obesity.

The increased prevalence of obesity has multiple potential causes. As already discussed, energy imbalance is the final common pathway for all of these causes. Recent significant scientific advances, however, have led to more sophisticated understandings of what contributes to this energy imbalance. Predisposing factors for energy imbalance include genetics, epigenetics, infections, smoking, poor sleep habits, gut microbiota, and multiple other factors, including endocrine disruptors, pharmaceutical agents, and ambient temperature control (18–27).

12.3 THE PATHOPHYSIOLOGY OF OBESITY

The final common pathway for obesity is that it results from an imbalance between energy intake and expenditure. Energy balance is regulated by a complex physiologic system that requires integration of multiple peripheral signals and coordination with the brain. As already indicated, multiple underlying factors contribute to the development of obesity, including interaction with the environment and genetic factors, which can also contribute to disorders in energy balance. Energy balance is exquisitely regulated. Even in some societies where obesity is very prevalent, the average weight gain is only about 2.2 pounds per year (18). This reflects an energy excess of about 20 kcal per day, or less than 1% of daily energy expenditure.

Human beings have a complicated and sophisticated system for regulating energy balance and fat storage that interacts with adipocytes. Obesity develops when energy intake exceeds energy output, which leads to an accumulation of adipose tissue.

Control of Appetite and Metabolism Maintains Energy Balance: Appetite regulation is in itself complex and affected by the integration of both peripheral and central signals. In the gastrointestinal tract, orexin, ghrelin, and decreasing concentrations of micronutrients (e.g., glucose, fatty acids, and amino acids) stimulate hunger (19–21). This is aided by the release of gastrointestinal peptides such as ghrelin, cholecystokinin (CCK), glucagon-like peptide-1 (GLP-1), and peptide YY-3–36 (as already noted, GLP-1 is the hormone that is being manipulated in the new GLP-1 anti-obesity pharmaceuticals) (22).

Food Intake: Food intake is under both short- and long-term control. Short-term hunger develops in response to decreased circulating levels of glucose, fatty acids, and amino acids.

Long-term control depends on signals from the magnitude of energy stores and includes the adipose tissue hormone leptin.

The discovery of the obesity (OB) gene and its products has led to major advances in understanding the physiologic systems regulating energy balance (23). The OB gene encodes the leptin hormone, which is secreted by adipocytes in proportion to the level of body adipose tissue. Low leptin levels trigger events that lead to increased energy intake, whereas high leptin levels in response to increased fat deposits result in negative energy balance (24).

Energy Expenditure: With regard to energy expenditure, a complex system also exists. Contributors to energy expenditure include resting metabolic rate (RMR), exercise-induced thermogenesis (physical activity), and food-induced thermogenesis (25,26). RMR contributes 60%–75% of total energy expenditure and is a function of lean body mass, energy intake, physical fitness, and other factors, including age, height, stress, and environmental temperature. Dietary thermogenesis represents the energy required to digest and store food. It is greatest with protein-rich foods. Physical activity is also influenced by behavioral and environmental factors. The adrenergic system also plays a major role in regulating energy expenditure. As discussed in Chapter 4, adipose tissue plays a central role in energy homeostasis and demonstrates complex interactions with the brain and peripheral organs. Adipose tissue constantly communicates with other tissues through the release of secretagogues such as leptin, adiponectin, and visfatin, all of which, along with insulin, play important roles in regulating body fat mass (27–29).

Causes of Obesity: Multiple underlying causes contribute to obesity, including genetics, environment, lower density of food intake, and physical inactivity. All of these are discussed in more detail in Chapter 4.

As already indicated, the system that controls energy balance is exquisitely fine-tuned. It can be disrupted, however, by mechanisms in the environment that promote energy intake and decrease physical activity. The genetic component of obesity is estimated at 30%–50%. This genetic component, however, does not explain the dramatic increases in obesity in the United States and worldwide over the last 40 years. Clearly, susceptibility to weight gain and overweight or obesity responds dramatically to lifestyle habits and practices, including paying attention to energy density, consumption of high-calorie foods, and decreased physical activity (30–32). Thus, multiple components of lifestyle factors play a very significant role in weight gain, overweight, and obesity. Therefore, an optimum approach to obesity prevention and treatment involves the use of multiple lifestyle medicine modalities.

12.4 THE ROLE OF LIFESTYLE MODALITIES IN THE PREVENTION AND TREATMENT OF OBESITY

Obesity is a quintessential condition in which lifestyle modalities can play a very significant role, particularly when used in combination with each other. In this section, we will explore how various lifestyle modalities interact with each other to either treat or prevent weight gain, overweight, or obesity.

12.4.1 Physical Activity

As outlined in numerous chapters in this book, regular physical activity is associated with multiple health benefits. In the area of weight gain, overweight, and obesity, numerous benefits are derived from physical activity. Physical activity is supported by considerable evidence to assist in the prevention of weight gain. Numerous cross-sectional studies have supported an inverse relationship between physical activity and BMI, as well as body fat measures.

Multiple epidemiological studies, including National Health & Nutrition Examination Survey (NHANES) I, The Aerobic Center for Longitudinal Studies (33), The Women's Health Initiative (34), and the Harvard Alumni Study (35), all support the importance of physical activity in the prevention of weight gain. It appears that the amount of physical activity needed to prevent weight gain is somewhat higher than that required for general health (36). The goal of 150 minutes of moderate-intensity physical activity per week, as recommended by the Physical Activity Guidelines for Americans 2018 (37), has been supported by numerous other organizations such as the American Heart Association (AHA) (38), the American College of Sports Medicine (ACSM) (39), and the Dietary Guidelines for Americans 2020–2025 (DAGs) (40). It appears that to prevent weight gain of at least 5% of current body weight, between 150 and 250 minutes a week are necessary.

In contrast, the effects of physical activity on weight loss, when not coupled with a concurrent reduction of energy intake, appear to be modest. Weight loss averaging between 1% and 2% in studies of physical activity alone for weight loss, lasting between 16 and 18 months, has been reported.

According to data reported by ACSM, no significant change in body weight typically occurs in response to less than 150 minutes per week. In one study, however, three kilograms of weight loss was observed with activity greater than 150 minutes per week, and 5–7.5 kg for amounts between 225 and 420 minutes of moderate-intensity physical activity per week. It should be emphasized that these high levels of physical activity are based on using physical activity alone without energy restriction (40). Systematic reviews in the area of resistance exercise suggest that resistance exercise, in the absence of energy restriction, results in very modest weight loss.

Numerous organizations have now suggested potential benefits from what has been called "lifestyle" activity. Most of these studies utilize pedometers. The most persuasive studies of lifetime physical activity for weight loss involve walking at least 10,000 steps per day. This is equivalent to walking approximately five miles per day.

The duration of physical activity bouts has been under study for the last two decades (37,40). Initially, it was thought that sessions of 8–10 minutes of physical activity were necessary in order to achieve the most benefits, particularly in the area of weight loss. Recent data from PAGA 2018 suggest that even shorter bouts of physical activity may yield benefits. Most data, however, support physical activity sessions of at least 10 minutes in duration as desirable for weight loss (37).

The most common form of weight loss recommendation involves physical activity in combination with the reduction of energy intake. In this area, physical activity is particularly valuable for the maintenance of weight loss. It should be noted, however, that improved weight loss has been achieved in some studies with 200–300 minutes of moderate intensity physical activity per week (40).

It is also important to note that there is considerable variability in weight loss in response to physical activity. In one study, in response to highly controlled exercise, weight loss ranges of approximately 3–12 kg were reported (41). This high level of variability may be a result of factors such as underlying biological differences or the influence of physical activity on energy intake. Some individuals find that physical activity causes them to consume more calories. In addition, multiple factors may influence adherence to physical activity (42).

Several additional issues related to physical activity for obese individuals are important to mention. The level of cardiorespiratory fitness is associated with reduced mortality in obese individuals, even when adjusted for the level of adiposity (43). This has led to a debate that has been characterized as "fit versus fat" (44). Nonetheless, high levels of cardiorespiratory fitness do not completely ameliorate the risk of a high BMI or body fat. It should be pointed out that cardiorespiratory fitness may impact other risk factors. Physical activity helps with the control of blood pressure even in individuals who are overweight or obese (45). Obesity represents a significant risk factor for hypertension.

Dyslipidemia is also a significant risk factor for heart disease. Physical activity appears to have only a very modest influence on blood lipids in individuals who are overweight or obese (46).

It has also been suggested that overweight and obesity result in increased total body inflammation (47). It has been suggested that increased physical activity may result in decreased inflammation; however, initial studies in this area have not yielded this finding (48,49).

12.4.2 Nutrition

Nutritional modifications are key behavioral interventions in weight management (50). Specifically, appropriate dietary modification allows essential nutrients to maintain optimal nutritional status while simultaneously creating an energy deficit to yield reasonable weight loss. It is important to balance eating enjoyment with reductions in energy consumption to provide sustainable eating patterns. It may be valuable for clinicians to engage registered dietitian nutritionists (RDNs) who can provide detailed assessment and recommendations for proper nutrition patterns to help individuals lose weight (51). The typical energy deficit for weight loss is 500–750 kcal per day. RDNs may specifically determine that by assessing basal energy expenditure, the thermoeffect food, and an adjustment factor for physical activity level.

Typically, the equation utilized to derive these results involves computation of resting energy expenditure (REE). This applies to both males and females utilizing the equation called the Mifflin-St. Jeor equation, which is highly accurate in determining resting metabolic rate within 10% in most individuals (52).

$$\text{For females, REE} = 10 \times \text{weight (kg)} + 6.25 \times \text{height (cm)} - 5 \times \text{age (y)} - 161$$
$$\text{For males, REE} = 10 \times \text{weight (kg)} + 6.25 \times \text{height (cm)} - 5 \times \text{age (y)} + 5$$

A physical activity level determination is necessary to fine-tune the energy expenditure equation. The activity factor for a sedentary individual is REE × 1.2. For low to moderate activity, it is ×1.4, and for an active person, it is REE × 1.6.

Multiple dietary intake assessment methods are available. The ones most frequently used are either the 24-hour food recall or food frequency questionnaire. Utilizing these tools may be more than the typical clinician will want to undertake. They are, however, standard tools in use by RDNs.

It is also important to determine a person's eating environment and their readiness for a weight loss regimen. Motivational interviewing (MI) helps determine the individual's goals and is useful in this area.

Dietary intervention should start with as little as 3%–5% weight loss and ultimately aim for 5%–10% weight loss to improve various risk factors, including those for CVD (53).

While many different dietary approaches exist, no one is ideal. The key is finding one that will fit best in the individual's life. Eating foods with low energy density and high nutrient density is important. As indicated in multiple chapters in this book, the dietary strategies involved with the Mediterranean diet (54), the DASH diet (55), and the US-Style Eating Pattern (40) are all very effective in terms of supplying adequate nutrients. Each of these plant-forward diets should be geared to create a 500–750 kcal per day deficit to achieve weight loss (56).

12.4.3 Sleep Hygiene

Sleep is one of the key components of lifestyle medicine and is an important component of maintaining a healthy weight or losing weight if an individual is obese (57).

Multiple sleep disorders exist. These are discussed in detail in Chapter 6. In the area of obesity, some data suggest that healthy sleep is associated with reduced adiposity, improved quality of life, and improved nutritional habits. Sleep deprivation has been associated with an increased likelihood of consuming high-calorie foods. The hypothesized mechanism for increased consumption of high-calorie foods associated with sleep deprivation may be changes in hormones such as leptin and ghrelin based on inadequate sleep. For adults, between seven and nine hours of sleep is recommended nightly. Details about sleep hygiene can be found in Chapter 6. It should also be noted that obesity is associated with a four to five times increased likelihood of obstructive sleep apnea, which can be another cause of disruption to healthy sleep.

12.5 BEHAVIORAL MANAGEMENT

Behavioral management is essential to effective weight loss and management of obesity. For this reason, it is advocated in the guidelines from the American Heart Association/American College of Cardiology/The Obesity Society (AHA/ACC/TOS) as one of the key components (53). Behavioral management according to the AHA/ACC/TOS guidelines, includes counseling sessions on a weekly basis for six months, followed by monthly sessions for another 12 months. The reason that the AHA/ACC/TOS guidelines recommend behavior modification for all patients receiving obesity treatment is that behavioral strategies will help patients overcome challenges as they strive to achieve a healthier lifestyle.

For the health care provider to be effective in counseling behavioral change, it is important that he or she has a "toolbox" of strategies based on the unique needs of each patient with obesity. Multiple behavioral strategies are available, which are aimed at helping patients develop, for themselves, the skills needed to achieve and maintain a healthier lifestyle. The following management strategies are all appropriate:

- *Setting Goals*: It is important to emphasize to patients that achieving a 5%–10% weight loss will result in significant health benefits. Some patients tell providers they want to lose 20% or more of their current weight, which, for the vast majority of individuals, is unrealistic and not necessary to achieve health benefits.
- *Raising Awareness*: It is important for patients to self-monitor their behavior and raise awareness of the behaviors that need to be changed (58,59).
- *Confronting Barriers*: It is important to help the obese patient understand and explore the barriers that are preventing them from healthy eating and exercising regularly. The technique of motivational interviewing is very valuable in this area.
- *Restructuring Beliefs*: Oftentimes, patients' beliefs, attitudes, thoughts, and negative feelings about themselves will determine whether or not a behavioral intervention will succeed. Cognitive restructuring using techniques such as cognitive behavioral therapy is very valuable in helping restructure beliefs (60).
- *Managing Stress*: Stress, tension, anxiety, depression, anger, boredom, loneliness, and other negative affective states can interfere with a healthy lifestyle. Stress, in particular, can contribute to overeating and under-exercising (61,62). It is important to help patients with obesity use behavioral strategies to help them manage stress. Physical activity is a particularly useful strategy for managing stress. Other stress-reducing modalities such as daily meditation and progressive muscle relaxation may also be helpful.
- *Preventing Relapse*: Once realistic goals have been agreed upon, identifying potential barriers is useful to help patients recognize that there will be times when it is challenging to remain in a weight loss program (62,63). The goal is not to prevent all lapses but to help a patient understand that these may occur and prevent them from becoming either relapses or total collapses (64).
- *Providing Support*: Strong support from a variety of individuals, such as family members, close friends, neighbors, colleagues at work, physicians, registered dietitians, counselors, and other care providers, can be very powerful for patients trying to lose weight or maintain weight loss and make other healthy lifestyle changes (65). This, of course, is a major pillar of lifestyle medicine.
- *Pharmaceutical Management*: A variety of pharmaceutical agents are available to help individuals lose weight (65). These are discussed in more detail in Chapter 4.
- *Bariatric Surgery*: Individuals who have a body mass index of >40 or >35 kg/m^2 with an obesity-related comorbidity are potentially eligible for bariatric surgery (66). Bariatric surgery is discussed in more detail in Chapter 4. These agents are invariably recommended for use in conjunction with lifestyle activities such as healthy nutrition and regular physical activity.

12.6 OBESITY AND SPECIFIC MEDICAL CONDITIONS

Obesity and Cardiovascular Disease: Overweight and obesity represent significant risk factors for CVD (67,68). The AHA lists obesity as a major risk factor for CVD both because of its association with other risk factors (e.g., T2DM, dyslipidemia, elevated blood pressure, and the MetS). Obesity also serves as an independent risk factor. As already indicated in Chapter 4, the distribution of body fat is also important since abdominal obesity represents a separate and additional risk factor for CVD.

Obesity is strongly associated with hypertension, as is adult weight gain (69). A 20-pound weight gain is associated with 3 mm Hg higher diastolic blood pressure, which results in a 12% increase in risk of coronary heart disease (CHD) and a 24% increase in risk of stroke.

Body weight correlates strongly with glucose intolerance and T2DM. The link between T2DM appears to be mediated by hyperinsulinemia. Individuals who gain between 5 and 20 kg during adult years increase their risk of developing diabetes between 4- and 12-fold.

Multiple lipid abnormalities are associated with obesity, including higher triglyceride levels and lower HDL (70). LDL cholesterol is also related to BMI. Obesity is strongly associated with the development of the MetS, which is handled in detail in the next chapter of this book.

It should be pointed out that many of the pillars of lifestyle medicine act synergistically to help control the likelihood of adult weight gain and also help with weight loss. These include healthy nutrition, regular physical activity, stress reduction, and avoiding cigarette smoking or discontinuing it if already smoking. Developing positive connections with other individuals is also important.

As already indicated in Chapter 4, obesity is also strongly associated with T2DM, MetS (71,72), cancer, and arthritis. More details about all of these medical conditions are outlined in Chapter 4. It should be pointed out that lifestyle medicine modalities, including regular physical activity, healthy nutrition, stress reduction, discontinuing cigarettes, and obtaining support from other individuals, are all key lifestyle medicine modalities and act synergistically to help combat obesity and/or lower the risk of weight gain in the first place.

12.7 THE ROLE OF THE PHYSICIAN IN WEIGHT MANAGEMENT AND OBESITY

Physicians can play a significant role in not only helping individuals understand the importance of not gaining weight during adult years, but also in weight management for individuals who are currently overweight or obese. One important action that a physician can take is to open a positive and non-judgmental conversation with overweight or obese patients. It is very important not to shame an individual who is overweight or obese. Often, these individuals will feel very self-conscious about their weight. As already indicated in this chapter, overweight and obesity are classic situations where virtually every one of the lifestyle medicine modalities can be employed. Of course, energy balance should be addressed with both increased physical activity and healthy nutrition.

In addition, avoiding tobacco, managing stress, reaching out to other individuals for support, and getting healthy, restorative sleep are also important. Thus, obesity treatment is the classic situation for employing multiple components of lifestyle medicine.

In addition, if a physician himself or herself is overweight or obese, personally following these steps can set a positive example and serve as a role model for other individuals. We have provided a six-day starter program based on the plant-forward Full Plate Living Weight Loss Program (73), which can assist physicians, and also patients who have overweight or obesity, to get started with healthy nutrition. We have also included walking programs in Appendix B, which will be very helpful to get an individual started on increased physical activity.

12.8 USE OF ANCILLARY PROFESSIONALS

The AHA/ACC/TOS guidelines recommend that the most effective weight management programs involve team approaches with not only physicians, but RDNs, exercise physiologists, if they are available, and nurses (53). All of these individuals bring their own unique skills, perspectives, and backgrounds and will be important contributors to helping overweight or obese patients lose weight.

12.9 RESOURCES

As indicated in other chapters in this book, multiple healthy nutritional plans are available including the Mediterranean diet, DASH diet, and US-Style Eating Pattern. If the goal is to lose weight, simply reducing calories by 500–750 kcal per day using one of these plant-forward, healthy plans is the research-proven method for helping with weight loss. The good news is that these diets are all anti-inflammatory and all contribute to reducing the risk of multiple other metabolic conditions.

12.10 CLINICAL APPLICATIONS

Adult weight gain, overweight, and obesity are endemic in the United States and around the world. These are classic situations where multiple components of daily lifestyle habits and actions contained in the field of lifestyle medicine can play a very important role in reducing adverse consequences. Clinicians should become knowledgeable about all of these factors and endeavor to counsel all patients at every visit about the importance of weight management.

For individuals who are currently in the healthy weight range, this counseling should focus on those daily habits and actions to lower the risk of gaining weight during the adult years. It is also important to help individuals understand that relatively modest amounts of weight loss, 5–10% of initial weight, if the individual is overweight or obese, can result in significant risk factor reduction.

The relationship of obesity to CVD, T2DM, MetS, and cancer should be emphasized to all patients to provide a strong impetus to engage in healthy weight management.

REFERENCES

1. Rippe JM, Foreyt JP. *Lifestyle Medicine: Obesity Prevention and Treatment: A Practical Guide*. Boca Raton, FL: CRC Press, 2021.
2. US Obesity Forecasting Collaborators. National-level and state-level prevalence of overweight and obesity among children, adolescents, and adults in the USA, 1990–2021, and forecasts up to 2050. *Lancet*. 2024;404(10469):2278–2298.
3. Faries MD, Kephart WC, Graham D. The intention-behavior gap. In Rippe JM (ed), *Lifestyle Medicine* (4th ed). Boca Raton, FL: CRC Press, 2024.
4. American Society of Nutrition Statement on Metabolism. https://nutrition.org/publications/fact-sheets-and-position-papers/. Accessed February 26, 2025.
5. Foreyt JP, Johnston CA. Behavior modification and cognitive therapy. In Mechanick J, Kushner R (eds.) *Lifestyle Medicine: A Manual for Clinical Practice*. New York: Springer, 2016, pp. 129–134.
6. D'Agostino R, Hamman R, Karter A, et al. Cardiovascular disease risk factors predict the development of type 2 diabetes: the insulin resistance atherosclerosis study. *Diabetes Care*. 2004;27(9):2234–2240.
7. Katzmarzyk P, Janssen I, Ardern C. Physical inactivity, excess adiposity and premature mortality. *Obes Rev*. 2003;4(4):257–290.
8. Kenchaiah S, Gaziano J, Vasan R. Impact of obesity on the risk of heart failure and survival after the onset of heart failure. *Med Clin North Am*. 2004;88(5):1273–1294.
9. Guh D, Zhang W, Bansback N, et al. The incidence of co-morbidities related to obesity and overweight: a systematic review and meta-analysis. *BMC Public Health*. 2009;9:88.
10. Wang Y, McPherson K, Marsh T, et al. Health and economic burden of the projected obesity trends in the USA and the UK. *Lancet*. 2011;378(9793):815–825.
11. Renehan A, Tyson M, Egger M, et al. Body-mass index and incidence of cancer: a systematic review and meta-analysis of prospective observational studies. *Lancet*. 2008;371(9612):569–578.
12. The Diabetes Prevention Program Research Group. The diabetes prevention program (DPP): description of lifestyle intervention. *Diabetes Care*. 2002;25(12):2165–2171.
13. Look Ahead Research Group, Wadden TA, West DS, et al. The look AHEAD study: a description of the lifestyle intervention and the evidence supporting it. *Obesity*. 2006;14(5):737–752.

14. Anonymous. Clinical guidelines on the identification, evaluation, and treatment of overweight and obesity in adults – the evidence report. *National Institutes of Health. Obes Res.* 1998;6(Suppl 2):51S–209S.
15. Ng M, Fleming T, Robinson M, et al. Global, regional, and national prevalence of overweight and obesity in children and adults during 1980–2013: a systematic analysis for the Global Burden of Disease Study 2013. *Lancet.* 2014;384(9945):766–781.
16. Via M. Adiposity-based chronic disease: a new diagnostic term. In Rippe JM (ed.) *Lifestyle Medicine* (3rd ed). Boca Raton, FL: CRC Press, 2019.
17. Jensen MD, Ryan DH, Apovian CM, et al. Guideline for the management of overweight and obesity in adults: a report of the American College of Cardiology/American Heart Association Task Force on Practice Guidelines and The Obesity Society. *Circulation.* 2014;129(25 Suppl 2):S102–S138.
18. Hall K, Sacks G, Chandramohan D, et al. Quantification of the effect of energy imbalance on bodyweight. *Lancet* 2011:378(9793):826–837.
19. Hall K, Chow C. Estimating the quantitative relation between food energy intake and changes in body weight. *Am J Clin Nutr.* 2010;91(3):816; Author Reply 817.
20. Hall KD, Sacks G, Chandramohan D, et al. Quantification of the effect of energy imbalance on bodyweight. *Lancet.* 2011;378(9793):826–837.
21. McAllister E, Dhurandhar N, Keith S., et al. Ten putative contributors to the obesity epidemic. *Crit Rev Food Sci Nutr.* 2009;49(10):868–913.
22. Emanuel EJ, Dellgren JL, McCoy MS, et al. Fair allocation of GLP-1 and dual GLP-1–GIP receptor agonists. *N Engl J Med.* 2024;390(20):1839–1842.
23. Zhang Y, Proenca R, Maffei M, et al. Positional cloning of the mouse obese gene and its human homologue. *Nature.* 1994;372(6505):425–432.
24. Green ED, Maffei M, Braden VV, et al. The human obese (OB) gene: RNA expression pattern and mapping on the physical, cytogenetic, and genetic maps of chromosome 7. *Genome Res.* 1995;5(1):5–12.
25. Olefsky J. Obesity. In Isselbacher K, Braunwald E, Wilson J, et al. (eds.) *Harrison's Principles of Internal Medicine* (13th ed). New York: McGraw-Hill, 1994, pp. 446–452.
26. Zurlo F, Larson K, Bogardus C. et al. Skeletal muscle metabolism is a major determinant of resting energy expenditure. *J Clin Invest.* 1990;86:1423–1427.
27. Clemente J, Ursell L, Parfrey L. et al. The impact of the gut microbiota on human health: an integrative view. *Cell.* 2012;148(6):1258–1270.
28. Kershaw E, Flier J. Adipose tissue as an endocrine organ. *J Clin Endocrinol Metab.* 2004;89(6):2548–2556.
29. Ravussin E, Lillioja S, Knowler WC, et al. Reduced rate of energy expenditure as a risk factor for body-weight gain. *N Engl J Med.* 1988;318(8):467–472.
30. Neel J. Diabetes mellitus: a "thrifty" genotype rendered detrimental by progress? *Am J Hum Genet.* 1962;14:353–362.
31. Montague C, Farooqi I, Whitehead J, et al. Congenital leptin deficiency is associated with severe early-onset obesity in humans. *Nature.* 1997;387:903–908.
32. Farooqi I, O'Rahilly S. Monogenic obesity in Humans. *Ann Rev Med.* 2005;56:443–458.
33. DiPietro L, Dziura J, Blair S. Estimated change in physical activity level (PAL) and prediction of 5-year weight change in men: the aerobics center longitudinal study. *Int J Obes.* 2004;28:1541–1547.
34. Lee I, Djousse L, Sesso H, et al. Physical activity and weight gain prevention. *JAMA.* 2010;303:1173–1179.
35. Shiroma E, Sesso H, Lee I. Physical activity and weight gain prevention in older men. *Int J Obes.* 2012;36:1165–1169.
36. Donnelly JE, Blair SN, Jakicic JM, et al. American College of Sports Medicine Position Stand. Appropriate physical activity intervention strategies for weight loss and prevention of weight regain for adults. *Med Sci Sports Exerc.* 2009;41(2):459–471.
37. Physical Activity Guidelines Advisory Committee. 2018 Physical Activity Guidelines Advisory Committee. 2018 Physical Activity Guidelines Advisory Committee Scientific Report. Washington, DC: U.S. Department of Health and Human Services, 2018.
38. Lloyd-Jones DM, Allen NB, Anderson CAM, et al. Life's essential 8: updating and enhancing the American Heart Association's construct of cardiovascular health: a presidential advisory from the American Heart Association. *Circulation.* 2022;146(5):e18–e43.
39. Jakicic JM, Rogers RJ, Davis KK, et al. Role of physical activity and exercise in treating patients with overweight and obesity. *Clin Chem.* 2018;64(1):99–107.
40. Jakicic J. Exercise management for the patient with obesity. In: Rippe J (ed.) *Lifestyle Medicine* (4th ed). Boca Raton, FL: CRC Press, 2024.
41. Bouchard C, Tremblay A, Despres J, et al. The response to exercise with constant energy intake in identical twins. *Obes Res.* 1994;2:400–410.

42. Finlayson G, Bryant E, Blundell J, et al. Acute compensatory eating following exercise is associated with implicit hedonic wanting for food. *Physiol Behav.* 2009;97:62–67.
43. Ross R, Dagnone D, Jones P, et al. Reduction in obesity and related comorbid conditions after diet-induced weight loss or exercise-induced weight loss in men. *Ann Intern Med.* 2000;133:92–103.
44. Stevens J, Cai J, Evenson K, et al. Fitness and fatness as predictors of mortality from all causes and from cardiovascular disease in men and women in the lipid research clinics study. *Am J Epidemiol.* 2002;156:832–841.
45. Rankinen T, Church T, Rice T, et al. Cardiorespiratory fitness, BMI, and risk of hypertension: the hypgene study. *Med Sci Sports Exerc.* 2007;39:1687–1692.
46. Kelley G, Kelley K, Tran Z. Aerobic exercise, lipids and lipoproteins in overweight and obese adults: a meta-analysis of randomized controlled trials. *Int J Obes.* 2005;29:881–893.
47. Van Gaal L, Mertens I, DeBlock C. Mechanisms linking obesity with cardiovascular disease. *Nature.* 2006;444:875–880.
48. Church T, Earnest C, Thompson A, et al. Exercise without weight loss does not reduce C-reactive protein: the inflame study. *Med Sci Sports Exerc.* 2010;42:708–716.
49. Nicklas B, Ambrosius W, Messier S, et al. Diet-induced weight loss, exercise, and chronic inflammation in older, obese adults: a randomized controlled clinical trial. *Am J Clin Nutr.* 2004;79:544–551.
50. Crowley N, Arlinghaus KR. Dietary management of overweight and obesity. In Rippe J (ed.) *Lifestyle Medicine* (4th ed). Boca Raton, FL: CRC Press, 2024.
51. Academy of Nutrition and Dietetics Evidence Analysis Library. Adult Weight Management: Executive Summary of Recommendations 2014. Academy of Nutrition and Dietetics. https://www.andeal.org/topic.cfm?menu=5276&cat=4690. Accessed February 14, 2025.
52. Mifflin MD, St Jeor ST, Hill LA, et al. A new predictive equation for resting energy expenditure in healthy individuals. *Am J Clin Nutr.* 1990;51(2):241–247.
53. Jensen MD, Ryan DH, Apovian CM, et al. 2013 AHA/ACC/TOS guideline for the management of overweight and obesity in adults: a report of the American College of Cardiology/American Heart Association Task Force on Practice Guidelines and The Obesity Society. *J Am Coll Cardiol.* 2014;63 (25 Pt B):2985–3023.
54. Estruch R, Ros E, Salas-Salvado J, et al. Primary prevention of cardiovascular disease with a mediterranean diet. *N Engl J Med.* 2013;368(14):1279–1290.
55. Sacks FM, Svetkey LP, Vollmer WM, et al. Effects on blood pressure of reduced dietary sodium and the Dietary Approaches to Stop Hypertension (DASH) diet. DASH-Sodium Collaborative Research Group. *N Engl J Med.* 2001;344(1):3–10.
56. Raynor HA, Champagne CM. Position of the academy of nutrition and dietetics: interventions for the treatment of overweight and obesity in adults. *J Acad Nutr Diet.* 2016;116(1):129–147.
57. Patel S, Hu F. Short sleep duration and weight gain: a systematic review. *Obesity.* 2008;16(3):643–653.
58. Baker RC, Kirschenbaum DS. Self-monitoring may be necessary for success weight control. *Behav Ther.* 1993;24:377–394.
59. Wing RR, Tate DF, Gorin AA, et al. A self-regulation program for maintenance of weight loss. *N Engl J Med.* 2006;355(15):1563–1571.
60. Foreyt JP. Behavioral management for the patient with obesity. In Rippe J, Foreyt J (eds.) *Obesity Prevention and Treatment: A Practical Guide.* Boca Raton, FL: CRC Press, 2021.
61. Fabricatore AN. Behavior therapy and cognitive-behavioral therapy of obesity: is there a difference? *J Am Diet Assoc.* 2007;107(1):92–99.
62. Berkel LA, Poston WSC, Reeves RS, et al. Behavioral interventions for obesity. *J Am Diet Assoc.* 2005;105:S35–S43.
63. Marlatt GA, Gordon JR. *Relapse Prevention.* New York: Guilford Press, 1985.
64. Anton SD., Foreyt JP, Perri MG. Preventing weight regain after weight loss. In Bray G, Bouchard C (eds.) *Handbook of Obesity: Clinical implications* (4th ed). New York: Taylor & Francis, 2009.
65. Garvey WT, Mechanick JI, Brett EM et al. American Association of Clinical Endocrinologists and American College of Endocrinology Comprehensive Clinical Practice Guidelines for Medical Care of Patients with Obesity. *Endocr Pract.* 2016;22(Suppl 3):1–203.
66. Kang, JH, Le, QA. Effectiveness of bariatric surgical procedures. A systematic review and network meta-analysis of randomized controlled trials. *Medicine.* 2017;96(46):e8632.
67. Lloyd-Jones D, Hong Y, Labarthe D, et al. American Heart Association Strategic Planning Task Force and Statistics Committee. Defining and setting national goals for cardiovascular health promotion and disease reduction: the American Heart Association's strategic impact goal through 2020 and beyond. *Circulation.* 2010;121:586–613.

68. Eckel R, Jakicic J, Ard J, et al. 2013 AHA/ACC guideline on lifestyle management to reduce cardiovascular risk: a report of the American College of Cardiology/American Heart Association Task Force on Practice Guidelines. *Circulation.* 2014;129(25 suppl 2):S76–S99.
69. Whelton PK, Carey RM, Aronow WS, et al. 2017 ACC/AHA/AAPA/ABC/ACPM/AGS/APhA/ASH/ASPC/NMA/PCNA guideline for the prevention, detection, evaluation, and management of high blood pressure in adults: executive summary: a report of the American College of Cardiology/American Heart Association Task Force on Clinical Practice Guidelines. *Hypertension.* 2018;71(6):1269–1324.
70. Grundy SM, Stone NJ, Bailey AL, et al. 2018 AHA/ACC/AACVPR/AAPA/ABC/ACPM/ADA/AGS/APhA/ASPC/NLA/PCNA guideline on the management of blood cholesterol: a report of the American College of Cardiology/American Heart Association Task Force on Clinical Practice Guidelines. *Circulation.* 2019;139(25):e1082–e143.
71. Sul H. Resistin/ADSF/FIZZ3 in obesity and diabetes. *Trends Endocrinol Metab.* 2004;15:247–249.
72. Goossens G. The role of adipose tissue dysfunction in the pathogenesis of obesity-related insulin resistance. *Physiol Behav.* 2008;94:206–218.
73. Full Plate Living. https://www.fullplateliving.org/. Accessed February 14, 2025.

13 The Metabolic Syndrome

13.1 INTRODUCTION

The metabolic syndrome (MetS) is a grouping of physiologic variables involving hypertension, dyslipidemia, hyperglycemia, and elevated adiposity, particularly central adiposity (1–9). The common underlying etiology for MetS is insulin resistance. Increased availability of tests to measure insulin, as well as other blood constituents, has led to increased diagnosis and better understanding of MetS.

The rising prevalence of MetS has correlated with a surge in obesity rates and suggests that obesity is a key underlying etiology, at least in some situations of MetS (1,2,8,9). Many individuals, however, who have MetS are not obese, and there are many individuals who are obese who do not have MetS. Nonetheless, MetS is an extremely important condition and is not diagnosed often enough by clinicians, despite the fact that it is a significant risk factor for both cardiovascular disease (CVD) and type 2 diabetes (T2DM) (1,10).

Of note, various lifestyle medicine modalities such as increased physical activity (11,12), healthy diet (13), weight loss (for those who are overweight or obese), restorative sleep, stress reduction, and positive interaction with others are all important components in the treatment of MetS and will be discussed in some detail in this chapter.

13.2 THE ELUSIVE DEFINITION OF METABOLIC SYNDROME

A number of different definitions have been utilized to describe the clustering of risk factors, which are components of MetS (14–21). Clinical characteristics of MetS include increased waist circumference, which reflects excess abdominal adiposity, impaired fasting glucose (IFG), elevated triglyceride concentration, low high-density lipoprotein (HDL) cholesterol, and high blood pressure. Despite the fact that many physicians do not routinely diagnose MetS, it is clearly an important diagnosis to make. MetS provides important underlying pathophysiologic linkage between obesity, T2DM, and CVD risk (1,8,9,22). In fact, the Third National Cholesterol Education Program (NCEP) Adult Treatment Panel III (ATP III) states that individuals with MetS should be treated as though they already have cardiovascular disease (21). Moreover, MetS is useful because once it is diagnosed, it emphasizes in clinical practice the importance of primary prevention strategies, particularly the key components of lifestyle habits and actions that can be utilized to treat all of the components of MetS.

While a variety of different definitions and criteria have been posed for MetS, the NCEP Panel III (NCEP-ATP III) published the criteria in 2001 that are most frequently used for determining MetS (21). The NCEP-ATP III criteria concluded that if three of five abnormalities were observed, then MetS was defined to be present. The five abnormalities are as follows:

- *Large Waist Circumference*: Greater than 102 cm (40 in) in men and greater than 88 cm (greater than 35 in) in women.
- *Impaired Fasting Glucose*: Greater than 100 mg/dL
- *Elevated Triglycerides*: Greater than 150 mg/dL
- *Elevated Blood Pressure*: Greater than or equal to 130/85 mm Hg
- *Low HDL Cholesterol*: Less than 40 mg/dL for men and less than 50 mg/dL for women

The clinical features of the metabolic syndrome are found in Table 13.1. These criteria are very similar to those issued shortly after the NCEP-ATP III Guidelines (21) by the American Heart Association (AHA) (1) and the National Heart, Lung, and Blood Institute (NHLBI) (1).

DOI: 10.1201/9781003630043-13

TABLE 13.1
Clinical Features of the Metabolic Syndrome

Risk Factor	Defining Level
Abdominal obesity (waist circumference)	
Men	>102 cm (>40 in)
Women	>88 cm (>35 in)
HDL cholesterol	
Men	<40 mg/dL
Women	<50 mg/dL
Triglycerides	>150 mg/dL
Fasting glucose	>100 mg/dL
Blood pressure (systolic/diastolic)	>130/>85 mmHg

Source: From National Cholesterol Education Program (NCEP) ATP III Criteria for the Metabolic Syndrome (MetS). US Department of Health and Human Services, NIH Document 01-3670. May 2001.

HDL, high density lipoprotein.

It should be noted that MetS is not an individual entity. Rather, it is a syndrome with multiple components. It is clear that MetS itself represents a significant risk factor for both atherosclerotic cardiovascular disease (ASCVD) and T2DM. The risk factors for these two conditions, however, have a significant overlap and may be slightly different. Patients with MetS are at increased risk for developing both T2DM and ASCVD (1). The underlying risk factors for those two diseases are based on metabolic risk factors. Both underlying risk factors and metabolic risk factors are relevant to the condition of MetS, although the fact that there are multiple risk factors and metabolic risk factors has led to some confusion and various definitions of what exactly MetS consists of.

13.3 EPIDEMIOLOGY OF THE METABOLIC SYNDROME IN THE UNITED STATES

The prevalence of MetS varies considerably depending on the definition used. Utilizing the NCEP-ATP III criteria, the prevalence of MetS increased from 23% to 27% in adult Americans aged 20 or over, based on National Health and Nutrition Examination Survey (NHANES) data (1988–1994 and 1999–2000) (21). Subsequently, Ford and Dietz estimated higher rates of MetS (34.5%–39%) in adults. This represents over 70 million adults living with MetS by NCEP-ATP III criteria (14,23).

Increases in overweight and obesity over the past 40 years have strongly correlated with the increased prevalence of MetS. Overweight and obesity greatly influence the prevalence of MetS since this condition occurs principally in individuals who are obese or overweight. It is important to point out, however, that not all individuals who are overweight or obese have MetS, and individuals who are not overweight or obese also may have MetS (24,25). For example, in 1999–2004 NHANES data, 23.5% of normal-weight individuals were found to have two or more cardiometabolic abnormalities compared to 49.7% of individuals who are overweight and 69.3% of adults with obesity (26). These data are important given that, according to Framingham data, the majority of heart disease occurs in individuals who have two or more risk factors (1).

MetS is also associated with age and ethnicity. MetS is estimated to occur in between 13% of men and 18% of women aged 20–39 years. Rates increase to 40% of men and 46% of women older than 60 years of age. MetS may also vary in some ethnic groups and is more prevalent in women than in men. A 57% higher prevalence of MetS was observed in African American women than in men, and 26% greater in Mexican American women compared to men of the same ethnicity (2).

MetS is more prevalent in those who engage in little or no physical activity and occurs more frequently with greater carbohydrate consumption and reduced fiber intake (11).

13.4 UNDERLYING RISK FACTORS FOR METABOLIC SYNDROME

The significant underlying risk factors for MetS appear to be abdominal obesity and insulin resistance (27–29). Other associated conditions include physical inactivity, aging, hormonal imbalance, and an atherogenic diet (e.g., a diet rich in saturated fat and cholesterol). While this diet enhances the risk of developing ASCVD in individuals who have MetS, the diet is not listed specifically as an underlying risk factor in the condition.

In addition, there is consensus that insulin resistance predisposes to hyperglycemia and T2DM (30). Some investigators have proposed that compensatory hyperinsulinemia in response to insulin resistance should be considered a component of MetS.

All of these different conditions are compounded by the recognition that people who are not obese are less insulin-resistant. Although insulin-resistant individuals may not be clinically obese, they nevertheless typically have abnormal fat distribution characterized by predominant upper body fat, which correlates strongly with insulin resistance (31,32). It has also been argued that the fat that is contained around the organs (visceral fat) is more strongly associated with insulin resistance than any other compartment that contains adipose tissue (33). A strong correlation exists between upper body obesity and the accumulation of lipid in other sites other than adipose tissue, including muscle and liver, which also predisposes to not only insulin resistance but also dyslipidemia (34–37).

Nonetheless, an association clearly exists between obesity as a driving force behind the rising prevalence of the metabolic syndrome. It may be abnormalities in adipose tissue metabolism, however, that are the key issue. It should also be pointed out that individuals who do not seem to have insulin resistance can develop the metabolic syndrome if they have marked abdominal obesity (32). This supports the concept that body fat distribution, particularly excess abdominal fat, is a central component of the etiology of MetS.

It should also be noted that a strong association exists between MetS and chronic low-grade inflammation (38). This is thought to be caused by inflammatory cytokines generated by adipocytes, which contribute to insulin resistance. Of note, insulin-resistant people can have low-grade inflammation even without an increase in body fat. It should also be noted that individual and ethnic variations occur in the clinical pattern of risk factors in obese/insulin-resistant patients. For example, many South Asians appear to be inherently insulin resistant (39). A further complication arises in that even though MetS is a significant risk factor for T2DM, T2DM is a significant risk factor for ASCVD (40).

13.5 METABOLIC RISK FACTORS, ASCVD, T2DM

One of the key components of MetS is atherogenic dyslipidemia, including elevated serum triglycerides, increased small LDL particles, and reduced levels of HDL. A number of studies have suggested that small LDL particles are particularly atherogenic (41). The other metabolic risk factors, such as hypertension and elevated plasma glucose, as well as a prothrombotic state and proinflammatory state, are also metabolic risk factors. In addition, elevated plasma glucose may also promote atherosclerosis and, as already mentioned, the development of T2DM makes MetS an even higher risk for ASCVD.

13.6 CONTROVERSIES IN METS IN SCIENCE AND MEDICINE

Controversies exist concerning MetS as to whether or not insulin resistance can be seen as the unifying cause of the syndrome (24,42,43). It has been estimated that only 48% of people with insulin resistance have MetS. This may be a result of the ability of physiologic processes to compensate for impaired insulin or glucose uptake. On the other hand, 78% of patients who meet criteria for MetS diagnosis have insulin resistance (43,44). These data suggest that the underlying causes of MetS are more complicated than simply insulin resistance or compensatory hyperinsulinemia.

With regard to obesity, there are between 29% and 35% of individuals with obesity who do not qualify for MetS and between 21% and 30% of normal-weight individuals who would be classified as having MetS (24,43). These data suggest that although obesity does increase cardiometabolic risk, it does not necessarily result in metabolic dysfunction.

13.7 PATHOPHYSIOLOGY

Location and types of fat are strongly related to insulin resistance. Some fat deposits, such as gynoid or subcutaneous adipose tissue, may actually prevent the development of insulin resistance and MetS (44).

Visceral fat, however, which is the type of fat found around the internal organs, is associated with insulin resistance and development of cardiovascular and metabolic dysfunction (45–47). In addition, excess fat may accumulate in sites not well suited to store fat, such as the liver, skeleton, cardiac muscle, pancreas, and kidney (34,25,48). These ectopic fat deposits greatly contribute to insulin resistance and also disturb glucose and lipid metabolism, contributing to inflammation and heightened oxidative stress.

This type of metabolic reaction also occurs in visceral fat. In adipose tissue, insulin creates expression of non-esterified fatty acids (NEFAs) mobilization and secretion is dampened, which results in systemic metabolic dysfunction and compensatory hyperinsulinemia, hyperglycemia, elevated NEFAs, and chronic low-grade inflammation. The oversupply of NEFAs also facilitates triglyceride synthesis and enhanced production of triglyceride-rich very-low-density-lipoprotein (VLDL). Ectopic liver fat also potentiates the transfer of triglycerides from VLDL to HDL and results in the formation of small dense LDL, which readily penetrates the vascular endothelium (49,50). The reduction in HDL and altered HDL composition further impairs reverse cholesterol transport and contributes to dyslipidemia, vascular dysfunction, and ASCVD. Thus, the molecular pathophysiology of obesity, insulin resistance, and MetS is related to adverse cardiovascular risk factors and health outcomes and is quite complex.

13.8 RELATIONSHIP OF METS TO OTHER CHRONIC DISEASES

There is widespread scientific agreement that MetS predicts high risk of CVD and T2DM. In a meta-analysis of 87 studies involving 951,083 patients, overall CVD risk was 2.3 times greater in those with MetS (51). Another meta-analysis of 37 longitudinal studies involving 172,573 patients reported a greater risk of CVD in participants with MetS than in those without this syndrome (52).

In an analysis of 16 cohorts involving 42,419 patients with MetS, there was a consistently strong association with T2DM (53). Whether or not the grouping of metabolic factors in MetS is superior to predicting future CVD and T2DM than these individual components remains elusive and is subject to ongoing debate.

- *Non-alcoholic Fatty Liver Disease*: A similar pathophysiology that links MetS to obesity is also involved in non-alcoholic fatty liver disease (NAFLD). NAFLD has risen dramatically in the past 20 years in both obesity and MetS (54). NAFLD is now the leading cause of liver failure and liver transplantation in the world. Greater than 5% of the volume of fat in the liver defines steatosis, and 30% fat is the cutoff for liver transplantation donors (55). The presence of fatty liver in persons with a Body Mass Index (BMI) greater than 30 kg/m^2 is estimated to be twice that of the general population (56,57). Visceral adiposity, as already indicated, interacts through a complex series of physiologic changes and is correlated with hepatic fat since the liver is one of the ectopic locations of excess fat deposition. NAFLD is also clearly associated with T2DM.

How NAFLD develops is not completely understood, but it has been posited that dysregulation of fatty acid metabolism (resulting in lipotoxicity by hepatocyte necrosis), followed by oxidative stress and an increase in inflammatory markers (58), underlies NAFLD. Visceral adipose tissue accounts for the state of low-grade inflammation in 75% of patients (59). Blood triglyceride levels greater than 150 mg/dL are often present in NAFLD. The underlying pathophysiology in NAFLD is that the hepatic portal vein collects venous blood from the stomach, small intestines, pancreas, spleen, and drains the omental and mesenteric adipose tissue associated with these organs (60). Thus, the tendency of visceral abdominal fat to store triglycerides and release fatty acids directly affects the liver.

13.9 THE ROLE OF LIFESTYLE MODALITIES IN THE TREATMENT AND MANAGEMENT OF METABOLIC SYNDROME

The goal of managing MetS is to reduce the global risk of ASCVD, T2DM, and other metabolic diseases. Thus, the goal should be the reduction of the severity and number of traditional risk factors for ASCVD and T2DM. There is no specific pharmaceutical therapy available for MetS. However, a cluster of lifestyle behaviors, including a healthy diet, increased physical activity, and weight loss, can act synergistically to lower the risk of MetS evolving into ASCVD and T2DM and also reduce the likelihood of fat accumulation in the liver turning into NAFLD (61–64).

For all these reasons, therapy for individuals with MetS includes regular physical activity, consumption of a heart-healthy diet, weight loss, and prevention of weight regain after weight loss. MetS itself can be mitigated with these lifestyle behaviors when they are consistently practiced. In addition, efforts should be made to quit smoking, improve stress management, and practice behavioral strategies to enhance lifelong adherence to these healthy lifestyle changes.

In this book and in the embedded curriculum, we have emphasized throughout the importance of following the recommendations from the Physical Activity Guidelines for Americans 2018 (PAGA 2018), which involve accumulating 30 minutes of moderate-intensity physical activity on at least five out of seven days (12). In addition, we have focused attention on healthy diets. These include the Mediterranean diet (65), DASH diet (66), and US Healthy Eating Style (13). All of these are anti-inflammatory diets. They all contain abundant fruits and vegetables, whole grain, fish, fiber, and nuts, and all have been shown to lower the risk of cardiovascular disease. These diets should be followed in the overall treatment of MetS.

Since obesity is implicated in many individuals who have MetS, healthy weight loss is also critically important, as is quitting smoking and lowering stress, utilizing the techniques outlined in Chapter 4. Following the behavioral recommendations to enhance adherence to these healthy lifestyle patterns, which we have outlined in Chapter 4, is also very important.

It should be emphasized that MetS carries both enhanced inflammatory potential and prothrombotic potential. As we have emphasized in multiple chapters throughout this book, inflammation is emerging as the underlying common denominator for many metabolic diseases, including ASCVD, T2DM, obesity, and even cancer and cognitive decline. MetS is also a proinflammatory condition, which is a major reason why it is such a prominent risk to evolve into ASCVD and T2DM (59). In addition, the issue of healthy sleep, which plays a prominent role in both ASCVD and T2DM, is an important component of the management of MetS and interacts with both regular physical activity and healthy nutrition (67).

13.10 CONCLUSIONS/CLINICAL APPLICATIONS

The metabolic syndrome is a clustering of risk factors with an underlying etiology involving components of obesity, particularly upper-body (abdominal) obesity, insulin resistance, hyperglycemia, and atherogenic risk factors such as low HDL and elevated triglycerides. MetS is a significant risk factor for both ASCVD and T2DM. Lifestyle modalities such as increased physical activity, a healthy diet, weight loss (if necessary), healthy sleep, and stress reduction are all key components of treating MetS itself and lowering its risk of advancing into other metabolic conditions such as ASCVD, T2DM, and NAFLD. Strategies for maintaining these healthy lifestyle practices are found throughout this book and in the embedded curriculum.

REFERENCES

1. Grundy SM, Cleeman JI, Daniels SR, et al. Diagnosis and management of the metabolic syndrome. *Circulation*. 2005;112(17):2735–2752.
2. Walton C, Lees B, Crook D, Godsland IF, Stevenson JC. Relationships between insulin metabolism, serum lipid profile, body fat distribution and blood pressure in healthy men. *Atherosclerosis*. 1995;118(1):35–43.
3. Eckel RH, Grundy SM, Zimmet PZ. The metabolic syndrome. *Lancet*. 2005;365(9468):1415–1428.
4. Mohamed SM, Shalaby MA, El-Shiekh RA, et al. Metabolic syndrome: risk factors, diagnosis, pathogenesis, and management with natural approaches. *Food Chem Adv*. 2023;3:100335.
5. Neeland IJ, Lim S, Tchernof A, et al. Metabolic syndrome. *Nat Rev Dis Primers*. 2024;10(1):77.
6. Fahed G, Aoun L, Bou Zerdan M, et al. Metabolic syndrome: updates on pathophysiology and management in 2021. *Int J Mol Sci*. 2022;23(2):786.
7. Grandjean P. Obesity and the metabolic syndrome. In Rippe J, Angelopoulos T (eds.) *Obesity: Prevention and Treatment* (1st ed). Boca Raton, FL: CRC Press, 2012, pp. 311–341.
8. Rippe J. Beyond subcutaneous fat. In Rippe J, Angelopoulos T (eds.) *Obesity: Prevention and Treatment* (1st ed). Boca Raton, FL: CRC Press, 2012.
9. Rippe J. Obesity and the metabolic syndrome. In Rippe J, Angelopoulos T (eds.) *Obesity: Prevention and Treatment* (1st ed). Boca Raton, FL: CRC Press, 2012.
10. Rippe JM. Lifestyle medicine and GLP-1 therapy for obesity: time to get real. *Am J Lifestyle Med*. 2025 (in press).
11. Chomiuk T, Niezgoda N, Mamcarz A, Sliz D. Physical activity in metabolic syndrome. *Front Physiol*. 2024;15:1365761.
12. Physical Activity Guidelines Advisory Committee. 2018 Physical Activity Guidelines Advisory Committee. 2018 Physical Activity Guidelines Advisory Committee Scientific Report. Washington, DC: U.S. Department of Health and Human Services, 2018.
13. U.S. Department of Health and Human Services and U.S. Department of Agriculture. 2020–2025 Dietary Guidelines for Americans. 9th edition. 2020, p. 164.
14. Ford E. Increasing prevalence of the metabolic syndrome among U.S. adults. *Diabetes Care*. 2004;27:2444–2449.
15. Ford E. Prevalence of the metabolic syndrome defined by the International Diabetes Federation among adults in the U.S. *Diabetes Care*. 2005;28:2745–2749.
16. Ford E, Zhao G. Prevalence and correlates of metabolic syndrome based on a harmonious definition among adults in the U.S. *J Diabetes*. 2010;3:180–193.
17. Rasouli N, Molavi B, Elbien S, et al. Ectopic fat accumulation and metabolic syndrome. *Diabetes Obes Metab*. 2007;9:1–10.
18. Koh K, Han S, Quon M. Inflammatory markers and the metabolic syndrome. *Insights from therapeutic interventions. J Am Coll Cardiol*. 2005;46:1978–1985.
19. Alberti K, Eckel R, Grundy S, et al. Harmonizing the Metabolic Syndrome. A joint interm statement of the International Diabetes Federation Task Force on Epidemiology and Prevention; National Heart, Lung, Blood Institute; American Heart Association; World Heart Federation; International Atherosclerosis Society; and International Association for the Study of Obesity. *Circulation*. 2009;120:1640–1645.
20. Alberti K, Zimmet P, Shaw J. Metabolic syndrome: a new worldwide definition. A consensus statement from the International Diabetes Federation. *Diabet Med*. 2006;23:469–480.
21. National Cholesterol Education Program. Executive Summary of the Third Report of the National Cholesterol Education Program (NCEP) Expert Panel on Detection, Evaluation and Treatment of High Blood Cholesterol in Adults (Adult Treatment Panel III). *JAMA*. 2001;285:2486–2497.
22. Grundy SM. Obesity, metabolic syndrome, and cardiovascular disease. *J Clin Endocrinol Metab*. 2004;89(6):2595–600.
23. Ford E, Giles W, Dietz W. Prevalence of the metabolic syndrome among U.S. adults. Findings from the third National Health and Nutrition Examination Survey. *JAMA*. 2002;287:356–359.

24. Stefan N, Kantartzis K, Machann J, et al. Identification and characterization of metabolically benign obesity in humans. *Arch Intern Med.* 2008;168:1609–1616.
25. Wildman R, Munter P, Reynolds K, et al. The obese without cardiometabolic risk factor clustering and the normal weight with cardiometabolic risk factor clustering. *Arch Intern Med.* 2008;168:1617–1624.
26. Park Y, Zhu S, Palaniappan L, et al. The metabolic syndrome: prevalence and associated risk factor findings in the U.S. population from the third National Health and Nutrition Examination Survey, 1988–1994. *Arch Intern Med.* 2003;163:427–436.
27. Miyazaki, Y., DeFronzo, R.A. Visceral fat dominant distribution in male type 2 diabetic patients is closely related to hepatic insulin resistance, irrespective of body type. *Cardiovasc Diabetol.* 2009;8:44. doi:10.1186/1475-2840-8-44.
28. Carr DB, Utzschneider KM, Hull RL, et al. Intra-abdominal fat is a major determinant of the National Cholesterol Education Program Adult Treatment Panel III criteria for the metabolic syndrome. *Diabetes.* 2004;53(8):2087–2094.
29. Reaven G. The metabolic syndrome or the insulin resistance syndrome? Different names, different concepts, and different goals. *Endocrinol Metab Clin North Am.* 2004;33(2):283–303.
30. Le Roith D, Zick Y. Recent advances in our understanding of insulin action and insulin resistance. *Diabetes Care.* 2001;24:588–597.
31. Lakka T, Lakka H, Salonen R, et al. Abdominal obesity is associated with accelerated progression of carotid atherosclerosis in men. *Atheroscler.* 2001;154:497–504.
32. Despres J, Lemieux I. Abdominal obesity and metabolic syndrome. *Nature.* 2006;444:881–887.
33. Despres J. Cardiovascular disease under the influence of excess visceral fat. *Crit Pathways Cardiol.* 2007;6:51–59.
34. Eckhardt K, Taube A, Eckel J. Obesity-associated insulin resistance in skeletal muscle: role of lipid accumulation and physical inactivity. *Rev Endocr Metab Disord.* 2011;12(3):163–172.
35. Meijer R, Serne E, Smulders Y, et al. Perivascular adipose tissue and its role in type 2 diabetes and cardiovascular disease. *Curr Diab Rep.* 2011;11:211–217.
36. Lakka H, Laaksonen DE, Lakka TA, et al. The metabolic syndrome and total and cardiovascular disease mortality in middle-aged men. *JAMA.* 2002;288(21):2709–2716.
37. DeFronzo RA. Pathogenesis of type 2 diabetes mellitus. *Med Clin North Am.* 2004;88(4):787–835.
38. Bremer AA, Devaraj S, Afify A, et al. Adipose tissue dysregulation in patients with metabolic syndrome. *J Clin Endocrinol Metab.* 2011;96(11):E1782–E1788.
39. Hill J, Sidney S, Lewis C, et al. Racial differences in amounts of visceral adipose tissue in young adults: the CARDIA (Coronary Artery Risk Development in Young Adults) Study. *Am J Clin Nutr.* 1999;69(3): 381–387.
40. Wilson PW, D'Agostino RB, Parise H, et al. Metabolic syndrome as a precursor of cardiovascular disease and type 2 diabetes mellitus. *Circulation.* 2005;112(20):3066–3072.
41. Stolar M. Metabolic syndrome: controversial but useful. *Cleveland Clin J Med.* 2007;74:199–208.
42. Kim S, Reaven G. The metabolic syndrome: one step forward, two steps back. *Diabetes Vasc Dis Res.* 2004;2:68–75.
43. McLaughlin T, Allison G, Abbasi F, et al. Prevalence of insulin resistance and associated cardiovascular disease risk factors among normal weight, overweight, and obese individuals. *Metabolism.* 2004;53:495–499.
44. Aguilera CM, Gil-Campos M, Canete R, et al. Alterations in plasma and tissue lipids associated with obesity and metabolic syndrome. *Clin Sci.* 2008;114(3):183–193.
45. Walton C, Lees B, Crook D, et al. Relationships between insulin metabolism, serum lipid profile, body fat distribution and blood pressure in healthy men. *Atherosclerosis* 1995;118(1):35–43.
46. Kahn B, Flier J. Obesity and insulin resistance. *J Clin Invest.* 2000;106(4):473–481.
47. Miyazaki Y, DeFronzo R. Visceral fat dominant distribution in male type 2 diabetic patients is closely related to hepatic insulin resistance, irrespective of body type. *Cardiovasc Diabetol.* 2009;(5)8:44.
48. Ohman MK, Wright AP, Wickenheiser KJ, et al. Visceral adipose tissue and atherosclerosis. *Curr Vasc Pharmacol.* 2009;7(2):169–179.
49. Adiels M, Taskinen M, Packard C, et al. Overproduction of VLDL particles is driven by increased liver fat content in man. *Diabetologia.* 2006;49:755–765.
50. Seppala-Lindroos A, Vehkavaara S, Hakkinen A, et al. Fat accumulation in the liver is associated with defects in insulin suppression of glucose production and serum free fatty acids independent of obesity in normal men. *J Clin Endocrinol Metab.* 2002;87:3023–3028.
51. Mottillo S, Filion K, Genest J, et al. The metabolic syndrome and cardiovascular risk. *J Am Coll Cardiol.* 2010;56:1113–1132.

52. Gami A, Witt B, Howard D, et al. Metabolic syndrome and risk of incident cardiovascular events and death. *J Am Coll Cardiol.* 2007;49:403–414.
53. Ford ES, Li C, Sattar N. Metabolic syndrome and incident diabetes: current state of the evidence. *Diabetes Care.* 2008;31(9):1898–1904.
54. Ludwig J, Viggiano T, McGill D, et al. Nonalcoholic steatohepatitis: Mayo Clinic experiences with a hitherto unnamed disease. *Mayo Clin Proc.* 1980;55(7):434–438.
55. Busuttil R, Tanaka K. The utility of marginal donors in liver transplantation. *Liver Transpl.* 2003;9(7):651–663.
56. Scheen AJ, Luyckx FH, Desaive C, et al. Severe/extreme obesity: a medical disease requiring a surgical treatment? *Acta Clin Belg.* 1999;54(3):154–161.
57. Gholam PM, Flancbaum L, Machan JT, et al. Nonalcoholic fatty liver disease in severely obese subjects. *Am J Gastroenterol.* 2007;102(2):399–408.
58. Buechler C, Wanninger J, Neumeier M, et al. A key adipokine in obesity related liver diseases. *World J Gastroenterol.* 2011;17(23):2801–2811.
59. Farb M, Bigornia S, Mott M, et al. Reduced adipose tissue inflammation represents an intermediate cardiometabolic phenotype in obesity. *J Am Coll Cardiol.* 2011;58(3):232–237.
60. Shah V, Kamath P. Portal hypertension and gastrointestinal bleeding. In Feldman M, Friedman LS, Brandt LJ (eds.) *Sleisenger and Fordtran's Gastrointestinal and Liver Disease: Pathophysiology, Diagnosis, Management.* Philadelphia, PA: Saunders Elsevier, 2010.
61. Busuttil RW, Tanaka K. The utility of marginal donors in liver transplantation. *Liver Transpl.* 2003;9(7):651–663.
62. Sagi R, Reif S, Neuman G, et al. Nonalcoholic fatty liver disease in overweight children and adolescents. *Acta Paediatrica.* 2007;96(8):1209–1213.
63. Day CP, James OF. Steatohepatitis: a tale of two "hits"? *Gastroenterology.* 1998;114(4):842–845.
64. Look Ahead Research Group, Wing RR. Long-term effects of a lifestyle intervention on weight and cardiovascular risk factors in individuals with type 2 diabetes mellitus: four-year results of the Look AHEAD trial. *Arch Intern Med.* 2010;170(17):1566–1575.
65. Estruch R, Ros E, Salas-Salvado J, et al. Primary prevention of cardiovascular disease with a mediterranean diet. *N Engl J Med.* 2013;368(14):1279–1290.
66. Sacks FM, Svetkey LP, Vollmer WM, et al. Effects on blood pressure of reduced dietary sodium and the Dietary Approaches to Stop Hypertension (DASH) diet. DASH-Sodium Collaborative Research Group. *N Engl J Med.* 2001;344(1):3–10.
67. Bonnet MH, Berry RB, Arand DL. Metabolism during normal, fragmented, and recovery sleep. *J Appl Physiol.* 1991;71(3):1112–1118.

14 Brain Health, Cognitive Function, Dementia Prevention

14.1 INTRODUCTION

A healthy brain is essential for a fulfilling life. Recent interest has emerged in ways to optimize brain health (1–10). Many lifestyle measures play an important role in maintaining brain health and avoiding decline or dementia.

The American Heart Association (AHA) and the American Stroke Association (ASA) have taken this a step further and issued a Presidential Advisory entitled "Optimizing Brain Health" (8). Many components of brain health and avoiding cognitive decline will be discussed in this chapter.

Cognitive function, a key component of brain health, is essential for maintaining a good quality of life and functional independence. Good cognitive function is also an important component of healthy aging. As life expectancy continues to increase in developed countries, the number of individuals over the age of 65 will increase dramatically over the next 15–20 years. This makes maintaining good brain health a worldwide health imperative. Currently, there are an estimated 50 million people with dementia worldwide, and this is projected to increase to 75 million individuals by 2030 and 131 million individuals by 2050 (11). Linkages between brain health and cardiovascular health are very strong. The same measures that promote good cardiovascular health also play a vital role in maintaining good brain health. This is the central synergy that is underscored and articulated by the Presidential Advisory on "Defining Optimal Brain Health in Adults."

Positive lifestyle measures play central roles in maintaining a healthy brain and good cognitive function for a lifetime. The same lifestyle factors that compromise cardiovascular health may also compromise brain health. These include uncontrolled hypertension, type 2 diabetes mellitus (T2DM), obesity, physical inactivity, smoking, and depression (12). All of these can be potentially ameliorated by the seven components of healthy lifestyle medicine, which we have discussed in this book. These are also among those measures included in the Presidential Advisory from the AHA and ASA (8).

It should also be noted that many of the manifestations of the spectrum of cognition, ranging from good cognition to diminished cognition and dementia, occur in individuals in their 50s and 60s and beyond. Most research now suggests that paying close attention to risk factors throughout a lifetime is important to lessen the likelihood of cognitive decline in individuals in their 50s and 60s and beyond.

Among these measures, regular physical activity (7,9,13) and healthy nutrition (6) play particularly prominent roles. The benefits of both regular physical activity and healthy, plant-forward nutrition are prominent throughout the lifespan and will be emphasized in this chapter.

Lifestyle measures that we focus on in this book and in the embedded curriculum include weight management, stress reduction, avoiding addictive substances such as cigarettes and alcohol, and engaging in positive relationships with other people. All of these have been shown to be relevant for maintaining brain health and diminishing the likelihood of cognitive decline.

14.2 DEFINITION OF BRAIN HEALTH

An agreed-upon definition of brain health has been elusive (14,15). At the current time, there is a major bias in the scientific literature toward brain injury and disease. Part of the problem with discussing brain health is that there are multiple definitions. Perhaps the one most widely used comes

DOI: 10.1201/9781003630043-14

from the World Health Organization (WHO), which defines brain health as the "promotion of optimal brain development, cognitive health, and well-being across the life course" (16). Some investigators have included the element of connectedness to other people and life purpose and emphasize that brain health is a continuous process rather than a fixed state, which incorporates the evidence of lifelong neuroplasticity.

The relationship between brain health and mental health creates further confusion. Brain health includes mental health but does not replace it (17). Unlike brain health, mental health does not usually embrace cognitive and social connections.

Brain health is highly relevant to the issues of lifestyle medicine that are discussed in this book and the embedded curriculum. This is due to the fact that many lifestyle factors impact the risk of cognitive decline and are also important in maintaining brain health. Thus, we will utilize the WHO definition of brain health in this chapter.

14.3 OPTIMAL BRAIN HEALTH

The Presidential Advisory from the AHA and ASA defines optimal brain health as "the optimal capacity to function adaptively in an environment" (8). This advisory goes on to state that optimum brain health can be assessed in competencies across the domains of "thinking, moving, and feeling" and can be operationally defined and measured. Optimal brain health may be affected by the environment, behaviors and disease, which are potentially modifiable if changes are detected early enough. The AHA/ASA Presidential Advisory goes on to state that optimal brain health should be viewed as the equivalent of "vital signs of the brain." It is important to emphasize that this definition of optimal brain health is broader than the mere absence of overt vascular or neurodegenerative injury and is analogous to the emerging definition of optimal cardiovascular health. Indeed, the two concepts share many of the same risk factors.

14.4 COGNITIVE DECLINE AND DEMENTIA

In contrast to optimal brain health, cognitive impairment can ultimately be a function of poor brain health, which can be manifested as cognitive impairment or dementia. These underlying disorders include Alzheimer's disease (AD), stroke, other causes of vascular impairment, brain trauma, and other neurodegenerative disorders (5).

In the United States, it has been estimated that 6.9 million people are living with AD. The total number of people living with all forms of dementia is difficult to quantify but is likely to be much higher. Modifiable risk factors for dementia are similar to those for poor cardiovascular health and include uncontrolled hypertension, T2DM, obesity, physical inactivity, smoking, and depression.

Cognitive impairment is much more prevalent than dementia. It has been estimated that one in eight adults over the age of 60 has memory loss, and approximately 35% of individuals in this age range report functional difficulties. In addition, it is estimated that there are 6.9 million individuals in the United States over the age of 65 who have AD (18). This is predicted to rise to 13.2 million by 2050 (19).

14.5 DEMENTIA AND ALZHEIMER'S DISEASE

There are several types of dementia, including Parkinson's dementia, vascular dementia, frontal temporal dementia, dementia with Lewy bodies, Huntington's dementia, and dementia secondary to underlying conditions such as traumatic brain injury (TBI). The most common type of dementia is AD, representing 60%–80% of all dementias (18,19). The exact cause of AD is not known. Early onset pathology seems to play an important role in the onset of this disease. Amyloid beta-peptide and hyperphosphorylated tau (P-tau) are often present. There are many risk factors for AD, including insulin resistance, high cholesterol, elevated blood pressure, and high body mass index, as well as inflammation.

Early diagnosis of risk factors and comprehensive lifestyle change are the most powerful approaches to reducing mortality and the incidence of dementia. Included in these lifestyle factors are healthy nutrition, regular physical activity, stress management, restorative sleep, and social optimization.

14.6 PARALLELS BETWEEN CARDIOVASCULAR AND CEREBRAL VASCULAR HEALTH AND BRAIN HEALTH

Multiple factors act on all organ systems involved in aging. Aging has a profound impact on the structure and function of the cerebrovascular system and acts in concert with other cardiovascular risk factors to further compromise brain health (20–26). Age-related alterations in organs such as the liver, kidney, and the endocrine and immune systems may cause secondary adverse effects on the brain. In turn, brain dysfunction can cause systemic diseases. Vascular risk factors that lead to adverse effects on the cardiovascular system by altering neurohumoral mechanisms controlling the heart, blood vessels, and metabolism, and promoting cardiac damage and hypertension, also affect the brain. Therefore, the health of the brain is inextricably linked to cardiovascular and cerebrovascular health. Interventions aimed at promoting cardiovascular health will also promote brain health and vice versa.

14.7 CARDIOVASCULAR AND STROKE RISK AND BRAIN HEALTH

Cardiovascular disease (CVD) remains the leading cause of mortality in the United States. Risk factors for CVD and stroke are very similar to risk factors for cognitive decline. These risk factors include T2DM, obesity, smoking, an inactive lifestyle, dyslipidemia, and hypertension (27). Since these modifiable risk factors are shared by heart disease and stroke and can decrease brain function, strategies to ameliorate these risk factors can play a significant role in brain health.

14.8 BRAIN HEALTH ACROSS THE LIFESPAN

Both cardiovascular disease and brain disorders tend to be manifested later in life. The risk factors for both cardiovascular and brain disorders are established throughout the life course, which makes interventions focused on modifiable risk factors and protective factors important, even in young adulthood and perhaps as far back as childhood. Prominent among these risk factors are poor nutrition and an inactive lifestyle.

14.9 LIFESTYLE FACTORS AND BRAIN HEALTH

The seven major components of a healthy lifestyle, which we have discussed in this book and in the embedded curriculum, are all relevant to maintaining brain health.

14.9.1 Physical Activity

Regular physical activity has been demonstrated to play a significant role in maintaining healthy cognition. Several studies have shown that levels of physical activity are strongly associated with cognitive health outcomes (7). In addition, there is evidence that acute responses to vigorous physical activity can improve cognition and memory. The most dramatic improvements in cognitive function associated with physical activity have been shown to involve executive function (7,13). The Physical Activity Guidelines for Americans 2018 (PAGA 2018) reported that regular physical activity improves cognition. A relationship also exists between regular physical activity and improved quality of life (28,29). In addition, physical activity has been demonstrated to be beneficial for affect, anxiety, and depression.

In addition, regular physical activity improves restorative sleep (7). Regular physical activity has been shown to lower the risk of both dementia and, in particular, AD.

The amount of physical activity recommended to maintain brain health and lower the risk of cognitive decline is the same as recommended in the PAGA 2018 for general and cardiovascular health, namely, 150 minutes of moderate-intensity physical activity per week. Physical activity has also been shown to increase multiple aspects of cognition. In particular, physical activity helps maintain brain volume and enhances neurotransmitters and neurotrophic factors, which allow for increased growth and survival of neurons.

Physical activity enhances connections between neurons, called synaptogenesis, and also stimulates growth of new neurons (neurogenesis) and increased cerebral blood flow (angiogenesis) (30–32). It has been speculated that physical activity also enhances a concept which has been called "cognitive reserve," which supports the idea that physical activity and healthy lifestyle factors play important roles throughout the lifespan and, indeed, promote resilience against cognitive decline in old age (13,30–32).

14.9.2 Nutrition

A variety of observational studies have linked healthy dietary patterns to cognitive benefits, although nutritional interventions have, at best, demonstrated small effects on cognitive outcomes (1,6). This may be due to methodological limitations and remains an area of active investigation.

A number of dietary patterns have been shown to enhance cognitive health in observational clinical trials. Perhaps the most studied is the Mediterranean diet (MedDiet). Studies have suggested an association between higher adherence to this diet with slower rates of global cognitive decline, as well as decline in specific cognitive measures, and a lower risk of mild cognitive impairment and dementia. Several sub-studies of the PREDIMED study, which followed subjects for between 4.1 and 6.5 years, also corroborated these observational findings (33). It should be noted that these trials were performed in individuals with high cardiovascular risk without cardiovascular disease at baseline.

A meta-analysis of observational data from 26 prospective cohort studies reported that higher adherence to the MedDiet was associated with lower risk of mild cognitive impairment and Alzheimer's disease.

The DASH diet alone did not result in improvement in cognitive performance measures (34–37). However, in one study, the DASH diet combined with aerobic exercise demonstrated significant improvements in global executive function and global cognitive function (38).

The MIND diet is a combination of the Mediterranean and DASH diets, specifically designed to reduce neurodegeneration (39). The association of the MIND diet with cognitive function has been mixed. There has also been an attempt to generate an anti-inflammatory diet. Six observational studies have examined the association between anti-inflammatory diets and cognitive outcomes (40–45). Five of these studies assessed the inflammatory potential of the diet using the dietary inflammatory index. While no specific data are yet available from these studies, the suggestion that inflammation is a key component of cognitive decline may provide a linkage between brain health and heart health and is an area of active investigation.

A number of mechanisms have been proposed for why healthy diets may lower the risk of cognitive decline. These diets may help delay or halt underlying neurodegenerative processes that ultimately lead to cognitive decline. These diets have been demonstrated in multiple studies to be associated with better cardiovascular health, which would have implications for brain health as well. In addition, it is well known that aging is accompanied by an increase in cellular production of proinflammatory cytokines and mediators, which lead to low-grade systemic inflammatory states in older individuals. This area is known as "inflammaging." This is another area where a less inflammatory diet, such as the MedDiet and the DASH diet, may yield less inflammation resulting in less cognitive decline (33,34).

In addition, some investigators have proposed that epigenetics plays a key role in cognitive decline. DNA methylation of cysteine bases has been suggested to play a potential role in the development of AD. Nutrition and diet are the main environmental factors that influence epigenetics. One trial that looked at genetic biomarkers of aging involved a 12-month Mediterranean-like diet in 120 healthy older adults and observed trends toward epigenetic rejuvenation (46–48).

While a variety of issues remain to be resolved concerning the linkage between nutrition and healthy brain aging, it is an area where there already exists intriguing evidence and ongoing active research is in progress.

14.9.3 Obesity

The role of obesity as a risk factor for AD development remains uncertain. One meta-analysis demonstrated that a BMI of >30 kg/m^2 was significantly and independently associated with AD development. Other studies, however, have suggested that obesity in middle age is associated with increased AD risk but not in later years (5). It is certainly plausible that obesity would be related to AD, given that obesity is strongly and independently related to CVD and T2DM and also carries an inflammatory component.

14.9.4 Diabetes and Insulin Resistance

The brain is extremely glucose sensitive and therefore is an insulin-dependent organ. Multiple aspects of the brain are impacted by insulin resistance and hyperinsulinemia (5,49). For this reason, AD is sometimes referred to as "type 3 diabetes." This is the result of peripheral hyperglycemia causing glial-mediated inflammation and leading to increased neural insulin resistance. Insulin signaling is often impaired in the brains of patients with diabetes and AD as a result of hyperinsulinemia.

14.9.5 Stress

Stress increases systemic cortisol production and, in turn, also regulates the production of pro-inflammatory cytokines. These factors, in turn, cause the release of multiple pituitary hormones, including Adrenocorticotropic Hormone (ACTH) (50,51). This flood of steroid hormones results in the dampening of higher cognitive processing. The sympathetic nervous system pathway also activates a similar response and perpetuates systemic vasoconstriction, which can result in neuron loss, particularly in the prefrontal cortex (52).

14.9.6 Avoidance of Risky Substances

Alcohol consumption, particularly "heavy" alcohol use (an average of more than four standard drinks daily), has been shown to have deleterious effects on cognitive function as well as CVD and cancer. Some studies have shown that even one standard drink daily can result in damage to the frontal lobe, hippocampus, and cerebellum (53–55). Therefore, it is no longer accurate to suggest that any level of alcohol consumption is either irrelevant or beneficial to brain health. This remains a topic of considerable debate.

Smoking also exerts significant deleterious effects on brain health. These effects appear to be mediated by the increase in inflammation caused by cigarette smoking. Cigarette smoking also results in increased production of superoxide radicals and hydrogen peroxide (56,57). A number of epidemiologic studies have demonstrated that there is a dependent but increased risk of AD and other forms of dementia in association with cigarette smoking. These risks have been shown to persist even after years of tobacco cessation.

14.9.7 Sleep

Inadequate sleep has been shown to adversely affect memory consolidation, cognition, and appetite. Sleep is also an anti-inflammatory process (56–58). This is particularly true of non-REM sleep. The relationship between brain health and sleep is bidirectional. Sleep deprivation harms brain health through a variety of mechanisms, while poor brain health results in difficulties with sleep. Further information about sleep may be found in Chapter 6.

14.9.8 Positive Social Relations

A wide variety of studies have shown that social isolation and, in particular, loneliness are associated with multiple adverse health consequences (59). However, the linkage between social isolation and loneliness and brain health remains controversial. There are some studies showing no beneficial effect of social relationships on brain health (4,60–64). These studies, however, have been criticized for methodological problems. This is an area of active ongoing research.

A number of other risk factors are associated with cognitive decline, dementia, and AD. For example, a number of studies have shown that genetics plays an important role. The Swedish Twin Study reported that 60%–80% of cognitive decline may be somewhat attributable to genetic effects (5). In addition, sex is also an important contributor to cognitive decline. One study demonstrated that after the age of 85, the incidence of AD is more prevalent in women than in men.

One modifiable risk factor involves diminished hearing. In a meta-analysis conducted in 2018, hearing loss was demonstrated to affect clinical outcomes of dementia. Hearing loss is easily amenable to hearing aids, yet only one in five Americans with hearing loss acquires these devices (65). In addition, both dyslipidemia (66) and high blood pressure (8) are associated with cognitive decline. Both of these are treatable through other lifestyle measures such as healthy nutrition, weight management, and regular physical activity (see Chapters 2 and 3).

14.10 TRIALS OF MULTIPLE COMPONENTS OF LIFESTYLE FACTORS IN COMBINATION WITH BRAIN HEALTH

Studies are beginning to emerge that combine various lifestyle medicine modalities to assess their role in potentially preserving cognitive health. Perhaps the most prominent study in this area was the FINGER Study (1). This was a two-year multi-domain intervention utilizing diet, exercise, cognitive training, and vascular risk monitoring versus control to prevent cognitive decline in elderly people. This study enrolled over 2,000 individuals at risk for cognitive decline and randomly assigned 1,062 individuals to either the intervention group (n = 631) or the control group (N = 629). The findings in this large, randomized controlled trial suggested that multi-domain interventions in the areas of diet, exercise, and cognitive training improve or maintain cognitive function in at-risk elderly people in the general population. This study has stimulated worldwide work in similar trials to begin. These trials should provide useful information on lifestyle medicine modalities and their role in slowing down or improving cognitive function in elderly individuals.

14.11 METRICS FOR DEFINING OPTIMAL BRAIN HEALTH/LIFE'S ESSENTIAL EIGHT

As already indicated, the Presidential Advisory from the AHA and ASA for defining and improving "Optimal Brain Health" utilized the framework of the AHA's "Life's Simple Seven" (5,67). Subsequently, this framework added healthy sleep, and it was changed to "Life's Essential Eight" (68). The following seven factors are listed in the AHA/ASA framework components of optimal brain health. They are the following:

- Manage blood pressure
- Control cholesterol

- Reduce blood sugar
- Get active
- Eat better
- Lose weight
- Stop smoking

The AHA then added #8, which is Obtaining Healthy Sleep (68). As can be seen from this list, these are largely lifestyle medicine modalities to improve brain health endorsed in this framework by both the AHA and the ASA.

Brain Training – As already indicated, a number of initiatives are now being considered to enhance healthy brain function and lower the risk of cognitive decline. While the FINGER Study provided important evidence on multi-modal approaches, it was labor-intensive and not scalable to a large number of people. The ability to offer scalable "brain training" is being researched in a number of settings. The US National Academy of Sciences published an expert review of the most promising messages for preventing cognitive decline (69) and improving brain health, and listed the following factors:

- Blood pressure control
- Increase physical activity
- Cognitive training

The expert panel concluded that the evidence was strongest for cognitive training.

The leading research group in exploring brain training is the Center for Brain Health at the University of Texas at Dallas (3). These researchers focus on a variety of methods, including

A. Strategic and tactical control of tension
B. Use of everyday materials in training
C. Proven ability to improve cognitive health, well-being, connectedness, and real-life functions.

They call their approach Strategic Memory Advanced Reasoning Training (SMART). The research in this area follows a 12-week online training program enrolling individuals between 18 and 87 years of age. More information about this training initiative may be found in the chapter written by the Center for Brain Health faculty under the direction of Dr. Sandra Bond Chapman, entitled "The Neuro Science for Brain Health," and may be found in the 4th edition of the *Lifestyle Medicine* textbook that Dr. Rippe edits.

14.12 CONCLUSIONS/CLINICAL APPLICATIONS

The area of brain health, cognitive function, and delaying decreases in cognitive function is critically important to helping individuals lead healthy and fulfilling lives. These issues are particularly important as the population continues to age.

Multiple lifestyle medicine modalities have clearly been shown to assist in the process of maintaining cognitive function and thereby maintaining brain health. Studies suggest that these modalities should be initiated at the earliest possible time and become lifelong strategies to lower the risk of cognitive decline in general and particularly Alzheimer's disease in later years. Research is now beginning to demonstrate the value of combining these modalities and also including "brain training" in an overall approach to maintaining cognitive function and improving brain health. These should be topics of discussion for all physicians in their regular consultations with adult patients of all ages.

REFERENCES

1. Ngandu T, Lehtisalo J, Solomon A, et al. A 2 year multidomain intervention of diet, exercise, cognitive training, and vascular risk monitoring versus control to prevent cognitive decline in at-risk elderly people (FINGER): a randomised controlled trial. *Lancet.* 2015;385(9984):2255–2263.
2. Jamall S, Thiagarajan S, Sherzai D. Alzheimer's disease: pathophysiology and prevention. In Rippe JM (ed.) *Lifestyle Medicine* (4th ed). Boca Raton, FL: CRC Press, 2024.
3. Bond Chapman S., Robertson I., Zientz J. et al. The neuroscience of brain health. In Rippe JM (ed.) *Lifestyle Medicine* (4th ed). Boca Raton, FL: CRC Press, 2024.
4. Piolatto M, Bianchi F, Rota M, et al. The effect of social relationships on cognitive decline in older adults: an updated systematic review and meta-analysis of longitudinal cohort studies. *BMC Public Health.* 2022;22(1):278.
5. Silva MVF, Loures CMG, Alves LCV, et al. Alzheimer's disease: risk factors and potentially protective measures. *J Biomed Sci.* 2019;26(1):33.
6. Charisis S, Yannakoulia M, Scarmeas N. Diets to promote healthy brain ageing. *Nat Rev Neurol.* 2025;21(1):5–16.
7. Brain Health. Part F. Chapter 3. 2018 Physical Activity Guidelines Advisory Committee Scientific Report. Washington, DC: U.S. Department of Health and Human Services, 2018.
8. Gorelick PB, Furie KL, Iadecola C, et al. Defining optimal brain health in adults: a presidential advisory from the American Heart Association/American Stroke Association. *Stroke.* 2017;48(10):e284–e303.
9. Iso-Markku P, Aaltonen S, Kujala UM, et al. Physical activity and cognitive decline among older adults: a systematic review and meta-analysis. *JAMA Network Open.* 2024;7(2):e2354285.
10. Bloomberg M, Muniz-Terrera G, Brocklebank L, et al. Healthy lifestyle and cognitive decline in middle-aged and older adults residing in 14 European countries. *Nat Commun.* 2024;15(1):5003.
11. Winblad B, Amouyel P, Andrieu S, et al. Defeating Alzheimer's disease and other dementias: a priority for European science and society. *Lancet Neurol.* 2016;15(5):455–532.
12. Gorelick PB, Scuteri A, Black SE, et al. Vascular contributions to cognitive impairment and dementia: a statement for healthcare professionals from the American Heart Association/American Stroke Association. *Stroke.* 2011;42(9):2672–713.
13. Rippe JM., Petruzzello SJ. Influence of physical activity on brain aging and cognition. In Rippe JM (ed.) *Lifestyle Medicine* (4th ed). Boca Raton, FL: CRC Press, 2024.
14. Hachinski V, Avan A, Gilliland J, et al. A new definition of brain health. *Lancet Neurol.* 2021; 20(5):335–336.
15. Chapman SB, Mudar RA. Enhancement of cognitive and neural functions through complex reasoning training: evidence from normal and clinical populations. *Front Syst Neurosci.* 2014;8:69.
16. Brain Health. World Health Organization. 2022. https://www.who.int/publications/i/item/9789240054561. Accessed April 21, 2025.
17. Chapman SB, Aslan S, Spence JS, et al. Neural mechanisms of brain plasticity with complex cognitive training in healthy seniors. *Cerebral Cortex.* 2015;25(2):396–405.
18. World Health Organization and Alzheimer's Disease International. Dementia: A Public Health Priority. Paper presented at: World Health Organization; April 11, 2012; Geneva, Switzerland. Dementia: a public health priority. Accessed April 16, 2025.
19. Alzheimer's Association. 2013 Alzheimer's disease facts and figures. *Alzheimer's Dement.* 2013; 9(2):208–245.
20. Pal S, Tyler JK. Epigenetics and aging. *Sci. Adv.* 2016;2(7):e1600584.
21. Kaeberlein M, Rabinovitch PS, Martin GM. Healthy aging: the ultimate preventative medicine. *Science.* 2015;350(6265):1191–1193.
22. Zahn LM. Aging and variability among immune cells. *Science.* 2017;355(6332):1386–1387.
23. Labbadia J, Morimoto RI. The biology of proteostasis in aging and disease. *Annu Rev Biochem.* 2015; 84:435–464.
24. Farkas E, Luiten PG. Cerebral microvascular pathology in aging and Alzheimer's disease. *Prog Neurobiol.* 2001;64(6):575–611.
25. Tahsili-Fahadan P, Geocadin RG. Heart-brain axis: effects of neurologic injury on cardiovascular function. *Circ Res.* 2017;120(3):559–572.
26. Young CN, Davisson RL. Angiotensin-II, the brain, and hypertension: an update. *Hypertension.* 2015;66(5):920–926.
27. Faraci FM. Protecting against vascular disease in brain. *Am J Physiol Heart. Circ Physiol.* 2011; 300(5):H1566–H1582.

28. Marquez DX, Aguinaga S, Vasquez PM, et al. A systematic review of physical activity and quality of life and well-being. *Transl Behav Med.* 2020;10(5):1098–1109.
29. Kline CE, Hillman CH, Bloodgood Sheppard B, et al. Physical activity and sleep: an updated umbrella review of the 2018 physical activity guidelines advisory committee report. *Sleep Med Rev.* 2021; 58:101489.
30. Stern Y. What is cognitive reserve? Theory and research application of the reserve concept. *J Int Neuropsychol Soc.* 2002;8(3):448–460.
31. Ajmani RS, Metter EJ, Jaykumar R, et al. Hemodynamic changes during aging associated with cerebral blood flow and impaired cognitive function. *Neurobiol Aging.* 2000;21(2):257–269.
32. Anderson BJ, Greenwood SJ, McCloskey D. Exercise as an intervention for the age-related decline in neural metabolic support. *Front Aging Neurosci.* 2010;2:30.
33. Estruch R, Ros E, Salas-Salvado J, et al. Primary prevention of cardiovascular disease with a mediterranean diet. *N Eng J Med.* 2013;368(14):1279–1290.
34. Sacks FM, Svetkey LP, Vollmer WM, et al. Effects on blood pressure of reduced dietary sodium and the Dietary Approaches to Stop Hypertension (DASH) diet. DASH-Sodium Collaborative Research Group. *N Engl J Med.* 2001;344(1):3–10.
35. Wengreen, H. et al. Prospective study of dietary approaches to stop hypertension- and mediterranean-style dietary patterns and age-related cognitive change: the Cache County Study on memory, health and aging. *Am J Clin Nutr.* 2013;98:1263–1271.
36. Berendsen AAM, Kang JH, van de Rest O, et al. The dietary approaches to stop hypertension diet, cognitive function, and cognitive decline in american older women. *J Am Med Dir Assoc.* 2017;18(5):427–432.
37. Haring B, Wu C, Mossavar-Rahmani Y, et al. No association between dietary patterns and risk for cognitive decline in older women with 9-year follow-up: data from the women's health initiative memory study. *J Acad Nutr Diet.* 2016;116:921–930.e1.
38. Blumenthal JA, Smith PJ, Mabe S, et al. Lifestyle and neurocognition in older adults with cognitive impairments: a randomized trial. *Neurology.* 2019;92(3):e212–e223.
39. Hosking DE, Eramudugolla R, Cherbuin N, et al. MIND not Mediterranean diet related to 12-year incidence of cognitive impairment in an Australian longitudinal cohort study. *Alzheimer's Dement.* 2019;15, 581–589.
40. Zhang X, Wang Y, Liu W, et al. Diet quality, gut microbiota, and microRNAs associated with mild cognitive impairment in middle-aged and elderly Chinese population. *Am J Clin Nutr.* 2021;114:429–440.
41. Hayden KM, Beavers DP, Steck SE, et al. The Association between an inflammatory diet and global cognitive function and incident dementia in older women: the women's health initiative memory study. *Alzheimer's Dement.* 2017;13(11):1187–1196.
42. Shi Y, Lin F, Li Y. et al. Association of pro-inflammatory diet with increased risk of all-cause dementia and Alzheimer's dementia: a prospective study of 166,377 UK Biobank participants. *BMC Med.* 2023;21:266.
43. Ozawa M, Shipley M, Kivimaki M, et al. Dietary pattern, inflammation and cognitive decline: the whitehall II prospective cohort study. *Clin Nutr.* 2017;36:506–512.
44. Charisis S, Ntanasi E, Yannakoulia M, et al. Diet inflammatory index and dementia incidence: a population-based study. *Neurology.* 2021;97:e2381–e2391.
45. van Lent DM, Mesa HG, Short MI, et al. Association between dietary inflammatory index score and incident dementia. *Alzheimer's Dement.* 2025; 21(1):e14390.
46. Valls-Pedret C, Sala-Vila A, Serra-Mir M, et al. Mediterranean diet and age-related cognitive decline: a randomized clinical trial. *JAMA Intern Med.* 2015;175:1094–1103.
47. Knight A, Bryan J, Wilson C, et al. The mediterranean diet and cognitive function among healthy older adults in a 6-month randomised controlled trial: the MedLey study. *Nutrients.* 2016;20;8(9):579.
48. Fu J, Tan L, Lee J, et al. Association between the Mediterranean diet and cognitive health among healthy adults: a systematic review and meta-analysis. *Front Nutr.* 2022;9:946361.
49. Lee HJ, Seo HI, Cha HY, et al. Diabetes and Alzheimer's disease: mechanisms and nutritional aspects. *Clin Nutr Res.* 2018;7(4):229–240.
50. Avila-Villanueva M, Gomez-Ramirez J, Maestu F, et al. The role of chronic stress as a trigger for the Alzheimer disease continuum. *Front Aging Neurosci.* 2020;12:561504.
51. Justice NJ, Huang L, Tian JB, et al. Posttraumatic stress disorder-like induction elevates beta-amyloid levels, which directly activates corticotropin-releasing factor neurons to exacerbate stress responses. *J Neurosci.* 2015;35(6):2612–2623.
52. Miranda M, Morici JF, Zanoni MB, et al. Brain-derived neurotrophic factor: a key molecule for memory in the healthy and the pathological brain. *Front Cell Neurosci.* 2019;13:363.

53. Daviet R, Aydogan G, Jagannathan K, et al. Associations between alcohol consumption and gray and white matter volumes in the UK Biobank. *Nat Commun.* 2022;13(1):1175.
54. Wei J, Qin L, Fu Y, et al. Long-term consumption of alcohol exacerbates neural lesions by destroying the functional integrity of the blood-brain barrier. *Drug Chem Toxicol.* 2022;45(1):231–238.
55. Topiwala A, Wang C, Ebmeier KP, et al. Associations between moderate alcohol consumption, brain iron, and cognition in UK Biobank participants: observational and Mendelian randomization analyses. *PLoS Med.* 2022;19(7):e1004039.
56. Wallin C, Sholts SB, Osterlund N, et al. Alzheimer's disease and cigarette smoke components: effects of nicotine, PAHs, and Cd(II), Cr(III), Pb(II), Pb(IV) ions on amyloid-beta peptide aggregation. *Sci Rep.* 2017;7(1):14423.
57. Tsuang D, Larson EB, Li G, et al. Association between lifetime cigarette smoking and lewy body accumulation. *Brain Pathol.* 2010;20(2):412–418.
58. Swift KM, Gross BA, Frazer MA, et al. Abnormal locus coeruleus sleep activity alters sleep signatures of memory consolidation and impairs place cell stability and spatial memory. *Curr Biol.* 2018;28(22):3599–3609e4.
59. Vivek M, Office of the Surgeon General (OSG). Our Epidemic of Loneliness and Isolation: The U.S. Surgeon General's Advisory on the Healing Effects of Social Connection and Community. Washington, DC: US Department of Health and Human Services, 2023.
60. Perry BL, McConnell WR, Coleman ME, et al. Why the cognitive "fountain of youth" may be upstream: pathways to dementia risk and resilience through social connectedness. *Alzheimers Dement.* 2021;18(5):934–941.
61. Fratiglioni L, Marseglia A, Dekhtyar S. Ageing without dementia: can stimulating psychosocial and lifestyle experiences make a difference? *Lancet Neurol.* 2020;19(6):533–543.
62. Marseglia A, Wang H-X, Rizzuto D, et al. Participating in mental, social, and physical leisure activities and having a rich social network reduce the incidence of diabetes-related dementia in a cohort of Swedish older adults. *Diabetes Care.* 2019;42(2):232–239.
63. Haslam C, Cruwys T, Haslam SA. "The we's have it": Evidence for the distinctive benefits of group engagement in enhancing cognitive health in aging. *Soc Sci Med.* 2014;120:57–66.
64. Bourassa KJ, Memel M, Woolverton C, et al. Social participation predicts cognitive functioning in aging adults over time: comparisons with physical health, depression, and physical activity. *Aging Mental Health.* 2017;21(2):133–146.
65. Loughrey DG, Kelly ME, Kelley GA, et al. Association of age-related hearing loss with cognitive function, cognitive impairment, and dementia: a systematic review and meta-analysis. *JAMA Otolaryngol Head Neck Surg.* 2018;144(2):115–126.
66. Feringa FM, van der Kant R. Cholesterol and Alzheimer's disease; from risk genes to pathological effects. *Front Aging Neurosci.* 2021;13:690372.
67. Thacker EL, Gillett SR, Wadley VG, et al. The American Heart Association Life's simple 7 and incident cognitive impairment: the REasons for Geographic And Racial Differences in Stroke (REGARDS) study. *J Am Heart Assoc.* 2014;3(3):e000635.
68. Lloyd-Jones DM, Allen NB, Anderson CAM, et al. Life's essential 8: updating and enhancing the American Heart Association's construct of cardiovascular health: a presidential advisory from the American Heart Association. *Circulation.* 2022;146(5):e18–e43.
69. Brain Health across the Lifespan: A Workshop. National Academies Sciences Engineering Medicine. https://www.nationalacademies.org/our-work/brain-health-across-the-lifespan-a-workshop. Accessed April 16, 2025.

15 Aging

15.1 INTRODUCTION

Primary care physicians (particularly those practicing in the area of lifestyle medicine), as well as family practitioners, will see a large number of individuals over the age of 65. At the current time, individuals over the age of 65 comprise approximately 13% of the US population, and these numbers are projected to increase to 19% of the total population (72.1 million) by the year 2030 (1). This group is the most rapidly growing of all population segments in the United States.

An enormous and persuasive body of scientific information supports the concepts of a variety of lifestyle measures to yield multiple health and quality-of-life benefits in people over the age of 65 (1,2). Cost-effective mechanisms for improving health and forestalling disabilities in this age group assume great importance. Thus, the role of lifestyle medicine plays not only into clinical concerns but also into overall health, well-being, and quality of life, and assumes great importance. Lifestyle measures are also cost-effective. This chapter will explore the role of lifestyle-related measures both individually and as a group for people over the age of 65.

Cognitive decline is a significant concern in people over the age of 65, as is frailty, loneliness, and social isolation. These considerations will be discussed in this chapter. In addition, the concept of "successful aging" will be considered, given that increasing interest has risen in promoting this concept in people over the age of 65 (3).

Much of the information contained in this chapter comes from the superb section on geriatrics edited by Dr. Susan Friedman in the 4th edition of Dr. Rippe's *Lifestyle Medicine* textbook and the book on *Lifestyle Medicine and Geriatrics* that she has edited in the *Lifestyle Medicine Series* that Dr. Rippe edits (4). Geriatricians treat many of the individuals over the age of 65 and share many of the fundamental principles of lifestyle medicine (5). Some of these overlapping philosophies will also be considered.

15.2 NORMAL AGING OF THE BRAIN

Since age-related cognitive decline represents a critically important issue in people over the age of 65, it is important to start with the consideration of how the normal aging process impacts the brain (6–9). As the brain ages, changes are wide-ranging and occur in a variety of structures and include molecular, cellular, vascular, and structural levels. It has been documented that the brain loses volume at a rate of about 5% per decade from age 40. This volume loss is primarily from the gray matter and also the myelin from nerve sheaths within the white matter (7).

In addition, it is also important to understand the concept of cerebrovascular aging. The brain receives about 15% of total cardiac output and is highly dependent on the vascular system both for the delivery of nutrients and the removal of waste products (10). The cerebral vasculature is protected by the blood-brain barrier (BBB), which is designed to prevent harmful molecules from entering the brain (11). The regulation of blood flow to the brain is achieved through smooth muscle control of arteries, long permeating arterioles, and capillary beds in response to carbon dioxide pressure in the blood ($PaCO_2$). In addition, input from the autonomic nervous system helps regulate blood flow to the brain.

As the brain ages, there is a loss of compliance of the arteries. This process may be accelerated by chronic oxidative stress, which is related to the concept of inflammaging. The consequence of these changes results in the diminishment of the blood-brain barrier and of the brain's ability to autoregulate, which ultimately causes normal cognitive aging to be superseded by cognitive impairment or dementia.

DOI: 10.1201/9781003630043-15

15.3 AGE-ASSOCIATED COGNITIVE DECLINE

To discuss cognitive decline, it is important to understand a few key definitions.

- *Cognitive Domains*: Cognition in the brain is organized into functional "domains," which are often handled by distinct parts of the brain. These domains include regulating a variety of motor skills, as well as memory, executive function, processing speed, language, and verbal skills. Executive function involves the tasks of planning and problem solving, and involves coordination of input from the other cognitive domains.
- *Age-Associated Memory Impairment*: Most individuals will experience age-associated memory impairment (AAMI) through normal aging. This is thought to be primarily due to changes within the hippocampus and the frontal and temporal lobes of the cerebral cortex (12). There are four types of memory: episodic, semantic, procedural, and working memory. Episodic memory refers to memories associated with events in personal experience. Semantic memory refers to general accumulated knowledge. Procedural memory is a form of long-term memory involved in the performance of actions and skills (12). Working memory facilitates the performance of complex tasks.
- *Mild Cognitive Impairment*: Mild cognitive impairment (MCI) is defined as more severe changes than those expected with normal aging but with an absence of functional impairment (13,14). The incidence of MCI increases with each decade after age 60 and is associated with a 15% risk of progression to dementia.
- *Age-Associated Cognitive Decline*: Just as there are age-related effects of various organ systems, so too the brain experiences age-related changes (15). In addition to loss of volume as already discussed, the brain experiences a gradual reduction in the ability to replace lost neurons in the process of neurogenesis. Synapses and networks also show age-related decline, as well as neurotransmitter activity at synapses. In addition, vascular changes reduce cerebral blood flow, which also occurs with aging (16). The changes in the brain may be associated with a decline in cognitive processes, including memory, learning ability, problem-solving, and executive control. These may range from relatively minor changes in age-related memory (ARMI), MCI, or various forms of dementia, including Alzheimer's disease (AD).

Lifestyle measures may have a salutary effect on all of these processes. For example, controlling blood pressure, type 2 diabetes (T2DM), and dyslipidemia all play roles in slowing cognitive decline and are influenced by the lifestyle measures discussed in this book.

Physical activity, particularly at the level recommended by the Physical Activity Guidelines for Americans 2018 (17) and the Centers for Disease Control (CDC), has been repeatedly shown to improve cognitive function in the elderly population. The recommended doses of physical activity may need to be adjusted for the elderly population, particularly those who are sedentary or very unfit. These levels of physical activity have been shown to reduce the risk of MCI and dementia.

The precise mechanisms for the improvement in cognitive function are not completely understood. However, as indicated in Chapter 20, lifestyle measures in combination may increase the level of "cognitive reserve." Cognitive reserve can also be enhanced by brain training and encouraging the elderly population to be involved in volunteer work and social work engagements.

15.4 REDUCING AGE-RELATED COGNITIVE DECLINE BY LIFESTYLE MEASURES

- *Physical Activity*: Regular physical activity at levels recommended by the PAGA 2018 is one of the most powerful tools to combat long-term cognitive decline. It also exerts a positive impact on improving mood and enhancing cognition. One study of older adults aged 60–74 who participated in either a walking program or a stretching and toning program found that only the walking program showed improvement in cognitive tasks related to executive function after six months (18). Other randomized controlled trials have corroborated these findings (19). Regular physical activity improves angiogenesis, neurogenesis, and synaptogenesis (20). In addition to its role in the primary prevention of cognitive decline, regular physical activity has also been shown to improve cognition in individuals with mild cognitive impairment (21). Of course, regular physical activity, as outlined in numerous chapters in this book, also lowers the risk of various chronic diseases, particularly CVD and T2DM.

- *Nutrition*: Healthy nutrition has been shown in numerous observational trials to slow cognitive decline (22). As already indicated in Chapter 20, the Mediterranean Diet is the most studied (23). In addition, the DASH Diet (24) and the Mediterranean-DASH Intervention for Neurodegenerative Delay (MIND) diet have been shown in observational studies to reduce cognitive decline (25). In contrast, the standard American diet appears to accelerate cognitive aging in a number of ways (26). This has been shown in a variety of studies, including the Honolulu Aging Study, where Japanese Americans who lived in Hawaii had considerably higher rates of cognitive impairment than inhabitants of mainland Japan (27).

  A variety of dietary and lifestyle guidelines were studied in a 2018 review in the journal *Neurobiology of Aging,* which focused on decreasing intake of saturated and trans fats and increasing vegetables, legumes, fruits, and whole grains while minimizing red meat and dairy to slow the process of cognitive decline (22).
- *Stress Reduction*: Stress reduction has gained recognition as a factor in slowing cognitive aging (28,29). It has been hypothesized that chronic stress leads to dysregulation of the hypothalamic-pituitary-adrenal (HPA) axis and glucocorticoid release. Glucocorticoid excess can lead to increased insulin resistance and a variety of adverse epigenetic changes.
- *Avoidance of Risky Substances*: Both alcohol and cigarette smoking can contribute to cognitive decline. The multiple health hazards of cigarette smoking have been documented in a number of chapters in this book. Cigarette smoking also contributes to cognitive decline (30). This is discussed in detail in Chapter 14.

  Alcohol can also contribute to cognitive decline (31–33). It used to be thought that heavy drinking (greater than four alcoholic beverages per day) resulted in cognitive decline. Some recent evidence, however, suggests that even one alcoholic drink per day can contribute to cognitive decline. This latter finding has sparked intense debate. This is discussed in detail in Chapter 14.
- *Sleep*: Sleep disorders are very common in the United States. The CDC estimates that 35% of all adults and 26% of those above the age of 65 get insufficient sleep, which is defined as seven hours nightly on average (34). This is clearly a bidirectional issue. Disrupted sleep is both a cause and consequence of cognitive decline (35). In particular, adequate sleep is critical for memory formation and is thought to increase cognitive reserve. One meta-analysis found a 53% increased risk of all-cause dementia for those with insomnia (36).
- *The Roles of Relationships*: The role of positive relationships and socialization has been shown to improve cognitive reserve. A 2020 meta-analysis explored the link between social relationships and cognitive decline and found that poor social relationships increased the risk of cognitive decline (37). A 2022 analysis of Framingham Study cohort data found a hazard ratio of 1.54 for ten-year dementia risk for those who reported loneliness at least three days per week (38). Thus, components of lifestyle discussed in multiple chapters in this book are all relevant to the healthy brain, normal aging of the brain, and also reducing the risk of cognitive decline.

15.5 REDUCING THE AGE-RELATED RISK OF SARCOPENIA AND FRAILTY

Skeletal muscle declines with age. Skeletal muscle is key to functioning for people of all ages, but particularly for those over the age of 65. Skeletal muscle is the largest soft tissue mass in the human body, constituting about 40% of total lean body mass on average in healthy young men and about 25% in comparably aged young women (39). Skeletal muscle mass and strength generally peak in the mid-20s to 30 years old. Between the ages of 30 and 50 there is a progressive decline in skeletal muscle of about 1% per year. After the age of 70, the rate of loss is accelerated to about 3% per year (40).

When a significant amount of muscle is lost, it can lead to frailty. This condition is commonly denoted by the term "sarcopenia," which is defined as loss of two or more standard deviations of muscle mass below the mean (20–30-year-old) of the same sex and ethnicity. Sarcopenia can also result in a significant decline in metabolism and frailty and lead to significant functional decline. It is currently estimated that 13%–24% of adults over the age of 70, and 50% of those over the age of 80, have sarcopenia (41).

A variety of biological mechanisms appear to underlie sarcopenia. These include a reduction in muscle fiber size as well as molecular and biochemical changes. Cell death (apoptosis), inflammation, accumulation of muscle protein, reduced anabolic hormone activities, and reduced levels of blood supply also contribute to sarcopenia.

A sedentary lifestyle contributes to both sarcopenia and frailty. In contrast, exercise training, even in older, physically frail individuals, has been shown in numerous research studies to improve muscle mass and strength, as well as muscular and cardiorespiratory endurance. Regular physical activity throughout the life span can also forestall sarcopenia. Regular exercise in individuals over the age of 40 can also combat sarcopenia.

The recommendations for physical activity over the age of 70 are the same as for younger individuals, according to the PAGA 2018 (17). These include moderate aerobic activity at 150 minutes per week and two to three sessions per week of strength training. Low-impact exercise, in particular, such as walking, stationary cycling, or swimming, is recommended. In addition, flexibility and balance training are important and can be conducted as a component of warming up and cooling down. These have been shown to lower the risk of falls and associated injuries.

In addition, as already documented in multiple chapters in this book, regular physical activity, even for people in their 1970s and 1980s, contributes to lowering the risk of CVD and T2DM.

With regard to age-related loss of muscle, a variety of recommendations have been made, including the following:

- Follow the national guidelines for a healthy, balanced diet
- Ensure adequate food intake
- Meet the requirement for good-quality protein
- Maintain an adequate circulating vitamin D level from sun exposure, diet, and supplements
- Obtain adequate intake of food sources with exogenous antioxidants

15.6 AGING SUCCESSFULLY: PREDICTORS AND PATHWAYS

As we learn more about ways to enhance and improve the quality of life in individuals over the age of 65, the concept of "successful aging" (SA) has achieved prominence. Currently in the United States (3), an alarmingly low percentage of individuals over the age of 65 are aging successfully. The Health and Retirement Study showed that only 11.9% of older adults could be categorized as aging successfully. Other studies have shown similarly low percentages.

A number of definitions and models of successful aging have been proposed. The one that is most commonly utilized was developed by Rowe and Kahn (3). They used three key characteristics as a basis of their SA model: low risk of disease and disease-related disability, high mental and physical function, and active engagement with life. To be considered as aging successfully, older adults need to display high levels in all three of these characteristics.

It is also clear that these factors should be engaged at a much earlier stage in life. Perhaps the most important single component of SA is regular physical activity. Physical activity can serve as a primary vehicle for enhancing and maintaining all of the key characteristics of SA defined by Rowe and Kahn. In addition, inactivity has been clearly shown to increase the risk of chronic medical conditions. Other lifestyle practices also play an important role in SA. These include the other lifestyle habits and factors emphasized throughout this book, including cognitive training, a healthy non-inflammatory diet, healthy restorative sleep, avoiding risky substances, and active, positive engagement with other people (41).

Physicians can play a very important role in urging older adults to practice these key components of a healthy lifestyle. Numerous studies have shown that physician-based counseling, in as little as three to five minutes, can enhance individuals' likelihood of engaging in positive lifestyle-related habits and actions. Thus, the high number of individuals who see their primary care physician on at least an annual basis can be helped to achieve the underlying concepts behind SA.

15.7 THE ROLE OF PHYSICAL ACTIVITY IN WELL-BEING FOR OLDER ADULTS

As already indicated, physical activity is associated with multiple benefits for individuals over the age of 65 (17). Physical activity has been routinely shown to yield multiple benefits, including improving cognitive function and lowering cognitive decline. In addition, regular physical activity lowers the risk of age-related sarcopenia and frailty and improves physical function.

The PAGA 2018 Scientific Report demonstrated that the volume of aerobic physical activity has a strong relationship to physical function in patients in the aging population. This is important since the National Health Review Survey conducted from 2001 to 2007 showed that almost 23% of older individuals reported limitations or the inability to do normal tasks of life (e.g., walk a quarter mile or lift a 10-pound bag of groceries) (17). The same is true of almost 43% of adults aged 80 or older. Multiple cohort studies on physical activity have shown that there is a 50% reduction in functional limitations for individuals who are physically active who are over the age of 65.

In addition, regular physical activity significantly lowers the risk of falls as well as reduces the risk of injury from severe falls, which may result in bone fractures, head trauma, or open wounds. Regular physical activity has been shown to reduce the likelihood of trauma to the bones by between 32% and 40% and bone fractures by between 40% and 66%. These are important benefits since up to 25% of individuals over the age of 65 experience a fall in the United States every year (17). Falls are the leading cause of fatal injury and the most common cause of non-fatal trauma-related hospital admissions for older individuals. Thus, physical activity is a cost-effective way of approaching fall prevention.

15.8 NUTRITION FOR OLDER ADULTS

Individuals over the age of 70 may have significant difficulty in obtaining adequate nutrition (42). There are significant shortfalls that were addressed by the Food and Nutrition Board and the Institute of Medicine starting in 1999 (43), which recommended that vitamin D, calcium, and vitamin B6 should be higher for individuals over the age of 70. The Dietary Reference Intake (DRI) for Vitamin D increased from 600 IU for females and males ages 51–70 to 800 IU per day for both females and males above the age of 80 (43–45). The DRI for calcium increased from 1,000 to 1,200 mg per day for both males and females between the ages of 51 and 70, and to 1,200 mg per day for both males and females over the age of 70. The DRI for vitamin B6 increased from 1.3 mg per day for females and males, respectively, between the ages of 50 and 70 to 1.5 and 1.7 mg for both males and females, respectively, over the age of 70 (46).

Individuals over the age of 60 may experience a variety of challenges in obtaining adequate nutrition. For example, changes in sensory perception and the onset of chronic diseases may necessitate added attention to diet composition, whereas alterations in living situations may complicate both obtaining and preparing food.

In the 2020–2025 Dietary Guidelines for Americans Advisory Committee Report, vitamin D, calcium, potassium, and fiber were all considered nutrients of concern for older adults (2). There was also concern about overconsumption of sodium, saturated fat, and added sugar (2,47).

Other factors that may impact adequate nutrition include diminished taste and smell in older individuals as well as diminished vision, dexterity, and mobility, which may make food acquisition and preparation difficult (48–50). Arthritis may also make it difficult for older individuals to open containers. Loss of teeth and other dental problems may make it difficult to chew food adequately.

Since the amount of food consumed in older individuals may decrease, it is particularly important to emphasize nutrient density. Also, the considerations of healthy diets such as the Mediterranean Diet and the DASH Diet remain relevant to elderly individuals.

15.9 HEARING LOSS

Diminished hearing is a modifiable risk factor that has been linked to cognitive decline and dementia. This has been demonstrated in a 2018 meta-analysis by Loughrey et al. Diminished hearing is easily fixable with hearing aids, although only one in five Americans with hearing loss acquire these devices (51). Diminished vision is also a significant, typically modifiable condition which can lead to decreased mobility, increased cognitive decline, and the potential for falls.

15.10 MEDICATION MANAGEMENT

Medication management in the elderly population is a vitally important and often neglected part of the overall approach to healthy aging. This clearly is an area where lifestyle medicine issues play an important role. Unfortunately, this is an area where there is limited guidance from medical societies. One area where lifestyle medicine plays an important role is that of deprescribing.

In an article by Scott et al., the goal of reducing polypharmacy, the following definition was given (52): "The systematic process of identifying and discontinuing drugs in instances in which existing or potential harms outweigh existing or potential benefits." Deprescribing is supervised by health care professionals with the intent of reducing polypharmacy and improving outcomes. It is not denying care but rather a patient-centered risk mitigation strategy where thoughtful discussion occurs between the care team and patients and their caregivers on the balance regarding the risks or harms of continuing certain medications compared to stopping them.

The problem of polypharmacy in elderly patients relates to multiple caregivers often adding medicines without carefully considering other medicines that may already have been prescribed for other chronic conditions. Polypharmacy is defined as greater than five chronic medicines, while hyperpolypharmacy is defined as greater than ten chronic medications for greater than 90 days. Individuals who take more than four medications and greater than ten medications are 21% and 50% more likely to experience falls as well as a high risk of avoidable health care utilization such as emergency care, hospitalizations, re-hospitalizations, or long-term care, as well as mortality (53). The use of automatic refill systems, while beneficial in many respects, has further exacerbated this problem.

Polypharmacy is a major cause of medical errors. A 2016 study of medical errors reported that they contributed to more than 250,000 annual deaths (54,55). This makes medical errors the third leading cause of death. While details about polypharmacy are beyond the scope of this chapter, a good general rule for primary care physicians is to perform a thorough reconciliation so that all medicines are appropriately accounted for in all patients, but particularly those over the age of 65.

Also, the American Geriatrics Society has available a good questionnaire called "ASK-12," which stands for Adherence Starts with Knowledge. There is also a questionnaire called STOPP, which stands for the Screening Tool for Older Person's Prescriptions (56–58).

15.11 LIFESTYLE MEDICINE AND PALLIATIVE CARE

Primary care physicians and individuals who practice lifestyle medicine may, on occasion, be called upon to co-manage an individual who is referred to palliative care. Palliative care is designed to improve quality of life consistent with patients' specific goals of care in individuals with severe chronic and terminal illness.

In a sense, the philosophy of palliative care is very consistent with the goals and philosophy of lifestyle medicine. Often, individuals who have multiple chronic illnesses or terminal illnesses will require palliative care. Just as in lifestyle medicine, palliative care at its best focuses on the whole person and concerns itself with what matters to the patient. Here is the official definition of quality palliative care in case lifestyle physicians are not familiar with specific aspects of this very important care. This definition comes from the National Coalition for Hospice and Palliative Care, Clinical Practice Guidelines for Quality Palliative Care, 4th edition, 2018, "Palliative care focuses on expert assessment and management of pain, other symptoms, assessment and supportive caregiver needs, and coordination of care. Palliative care attends to physical, functional, psychological, practical, and spiritual consequences of serious illness. It is a person- and family-centered approach to care, providing people living with serious illness relief from the symptoms and stress of an illness. Through early integration into the care plan for the seriously ill, palliative care improves quality of life for the patient and the family" (59).

It is important for primary care physicians and those practicing in lifestyle medicine to understand the expertise and compassionate philosophy of palliative care. Lifestyle medicine principles and practices in the hands of compassionate physicians can create a smooth working relationship with physicians who deliver palliative care.

15.12 THE IMPACT OF LONELINESS AND SOCIAL ISOLATION

We have discussed in detail in Chapter 7 the pillar of lifestyle medicine that deals with the profound importance of positive relationships with others. This importance is underscored by a recent Surgeon General's Advisory entitled "The Healing Effects of Social Connection and Community." In this Surgeon General's Advisory (60), Dr. Vivek Murthy focuses on the adverse health impacts of social isolation and loneliness.

It is important to remember that loneliness and isolation are increasingly part of the experience of growing old. There are many reasons why this has emerged in the elderly population. Perhaps it is due to reduced intergenerational living, greater geographical mobility, or the rise in one-person households. All of these conditions can increase the vulnerability of older adults to social isolation. As described in Chapter 7, it is important to understand that loneliness and social isolation are different concepts (61). Loneliness has to do with the response to being isolated, whereas some people can be socially isolated and not experience the feeling of loneliness (61–66).

Social isolation and loneliness have been clearly recognized as having deleterious effects on the health of older individuals. These adverse health effects rival risk factors such as heart disease, T2DM, and cancer, which are well recognized by the medical community (60,67–69). There is currently evidence that 25%–29% of adults over the age of 70 report feeling lonely, and up to half of individuals in this age group have only one person or no people to discuss personal matters with.

For the primary care physician or lifestyle medicine practitioner, it is important to discuss with all patients, but particularly older patients, about loneliness. One useful way of doing this is to utilize the UCLA 3-Item Loneliness Scale (70). This scale is comprised of three questions that measure three dimensions of loneliness: relational connectedness, social connectedness, and self-perceived isolation. This loneliness scale is found in Table 15.1.

There are many reasons why individuals in this age group may be particularly vulnerable to loneliness. The loss of one's partner or friends through death, deteriorating health, or

TABLE 15.1
UCLA Three-Item Loneliness Scale

This scale is comprised of three questions that measure three dimensions of loneliness: relational connectedness, social connectedness, and self-perceived isolation.

How often do you feel that you lack companionship?
How often do you feel left out?
How often do you feel isolated from others?
The scale generally uses three response categories:

Response	Score
Hardly ever	1
Some of the time	2
Often	3

Scoring
Least lonely 1 2 3 4 5 6 7 8 9 Most lonely

Source: Adapted from: Hughes ME, Waite LJ, Hawkley LC, Cacioppo JT. A short scale for measuring loneliness in large surveys: results from two population-based studies. *Res Aging*. 2004;26(6):655–672.

institutionalization, or changes in social roles through retirement, are common experiences for older adults.

There may also be community factors that increase vulnerability to social isolation and loneliness. These may include a lack of good opportunities to participate in social activities, high levels of neighborhood crime, or even social discrimination, and the expectation that older patients should be discouraged from physical activity (69).

Because of the adverse physical and mental consequences of loneliness, it is important for primary care and lifestyle medicine physicians to engage in conversations with all patients, particularly those over the age of 65, about this and to counsel patients on ways to increase social interaction and positive connections with other individuals.

15.13 CAREGIVERS

It is likely that physicians practicing primary care and lifestyle medicine will have individuals within their practice who are caregivers to other people. One in six Americans can be classified as a caregiver to individuals over the age of 50 (71). Significantly, one-third of these caregivers describe the high burden of care referred to as "caregiver burden" (72,73), which is defined as the extent to which caregivers perceive that caregiving has had an adverse effect on their emotional, social, financial, physical, and/or spiritual functioning. The health outcomes of caregiver burden include an increased risk of depression, anxiety, and even death. The average age for a caregiver is 50.1 years old, and 56% are over 50 years old, and 20% are over the age of 65 (71). With baby boomers entering the sixth and seventh decades of life, it is likely that the role of caregiving will accelerate. Risk factors for caregiver burden include a variety of factors, including a lower level of education, female sex, residing with the care recipient, and low income level. The average caregiver with a household income of less than $50,000 is more likely to suffer caregiver burden than higher-income individuals (70). Caregivers of color also report higher weekly hours of care than those of white caregivers. A wide variety of conditions are likely to have the need for caregivers. They include dementia, cancer, and other chronic conditions.

Unfortunately, only one-third of caregivers recalled being asked by their physician about this role, and even fewer about what kind of help they need themselves. To partially ameliorate this problem, a screening questionnaire has been developed by the American Geriatrics Society, which includes the following four screening questions (74):

1. Do you provide care for another adult loved one? Who is the person? (friend, spouse, etc.).
2. Do you feel strained when you are around your loved one?
3. Do you feel you have lost control of your life since you started providing care for your loved one?
4. How burdened do you feel caring for your loved one?

Addressing whether or not individuals in your practice are functioning as caregivers and starting a dialogue using this type of screening instrument can be very helpful to increase the likelihood that caregivers will receive adequate support and to, to some degree, alleviate the issue of caregiver burden. This can help mitigate the problem that caregivers often experience, which has been called being "the invisible patient."

15.14 CONCLUSIONS/CLINICAL APPLICATIONS

Multiple physiological and mental changes occur as individuals age. These include age-related declines in cognition, risk of sarcopenia and frailty, multiple chronic diseases that occur later in life, including CVD, T2DM, and cancer. In addition, older individuals are particularly susceptible to polypharmacy as clinicians try to treat multiple chronic conditions, oftentimes without clearly understanding the interface between new medicines being prescribed and the ones elderly patients are currently taking.

This age group, over the age of 65, is increasingly common in the United States and other advanced countries, and it is very important that the principles of lifestyle medicine be applied to these individuals. Many of the problems associated with aging can be somewhat ameliorated by healthy nutrition, regular physical activity, techniques for stress reduction, helping individuals obtain restorative sleep, counseling elderly patients about the adverse effects of risky substances such as cigarettes and alcohol, and the importance of establishing positive relationships with others. For all these reasons, we focus attention on the embedded curriculum in this book on the importance of lifestyle medicine modalities to help with the ongoing health of our increasingly aging population.

REFERENCES

1. Centers for Disease Control and Prevention. Healthy Aging at Any Age. Healthy Aging| CDC. https://www.cdc.gov/healthy-aging/about/index.html. Accessed March 21, 2025.
2. U.S. Department of Agriculture and U.S. Department of Health and Human Services. U.S. Department of Agriculture and U.S. Department of Health and Human Services. Dietary Guidelines for Americans, 2020–2025. 9th Edition. December 2020. Available at DietaryGuidelines.gov. 2020; https://www.dietaryguidelines.gov/resources/2020-2025-dietary-guidelines-online-materials.
3. Rose D. Aging successfully predictors and pathways. In Rippe JM (ed.) *Lifestyle Medicine* (3rd ed). Boca Raton, FL: CRC Press, 2019.
4. Friedman SM. *Geriatrics, Lifestyle Medicine and Healthy Aging: A Practical Guide.* Boca Raton, FL: CRC Press, 2025 (in press).
5. Muniak JD. How geriatrics principles and paradigms can inform lifestyle medicine practice. In Rippe JM (ed.) *Lifestyle Medicine* (4th ed). Boca Raton, FL: CRC Press, 2023.
6. Shehata M, Friedman SM. Reducing cognitive decline through lifestyle medicine. In Rippe JM (ed.) *Lifestyle Medicine* (4th ed). Boca Raton, FL: CRC Press, 2023.
7. Svennerholm L, Boström K, Jungbjer B. Changes in weight and compositions of major membrane components of human brain during the span of adult human life of Swedes. *Acta Neuropathol.* 1997;94(4):345–352.
8. Raz N. The aging brain: structural changes and their implications for cognitive aging. In Dixon R, Backman L, Nilsson LG (eds.) *New Frontiers in Cognitive Aging.* Oxford: Oxford Academic, 2004. Accessed March 21, 2025. doi:10.1093/acprof:oso/9780198525691.003.0006.

9. Fjell AM, Walhovd KB. Structural brain changes in aging: courses, causes and cognitive consequences. *Rev Neurosci.* 2010;21(3):187–221.
10. Purves D, Augustine GJ, Fitzpatrick D, et al. (eds.). *Neuroscience* (2nd ed). Sunderland, MA: Sinauer Associates, 2001. The Blood Supply of the Brain and Spinal Cord.
11. Yang T, Sun Y, Lu Z, et al. The impact of cerebrovascular ageing on vascular cognitive impairment and dementia. *Aging Res Rev.* 2017;34:15–29.
12. Peters R. Ageing and the brain. *Postgrad Med J.* 2006;82(964):84–88.
13. Lopez OL, Jagust WJ, DeKosky ST, et al. Prevalence and classification of mild cognitive impairment in the cardiovascular health study cognition study: part 1. *Arch Neurol.* 2003;60(10):1385–1389.
14. Harvey PD. Domains of cognition and their assessment. *Dialogues Clin Neurosci.* 2019;21(3):227–237.
15. Olivari BS, Baumgart M, Taylor CA, et al. Population measures of subjective cognitive decline: a means of advancing public health policy to address cognitive health. *Alzheimers Dement.* 2021;7(1):e12142.
16. Livingston G, Huntley J, Sommerlad A, et al. Dementia prevention, intervention, and care: 2020 report of the Lancet commission. *Lancet.* 2020;396(10248):413–446.
17. Physical Activity Guidelines Advisory Committee. 2018 Physical Activity Guidelines Advisory Committee. 2018 Physical Activity Guidelines Advisory Committee Scientific Report. Washington, DC: U.S. Department of Health and Human Services, 2018.
18. Aichberger MC, Busch MA, Reischies FM, et al. Effect of physical inactivity on cognitive performance after 2.5 years of follow-up: longitudinal results from the survey of health, ageing, and retirement (SHARE). *GeroPsych.* 2010;23(1):7–15.
19. Kramer AF, Hahn S, Cohen NJ, et al. Ageing, fitness and neurocognitive function. *Nature* 1999;400(6743):418–419.
20. Bherer L, Erickson KI, Liu-Ambrose T. A review of the effects of physical activity and exercise on cognitive and brain functions in older adults. *J Aging Res.* 2013;2013:657508.
21. Law CK, Lam FM, Chung RC, et al. Physical exercise attenuates cognitive decline and reduces behavioural problems in people with mild cognitive impairment and dementia: a systematic review. *J Physiother.* 2020;66(1):9–18.
22. Barnard ND, Bush AI, Ceccarelli A, et al. Dietary and lifestyle guidelines for the prevention of Alzheimer's disease. *Neurobiol Aging.* 2014;35(Suppl. 2):S74–S78.
23. Petersson SD, Philippou E. Mediterranean diet, cognitive function, and dementia: a systematic review of the evidence. *Adv Nutr.* 2016;7(5):889–904.
24. Sacks FM, Svetkey LP, Vollmer WM, et al. Effects on blood pressure of reduced dietary sodium and the Dietary Approaches to Stop Hypertension (DASH) diet. DASH-Sodium Collaborative Research Group. *N Engl J Med.* 2001;344(1):3–10.
25. Morris MC, Tangney CC, Wang Y, et al. MIND diet slows cognitive decline with aging. *Alzheimer's Dement.* 2015;11(9):1015–1022.
26. Hargrave SL, Davidson TL, Zheng W, et al. Western diets induce blood-brain barrier leakage and alter spatial strategies in rats. *Behav Neurosci.* 2016;130(1):123–135.
27. Gelber RP, Launer LJ, White LR. The Honolulu-Asia aging study: epidemiologic and neuropathologic research on cognitive impairment. *Curr Alzheimer Res.* 2012;9(6):664–672.
28. Luders E, Kurth F, Toga AW, et al. Meditation effects within the hippocampal complex revealed by voxel based morphometry and cytoarchitectonic probabilistic mapping. *Front Psychol.* 2013;9;4:398.
29. Marciniak R, Sheardova K, Cermáková P, et al. Effect of meditation on cognitive functions in context of aging and neurodegenerative diseases. *Front Behav Neurosci.* 2014:27;8:17.
30. Sabia S, Elbaz A, Dugravot A, et al. Impact of smoking on cognitive decline in early old age: the Whitehall II cohort study. *Arch Gen Psychiatry.* 2012;69(6):627–635.
31. Sabia S, Elbaz A, Britton A, et al. Alcohol consumption and cognitive decline in early old age. *Neurology.* 2014;82(4):332–339.
32. Koch M, Fitzpatrick AL, Rapp SR, et al. Alcohol consumption and risk of dementia and cognitive decline among older adults with or without mild cognitive impairment. *JAMA Netw Open.* 2019;2(9):e1910319.
33. Wiegmann C, Mick I, Brandl EJ, et al. Alcohol and dementia – what is the link? A systematic review. *Neuropsychiatr Dis Treat.* 2020;16:87–99.
34. Palmer K, Mitolo M, Burgio F, et al. Sleep disturbance in mild cognitive impairment and association with cognitive functioning. A case-control study. *Front Aging Neurosci.* 2018;10:360.
35. Song D, Yu DSF, Sun Q, et al. Correlates of sleep disturbance among older adults with mild cognitive impairment: a cross-sectional study. *Int J Environ Res Public Health.* 2020;17(13):4862.
36. de Almondes KM, Costa MV, Malloy-Diniz LF, et al. Insomnia and risk of dementia in older adults: systematic review and meta-analysis. *J Psychiatr Res.* 2016;77:109–115.

37. Piolatto M, Bianchi F, Rota M. et al. The effect of social relationships on cognitive decline in older adults: an updated systematic review and meta-analysis of longitudinal cohort studies. *BMC Public Health.* 2022;22(1):278.
38. Salinas J, Beiser AS, Samra JK, et al Association of loneliness with 10-year dementia risk and early markers of vulnerability for neurocognitive decline. *Neurology* 2022;98(13):e1337–e1348.
39. Leon A. Reducing aging-associated risk of sarcopenia. In Rippe JM (ed.) *Lifestyle Medicine* (3rd ed). Boca Raton, FL: CRC Press, 2019.
40. Leon AS. Attenuation of adverse effects of aging on skeletal muscle by regular exercise and nutritional support. *Am J Lifestyle Med.* 2016;11(1):4–16.
41. American College of Lifestyle Medicine. https://lifestylemedicine.org/. Accessed March 21, 2025.
42. de Groot LC, van Staveren WA, Burema J. Survival beyond age 70 in relation to diet. *Nutr Rev.* 1996;54(7):211–212.
43. Institute of Medicine (US) Food and Nutrition Board. How Should the Recommended Dietary Allowances Be Revised? Washington, DC: National Academies Press (US), 1994. 2, Concepts Underlying the Recommended Dietary Allowances. https://www.ncbi.nlm.nih.gov/books/NBK231420/. Accessed March 21, 2025.
44. Institute of Medicine (US) Standing Committee on the Scientific Evaluation of Dietary Reference Intakes. Calcium, Phosphorus, Magnesium, Vitamin D and Fluoride. Washington, DC: National Academy of Sciences, 1997.
45. Institute of Medicine (US) Committee to Review Dietary Reference Intakes for Vitamin D and Calcium, Ross AC, Taylor CL, Yaktine AL, et al. (eds.). Dietary Reference Intakes for Calcium and Vitamin D. Washington, DC: National Academies Press, 2011. The National Academies. https://www.ncbi.nlm.nih.gov/books/NBK56064/
46. Institute of Medicine (US) Standing Committee on the Scientific Evaluation of Dietary Reference Intakes and its Panel on Folate, Other B Vitamins, and Choline. Dietary Reference Intakes for Thiamin, Riboflavin, Niacin, Vitamin B6, Folate, Vitamin B12, Pantothenic Acid, Biotin, and Choline. Washington, DC: National Academies Press (US), 1998.
47. Malik VS, Pan A, Willett WC, et al. Sugar-sweetened beverages and weight gain in children and adults: a systematic review and meta-analysis. *Am J Clin Nutr.* 2013;98(4):1084–1102.
48. Lipson LG, Bray GA. *Nutritional Aspects of Aging*, Vol. I, Chen LH (ed.). Boca Raton, FL: CRC Press, 1986.
49. Griep MI, Collys K, Mets TF, et al. Sensory detection of food odour in relation to dental status, gender and age. *Gerodontology.* 1996;13(1):56–62.
50. Griep MI, Verleye G, Franck AH, et al. Variation in nutrient intake with dental status, age and odour perception. *Eur J Clin Nutr.* 1996;50(12):816–825.
51. Loughrey DG, Kelly ME, Kelley GA, et al. Association of age-related hearing loss with cognitive function, cognitive impairment, and dementia: a systematic review and meta-analysis. *JAMA Otolaryngol Head Neck Surg.* 2018;144(2):115–126.
52. Scott IA, Hilmer SN, Reeve E, et al. Reducing inappropriate polypharmacy: the process of deprescribing. *JAMA Intern Med.* 2015;175(5):827–834.
53. Halli-Tierney AD, Scarbrough C, Carroll D. Polypharmacy: evaluating risks and deprescribing. *Am Fam Physician.* 2019;100(1):32–38.
54. NORC at the University of Chicago and Lucian Leape Institute. American's Experiences with Medical Errors and views on Patient Safety. Cambridge, MA: Institute for Healthcare Improvement and NORC at the University of Chicago, 2017. Americans' Experiences with Medical Errors and Views on Patient Safety|Institute for Healthcare Improvement. https://www.ihi.org/resources/publications/americans-experiences-medical-errors-and-views-patient-safety. Accessed March 21, 2025.
55. Makary MA, Daniel M. Medical error-the third leading cause of death in the US. *BMJ.* 2016;353:i2139.
56. Hoel RW, Giddings Connolly RM, et al. Polypharmacy management in older patients. *Mayo Clin Proc.* 2021;96(1):242–256.
57. O'Mahony D, O'Sullivan D, Byrne S, et al. STOPP/START criteria for potentially inappropriate prescribing in older people: version 2. *Age Ageing.* 2015;44(2):213–218.
58. By the American Geriatrics Society Beers Criteria Update Expert Panel. American Geriatrics Society 2019 updated AGS beers criteria(r) for potentially inappropriate medication use in older adults. *J Am Geriatr Soc.* 2019;67(4):674–694.
59. National Consensus Project for Quality Palliative Care. *Clinical Practice Guidelines for Quality Palliative Care* (4th ed). Richmond, VA: National Coalition for Hospice and Palliative Care, 2018. https://www.nationalcoalitionhpc.org/ncp. Accessed April 16, 2025.

60. Our Epidemic of Loneliness and Isolation: The U.S. Surgeon General's Advisory on the Healing Effects of Social Connection and Community. Washington, DC, 2023.
61. Peplau LA, Perlman D. *Loneliness: A Sourcebook of Current Theory, Research and Therapy.* New York: John Wiley & Sons Incorporated, 1982.
62. Shiovitz-Ezra S, Leitsch SA. The role of social relationships in predicting loneliness: the national social life, health, and aging project. *Social Work Res.* 2010;34(3):157–167.
63. Wenger GC, Davies S, Shahtahmasebi S, et al. Social isolation and loneliness in old age: review and model refinement. *Ageing Soc.* 1996;16:333–358.
64. Hawkley LC, Cacioppo JT. Loneliness matters: a theoretical and empirical review of consequences and mechanisms. *Ann Behav Med.* 2010;40(2):218–227.
65. Smith KJ, Victor C. Typologies of loneliness, living alone and social isolation, and their associations with physical and mental health. *Ageing Soc.* 2019;39:1709–1730.
66. De Jong GJ, Van Tilburg TG, Dykstra PA. Loneliness and social isolation. In Perlman D, Vangelisti A (eds.) *The Cambridge Handbook of Personal Relationships.* Cambridge: Cambridge University Press, 2006.
67. Valtora N, Hanratty B. Loneliness, isolation and the health of older adults: do we need a new research agenda? *J R Soc Med.* 2012;105(12):518–522.
68. Cohen-Mansfield J, Hazan H, Lerman Y, et al. Correlates and predictors of loneliness in older-adults: a review of quantitative results informed by qualitative insights. *Int Psychogeriatr.* 2016;28(4):557–576.
69. National Academies of Sciences, Engineering, and Medicine. *Social Isolation and Loneliness in Older Adults: Opportunities for the Health Care System.* Washington, DC: The National Academies Press, 2020.
70. Hughes ME, Waite LJ, Hawkley LC, et al. A short scale for measuring loneliness in large surveys: results from two population-based studies. *Res Aging.* 2004;26(6):655–672.
71. National Alliance for Caregiving and AARP. Caregiving in the U.S. 2020: A Focused Look at Family Caregivers of Adults Age 50+. 2020.
72. Swartz K, Collins LG. Caregiver care. *Am Fam Physician.* 2019;99(11):699–706.
73. Adelman RD, Tmanova LL, Delgado D, et al. Caregiver burden: a clinical review. *JAMA.* 2014;311(10):1052–1060.
74. Harper GH, Lyons WL, Potter JF (eds.). *Geriatrics Review Syllabus* (11th ed). New York: American Geriatrics Society, 2022.

16 Women's Health

16.1 INTRODUCTION

A number of lifestyle factors play critically important roles in enhancing women's health. While many of these factors are highly relevant for men's health (1–11), there are some unique aspects of women's health that are important to emphasize for all primary care and lifestyle medicine physicians.

Physical activity, healthy nutrition, weight management, and avoiding tobacco products all profoundly impact lowering the risk of various chronic diseases in women, particularly cardiovascular disease (CVD), type 2 diabetes (T2DM), and even cancer and cognitive decline (12).

Despite the abundance of evidence for these powerful lifestyle-related modalities for women's health, less than half of physicians currently counsel women patients on the importance of lifestyle measures such as healthy, plant-forward nutrition, physical activity, and maintenance of a healthy body weight. Shockingly, only 20% of physicians recognize that heart disease is the leading cause of death in women (13).

Weight management and obesity are other areas where lifestyle factors play a central role in women's health throughout a lifetime (14). In addition to issues related to brain health and cognition (15), regular physical activity and proper nutrition are also critically important for bone health and osteoporosis (10). The other factors discussed in multiple chapters in this book, including stress reduction, avoidance of risky substances, and the power of personal relationships, are also important for lifetime health in women.

All of these factors, including physical activity, nutrition, and weight management, assume particular importance during pregnancy and also the post-natal period. There is increasing evidence that all of these factors play important roles in both the degree of symptoms such as hot flashes and their frequency during menopause.

16.2 EPIDEMIOLOGY

CVD is the leading cause of death among both men and women in the United States, accounting for literally half of all deaths and considerable morbidity (16). T2DM is also a significant risk factor for CVD and is a particularly potent risk factor for CVD in women. The prevalence of T2DM has increased dramatically in the last 20 years among women (17). Epidemiologic data indicate that CVD and T2DM are common risk factors and are largely preventable (18).

For all these reasons, it is important to pay particular attention to risk factors for CVD and T2DM in both men and women, but particularly in women (19,20). Historically, CVD was widely considered less of a health threat for women than men. There are a number of reasons to explain this. Coronary heart disease (CHD) tends to appear later in women than it does in men (10 years later for total CHD and 20 years later for most of the serious manifestations, such as myocardial infarction (MI) and sudden cardiac death).

CHD is the leading killer of US men by the age of 45 and women by the age of 65 (21). Once women develop CHD, they have a dramatically worse prognosis than men. Among those aged greater than or equal to 40, 43% of women but only 33% of men die within five years of their first MI (19). In addition, 64% of women and only 50% of men who die suddenly from CHD have no prior symptoms (19). Fortunately, in the past 20 years, the decline of CHD deaths in women has been less pronounced, particularly in women aged 35–54, than among similarly aged men (20). Unfortunately, a national survey of physician awareness of CVD prevention guidelines found that fewer than one in five physicians knew that more women than men die each year of CVD (13).

DOI: 10.1201/9781003630043-16

The incidence of T2DM, which is a major risk factor for CVD, has increased more sharply among women than men in the United States and now affects almost 13% of adult women. In addition, impaired fasting glucose levels (also called impaired glucose tolerance (IGT)) are now estimated to occur in 35% and 40% of women (22,23). T2DM is a particularly strong risk factor for CVD in women, increasing their risk of developing CHD by three- to sevenfold compared to a two- to threefold increase in men.

For all of these reasons, lowering lifestyle-related risk factors in women is critically important. It is clear that physicians need to focus on the importance of positive lifestyle behaviors, including regular physical activity, not smoking, maintaining a healthy weight, and eating a healthy diet, in order to lower the risk of CVD in women. All of these issues will be discussed in detail in this chapter.

16.3 THE COMBINED POWER OF LIFESTYLE MEDICINE MODALITIES

As we have emphasized in a number of chapters in this book, multiple positive lifestyle modalities act synergistically with each other. Regular physical activity and healthy nutrition are both critically important for maintaining a healthy body weight. Maintaining a healthy body weight, in turn, is critically important for maintaining a healthy blood pressure and lowering the risk of hypertension as well as lowering the risk of multiple cancers and cognitive decline. Studies that have shown combinations of lifestyle-related behaviors and their impact on health have shown very promising results. Perhaps the most prominent of these studies is the Nurses' Health Study, which includes women who have been followed for more than 20 years (18). When various lifestyle factors were considered, including regular physical activity (30 minutes, five times per week), healthy nutrition (more fruits and vegetables, whole grains, and avoidance of saturated and trans fats), healthy weight management (BMI >19 and <25), not smoking cigarettes, and, most controversially, consuming one alcoholic beverage per day the combination resulted in a decreased risk of CHD of 83% and a decreased risk of T2DM of 91% in women studied. While these are extremely positive results, it should be noted that even among these health care workers, less than 5% maintained all five of these healthy lifestyle factors.

These data are consistent with previous reports from the Behavioral Risk Factor Surveillance Study (24) and the AHA Presidential Advisory on Cardiovascular Health, which showed less than 5% of individuals exhibited all of these healthy lifestyle factors (25).

Clearly, we have a long way to go! We hope that by calling out these issues, particularly in women, in this book and in the embedded curriculum, we can move the needle in a positive direction to emphasize the critically important health-related benefits that women can achieve through positive lifestyle factors.

16.4 LIFESTYLE MEDICINE MODALITIES AND WOMEN'S HEALTH

In this section, we will look at each of the lifestyle modalities individually as they apply to women's health. In the next section, we will explore how these modalities interact synergistically to lower the risk of or assist in the treatment of various chronic diseases.

16.4.1 Physical Activity

Regular physical activity has been demonstrated in multiple studies to convey numerous benefits for women throughout their life span (18,26–28). These benefits include reducing the likelihood of dying from CHD, lowering the risk of weight gain and obesity, T2DM, and certain cancers. Cognition, affect, and other aspects of brain health have also been demonstrated to be improved in women through regular physical activity throughout the life span (29).

The vast database for the numerous benefits of physical activity for women is supported by recommendations from a number of organizations, including the American Heart Association

(AHA) (30), the Physical Activity Guidelines for Americans Scientific Statement 2018 (PAGA), and the American College of Sports Medicine (ACSM) (31). Guidelines from all of these organizations are very similar, not only for women but also for men. All of these guidelines recommend 150 minutes of moderate-intensity physical activity per week, divided typically into five sessions or more, and two strength training sessions per week. Unfortunately, only approximately 28% of women exercise enough to meet these basic recommendations and 41% engage in no physical activity at all (32–34). Thus, the key counseling issue for physicians is to discuss the multiple benefits of regular physical activity for women and explore ways to increase the likelihood that they will adopt this critically important health-promoting habit.

16.4.2 Nutrition

As discussed in multiple chapters in this book, recent studies have focused more on the whole diet and dietary patterns rather than single nutrients or individual foods. Healthy dietary pattern recommendations have been consistent from the AHA (11), the Dietary Guidelines for Americans 2020–2025 (DGA 2020–2025) (35), and the Academy of Nutrition and Dietetics (AND) (36). All of these organizations recommend plant-forward diets consisting of increased whole grains, an abundance of fruits and vegetables, unsaturated omega-3 fatty acids, nuts, legumes, fish (particularly fatty fish), and poultry, while reducing the intake of refined grains, sugar-sweetened beverages, and red meat. These dietary patterns have been shown to lower the risk of CVD and other conditions such as T2DM. Food patterns that fit with these recommendations include the Mediterranean diet (MedDiet) (37), the US Healthy Foods Diet (35), and the DASH diet (38). In the Nurses' Health Study, the "Prudent" diet was listed as one of the diets recommended by the AHA. Recommendations from the American Heart Association Dietary Guidelines (11) memorialized the benefits of a plant-forward diet that embodies the healthy dietary strategies outlined in the paragraph.

This diet also embodies similar recommendations to those mentioned above.

In contrast, in the Nurses' Health Study, women who followed the Western Dietary Pattern, which has higher intakes of red and processed meats, sweets and desserts, French fries, and refined grains, experienced a higher risk of CHD by 46% and T2DM by 49% over 14–16 years of observation (39).

16.4.3 Obesity and Weight Management

Overweight and obesity are very prevalent in both men and women in the United States. In 2006, it was estimated that 35% of women were obese and 62% of US women were overweight or obese (40,41). Excess weight represents a major risk factor for a variety of metabolic diseases, including CVD and T2DM (42). Obesity raises the risk of CVD partly through its effects on established risk factors such as hypercholesterolemia, hypertension, and hyperglycemia, but also serves as an independent risk factor for CVD and T2DM.

Adult weight gain in women also raises the risk of CVD. In the Nurses' Health Study, a weight gain of as little as 10 pounds during adult years is associated with a 37% increase in cardiovascular risk for women (18,43). In an observational study of 1,669 Israeli women aged 50–75 with a BMI > 27 and at least one other coronary risk factor, those who lost 10 pounds during six months of nutritional counseling were significantly less likely to develop CHD during a four-year follow-up than counterparts who did not lose that amount of weight (44–46).

16.4.4 Cigarette Smoking and Alcohol

Cigarette smoking is the leading preventable cause of death in the United States (47). While more men smoke than women, the gender gap has narrowed. For example, between 1965 and 2005, smoking prevalence among US men declined from 52% to 24%, whereas the prevalence among US women dropped from 34% to 18% (48–50).

Most disturbing is that smoking prevalence in US girls is now equivalent to that of boys, which will contribute substantially to the future burden of CHD in women.

Alcohol consumption remains an area of ongoing research and has engendered considerable controversy. Guidelines have historically recommended that women consume no more than one alcoholic beverage a day (51–53). According to these recommendations, men should not exceed two alcoholic beverages a day. Some recent data, however, now suggest that even one alcoholic drink a day for either men or women is associated with an increased incidence of cognitive decline and certain cancers. This topic has provoked considerable debate and is far from settled.

16.4.5 Stress

As indicated elsewhere in this book, chronic stress is associated with multiple adverse events, both mental and physical (54,55). It is important to consider stress within the context of a woman's health across a lifespan. Stress is heightened at times of significant hormonal change, such as puberty, childbirth, and menopause.

Differences in stress response between men and women are thought to be related to differences in the hypothalamic-pituitary-adrenal (HPA) and hypothalamic-pituitary-gonadal (HPG) axes (56–58). The interplay between the HPA and HPG axes in women is hypothesized to create enhanced glucocorticoid secretion (59,60) in response to various stressors, which may enhance the response to stress. After puberty, during the transition to adulthood, women become twice as likely as men to develop stress-related disorders such as depression, anxiety, and post-traumatic stress disorder.

16.4.6 Sleep

Healthy, restorative sleep is important for both men and women (61). Women face additional challenges in this area because of changes in sex hormones. Changes in sleep related to phases of menstrual cycles also occur (62). Pregnancy may also affect sleep quality and quantity (63). In addition, the transition to menopause may create challenges to restful sleep (64). A high percentage of women in menopause transition report poor quality sleep and nocturnal awakenings as they transition into menopause (40%–56% compared to 31% in premenopausal women).

These changes may be due to lower estradiol levels and higher Follicle-stimulating hormone (FSH) levels, so the frequency and severity of basal motor symptoms may correlate with sleep disturbances (65,66).

16.4.7 Positive Relations with Others

The role of positive relationships in both men and women is discussed in detail in Chapter 7 (67). It should be noted that in both men and women, there is a reciprocal relationship between positive emotions and healthy lifestyles (68–72). Thus, clinicians should explore in all encounters with both men and women the area of relationships with other individuals. This is discussed in detail in Chapter 7.

16.5 COMBINATION OF LIFESTYLE MODALITIES AND CHRONIC DISEASES

- *Cardiovascular Disease*: Both physical activity and nutrition play a substantial role in reducing the incidence of CHD in women. As already indicated, women experience serious manifestations of heart disease and suffer sudden cardiac death at a later age than men. Multiple studies have shown that 30 minutes per day of moderate-intensity physical activity substantially lowers the risk of CHD in women. This includes data from the Women's Health Initiative, where brisk walking for two hours per week or approximately 30 minutes five times per week resulted in a 30% reduction in cardiovascular events over a 3.2-year follow-up (73). Multiple other studies have shown similar reductions in CHD based on moderate-intensity physical activity (74–77). A healthy plant-based diet has also been shown to lower the risk of T2DM in women, as has healthy weight management.

- *Diabetes/Pre-diabetes*: Healthy nutrition and weight management both lower the risk of chronic disease in women, including both CVD and T2DM. In the Nurses' Health Study, excess body weight was by far the most predictive factor in the onset of T2DM (78). The risk of developing diabetes over 16 years of follow-up was 40-fold higher in women with a BMI > 35 kg/m^2 and 20-fold higher in women with a BMI > 30 compared to women with a BMI of <23. Even women in the healthy weight range (23.0–23.9) were at a threefold increased risk of diabetes compared to women with a BMI < 23 (78). Other studies have shown similar results (79).

  According to NHANES data, women who gained between 5.0 and 7.9 kg over the preceding decade doubled their risk of T2DM in a nine-year period compared to weight-stable counterparts (80). Intentional weight loss through calorie restriction combined with physical activity reduces the risk of T2DM in overweight individuals (81–84). This was shown in the Diabetes Prevention Program (DPP) (85) study and the Finnish Diabetes Study (FDS) (86).
- *Cancer*: Various lifestyle factors have been shown to interact with a number of gynecologic cancers (87,88). Obesity, inactivity, and poor diet can contribute to endometrial cancer (EC) and breast cancer. Approximately 50% of all new diagnoses of EC are attributed to obesity alone (87). Regular physical activity has been demonstrated to result in a 20%–30% risk reduction of EC in women who report moderate- to high-intensity exercise compared to non-exercisers (89,90). Cigarette smoking and alcohol have both been clearly associated with multiple cancers of the respiratory tract, GI tract, and also endocrine-responsive cancers such as breast and EC (91).
- *The Metabolic Syndrome*: As discussed in Chapter 10, the Metabolic Syndrome (MetS) is a significant risk factor for CVD (92,93). Gender differences in the prevalence of various components of MetS also affect CVD risk in women. For example, elevations in blood pressure, waist circumference, and triglycerides are responsible for most of the prevalence of CVD in women (43,94). Waist circumference also increases the risk of MetS in women to a higher degree than in men (95,96). Dyslipidemia is associated with a higher risk of CHD in women compared to men. Elevated triglyceride levels (particularly when combined with low HDL levels) have a greater impact on CHD risk in women than in men. Elevated fasting blood sugar is more common in women than in men.
- *Brain Health/Cognitive Decline/Dementia*: Cognitive decline and dementia are more common in women than in men (97). Lifestyle-related approaches such as whole food plant-based diets, regular physical activity, stress reduction, quality sleep, avoiding harmful substances, and continued positive relationships and socialization throughout the lifespan are known to optimize brain health and are particularly relevant given the high level of cognitive decline and dementia in women.

Psychiatric disorders are associated with a significant burden of morbidity and disability. Numerous studies suggest that gender is a significant determinant of mental health. Over 22% of adult women are estimated to suffer from a mental health disorder compared to 15.1% of men (98). The exact reasons for this disparity are not explicitly known and are likely to be multifactorial. There are potential contributions from hormones, social status, and exposure to mental health risks and other socioeconomic factors. Significantly, rates of depression are about two times higher in women than in men and may be more persistent in women.

Some psychiatric disorders are unique to women. These include disorders tied to hormonal changes such as pre- and post-natal depression, premenstrual dysphoric disorder, and perimenopausal-related depression (99,100). It has been argued that rather than viewing women's psychiatric health in each area, it may be more useful to determine women's psychiatric health comprehensively across the lifespan.

There are multiple ways that lifestyle modalities can prevent the onset of many psychiatric disorders in women. For example, studies suggest that a healthy diet may be associated with a lower incidence of depression compared to a Western Diet (101). In addition, a number of studies have reported that physical activity can ameliorate psychiatric disorders such as anxiety and depression in both men and women. This may be particularly appropriate for women, given the increased risk of these disorders in women (102). In addition, tobacco use cessation may have a particularly significant psychological health benefit for women than men. It has been shown in various research studies that patients with psychiatric disorders are more likely to smoke. For example, the prevalence of tobacco smoking in schizophrenic patients was 62%, while the prevalence of smoking in bipolar patients was lower (44%). Both of these are significantly higher than in the general population. Given these high levels of cigarette smoking in individuals with significant psychiatric disorders, it may be particularly relevant to counsel women about the important psychiatric benefits of smoking cessation.

Physical activity has been associated with multiple aspects of improved cognition and brain health throughout the lifespan in women. In 2009, a meta-analysis of 16 prospective studies reported that individuals at the highest level of physical activity experienced a 28% reduction in the risk of dementia and a 46% reduction in the risk of Alzheimer's disease compared to individuals at the lowest activity level (10).

16.6 SEXUAL HEALTH

Sexual health is clearly linked to overall health, with sexual dysfunction being common (103). A lifestyle medicine approach can support sexual health in women through various mechanisms, including improved vascular health and psychological well-being.

A plant-based, antioxidant-rich dietary pattern and regular physical activity support key measures of sexual health. Mindfulness-based stress reduction strategies can also be effective. Chronic stress, quality of social support, and other lifestyle factors can contribute to sexual health in women in a number of ways. Dietary composition affects sexual health through its association with reduced CVD, which, in turn, is related to sexual dysfunction. The MetDiet) has been studied, and adherence to the MetDiet results in better sexual function in a dose-dependent manner, regardless of menopausal or metabolic syndrome status (104,105).

Regular physical activity promotes sexual health in both short- and long-term ways (106). Short-term bouts of physical activity may stimulate the sympathetic nervous system and contribute to prompt physiological arousal. Regular physical activity also acts on a variety of hormones linked to sexual function, such as estrogen, testosterone, prolactin, oxytocin, and cortisol. Both the quality and quantity of sleep impact sexual desire, satisfaction, and function. The connections between stress and sexual health are multifaceted. Stress may influence sexual function physiologically through various hormonal pathways. Chronic stress is also associated with symptoms of anxiety and depression, which may also be linked to sexual dysfunction (107). Mindfulness-based stress reduction represents a promising approach to help women with sexual dysfunction.

The importance of positive social connections and high-quality relationships are key components of sexual health (108). Greater social support and intimacy result in a higher likelihood of sexual activity, desire, and satisfaction (109).

Substances such as alcohol, tobacco, and cannabis also impact female sexual health. Alcohol has a variety of effects on sexual function. Women who consume alcohol in moderation are more likely to be sexually active and may achieve higher levels of desire and satisfaction. High consumption of alcohol, however, is linked to sexual dysfunction. Cigarette smoking can contribute to sexual dysfunction and vascular dysfunction. There are also data showing that cigarette smokers are less likely to be sexually active and report more sexual dysfunction than non-smokers.

16.7 PREGNANCY AND POST-PARTUM

Multiple lifestyle measures carry a significant impact on both pregnancy and the post-partum period. Physical activity yields multiple benefits during both of these times. For this reason, the American College of Obstetricians and Gynecologists (ACOG) (110) and the PAGA 2018 Scientific Report recommend physical activity for women who are pregnant. The only caveat is to avoid contact activities or activities that increase the risk of falls. Other lifestyle behaviors during this period include the following:

- A healthy dietary pattern, such as the Mediterranean or DASH diet.
- Sleep disturbances are common during pregnancy so following proper sleep hygiene habits is essential (see also Chapter 6) (111).
- Stress, particularly chronic stress, can have an adverse impact on pregnancy outcomes (112).
- Nicotine, alcohol, and illicit substances raise the risk of maternal complications.
- Risky substances.

Women should also reduce the total burden of exposure to environmental and teratogenic substances during the reproductive years, but particularly during pregnancy. The various lifestyle medicine habits and practices discussed throughout this book and in the embedded curriculum are all highly relevant during pregnancy. Sleep disturbances were studied in one research trial with 2,000 women across the duration of their pregnancy. It was reported that 76% of women reported poor sleep quality, including frequent nighttime awakenings (111).

> The post-partum period is a particularly important time for both mental and physical recovery. This timeframe sets the stage for long-term health both for the woman and her infant. The risk is that the post-partum period is also a time when serious health risks may occur. The risk of maternal mortality peaks within 42 days of delivery, and it is 3–4 times higher for women of color compared to White women. There can also be a very real sense of abandonment, which can result in post-partum depression, which should be assessed and discussed at all post-partum visits.

16.8 MENOPAUSE

Multiple lifestyle medicine modalities can play an important role during menopause. Regular physical activity, for example, can play an important role in both physical and psychological well-being during menopause (113). In addition, as pointed out in multiple chapters in this book, regular physical activity is important for yielding multiple benefits, including lowering the risk of CVD and T2DM as well as lowering the risk of weight gain and obesity.

The onset of menopause can mean significant changes for women mentally, emotionally, and physically. Healthy lifestyle behaviors can help reduce adverse responses, including diet, physical activity, stress reduction, and positive relationships with other people. These can reduce menopausal symptoms (99). Eating a whole-food, plant-based diet for metabolic optimization may also improve menopausal symptoms. In addition, during the menopausal transition, many women experience weight gain and changes in body composition and distribution. Research studies have shown that women in midlife often gain an average of 1–1.5 pounds annually. Activity has not been shown to prevent age-related weight gain altogether, but it can protect against the development of obesity and the accumulation of metabolically harmful intra-abdominal fat.

Physical activity recommendations for postmenopausal women are the same as for other ages, as outlined by the PAGA 2018 Scientific Report, which contains the recommendation of 150 minutes of moderate-intensity physical activity on a weekly basis (10).

Stress reduction is also an important component of menopausal health. There is some evidence that stress is the precipitating or at least an aggravating factor in hot flashes (114). This is another reason to utilize physical activity to manage stress responses. In addition, menopause-related symptoms can disrupt interpersonal relationships. Postmenopausal women often experience a decrease in sexual activity, supportive partners, and positive workplace relationships, and good communication with the individual's physician can help ameliorate these issues.

Sleep disturbances are also common in menopause. As many as 26% of women experience significant sleep disorders during this period of time (115,116). These may be responsive to lifestyle modalities such as cognitive behavioral therapy and lifestyle-related strategies to address vasomotor symptoms. As in any other stage of a woman's life, counseling should be offered related to both alcohol and cigarette smoking. The study of women across the nation (SWAN) found that some individuals who had been previously heavy drinkers decreased their alcohol consumption during menopause, while others who had not been heavy drinkers increased their alcohol consumption. The SWAN study found no association between menopausal transition and smoking. However, both alcohol use and cigarette smoking should be assessed and counseled during clinical visits for women during menopause (117,118).

16.9 CONCLUSIONS/CLINICAL APPLICATIONS

Many of the recommendations regarding positive lifestyle habits and actions are similar for both men and women. However, there are a number of life stages, such as pregnancy and menopause, during which women can particularly benefit from positive lifestyle behaviors. In addition, it should be emphasized to all women patients that cardiovascular disease remains the leading cause of morbidity and mortality in women. This is a factor that is often not understood or recognized among physicians. The use of lifestyle medicine modalities can play a very important role throughout the entire lifespan of women to improve health and lower the risk of various chronic diseases.

REFERENCES

1. Tollefson M, Eriksen N, Pathak N. *Improving Women's Health across the Lifespan*. Boca Raton, FL: CRC Press, 2021.
2. Stone NJ, Robinson JG, Lichtenstein AH, et al. 2013 ACC/AHA guideline on the treatment of blood cholesterol to reduce atherosclerotic cardiovascular risk in adults. *Circulation*. 2014;129(25_suppl_2):S1–S45.
3. Lloyd-Jones DM, Allen NB, Anderson CAM, Black T, Brewer LC, Foraker RE, et al. Life's essential 8: updating and enhancing the American Heart Association's construct of cardiovascular health: a presidential advisory From the American Heart Association. *Circulation*. 2022;146(5):e18–e43.
4. Mozaffarian D, Appel LJ, Van Horn L. Components of a cardioprotective diet: new insights. *Circulation*. 2011;123(24):2870–2891.
5. Liu S, Stampfer MJ, Hu FB, et al. Whole-grain consumption and risk of coronary heart disease: results from the Nurses' Health Study. *Am J Clin Nutr.* 1999;70(3):412–419.
6. American Heart Association. Council on Lifestyle and Cardiometabolic Health. https://professional.heart.org/en/professional-membershipCounciles/ScientificCouncils. Accessed March 19, 2025.
7. Eckel RH, Jakicic JM, Ard JD, et al. 2013 AHA/ACC guideline on lifestyle management to reduce cardiovascular risk: a report of the American College of Cardiology/American Heart Association Task Force on Practice Guidelines. *Circulation*. 2014;129(25 Suppl 2):S76–S99.
8. Whelton PK, Carey RM, Aronow WS, et al. 2017 ACC/AHA/AAPA/ABC/ACPM/AGS/APhA/ASH/ASPC/NMA/PCNA guideline for the prevention, detection, evaluation, and management of high blood pressure in adults. A report of the American College of Cardiology/American Heart Association Task Force on Clinical Practice Guidelines, 2017.
9. U.S. Department of Agriculture and U.S. Department of Health and Human Services. U.S. Department of Agriculture and U.S. Department of Health and Human Services. Dietary Guidelines for Americans, 2020–2025 (9th ed). December 2020. Available at DietaryGuidelines.gov. 2020. https://www.dietaryguidelines.gov/resources/2020-2025-dietary-guidelines-online-materials.
10. Physical Activity Guidelines Advisory Committee. 2018 Physical Activity Guidelines Advisory Committee. 2018 Physical Activity Guidelines Advisory Committee Scientific Report. Washington, DC: U.S. Department of Health and Human Services, 2018.
11. Lichtenstein AH, Appel LJ, Vadiveloo M, et al. 2021 Dietary guidance to improve cardiovascular health: a scientific statement from the American Heart Association. *Circulation*. 2021;144(23):e472–e487.

12. Bassuk SS, Manson JE. Lifestyle and risk of cardiovascular disease and type 2 diabetes in women: a review of the epidemiologic evidence. *Am J Lifestyle Med.* 2008;2(3):191–213.
13. Mosca L, Linfante AH, Benjamin EJ, et al. National study of physician awareness and adherence to cardiovascular disease prevention guidelines. *Circulation.* 2005;111(4):499–510.
14. Committee on Accelerating Progress in Obesity Prevention; Food and Nutrition Board; Institute of Medicine; Glickman D, Parker L, Sim LJ, et al., (eds.). Accelerating Progress in Obesity Prevention: Solving the Weight of the Nation. Washington, DC: National Academies Press, 2012 May 8. doi: 10.17226/13275; https://www.ncbi.nlm.nih.gov/books/NBK201141/
15. Schwamm L, Fayad P, Acker JE, et al. Translating evidence into practice: a decade of efforts by the American Heart Association/American Stroke Association to reduce death and disability due to stroke. *Stroke.* 2010;41(5):1051–1065.
16. Virani SS, Alonso A, Aparicio HJ, et al. Heart disease and stroke statistics-2021 update: a report from the American Heart Association. *Circulation.* 2021;143(8):e254–e743.
17. American Diabetes Association. 2 classification and diagnosis of diabetes. Standards of medical care in diabetes 2018. *Diabetes Care.* 2018;41(suppl): S13–S27.
18. Liu S, Stampfer MJ, Hu FB, Giovannucci E, et al. Whole-grain consumption and risk of coronary heart disease: results from the Nurses' Health Study. *Am J Clin Nutr.* 1999;70:412–419.
19. Rosamond W., Flegal K., Friday G., et al. Heart disease and stroke statistics-2007 update: a report from the American Heart Association Statistics Committee and Stroke Statistics Subcommittee. *Circulation.* 2007;115:e69–e171.
20. Ford ES, Capewell S. Coronary heart disease mortality among young adults in the U.S. from 1980 through 2002: concealed leveling of mortality rates. *J Am Coll Cardiol.* 2007;50:2128–2132.
21. Rippe JM. Lifestyle strategies for risk factor reduction, prevention, and treatment of cardiovascular disease. *Am J Lifestyle Med.* 2018;13(2):204–212.
22. Centers for Disease Control and Prevention. Prevalence of diabetes and impaired fasting glucose in adults: United States, 1999–2000. *MMWR Morb Mortal Wkly Rep.* 2003;52:833–837.
23. Manson J, Spelsberg A. Risk modification in the diabetic patient. In Manson J, et al. (eds.) *Prevention of Myocardial Infarction* (online ed). New York: Oxford Academic, 1996. Accessed April 8, 2025.
24. Behavioral Risk Factor Surveillance study. National Center for Chronic Disease Prevention and Health Promotion, Division of Population Health. November 24, 2024.
25. AHA Presidential Advisory. Life's essential 8: updating and enhancing the American Heart Association's construct of cardiovascular health: a presidential advisory from the American Heart Association. *Circulation.* 2022;146:e18–e43.
26. CDC Benefits of Physical Activity. Centers for Disease Control and Prevention. Published September 11, 2020. Accessed March 19, 2025.
27. Hörder H, Johansson L, Guo X, et al. Midlife cardiovascular fitness and dementia: a 44-year longitudinal population study in women. *Neurology.* 2018;90(15):e1298–e1305.
28. Sallis R. Exercise is medicine: a call to action for physicians to assess and prescribe exercise. *Phys Sportsmed.* 2015;43(1):22–26.
29. Kramer AF, Erickson KI, Colcombe SJ. Exercise, cognition, and the aging brain. *J Appl Physiol.* 2006;101(4):1237–1242.
30. American Heart Association. American Heart Association Recommendations for Physical Activity in Adults and Kids. American Heart Association Recommendations for Physical Activity in Adults and Kids | American Heart Association. Accessed March 26, 2025.
31. American College of Sports Medicine. Physical Activity Guidelines. Physical Activity Guidelines – ACSM. Accessed March 26, 2025.
32. US Department of Health and Human Services. Physical Activity and Health: A Report of the Surgeon General. Atlanta, GA: US Dept of Health and Human Services, Centers for Disease Control and Prevention, National Center for Chronic Disease Prevention and Health Promotion, 1996.
33. Haskell WL, Lee IM, Pate RR, et al. Physical activity and public health: updated recommendation for adults from the American College of Sports Medicine and the American Heart Association. *Circulation.* 2007;116:1081–1093.
34. Barnes PM. Physical Activity among Adults: United States, 2000 and 2005. https://iiab.me/modules/en-cdc/www.cdc.gov/nchs/data/hestat/physicalactivity/physicalactivity.htm. Accessed March 19, 2025.
35. 2020–2025 US Department of Health and Human Services and US Department of Agriculture. 2020–2025 Dietary Guidelines for Americans (9th ed). 2020, p. 164.

36. Academy of Nutrition and Dietetics Evidence Analysis Library. Adult Weight Management: Executive Summary of Recommendations 2014. Academy of Nutrition and Dietetics. https://www.andeal.org/topic.cfm?menu=5276&cat=4690. Accessed March 19, 2025.
37. Estruch R, Ros E, Salas-Salvado J, et al. PREDIMED study investigators. Primary prevention of cardiovascular disease with a mediterranean diet. *N Eng J Med.* 2013;368:1279–1290.
38. Sacks FM, Svetkey LP, Vollmer WM, et al. Effects on blood pressure of reduced dietary sodium and the Dietary Approaches to Stop Hypertension (DASH) diet. *N Engl J Med.* 2001;344(1):3–10.
39. Satija A, Bhupathiraju SN, Spiegelman D, et al. Healthful and unhealthful plant-based diets and the risk of coronary heart disease in U.S. adults. *J Am Coll Cardiol.* 2017;70(4):411–422.
40. Ogden CL, Carroll MD, Curtin LR, et al. Prevalence of overweight and obesity in the United States, 1999–2004. *JAMA.* 2006;295:1549–1555.
41. Ogden CL, Carroll MD, McDowell MA, et al. Obesity Among Adults in the United States – No Change Since 2003–2004. NCHS Data Brief No. 1. Hyattsville, MD: National Center for Health Statistics, 2007.
42. Poirier P, Giles TD, Bray GA, et al. Obesity and cardiovascular disease: Pathophysiology, Evaluation, and effect of weight loss: An update of the 1997 American Heart Association Scientific Statement on Obesity and Heart Disease from the Obesity Committee of the Council on Nutrition, Physical Activity, and Metabolism. *Circulation.* 2006;113:898–918.
43. Wilson PW, Kannel WB, Silbershatz H, et al. Clustering of metabolic factors and coronary heart disease. *Arch Intern Med.* 1999;159:1104–1110.
44. Esposito K, Pontillo A, Di Palo C, et al. Effect of weight loss and lifestyle changes on vascular inflammatory markers in obese women: a randomized trial. *JAMA.* 2003;289(14):1799–1804.
45. Tchernof A, Nolan A, Sites CK, et al. Weight loss reduces C-reactive protein levels in obese postmenopausal women. *Circulation.* 2002;105:564–569.
46. Van Gaal LF, Wauters MA, De Leeuw IH. The beneficial effects of modest weight loss on cardiovascular risk factors. *Int J Obes Relat Metab Disord.* 1997;21(suppl 1):S5–S9.
47. Centers for Disease Control and Prevention. Smoking and Tobacco Use. Data and Statistics 2000. https://www.cdc.gov/tobacco/about/index.html. Accessed March 19, 2025.
48. Centers for Disease Control and Prevention. Tobacco use among adults – United States. 2005. *MMWR Morb Mortal Wkly Rep.* 2006;55:1145–1148.
49. Hennekens CH. Risk factors for coronary heart disease in women. *Cardiol Clin.* 1998;16:1–8.
50. Bolego C, Poli A, Paoletti R. Smoking and gender. *Cardiovasc Res.* 2002;53(3):568–576.
51. Di Castelnuovo A, Rotondo S, Iacoviello L, et al. Meta-analysis of wine and beer consumption in relation to vascular risk. *Circulation.* 2002;18;105(24):2836–44.
52. Stampfer MJ, Colditz GA, Willett WC, et al. A prospective study of moderate alcohol consumption and the risk of coronary disease and stroke in women. *N Engl J Med.* 1988;319(5):267–273.
53. Urbano-Márquez A, Estruch R, Fernández-Solá J, et al. The greater risk of alcoholic cardiomyopathy and myopathy in women compared with men. *JAMA.* 1995;274(2):149–154.
54. What is Stress? The American Institute of Stress. https://www.stress.org/what-is-stress/. Accessed March 19, 2025.
55. Avey H, Matheny KB, Robbins A, et al. Health care providers' training, perceptions, and practices regarding stress and health outcomes. *J Natl Med Assoc.* 2003;95(9):833,836–845.
56. Lewis KP, Barton RA. Amygdala size and hypothalamus size predict social play frequency in nonhuman primates: a comparative analysis using independent contrasts. *J Comp Psychol.* 2006;120(1):31–37.
57. McCorry LK. Physiology of the autonomic nervous system. *Am J Pharm Educ.* 2007;15;71(4):78.
58. Ulrich-Lai YM, Herman JP. Neural regulation of endocrine and autonomic stress responses. *Nat Rev Neurosci.* 2009;10(6):397–409.
59. Kuo T, McQueen A, Chen TC, et al. Regulation of glucose homeostasis by glucocorticoids. *Adv Exp Med Biol.* 2015;872:99–126.
60. Gupta S, Aslakson E, Gurbaxani BM, et al. Inclusion of the glucocorticoid receptor in a hypothalamic pituitary adrenal axis model reveals bistability. *Theor Biol Med Model.* 2007;4:8.
61. Mallampalli MP, Carter CL. Exploring sex and gender differences in sleep health: a Society for Women's Health Research Report. *J Women's Health.* 2014;23(7):553–562.
62. Baker FC, Lee KA. Menstrual cycle effects on sleep. *Sleep Med Clin.* 2022;17(2):283–294.
63. Sedov ID, Cameron EE, Madigan S, Tomfohr-Madsen LM. Sleep quality during pregnancy: a meta-analysis. *Sleep Med Rev.* 2018;38:168–176.
64. Baker FC, Lampio L, Saaresranta T, et al. Sleep and sleep disorders in the menopausal transition. *Sleep Med Clin.* 2018;13(3):443–456.

65. Hirotsu C, Tufik S, Andersen ML. Interactions between sleep, stress, and metabolism: from physiological to pathological conditions. *Sleep Sci.* 2015;8(3):143–152.
66. de Zambotti M, Trinder J, Colrain IM, et al. Menstrual cycle-related variation in autonomic nervous system functioning in women in the early menopausal transition with and without insomnia disorder. *Psychoneuroendocrinology.* 2017;75:44–51.
67. Peterson C. *A Primer in Positive Psychology* (Oxford Positive Psychology Series) (1st ed). Oxford: Oxford University Press, 2006.
68. Gardner MP, Wansink B, Kim J, et al. Better moods for better eating? How mood influences food choice. *J Consum Psychol.* 2014;24(3):320–335.
69. Van Cappellen P, Rice EL, Catalino LI, et al. Positive affective processes underlie positive health behaviour change. *Psychol Health.* 2018;33(1):77–97.
70. Kubzansky LD, Huffman JC, Boehm JK, et al. Positive psychological well-being and cardiovascular disease: JACC health promotion series. *J Am Coll Cardiol.* 2018;72(12):1382–1396.
71. Yeung JWK, Zhang Z, Kim TY. Volunteering and health benefits in general adults: cumulative effects and forms. *BMC Public Health.* 2017;18(1):8.
72. Kim ES, Strecher VJ, Ryff CD. Purpose in life and use of preventive health care services. *Proc Natl Acad Sci USA.* 2014;111(46):16331–16336.
73. Manson JE, Greenland P, LaCroix AZ, et al. Walking compared with vigorous exercise for the prevention of cardiovascular events in women. *N Engl J Med.* 2002;347:716–725.
74. Manson JE, Hu FB, Rich-Edwards JW, et al. A prospective study of walking as compared with vigorous exercise in the prevention of coronary heart disease in women. *N Engl J Med.* 1999;341: 650–658.
75. Lee IM, Rexrode KM, Cook NR, et al. Physical activity and coronary heart disease in women: is "no pain, no gain" passé? *JAMA.* 2001;285:1447–1454.
76. Sesso HD, Paffenbarger RS, et al. Physical activity and cardiovascular disease risk in middle-aged and older women. *Am J Epidemiol.* 1999;150:408–416.94.
77. Gregg EW, Cauley JA, Stone K, et al. Relationship of changes in physical activity and mortality among older women. *JAMA.* 2003;289:2379–2386.
78. Field AE, Coakley EH, Must A, et al. Impact of overweight on the risk of developing common chronic diseases during a 10-year period. *Arch Intern Med.* 2001;161(13):1581–1586.
79. Ford ES, Williamson DF, Liu S. Weight change and diabetes incidence: findings from a national cohort of US Adults. *Am J Epidemiol.* 1997;146:214–222.
80. Colditz GA, Willett WC, Rotnitzky A, et al. Weight gain as a risk factor for clinical diabetes mellitus in women. *Ann Intern Med.* 1995;122:481–486.
81. Pan XR, Li GW, Hu YH, et al. Effects of diet and exercise in preventing NIDDM in people with impaired glucose tolerance. The Da Qing IGT and Diabetes Study. *Diabetes Care.* 1997;20:537–544.
82. Tuomilehto J, Lindstrom J, Eriksson JG, et al. Prevention of type 2 diabetes mellitus by changes in lifestyle among subjects with impaired glucose tolerance. *N Engl J Med.* 2001;344:1343–1350.
83. Knowler WC, Barrett-Connor E, Fowler SE, et al. Reduction in the incidence of type 2diabetes with lifestyle intervention or metformin. *N Engl J Med.* 2002;346:393–403.
84. Ramachandran A, Snehalatha C, Mukesh B, et al. The Indian Diabetes Prevention Programme shows that lifestyle modification and metformin prevent type 2 diabetes in Asian Indian subjects with impaired glucose tolerance (IDPP-1). *Diabetologia.* 2006;49:289–297.85.
85. The Diabetes Prevention Program (DPP) Research Group. The Diabetes Prevention Program (DPP): description of lifestyle intervention. *Diabetes Care.* 2002;25(12):2165–2171.
86. Lindström J, Louheranta A, Mannelin M, et al. Finnish Diabetes Prevention Study Group. The Finnish Diabetes Prevention Study (DPS): lifestyle intervention and 3-year results on diet and physical activity. *Diabetes Care.* 2003:26(12):3230–3236.
87. Siegel RL, Miller KD, Jemal A. Cancer statistics, 2020. *CA Cancer J Clin.* 2020;70(1):7–30.
88. World Cancer Research Fund/American Institute for Cancer Research. Diet, Nutrition, Physical Activity and Cancer. A Global Perspective. Continuous Update Project Expert Report, 2018.
89. Irwin ML, Smith AW, McTiernan A, et al. Influence of pre- and postdiagnosis physical activity on mortality in breast cancer survivors: the health, eating, activity, and lifestyle study. *J Clin Oncol.* 2008;26(24):3958–3964.
90. Vainio H, Kaaks R, Bianchini F. Weight control and physical activity in cancer prevention: international evaluation of the evidence. *Eur J Cancer Prev.* 2002;11(Suppl 2):S94–S100.
91. World Health Organization. WHO Report on the Global Tobacco Epidemic. 2023. https://www.who.int/publications/i/item/9789240077164. Accessed March 24, 2025.

92. Grundy SM, Cleeman JI, Daniels SR, et al. Diagnosis and management of the metabolic syndrome: an American Heart Association/National Heart, Lung, and Blood Institute Scientific Statement. *Circulation.* 2005;112(17):2735–2752.
93. Ford ES, Giles WH, Dietz WH. Prevalence of the metabolic syndrome among US adults: findings from the Third National Health and Nutrition Examination Survey. *JAMA.* 2002;287(3):356–359.
94. Ashton WD, Nanchahal K, Wood DA. Body mass index and metabolic risk factors for coronary heart disease in women. *Eur Heart J.* 2001;22(1):46–55.
95. Bentley-Lewis R, Koruda K, Seely EW. The metabolic syndrome in women. *Nat Clin Pract Endocrinol Metab.* 2007;3(10):696–704.
96. Sarafidis PA, McFarlane SI, Bakris GL. Gender disparity in outcomes of care and management for diabetes and the metabolic syndrome. *Curr Diab Rep.* 2006;6:219–224.
97. 2020 Alzheimer's disease facts and figures. *Alzheimer's Dement.* 2020;16:391–460. doi: 10.1002/alz.12068. Accessed March 24, 2025.
98. Merlo G, Ryu H, Nikbin A. Psychiatric disorders in women. In Tollefson M, Eriksen N, Pathak N (eds.) *Improving Women's Health Across the Lifespan.* Boca Raton, FL: CRC Press, 2022.
99. Li RX, Ma M, Xiao XR, et al. Perimenopausal syndrome and mood disorders in perimenopause: prevalence, severity, relationships, and risk factors. *Medicine.* 2016:95(32):e4466.
100. Gibbs Z, Lee S, Kulkarni J. Factors associated with depression during the perimenopausal transition. *Women's Health Issues.* 2013:23(5):e301–e307.
101. Gaudlitz J, von Lindengerger B, Strohle A. Physical activity and anxiety. In Rippe JM (ed.) *Lifestyle Medicine* (3rd ed). Boca Raton, FL: CRC Press, 2019.
102. Fair K, Rethorst C. Physical activity and depression. In Rippe JM (ed.) *Lifestyle Medicine* (3rd ed). Boca Raton, FL: CRC Press, 2019.
103. World Health Organization (WHO) Sexual Health. https://www.who.int/health-topics/sexual-health#tab=tab_1. Accessed March 24, 2025.
104. Maiorino MI, Bellastella G, Caputo M, et al. Effects of Mediterranean diet on sexual function in people with newly diagnosed type 2 diabetes: The MÈDITA trial. *J Diabetes Complicat.* 2016;30(8):1519–1524.
105. Esposito K, Maiorino MI, Bellastella G, et al. Determinants of female sexual dysfunction in type 2 diabetes. *Int J Impot Res.* 2010;22(3):179–184.
106. Stanton AM, Handy AB, Meston CM. The effects of exercise on sexual function in women. *Sex Med Rev.* 2018;6(4):548–557.
107. Hamilton LD, Meston CM. Chronic stress and sexual function in women. *J Sex Med.* 2013;10(10):2443–2454.
108. McCool-Myers M, Theurich M, Zuelke A, et al. Predictors of female sexual dysfunction: a systematic review and qualitative analysis through gender inequality paradigms. *BMC Women's Health.* 2018;18(1):108.
109. Trompeter SE, Bettencourt R, Barrett-Connor E. Sexual activity and satisfaction in healthy community-dwelling older women. *Am J Med.* 2012:125(1):37–43.e1.
110. ACOG Committee Opinion No. 804. Physical activity and exercise during pregnancy and the postpartum period: correction. *Obstet Gynecol.* 2021;138(4):683.
111. Mindell JA, Cook RA, Nikolovski J. Sleep patterns and sleep disturbances across pregnancy. *Sleep Med.* 2015;16(4):483–488.
112. Woods SM, Melville JL, Guo Y, et al. Psychosocial stress during pregnancy. *Am J Obstet Gynecol.* 2010;202(1):61.e1–61.e7.
113. Warburton DE, Nicol CW, Bredin SS. Health benefits of physical activity: the evidence. *CMAJ.* 2006;174(6):801–809.
114. Dalal PK, Agarwal M. Postmenopausal syndrome. *Indian J Psychiatry.* 2015;57(Suppl 2):S222–S232.
115. Liu YZ, Wang YX, Jiang CL. Inflammation: the common pathway of stress-related diseases. *Front Hum Neurosci.* 2017;11:316.
116. Ginaldi L, Di Benedetto MC, De Martinis M. Osteoporosis, inflammation and ageing. *Immun Ageing.* 2005;2:14.
117. Ganry O, Baudoin C, Fardellone P. Effect of alcohol intake on bone mineral density in elderly women: The EPIDOS Study. Epidémiologie de l'Ostéoporose. *Am J Epidemiol.* 2000;151(8):773–780.
118. Ill PO, Alexandre C. Le tabac facteur de risque de l'ostéoporose. Mythe ou realité? [Tobacco as risk factor of osteoporosis, myth or reality?]. *Rev Rhum Ed Fr.* 1993;60(4):280–286. French. PMID: 8167625.

17 Lifestyle Medicine for Children

17.1 INTRODUCTION

While this book and the embedded curriculum are largely devoted to issues related to lifestyle medicine for adults, it is also important to emphasize that some of the same principles apply equally to children. Moreover, physicians who practice in a primary care, lifestyle medicine, or family practice environment will often need to make recommendations not only for adult patients but also for children. For this reason, understanding the role of lifestyle medicine modalities in the pediatric population is extremely important.

It is well known that many chronic diseases, which are ultimately manifested in adults, have their roots in childhood (1,2). Therefore, it is important to explore how lifestyle issues play a role in the health and well-being of children to reduce their risk of chronic diseases in later life.

Just as in the adult population, the various components of lifestyle medicine, which have been emphasized throughout this book, act synergistically in children to assist in developing positive habits that will carry them into adulthood and lower their risk of chronic disease (3). These include regular physical activity (4,5), proper nutrition, weight management, avoiding risky substances, obtaining adequate sleep, and developing strong relationships with other people. All of these are important and set the stage for children to enter adulthood with a healthy foundation.

These modalities will also help reduce risk factors for cardiovascular disease (CVD), diabetes (T2DM), hypertension, and dyslipidemia (6,7). There is even an emerging literature that shows that these lifestyle medicine modalities can improve academic performance as well as feelings of well-being (4). These benefits apply to both children and adults.

For example, physical inactivity is one of the major components of the World Health Organization (WHO) initiative to combat non-communicable diseases (8). This applies to both children and adults. There are some differences between recommendations in the area of lifestyle medicine modalities for children when compared to adults. For example, the current Physical Activity Guidelines from multiple sources call for children and youth to participate in at least 60 minutes of moderate or vigorous physical activity on a daily basis compared to 30 minutes daily of moderate or vigorous activity for adults (4).

Lifestyle modalities are extremely important to improve or maintain health for both children and adults. For example, a number of studies have shown that in the area of ideal cardiovascular health, only about 12%–18% is heritable (9). This means that 80%–85% of ideal cardiovascular health is related to the components of a healthy lifestyle, including healthy diet, physical activity, and many other factors that are emphasized throughout this book.

Unfortunately, an increasing proportion of children are exhibiting poor lifestyle behaviors. These can result in conditions previously seen only in adults and are now presenting in childhood. This includes CVD, T2DM, and obesity. Most current estimates indicate that fewer than 5% of individuals reach the age of 50 maintaining ideal cardiovascular health (6,10). Indeed, some studies suggest that only 1% achieve this standard (7). Clinicians should promote a healthy lifestyle not only in adults, but also in children, extending to fetuses and infants, as well as school-aged children and adolescents. We will focus on these issues in this chapter.

17.2 LIFESTYLE BEHAVIORS

As has been emphasized in multiple chapters in this book, multiple lifestyle behaviors, including regular physical activity, healthy nutrition, avoiding risky substances, weight management, and sleep, are critically important to the prevention or progression of non-communicable diseases,

DOI: 10.1201/9781003630043-17

including obesity, Coronary heart disease (CHD), cancer, obstructive sleep apnea, and T2DM. Optimal health outcomes, as we have noted, are most likely to result from maximizing the number of healthy lifestyle behaviors (7). These behaviors tend to act synergistically.

A good example of this is the strong evidence for using this synergistic methodology to improve childhood obesity by targeting multiple lifestyle behaviors and engaging both the children and their caregivers. Multiple models of behavior exist, which have been developed and studied as ways of changing lifestyle behavior. This reflects the fact that human behavior is complicated, with multiple factors contributing to any particular type of behavior.

Perhaps the most utilized and studied is the social ecological model (11). This model was founded on the principle that behaviors could only be understood by considering the context, which includes the child's immediate external environment (family members in the home environment), but is also influenced by peers and school environments. There are other levels of influence, such as the neighborhood, community, regions, and even governmental policies, which influence behavior. A detailed explanation of the social psychological model is beyond the scope of this book; however, further information on it will be included in the references.

A significant limitation of this model is that it does not directly identify interventions for modifying these impacts on particular behavior. One model that has been proposed to provide more specific recommendations for behavior change is called functional contextualism, which is based on learning theory and behavioral economics and uses psychotherapeutic practices, including acceptance and commitment therapy (12,13). This approach is also described in detail in the attached references.

With whatever model is used, it is important to adopt continual reinforcement. This is particularly important to reinforce positive behavior such as physical activity and healthy eating habits. Reinforcement can be emphasized by helping parents and children establish such behaviors as self-monitoring, goal setting, stimulus control, behavioral rehearsal, and regular feedback. These strategies are time-consuming and it will require the physician to share responsibilities with other members of their clinical staff, such as nurses, and, if available, nutritionists.

17.3 THE LIFE COURSE APPROACH TO PREVENTION OF CHRONIC DISEASE

Multiple lines of research have now clearly demonstrated that intrauterine exposure to a variety of maternal issues, such as nutritional deficiency, obesity, T2DM, and cigarette smoking, is associated with increased risk of chronic disease among offspring (14). Children who are exposed to these problems in the uterus are more likely to develop early signs of chronic disease. A variety of fetal exposures have been identified that carry adverse effects in childhood and throughout the adult lifecycle. A summary of some of these intrauterine experiences is found in Table 17.1.

TABLE 17.1
Early Life Exposures and Associated Outcomes

Exposures and Associated Outcomes		
Fetal undernutrition	Total calories	
		Atherogenic lipid profile
		Disturbed blood coagulation
		Obesity
		Breast cancer
		Insulin resistance
		Obstructive airway disease
		Microalbuminuria
	Folic acid	
		Neural tube defects

(*Continued*)

TABLE 17.1 (*Continued*)
Early Life Exposures and Associated Outcomes

Exposures and Associated Outcomes		
	Iron	
		Obesity
		Hypertension
		Impaired kidney development
	Calcium	
		Hypertension
	Vitamin D	
		Increased adiposity
Fetal overnutrition	Maternal diabetes	
		Obesity
		Glucose intolerance, type 2 diabetes
		Increased blood pressure
		Endothelial dysfunction
		Atherogenic lipid profile
		Metabolic syndrome
	Maternal obesity	
		Increased birthweight, obesity, adiposity
		Increased blood pressure
		Metabolic syndrome
	Sub-optimal macronutrient profile	
		Obesity, increased adiposity
		Increased blood pressure
	Methyl donors	
		Increased weight
		Metabolic syndrome
Other intrauterine exposures	Physical activity (protective)	
		Reduced fat mass at birth
	Smoking	
		Obesity, increased adiposity
		Increased blood pressure
		Asthma
		Attention-deficit hyperactivity disorder
	Endocrine-disrupting chemicals	
		Obesity
		Metabolic syndrome
		Asthma, respiratory tract infections
Post-natal exposures	Breastfeeding (protective)	
		Reduced obesity, adiposity
		Fewer infections
		Lower blood pressure
		Less type 2 diabetes
		Improved cognitive development
	Shared environment	
		Child diet follows maternal diet
		Parental support increases child activity

Source: Sauder K, Dabelia D. Life course approach to prevention of chronic disease. In Rippe JM (ed.) *Lifestyle Medicine* (3rd ed). Boca Raton, FL: CRC Press, 2019. Used with permission of the editor, James M. Rippe, MD.

17.4 IDEAL CARDIOVASCULAR HEALTH

The American Heart Association has been a leading organization in a new construct to help individuals avoid risk factors in the first place. This has been called "Primordial Prevention." This initiative began in 2010 when the AHA issued a special report on defining and setting national goals for cardiovascular health promotion and disease reduction as part of its 2020 Strategic Plan (6). The AHA defined a new construct called "Ideal Cardiovascular Health" (CVD), which they defined as:

1. The simultaneous presence of four favorable health behaviors abstinence from smoking within the past year, ideal body mass index [BMI], physical activity to goal, and consumption of a dietary pattern that promotes cardiovascular health.
2. The simultaneous presence of three favorable health factors, including behaviors abstinence from smoking within the past year, untreated total cholesterol less than 200 mg/dL, untreated blood pressure less than 120/80 mm Hg, and absence of T2DM.
3. Absence of clinical CVD (including CHD, stroke, heart failure, etc.).

These components to establish ideal cardiovascular health were then elaborated in more detail in the Presidential Advisory in 2022 and in addition, an eighth criterion was added in the area of healthy sleep (7).

The AHA emphasized that it was never too early to realize benefits from improved cardiovascular disease (CVH) and emphasized that the earlier CVH is optimized, the better the outcomes are. For this reason, it is a very important concept to emphasize to families, with a particular emphasis on children achieving ideal cardiovascular health. The AHA has estimated that less than 5% of individuals meet the criteria for ideal cardiovascular health, and some estimates have indicated that as few as 1% of individuals achieve this criterion. These abysmally low numbers underscore the reason why it is so important to emphasize CVH for children.

17.5 LIFESTYLE MODALITIES IN CHILDREN

17.5.1 Physical Activity

Physical activity is a key habit and practice that should be encouraged in all children. Multiple studies have demonstrated that regular physical activity reduces risk factors for CVD, including improving lipids, blood pressure, and blood glucose (4,15). Regular physical activity can also lower the risk of weight gain and obesity and, in general, improve body composition, aerobic fitness, muscular strength, motor skills, and bone health (16). Both the PAGA 2018 Scientific Report (4) and the American College of Sports Medicine (ACSM) (16) recommend that youth participate in at least 60 minutes of moderate or vigorous physical activity on a daily basis. Unfortunately, by the time children are adolescents, 80% do not achieve these recommended levels. In 2016, the US Report Card on Physical Activity in Children and Youth gave the overall performance grade for physical activity at D– (17,18). This report also listed that sedentary behaviors are prevalent and received a D–. School programs are not doing much better, and they were rated as D+.

In addition to the physiological improvements from regular physical activity, numerous studies have also demonstrated that cognitive function and academic achievement are improved with regular physical activity. It has been recommended that family, school, community, and government can all play roles in helping children become more physically active (19–22).

17.5.2 Nutrition

Healthy nutrition throughout childhood is very important to lower the risk of chronic disease and also to establish lifelong eating patterns, which are essential to maintaining good health and vitality

TABLE 17.2
Comparing the Nutritional Intervention Approaches in the Cardiovascular Health Integrated Lifestyle Diet-1 and 2 for LDL-Cholesterol and Non-HDL-Cholesterol Lowering in Children >2 Years of Age

Nutrient target for LDL-lowering	CHILD-1	CHILD-2
Total dietary fat	25%–30% of calories	25%–30% of calories
Saturated fat	<10% of daily calories	<7% of daily calories
Trans fat	Avoided	Avoided
Monounsaturated fat	Up to 10%–15% of calories	Up to 10%–15% of calories
Polyunsaturated fat	Up to 10% of calories	Up to 10% of calories
Cholesterol	300 mg or less	200 mg or less
Dietary fiber	Child's age +5 g up to 14 g/1,000 calories	Child's age +5 g up to 14 g/1,000 calories
Simple carbohydrates	Reduction of SSB	Reduction of SSB

Source: Hildebrandt J, Couch S. Cardiovascular risk and diet in children. In Rippe JM (ed.) *Lifestyle Medicine* (3rd ed). Boca Raton, FL: CRC Press, 2019. Used with permission of the editor, James M. Rippe, MD.

(23–26). Poor eating habits, in contrast, lead to the increasing prevalence of obesity in children as well as risk factors for CVD, T2DM, and hypertension.

It should also be noted that even in the United States, the wealthiest country in the world, hunger and malnutrition, as well as issues related to health equity, also apply significantly to children. It is also important to emphasize that pediatric CVD risk factors tend to track into adulthood, as do eating behaviors (27–29). A CVD-protective diet emphasizes unprocessed fruits and vegetables, whole grains, and the caloric intake based on metabolic needs. These have been recommended by the 2020–2025 Dietary Guidelines for Americans (DGA 2020–2025) (30), the American Academy of Pediatrics (AAP) (31), and the American Heart Association (AHA) (32). Multiple good nutrition patterns have been developed by the AAP. They are called the CHILD diet (Cardiovascular Health-Integrated Lifestyle Diet), which was specifically developed to help improve lipids in children. There are two CHILD diets: CHILD one and CHILD two (33). CHILD one is appropriate for most children, whereas CHILD two is more aggressive in terms of lipid management. These two diets are found in Table 17.2.

Other dietary patterns that we have recommended throughout this book for adults are also highly appropriate for children. These include the DASH diet (34) and the Mediterranean diet (35). These plant-forward diets have the added advantage of conveying health benefits to the entire family. More detailed information about these two diets is found in Chapter 3.

17.5.3 Body Weight/Childhood Obesity

Childhood obesity in the United States has increased significantly in the past three decades. The prevalence of obesity in 2- to19-year-olds in the United States is 18.5% and continues to rise in all age groups. Childhood overweight and obesity disproportionately affect Black, Hispanic, and other minority groups (36–38). Childhood obesity significantly increases the risk of comorbid conditions such as T2DM and CVD.

Clinicians should screen all children in primary care at least annually for excess weight gain using age- and sex-specific percentiles for weight (for children > 2 years old) or weight-to-length percentiles (for children <2 years old) (39). These are based on data from the WHO. It is also important to screen for lifestyle factors that can contribute to obesity. The Expert Committee from the

American Academy of Pediatrics recommended treatment to achieve a permanent healthy lifestyle, including the following (40):

- Patient/family early identification to help prioritize behaviors reflective of their values and preferences, and paired goal setting.
- Motivational interviewing.
- Implementation of self-monitored and planned reinforcement.
- Optimization of multidisciplinary expertise geared to physical and psychosocial needs of the family.
- Excellent communication with a primary care provider.

The nutritional interventions emphasize balanced, hypocaloric eating combined with physical activity and reduced sedentary behavior.

It has been clearly identified that sleep and stress are related to pediatric obesity. These will be addressed in subsequent sections.

17.5.4 Identification and Management of Children with Dyslipidemia

Lipid abnormalities underlie the process of atherosclerosis. These abnormalities are combined with inflammatory markers and start the process in the endothelium of atherosclerosis. It is well known that CVD has its roots in childhood. Therefore, it is critically important to identify and treat children with dyslipidemia. Optimal, borderline, and high lipid classifications for children are found in Table 17.3. Cholesterol screening recommendations are found in Table 17.4.

TABLE 17.3
Cholesterol Level Classification for Children and Adolescents (in md/dL)

Lipid Category	Optimal	Borderline-High	High	Low
TC	<170	170–199	>200	
LDL-C	<110	110–129	>130	
Non-HDL-C	<120	123–144	>145	
		TG		
0–9 years	<75	75–99	>100	
10–19 years	<90	90–129	>130	
HDL-C	>45	40–45		<40
Cholesterol Level Classification for Young Adults (20–24 years, in mg/dL) (7)				
TC	<190	190–224	>225	
LDL-C	<120	120–159	>160	
Non-HDL-C	<50	150–189	>190	
TG	<115	115–149	>150	
HDL-C	>45	40–45		<40

Source: Brothers J, Daniels S. Identification and management of children with dyslipidemia. In Rippe JM (ed.) *Lifestyle Medicine* (3rd ed). Boca Raton, FL: CRC Press, 2019. Used with permission of the editor, James M. Rippe, MD.

TC, total cholesterol; LDL-c, low-density lipoprotein cholesterol; non-HDL-c, nonhigh-density lipoprotein cholesterol; TG, triglycerides; HDL-c, high-density lipoprotein cholesterol.

TABLE 17.4
Cholesterol Screening Recommendations by Age

Age	Screening Recommendation	Labs to Obtain
<2 years	No screening	
2–8 years	No routine screening	
	Screening if:	
	• + family history of early heart disease	FLP×2*
	• Parent has TC>240mg/dL	
	• Family history is unknown	
	• High risk condition (see Table 17.5)	
9–11 years	Universal Screening	
	If non-HDL-c>145 or HDL-c<40	Non-FLP
	Then obtain	FLP×2*
	If LDL-c>130 or non-HDL-c>145 or	FLP
	HDL-c<40 or	
	TG>100 (age<10 years) or >130 (age>10 years)	
	Then obtain	Repeat FLP*
12–16 years	No routine screening	
	Screening if:	FLP×2*
	New knowledge of CVD risk, same as 2–8 years	
17–21 years	Universal screening	
	Ages 17–19:	
	If non-HDL-c>145 or HDL-c<40	Non-FLP
	Then obtain	FLP×2*
	If LDL-c>130 or non-HDL-c>145 or	FLP
	HDL-c<40 or	
	TG>100 (age<10 years) or >130 (age>10 years)	
	Then obtain	Repeat FLP*
	Ages 17–21:	
	If non-HDL-c>190 or HDL-c<40	Non-FLP
	Then obtain	FLP×2*
	If LDL-c>160 or non-HDL-c>190 or	FLP
	HDL-c<40 or TG>150	
	Then obtain	Repeat FLP*

Source: Brothers J, Daniels S. Identification and management of children with dyslipidemia. In Rippe JM (ed.) *Lifestyle Medicine* (3rd ed). Boca Raton, FL: CRC Press, 2019. Used with permission of the editor, James M. Rippe, MD.

*Second 1lipid profile should be obtained two weeks to three months after the first lipid profile obtained.

FLP, fasting lipid profile; non-FLP, non-fasting lipid profile; LDL-c, low-density lipoprotein cholesterol; HD122L-c, high-density lipoprotein cholesterol; non-HDL-c, non-high-density lipoprotein cholesterol (total cholesterol - high-density lipoprotein cholesterol); TG, triglycerides.

As noted in Table 17.4, it is recommended that all children and adolescents between the ages of 9 and 11 years and again between 17 and 21 years be screened at least once each for dyslipidemia (40). As already indicated, nutritional recommendations for any child with dyslipidemia should involve either the CHILD one or CHILD two diet, as well as weight loss if necessary, and increased physical activity and decreased sedentary time.

17.5.5 Diagnosis and Management of Children with Hypertension

Hypertension is very rare in children. In 2017, AAP listed evidence-based clinical practice guidelines for pediatric hypertension (41). For younger children aged 13 years or younger, persistent blood pressure above the 95th percentile is considered hypertension. For older children, the adult blood pressure thresholds are used (42). The definition of hypertension for children of various ages is found in Table 17.5.

Initial treatment of high blood pressure in children uses lifestyle interventions, including weight loss if necessary, healthy nutrition as outlined in multiple chapters in this book, and regular physical activity (41). Pharmacologic management is only recommended if target organ injury is detected or other cardiovascular risk factors are present.

17.5.6 Bone Health

The process of osteoporosis, which is a disorder of compromised bone strength, often begins in childhood. Bone accrual dramatically occurs during the first two decades of life and, to some extent, during the third decade of life until peak bone mass is achieved (42). The development of peak bone mass is important for lifelong bone health. Regular physical activity, particularly weight-bearing physical activity, is essential for optimizing bone health (4). Peak increases in bone mass occur during puberty. However, 40% of bone mass is achieved during the first four years, which offers an opportunity to maximize peak bone mass.

In addition to high levels of physical activity, adequate nutrient intake is important. Fruits, vegetables, and dairy food consumption are also associated with improved bone mass density. Both calcium and vitamin D are important for bone accrual (43,44). Some studies have shown that protein intake is important for bone mass in children and adolescents. Potassium, magnesium, vitamin C, vitamin K, and flavonoids are important for bone mass, and fruits and vegetables are rich sources of these micronutrients (45). In contrast, carbonated beverage intake has been associated with reduced bone mass in some studies, probably because of the displacement of dairy products. Tobacco use also exerts deleterious effects on bone mass (43).

17.5.7 Sleep

Considerable attention has been focused in the past decade on the issue of sleep and health in children and adolescents (46). There is now a well-established association between short sleep duration and obesity (47). Sleep duration in line with recommended amounts, in contrast, has been found to

TABLE 17.5
Definition of Hypertension in Children

For Children 1 to <13 Years of Age	For Children ≥13 Years of Age
Normal BP: <90th percentile	Normal BP: <120/<80 mm Hg
Elevated BP: ≥90th percentile to 95th percentile; or 120/80 mm Hg to <95th percentile (whichever is lower)	Elevated BP: 120/<80–129/<80 mm Hg
Stage 1 HTN: ≥95th percentile, or 130/80–139/89 mm Hg (whichever is lower)	Stage 1 HTN: 130/80–139/89 mm Hg
Stage 2 HTN: ≥95th percentile + 12 mm Hg or ≥140/90 mm Hg (whichever is lower)	Stage 2 HTN: ≥140/90 mm Hg

Source: Baker-Smith CM, Gidding S. Diagnosis, management and treatments of systemic hypertension in youth. In Rippe JM (ed.) *Lifestyle Medicine* (4th ed). Boca Raton, FL: CRC Press, 2024. Used with Permission of the Editor, Dr. James Rippe.

Note: Criteria for Hypertension in Children.

be protective against obesity. The National Sleep Foundation reported that children and adolescents are sleeping far less than the amount recommended, which results in the chronic problem of sleep deprivation (48).

Poor sleep patterns in childhood tend to persist into adulthood and develop into sleep problems (49–51). The link between sleep and obesity may be a function of the influence that sleep has on a variety of hormones, including leptin, ghrelin, insulin, cortisol, and growth hormone (51–53). In one study of 400 adolescents, the odds of obesity increased by 80% for each hour of sleep lost (54). Sleep also impacts dietary behaviors. One study showed that adolescents after five nights of sleep restriction have diets with a higher glycemic index compared to healthy sleep (55,56). In addition, adolescents who go to bed after midnight have been demonstrated to consume larger amounts of sugary and caffeinated beverages and tend to skip breakfast, consuming most of their meals late in the day. A relationship between physical activity levels and sleep also exists, although it is inconsistent (57–59). Sleep efficiency has been shown to improve with moderate to vigorous physical activity.

For all of these reasons, it is important for practitioners of lifestyle medicine or primary care to inquire about sleep. These counseling sessions should include both parents and the child. Clinical applications during sleep are found in Table 17.6.

17.5.8 Stress

Multiple issues may cause stress in children. For example, pain, injury, or illness are typical reasons that children can be under stress (60). Children can also experience stress by worrying about grades,

TABLE 17.6
Clinical Applications for Addressing Sleep Issues in Children

Presenting Problem	Possible Diagnoses	Recommended Treatment
	All Ages	
Snoring, pauses in breathing, gasping for air during sleep	Obstructive Sleep Apnea	Polysomnography; referral to pediatric sleep clinic
Irregular sleep/wake times	Poor sleep habits in the absence of a discrete sleep disorder	Scheduled, consistent, bed/wake times
Poor sleep habits (e.g., use of electronics at bedtime and/or to fall asleep)	Poor sleep habits in the absence of a discrete sleep disorder	Sleep hygiene recommendations
	Younger Children	
Difficulty falling asleep independently (need for parent presence to fall asleep or return to sleep after night wakings)	Insomnia	Behavioral treatments for independent sleep; referral to pediatric behavioral sleep medicine specialist
Bedtime resistance	Insomnia	Bedtime routine; positive reinforcement; referral to pediatric behavioral sleep medicine specialist
	Older Children/Adolescents	
Difficulty falling asleep	Insomnia	Cognitive-behavioral therapy for insomnia (CBT-I); referral to pediatric behavioral sleep medicine specialist
Frequent night wakings	Insomnia	CBT-I; referral to pediatric behavioral sleep medicine specialist

Source: Kaar J, Simon S. Sleep and obesity prevention in children and adolescents. In Rippe JM (ed.) *Lifestyle Medicine* (3rd ed). Boca Raton, FL: CRC Press, 2019. Used with permission of the editor, James Rippe, MD.

juggling responsibilities, or problems with friends (bullying) or peer group pressure. Changing schools or dealing with housing problems or homelessness can also cause stress. Having negative feelings about themselves can also cause stress in children. It is important to point out that stress can actually be positive. When children get proper support, it can help them rise to a challenge and push them toward goals and meet deadlines, etc. This kind of positive stress allows children to build inner strength and skills, which results (61) in resilience. It is particularly important that parents play a supportive role by helping children deal with stress in a positive manner. Experts have recommended that doing too much for kids can actually be harmful. Parents should help children develop the skills that they need to manage stress, which will prepare them for subsequent challenges in their adult lives. It should also be noted that some strategies, such as regular physical activity, are potent stress reducers in children as they are in adults (62).

17.5.9 The Use of Risky Substances

While cigarette smoking is relatively uncommon among middle and high school students, the health consequences can be very significant. Approximately 8% of middle and high school students have used any tobacco product, and an additional 6% have used e-cigarettes. Nicotine pouches are also occasionally used by about 2% of students in this age group (63).

Unfortunately, the consequences of cigarette smoking are significant. Tobacco product use is started and established usually during adolescence. In fact, nine out of ten adults who smoke cigarettes daily started smoking by age 18. Flavoring of tobacco products can make them more appealing to youth. For all these reasons, it is important to counsel children to avoid tobacco products and if already started, to help them discontinue using them.

Alcohol consumption can also lead to a variety of significant health problems (64). Young people who drink alcohol are more likely to engage in risky behaviors, which can lead to serious injuries and other health conditions. In addition, alcohol consumption among high school students leads to more school absences and lower grades. Drinking and driving can also be a problem. In addition, people who start drinking earlier in life have a higher risk of developing alcohol use disorder later in life. For all of these reasons, it is important to ascertain whether children are utilizing alcohol and, if so, to have counselling sessions with them about the potential dangers of this risky act.

Unfortunately, alcohol consumption is relatively common among high school students. Alcohol is the most commonly used drug among young people. Twenty percent of high school students have, at least occasionally, consumed alcohol (65,66). Thus, this is a common issue and one that bears vigilance and, if alcohol use is present, counseling with the children and/or the family should occur to discuss the dangers of alcohol consumption.

17.6 THE ROLE OF FAMILY

Family support is an example of the final component of positive lifestyle measures that we have discussed, which is developing positive relationships with others. Family appears to be the key here for children. Having a supportive, loving family can make an enormous difference not only in a child's life but also prepare them for future challenges as an adult. Positive relationships with other adults, such as supportive teachers, coaches, and adult friends, can also make an enormous difference. Parents can often guide their children in ways that can enable them to establish positive relationships with a wide variety of peers and adults.

17.7 CONCLUSIONS/CLINICAL APPLICATIONS

While this book and the embedded curriculum are mostly geared toward adults, it is important to emphasize that many of the chronic conditions that occur during adulthood have their roots in childhood. The good news is that these same types of lifestyle modalities, which can yield multiple synergistic benefits in adults, can also yield these benefits in children. It is important that habits established in childhood be positive ones, since these habits tend to carry over into adulthood, making lifestyle medicine issues for children particularly important.

REFERENCES

1. Miller J, Boles R, Daniel S. Pediatric lifestyle medicine. In Rippe JM (ed.) *Lifestyle Medicine* (3rd ed). Boca Raton, FL: CRC Press, 2019.
2. Boles R, Miller J, Daniels S. Pediatric preventive medicine: an introduction. In Rippe JM (ed.) *Lifestyle Medicine* (4th ed). Boca Raton, FL: CRC Press, 2024.
3. Eriksson J, et al. Early growth and coronary heart disease in later life: longitudinal study. *BMJ*. 2001;322(7292):949–953.
4. Physical Activity Guidelines Advisory Committee. 2018 Physical Activity Guidelines Advisory Committee Scientific Report, Washington, DC: U.S. Department of Health and Human Services, 2018.
5. U.S. Department of Health and Human Services. Physical Activity Guidelines for Americans (2nd ed). Washington, DC: U.S. Department of Health and Human Services, 2018. Chapter 3: Active children and adolescents, pp. 46–55.
6. Lloyd-Jones D, et al. Defining and setting national goals for cardiovascular health promotion and disease reduction: The American Heart Association's strategic impact goal through 2020 and beyond. *Circulation*. 2010;121(4):586–613.
7. Lloyd-Jones DM, Allen NB, Anderson CAM, et al. Life's essential 8: updating and enhancing the American Heart Association's construct of cardiovascular health: a presidential advisory from the American Heart Association. *Circulation*. 2022;146(5):e18–e43.
8. World Health Organization. Noncommunicable Diseases. https://www.who.int/news-room/fact-sheets/detail/noncommunicable-diseases. Accessed March 26, 2025.
9. Allen N. Abstract 17245: the heritability of ideal cardiovascular health: the Framingham heart study. *Circulation*. 2018;122(suppl 21).
10. Bambs C, et al. Low prevalence of "Ideal Cardiovascular Health" in a community based population the heart strategies concentrating on risk evaluation (Heart SCORE) study. *Circulation*. 2011;123(8):850–857.
11. Bronfenbrenner U. *The Ecology of Human Development*. Cambridge, MA: Harvard University Press, 1979.
12. Biglan A, Hayes, SC. Should the behavioral sciences become more pragmatic? The case for functional contextualism in research on human behavior. *Appl Prev Psychol*. 1996;5(1):47–57.
13. Gifford EV, Hayes SC. Functional contextualism: A pragmatic philosophy for behavioral science. In O'Donohue W, Kitchener R (eds.) *Handbook of Behaviorism*. San Diego, CA: Elsevier, 1999, pp. 285–327.
14. Sauder K, Dabelea D. Life course approach to prevention of chronic disease. In Rippe JM (ed.) *Lifestyle Medicine* (3rd ed). Boca Raton, FL: CRC Press, 2019.
15. Rippe J. *Physical Activity: A Practical Guide*. Boca Raton, FL: CRC Press, 2020.
16. American College of Sports Medicine. Physical Activity Guidelines. https://acsm.org/education-resources/trending-topics-resources/physical-activity-guidelines/. Accessed March 27, 2025.
17. Tremblay M, LeBlanc A, Kho M, et al. Systematic review of sedentary behaviour and health indicators in school-aged children and youth. *Int J Behav Nutr Phys Act*. 2011;8:98.
18. 2008 Physical Activity Guidelines for Americans Advisory Committee Report, Washington, DC: U.S. Department of Health and Human Services, 2008.
19. Sun C, Pezic A, Tikellis G, et al. Effects of school-based interventions for direct delivery of physical activity on fitness and cardiometabolic markers in children and adolescents: a systematic review of randomized controlled trials. *Obes Rev*. 2013;14(10):818–838.
20. Larouche R, Saunders T, Faulkner G, et al. Associations between active school transport and physical activity, body composition, and cardiovascular fitness: a systematic review of 68 studies. *J Phys Act Health*. 2014;11(1):206–227.
21. Beets M, Beighle A, Erwin H, et al. After-school program impact on physical activity and fitness: a meta-analysis. *Am J Prev Med*. 2009;36(6):527–537.
22. American Academy of Pediatrics Council on Communications and Media. Policy statement – children, adolescents, obesity and the media. *Pediatrics*. 2011;128:201–208.
23. Benjamin-Neelon S. Position of the academy of nutrition and dietetics: benchmarks for nutrition in child care. *J Acad Nutr Diet*. 2018;118(7):1291–1300.

24. Murimi MW, Moyeda-Carabaza AF, Nguyen B, et al. Factors that contribute to effective nutrition education interventions in children: a systematic review. *Nutr Rev.* 2018;76(8):553–580.
25. Das J, Lassi Z, Hoodbhoy Z, et al. Nutrition for the next generation: older children and adolescents. *Ann Nutr Metab.* 2018;72(Suppl 3):56–64.
26. Clark H, Coll-Seck A, Banerjee A, et al. A future for the world's children? A WHO-UNICEF-Lancet Commission. *Lancet.* 2020;395(10224):605–658.
27. Kelly A, Barlow S, Rao G, et al. Severe obesity in children and adolescents: identification, associated health risks, and treatment approaches: a scientific statement from the American Heart Association. *Circulation.* 2013;128:1689–712.
28. Faulkner C, Couch S, Hemingway J. Cardiovascular risk and diet in children. In Rippe JM (ed.) *Lifestyle Medicine* (4th ed). Boca Raton, FL: CRC Press, 2024.
29. Berenson G, Srinivasan S, Bao W, et al. Association between multiple cardiovascular risk factors and atherosclerosis in children and young adults. The Bogalusa Heart Study. *N Engl J Med.* 1998;338(23):1650–1656.
30. U.S. Department of Agriculture and U.S. Department of Health and Human Services. U.S. Department of Agriculture and U.S. Department of Health and Human Services. Dietary Guidelines for Americans, 2020–2025. 9th Edition. December 2020. Available at DietaryGuidelines.gov. 2020; https://www.dietaryguidelines.gov/resources/2020-2025-dietary-guidelines-online-materials.
31. Kavey REW, Simons-Morton DG, de Jesus JM (supple eds). Expert panel on integrated guidelines for cardiovascular health and risk reduction in children and adolescents: summary report. *Pediatrics.* 2011;128(5):S213–S256.
32. Lichtenstein AH, Appel LJ, Vadiveloo M, et al. 2021 Dietary guidance to improve cardiovascular health: a scientific statement from the American Heart Association. *Circulation.* 2021;144(23):e472–e487.
33. Williams LA, Wilson DP. Nutritional management of pediatric dyslipidemia. 2023 Apr 30. In Feingold KR, Ahmed SF, Anawalt B, et al. (eds.) *Endotext [Internet].* South Dartmouth, MA: MDText.com, Inc., 2000. PMID: 27809443.
34. Estruch R, Ros E, Salas-Salvado J, et al. Primary prevention of cardiovascular disease with a mediterranean diet. *N Engl J Med.* 2013;368(14):1279–1290.
35. Sacks FM, Svetkey LP, Vollmer WM, et al. Effects on blood pressure of reduced dietary sodium and the Dietary Approaches to Stop Hypertension (DASH) diet. DASH-Sodium Collaborative Research Group. *N Engl J Med.* 2001;344(1):3–10.
36. Fryar CD, Carroll MD, Afful J. Prevalence of overweight, obesity, and severe obesity among adults aged 20 and over: United States, 1960–1962 through 2017–2018. NCHS Health E-Stats. 2020.
37. Ogden CL, Lamb MM, Carroll MD, et al. Obesity and socioeconomic status in children and adolescents: United States, 2005–2008. NCHS Data Brief, No. 51, December, 2010.
38. Barlow SE. Expert Committee recommendations regarding the prevention, assessment and treatment of child and adolescent overweight and obesity: summary report. *Pediatrics* 2007;120(Suppl 4):S164–S192.
39. CDC Growth Charts. https://www.cdc.gov/growthcharts. Accessed March 27, 2025.
40. Expert Panel on Integrated Guidelines for Cardiovascular Health and Risk Reduction in Children and Adolescents. Expert panel on integrated guidelines for cardiovascular health and risk reduction in children and adolescents: summary report. *Pediatrics.* 2011;128(Suppl 5):S213–S256.
41. Flynn JT, Kaelber DC, Baker-Smith CM, et al. Clinical practice guideline for screening and management of high blood pressure in children and adolescents. *Pediatrics*:2017;140(3):e20171904.
42. Kalkwarf H. Prevention of osteoporosis in children and adolescents. In Rippe JM (ed.) *Lifestyle Medicine* (3rd ed). Boca Raton, FL: CRC Press, 2019.
43. Rodrıguez-Martınez M, Garcıa-Cohen E. Role of Ca^{2+} and vitamin D in the prevention and treatment of osteoporosis. *Pharmacol Ther.* 2002;93(1):37–49.
44. Heaney R. Calcium, dairy products and osteoporosis. *J Am Coll Nutr.* 2000;19(sup2):83S–99S.
45. Stránský M, Rysava L. Nutrition as prevention and treatment of osteoporosis. *Physiol Res.* 2009;58:S7.
46. Kaar J, Simon S. Sleep and obesity prevention in children and adolescents. In Rippe JM (ed.) *Lifestyle Medicine* (3rd ed). Boca Raton, FL: CRC Press, 2019.
47. Gupta N, Mueller W, Chan W, et al. Is obesity associated with poor sleep quality in adolescents? *Am J Hum Biol.* 2002;14(6):762–768.
48. Wheaton AG, Claussen AH. Short sleep duration among infants, children, and adolescents aged 4 months–17 years – United States, 2016–2018. *MMWR Morb Mortal Wkly Rep.* 2021;70:1315–1321.
49. Beebe DW, Rausch J, Byars KC, et al. Persistent snoring in preschool children: Predictors and behavioral and developmental correlates. *Pediatrics.* 2012;130(3):382–389.

50. Byars KC, Yolton K, Rausch J, et al. Prevalence, patterns, and persistence of sleep problems in the first 3 years of life. *Pediatrics.* 2012;129(2):e276–e284.
51. Spruyt K, Molfese DL, Gozal D. Sleep duration, sleep regularity, body weight, and metabolic homeostasis in school-aged children. *Pediatrics.* 2011;127(2):e345–e352.
52. De Bernardi Rodrigues AM, da Silva Cde C, et al. Brazilian Metabolic Syndrome Study (BRAMS) investigators. Association of sleep deprivation with reduction in insulin sensitivity as assessed by the hyperglycemic clamp technique in adolescents. *JAMA Pediatr.* 2016;170(5):487–494.
53. Iglayreger HB, Peterson MD, Liu D, et al. Sleep duration predicts cardiometabolic risk in obese adolescents. *J Pediatr.* 2014:64(5):1085–1090.e1.
54. Nixon GM, Thompson JM, Han DY et al. Short sleep duration in middle childhood: risk factors and consequences. *Sleep.* 2008;31(1):71–78.
55. Beebe DW, Simon S, Summer S, et al. Dietary intake following experimentally restricted sleep in adolescents. *Sleep.* 2013; 1;36(6):827–34.
56. Simon SL, Field J, Miller LE, et al. Sweet/dessert foods are more appealing to adolescents after sleep restriction. *PLoS One.* 2015:23;10(2):e0115434.
57. Luo J, Cao M, Sun F, et al. Association between outdoor activity and insufficient sleep in Chinese school-aged children. *Med Sci Monit.* 2020;26:e921617.
58. Gong QH, Li H, Zhang XH, et al. Associations between sleep duration and physical activity and dietary behaviors in Chinese adolescents: results from the youth behavioral risk factor surveys of 2015. *Sleep Med.* 2017;37:168–173.
59. Stea TH, Knutsen T, Torstveit MK. Association between short time in bed, health-risk behaviors and poor academic achievement among Norwegian adolescents. *Sleep Med.* 2014;15(6):666–671.
60. Condon EM. Chronic stress in children and adolescents: a review of biomarkers for use in pediatric research. *Biol Res Nurs.* 2018;20(5):473–496.
61. Garner AS, Shonkoff JP, Committee on Psychosocial Aspects of Child and Family Health; Committee on Early Childhood Adoption, and Dependent Care, Section on Development and Behavioral Pediatrics. Early childhood adversity, toxic stress, and the role of the pediatrician: translating developmental science into lifelong health. *Pediatrics.* 2012;129(1):e224–e231.
62. Johnson SB, Riley AW, Granger DA, et al. The science of early life toxic stress for pediatric practice and advocacy. *Pediatrics.* 2013;131(2):319–327.
63. Healthychildren.org. Protecting Kids from Tobacco's Harms: AAP Policy Explained. https://www.healthychildren.org/English/health-issues/conditions/tobacco/Pages/AAP-Recommendations-on-Tobacco-E-Cigarettes.aspx. Accessed March 27, 2025.
64. Committee on Substance Abuse, Kokotailo PK. Alcohol use by youth and adolescents: a pediatric concern. *Pediatrics.* 2010;125(5):1078–1087.
65. Grant BF, Dawson DA. Age at onset of alcohol use and its association with DSM-IV alcohol abuse and dependence: results from the national longitudinal alcohol epidemiologic survey. *J Subst Abuse.* 1997;9:103–110.
66. National Institute on Alcohol Abuse and Alcoholism. Get the Facts About Underage Drinking. https://www.niaaa.nih.gov/publications/brochures-and-fact-sheets/underage-drinking. Accessed March 27, 2025.

18 Introduction to Lifestyle Medicine Education

History and Background

Lifestyle Medicine has been growing and evolving as a field for over 25 years. In 1999, Dr. James Rippe published the first textbook in the field, titled *Lifestyle Medicine*. This textbook, in its fourth edition, remains the defining and guiding text for lifestyle medicine. Research on the impact of exercise, diet, and lifestyle behaviors on major diseases, including heart disease, pulmonary disease, endocrine disorders, and cancer, is reviewed with a focus on the scientific evidence. Pioneers such as Denis Burkitt, Nathan Pritikin, John McDougall, T. Colin Campbell, Caldwell Esselstyn, Dean Ornish, Hans Diehl, and David Katz published articles on lifestyle medicine in the 1980s, 1990s, and 2000s. The Diabetes Prevention Program lifestyle medicine trial, titled "Reduction in incidence of type 2 diabetes with lifestyle intervention or metformin," was published in 2002 (1). The researchers reported that the lifestyle intervention resulted in a 58% reduction in the diagnosis of type 2 diabetes in a population with high fasting glucose and elevated post-load glucose at the start of the study, compared to placebo and metformin resulted in a 31% reduction compared to placebo. This type of data helps physicians acknowledge the power of lifestyle medicine.

In 2004, Mokdad and colleagues published their article on actual causes of death, identifying tobacco, poor diet, and physical inactivity as the top three actual causes of death in the United States in the year 2000 (2). These pioneers, this landmark research, and the science related to lifestyle medicine were so strong in the early 2000s that the American College of Lifestyle Medicine (ACLM) was founded in 2004. Over the past two decades, research has expanded, the science has become clearer, and ACLM membership has increased substantially to over 15,000.

The updated definition of lifestyle medicine from 2022, available on the ACLM's website, is

> Lifestyle medicine is a medical specialty that uses therapeutic lifestyle interventions as a primary modality to treat chronic conditions, including, but not limited to, cardiovascular diseases, type 2 diabetes, and obesity. Lifestyle medicine certified clinicians are trained to apply evidence-based, whole-person, prescriptive lifestyle change to treat and, when used intensively, often reverse such conditions. Applying the six pillars of lifestyle medicine—a whole-food, plant-predominant eating pattern, physical activity, restorative sleep, stress management, avoidance of risky substances and positive social connections—also provides effective prevention for these conditions (3).

This definition underscores the importance of medical education in the specialty of lifestyle medicine. To become certified in lifestyle medicine, a physician must be educated in the science and art of prescribing the six pillars of lifestyle medicine. The definition uses the term "specialty." The Association of American Medical Colleges (AAMC) recognized lifestyle medicine as a medical specialty in 2024 (4). When medical students search for medical specialties, they will find lifestyle medicine. The fact that lifestyle modification and the pillars of lifestyle medicine are listed as the primary modality to treat common chronic conditions such as cardiovascular disease, high blood pressure, type 2 diabetes, metabolic syndrome, and obesity emphasizes their importance for medical professionals. The American Heart Association, American Diabetes Association, and the Obesity Medicine Societies list lifestyle behaviors as first-line therapy. The term "evidence-based" is a critical component of the definition. Lifestyle medicine physicians follow the research and the science. The recommendations and guidelines for each pillar are based on research reported in

DOI: 10.1201/9781003630043-18

medical journal articles. In addition to the research, lifestyle medicine physicians and clinicians focus on the "whole-person," as the definition says. Physical, mental, social, and emotional health are considered for each patient.

The term "prescriptive" was explicitly used in this definition. As physicians prescribe pills with the name of the medicine, frequency, dose, and timing, lifestyle medicine physicians prescribe the pillars with frequency, intensity, time, and type (FITT). For example, for physical activity, the prescription may be five times a week, moderate intensity, 30 minutes of walking. For nutrition, the prescription may be two cups of green leafy vegetables at lunch or dinner, seven days a week. The word "treat" is used in this definition because lifestyle behaviors, such as aerobic exercise, can help lower blood pressure to a level comparable to that of some medications (5), as can dietary changes, such as following a DASH diet (6).

In its definition of lifestyle medicine, the ACLM used the term "reverse" to emphasize that these pillars, when used intensively at a defined dose and in combination, can help put chronic diseases such as diabetes and hypertension into remission. Remission means the patient no longer meets the diagnostic criteria and no longer requires medication. This point has implications for medical education, including the training of physicians, residents, and medical students in deprescribing medications. While the pillars are more intensively prescribed, such as exercise and a whole-food, plant-based eating pattern, a patient's blood pressure and blood glucose levels should be monitored more closely, as changes in physical activity and diet can lead to hypotension and hypoglycemia. For this reason, lifestyle medicine physicians need to learn to safely and effectively reduce medication doses while carefully monitoring patients.

Over the past two decades, there have been many advances in lifestyle medicine medical education, as depicted in Figures 18.1 and 18.2. One meaningful way to bring lifestyle medicine into medical education for preclinical medical students was introduced in 2008. This is a lifestyle medicine interest group (LMIG). The LMIG provides a parallel curriculum. In 2010, the core competencies of lifestyle medicine were delineated and reported in a JAMA article (7). In 2012, the American Medical Association (AMA) passed a resolution that all physicians should learn about lifestyle medicine (8). In 2013, the Ardmore Institute of Health (AIH) hosted a think tank for lifestyle medicine in medical education, and the LMEd Collaborative was formed. AIH funded LMEd to create curricula.

In 2014, a full bachelor's-level and master's-level course was created to teach the practices and principles of lifestyle medicine at Harvard Extension School in a hybrid format, allowing learning in person at Harvard in Cambridge and across the world to gain exposure to this burgeoning field (9). In

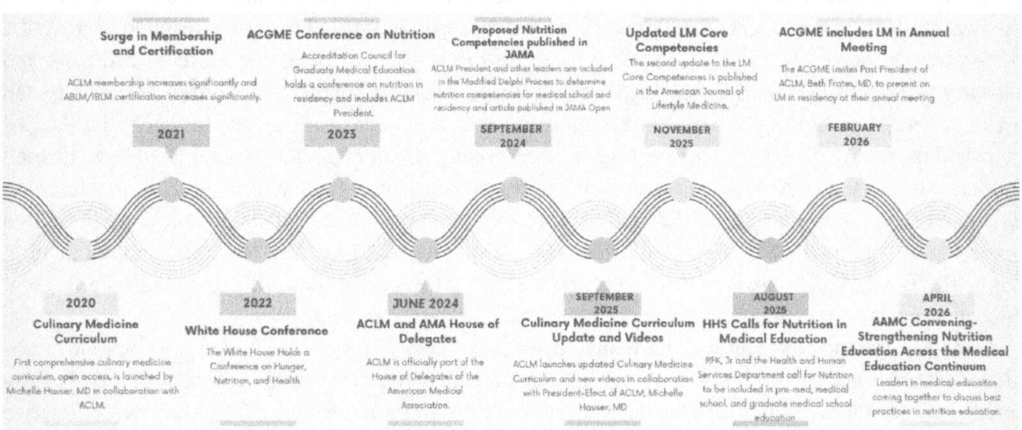

FIGURE 18.1 (Begins with 2020) Timeline of Advances in Medical Education from 2020 to 2026.

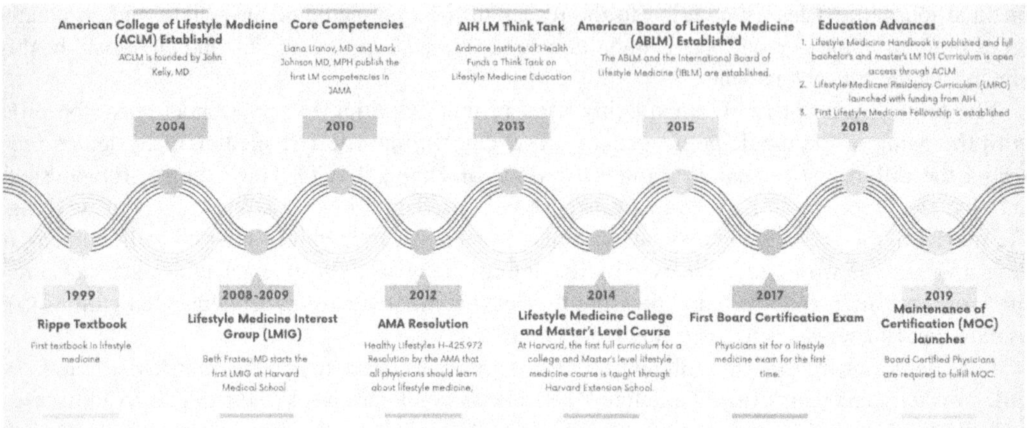

FIGURE 18.2 (Begins in 1999) Timeline of Advances in Medical Education from 1999 to 2019.

2015, the American Board of Lifestyle Medicine and the International Board of Lifestyle Medicine were created. The first board certification exam was successfully administered in 2017.

In 2018, the Lifestyle Medicine (LM) 101 Curriculum was co-created and shared via the ACLM as the first free, open-access lifestyle medicine curriculum. LM 101 was updated a couple of years later. It is currently available on the ACLM website and has been used by faculty and learners in the United States and worldwide. In 2018, the Lifestyle Medicine Residency Curriculum (LMRC) was introduced for the first time. It was created with significant funding and support from AIH. Over the years, the LMRC has been enhanced and updated many times. Another landmark for 2018 is the creation of the first lifestyle medicine fellowship. By 2019, the field had established Maintenance of Certification (MOC) for the Board. In 2020, the first comprehensive, open-source culinary medicine curriculum was published in collaboration with the ACLM. In 2022, LMEd Collaborative moved to Greenville, SC. The LMEd curricula are available free of charge via their website, thereby expanding the list of freely accessible resources for teaching lifestyle medicine (https://www.lifestylemedicinecurriculum.org/). In 2022, the 2010 lifestyle medicine core competencies were updated (10).

Landmark events at the federal and national level began in the United States in 2022. In September 2022, the White House held a conference on Hunger, Health, and Nutrition. In March 2023, the Accreditation Council for Graduate Medical Education (ACGME) held a conference on nutrition education in medical training. After this conference, medical educators from across the United States convened to participate in a modified Delphi process to determine proposed nutrition competencies for medical students and residents through a rigorous consensus strategy. This effort resulted in a JAMA publication in September 2024 titled Proposed Nutrition Competencies for Medical Students and Physician Trainees (11). In August 2025, the US Department of Health and Human Services issued a call for medical schools to incorporate nutrition education and assessment. In 2025, the ACLM launched the free Culinary Medicine Program, comprising 15 hours of video content and eight themed modules. In 2026, the ACGME invited Beth Frates, MD, the past-president of ACLM, to present at its annual meeting in February 2026 and to describe the importance of lifestyle medicine education for residents. In April 2026, AAMC hosted a convening on best practices for nutrition education in medical schools. The interest in this topic continues to grow. All of these lifestyle medicine medical education events are included in the timelines found in Figures 18.1 and 18.2.

Over the past quarter-century, there have been significant advances in the field of lifestyle medicine. Lifestyle medicine education is now at least acknowledged in most medical schools, is fully integrated across all four years in only a few, and provides a parallel curriculum with lifestyle medicine interest groups in over 120 of the almost 200 medical schools in the United States. There remains considerable room for growth. Most medical schools do not cover all six pillars of lifestyle medicine. Medical schools generally cover the pillar of risky substances and discuss tobacco, alcohol, opioids, and other substances. On average, medical schools provide 8 hours of physical activity, 14.3 hours of nutrition, and less than 2.5 hours of sleep; there are insufficient data to report the number of hours spent on stress resilience and social connection (12).

Journals such as the American Journal of Lifestyle Medicine, BMC Medical Education, Patient Education and Counseling, Circulation, Mayo Clinic Proceedings: Innovations, Quality, and Outcomes, and the American Journal of Preventive Medicine have published articles calling for increased education in lifestyle medicine for over a decade. Recent reviews and surveys demonstrate a gap between interest and action in lifestyle medicine education. Both medical students and educators acknowledge the importance of lifestyle medicine. Still, the journal articles indicate that most medical school curricula devote minimal time to these topics, with the majority of time and attention directed to nutrition and exercise. At the same time, the other pillars (such as sleep and stress) are often neglected (13–16).

US medical schools offer between 13 and 58 hours of lifestyle medicine content, with most delivered in lecture format rather than through practical or competency-based approaches (13,14). It is no surprise that tomorrow's doctors, the students, report low confidence in providing lifestyle counseling, particularly in exercise, sleep, and stress management (13,15). This must change. The time is now for lifestyle medicine education (17,18).

The American Heart Association and other professional societies recommend that lifestyle medicine be integrated comprehensively and longitudinally, emphasizing active learning, experiential approaches, and competency-based training in behavioral counseling, nutrition, and physical activity (19,20). Some medical schools have successfully developed dedicated lifestyle medicine themes or threads, or other innovative programs in lifestyle medicine, such as electives, but only a few schools are on that list (19–21). When medical schools have fully integrated lifestyle medicine into the curriculum, in most cases, medical school faculty, and even deans, have been aware of the science and research in lifestyle medicine and have often been strong advocates for it. For example, Dr. Phyllis MacGilvray serves as dean of the University of South Carolina School of Medicine Greenville, one of the first medical schools to fully integrate lifestyle medicine into its curriculum, and she is board-certified in lifestyle medicine (22).

SUMMARY

There is a concerning gap in medical education. The first 17 chapters of this book review the research and scientific evidence supporting the field of lifestyle medicine. Research in lifestyle medicine grows each year; the science of each of the six pillars and their effects on health and disease is becoming clearer; and medical school faculty members are increasingly advocating for greater integration of lifestyle medicine topics and patient cases into medical school curricula. There is more and more interest in lifestyle medicine, but still minimal action in most medical schools. The need for future physicians to be competent in prescribing nutrition, exercise, sleep, stress reduction, social connection, and the avoidance of harmful substances is increasing each year, and medical schools' actions must keep pace.

Raising awareness among medical school faculty and deans is a critical next step in the field's life, growth, and development (23). This is the reason this book was conceived, written, and published.

REFERENCES

1. Diabetes Prevention Program Research Group. Reduction in the incidence of type 2 diabetes with lifestyle intervention or metformin. *N Engl J Med.* 2002;346(6):393–403.
2. Mokdad AH, Marks JS, Stroup DF, Gerberding JL. Actual causes of death in the United States, 2000. *JAMA.* 2004;291(10):1238–1245. doi: 10.1001/jama.291.10.1238. Erratum in: *JAMA.* 2005;293(3):298. Erratum in: *JAMA.* 2005;293(3):293–294. doi: 10.1001/jama.293.3.293. PMID: 15010446.

3. American College of Lifestyle Medicine (ACLM). Definition at ACLM. www.lifestylemedicine.org. Accessed December 22, 2025.
4. AAMC Lifestyle Medicine as a Career. https://careersinmedicine.aamc.org/explore-options/specialty-profiles/lifestyle-medicine.
5. Lopes S, Mesquita-Bastos J, Alves AJ, Ribeiro F. Exercise as a tool for hypertension and resistant hypertension management: current insights. *Integr Blood Press Control.* 2018;11:65–71.
6. Sacks FM, Svetkey LP, Vollmer WM, et al. Effects on blood pressure of reduced dietary sodium and the Dietary Approaches to Stop Hypertension (DASH) diet. DASH-Sodium Collaborative Research Group. *N Engl J Med.* 2001;344(1):3–10.
7. Lianov L, Johnson M. Physician competencies for prescribing lifestyle medicine. *JAMA.* 2010;304(2):202–203. doi: 10.1001/jama.2010.903.
8. Healthy Lifestyles H-425.972. https://policysearch.ama-assn.org/policyfinder/detail/Healthy%20Lifestyles%20H-425.972?uri=%2FAMADoc%2FHOD.xml-0-3746.xml.
9. Frates EP, Xiao RC, Sannidhi D, McBride Y, McCargo T, Stern TA. A Web-based lifestyle medicine curriculum: facilitating education about lifestyle medicine, behavioral change, and health care outcomes. *JMIR Med Educ.* 2017;3(2):e14.
10. Lianov LS, Adamson K, Kelly JH, Matthews S, Palma M, Rea BL. Lifestyle medicine core competencies: 2022 update. *Am J Lifestyle Med.* 2022;16(6):734–739. doi: 10.1177/15598276221121580. PMID: 36389051; PMCID: PMC9644148.
11. Eisenberg DM, Cole A, Maile EJ, et al. Proposed nutrition competencies for medical students and physician trainees: a consensus statement. *JAMA Netw Open.* 2024;7(9):e2435425.
12. Frates B, Ortega HA, Freeman KJ, Co JPT, Bernstein M. Lifestyle medicine in medical education: maximizing impact. *Mayo Clin Proc Innov Qual Outcomes.* 2024;8(5):451–474.
13. Essa-Hadad J, Rudolf MC, Mani N, Malatskey L. Mapping lifestyle medicine in undergraduate medical education: a lever for enhancing the curriculum. *BMC Med Educ.* 2022;22(1):886. doi: 10.1186/s12909-022-03929-z.
14. Pasarica M, Boring M, Lessans S. Current practices in the instruction of lifestyle medicine in medical curricula. *Patient Educ Couns.* 2022;105(2):339–345. doi: 10.1016/j.pec.2021.05.042. Epub 2021 Jun 2. PMID: 34116891.
15. Sousa JR, Afreixo V, Carvalho J, Silva P. Nutrition and physical activity education in medical school: a narrative review. *Nutrients.* 2024;16(16):2809. doi: 10.3390/nu16162809. PMID: 39203945; PMCID: PMC11357297.
16. Stoutenberg M, Lewis LK, Jones RM, Portacio F, Vidot DC, Kornfeld J. Assessing the current and desired levels of training and applied experiences in chronic disease prevention of students during medical school. *BMC Med Educ.* 2023;23(1):54. doi: 10.1186/s12909-023-04044-3. PMID: 36690998; PMCID: PMC9872306.
17. Collings C, Frates EP, Shurney D. The time is now for lifestyle medicine: lesson from lifestyle medicine leaders. *Am J Lifestyle Med.* 2022;16(5):557–561,
18. Frates B. The evolution of lifestyle medicine education: what, why, how, who, and what now. *Am J Lifestyle Med.* 2025:15598276251359562.
19. Aspry KE, Van Horn L, Carson JAS, et al. Medical nutrition education, training, and competencies to advance guideline-based diet counseling by physicians: a science advisory from the American Heart Association. *Circulation.* 2018;137(23):e821–e841. doi: 10.1161/CIR.0000000000000563. Epub 2018 Apr 30. PMID: 29712711.
20. Hivert MF, Arena R, Forman DE, et al. Medical training to achieve competency in lifestyle counseling: an essential foundation for prevention and treatment of cardiovascular diseases and other chronic medical conditions: a scientific statement from the American Heart Association. *Circulation.* 2016;134(15):e308–e327. doi: 10.1161/CIR.0000000000000442. Epub 2016 Sep 6. PMID: 27601568.
21. Trilk J, Nelson L, Briggs A, Muscato D. Including lifestyle medicine in medical education: rationale for American College of Preventive Medicine/American Medical Association Resolution 959. *Am J Prev Med.* 2019;56(5):e169–e175. doi: 10.1016/j.amepre.2018.10.034. Erratum in: *Am J Prev Med.* 2019;57(1):134. doi: 10.1016/j.amepre.2019.05.002. PMID: 31003604.
22. Nation's First Lifestyle Medicine-Certified Medical School Dean Appointed at University of South Carolina School of Medicine Greenville by Sally Crocker. https://lifestylemedicine.org/nations-first-lifestyle-medicine-certified-dean/. Accessed on November 5, 2025.
23. Rippe JM, Frates B. Academic lifestyle medicine and physician education. *Am J Lifestyle Med.* 2025:15598276251355163.

19 Steps to Integrating Lifestyle Medicine into Medical School Education

Only a few medical schools in the United States have been able to dedicate significant time to providing lifestyle medicine education. To date, two of the approximately 200 medical schools (MD- and DO-granting schools) have demonstrated the ability to incorporate more than 100 hours of lifestyle medicine content over four years, divided into 40 hours of didactic material and 60 hours of application activities. That's approximately 1% of all medical schools in the country. More schools have been able to implement a lifestyle medicine theme or thread throughout the four years of medical school. Many medical schools offer lifestyle medicine electives during the pre-clinical or clinical years. At this time, at least 120 medical schools offer a lifestyle medicine interest group (LMIG), and 140 have been established over the years. That's the place to start, with an LMIG. That's a powerful seed.

Starting an LMIG is one of the first steps to bring the six pillars of lifestyle medicine into a medical school. An LMIG provides a parallel curriculum (1). In this way, faculty can teach the science and share research on the six pillars of lifestyle medicine during lunchtime or early evening, when students are not required to be in class. At these mealtimes, medical students can also actively engage with the nutrition pillar while learning about the foundation of healthy eating patterns. To encourage medical schools to offer medical students healthy, whole-food, plant-based meals, grants are available through the American College of Lifestyle Medicine (ACLM) under the Taste of Lifestyle Medicine program (https://lifestylemedicine.zendesk.com/hc/en-us/articles/35302043435931-Are-there-scholarships-and-grants-available-for-students-interested-in-lifestyle-medicine). Students need to be members of an LMIG and apply for the grant. These grants can provide $250–$500 in funding for the LMIG event.

To run a lifestyle medicine interest group, a dedicated faculty member with interest, experience, and, ideally, board certification in lifestyle medicine must commit to serving as the faculty advisor. Of course, there would be no interest group without the students. Identifying a student leader or leaders helps ensure that LMIG activities, workshops, and presentations are successfully marketed through announcements in class and online communications. The student leaders are champions for lifestyle medicine and are the engine that powers the LMIG.

The ACLM provides support to faculty and students interested in leading LMIGs at their medical schools. A standardized, formal training process has been in place for years to ensure that LMIGs across the country are consistent and use evidence-based practices to teach and inform medical students. In addition, the ACLM holds networking meetings for lifestyle medicine students and faculty throughout the academic year. This is an excellent opportunity to share ideas and brainstorm ways in which lifestyle medicine can be taught and incorporated into medical school curricula. Often, students in the lifestyle medicine interest group communicate with faculty from other courses and express interest in learning more about exercise, nutrition, sleep, stress resilience, social connection, and avoidance of risky substances. In many cases, students in the LMIG collaborate with faculty on the curriculum committee to initiate change and further bolster lifestyle medicine offerings. Additionally, students in the LMIG often assist faculty in mapping the curriculum to determine the extent of lifestyle medicine instruction and to identify opportunities within the curriculum to incorporate the six pillars of lifestyle medicine.

DOI: 10.1201/9781003630043-19

To sustain a lifestyle medicine interest group over the years, a dedicated faculty member is essential. Attending the annual medical student activities fair, collecting the names and email addresses of interested students, advertising upcoming lifestyle medicine events, and maintaining communication with the list of students ensures active participation in the LMIG each year. It is recommended that the faculty advisor and past student leaders attend the student activities fair. The ACLM can provide promotional items, such as pens, notepads, stress balls, computer screen cleaners, glass cleaners, and other giveaways, to distribute to students and to reinforce the importance of lifestyle medicine.

For some schools, there may be no faculty member who is comfortable or confident in their own education and experience in lifestyle medicine. If they have the interest and passion, they can still serve as the faculty advisor and identify other faculty members at the medical school with expertise in the six pillars of lifestyle medicine.

To assist medical school faculty members with limited experience, the ACLM has developed a video library. The video library contains recorded presentations on the six pillars of lifestyle medicine and counseling strategies. The presentations were delivered by faculty experts in the various pillars of lifestyle medicine from medical schools across the country, including Dr. Walter Willett of Harvard T.H. Chan School of Public Health. These videos are available to ACLM members via the Connect Platform at www.lifestylemedicine.org. They were produced by the ACLM Past President, Dr. Beth Frates, and the ACLM Past Secretary, Dr. Meagan Grega. As part of efforts to connect LMIGs nationwide during COVID-19, Dr. Frates invited LMIGs from across the country to the Harvard LMIG lecture on nature as medicine, featuring Dr. John La Puma, as a pilot program. Dr. Grega became involved immediately and assisted in recording the session. Over the years, Dr. Frates and Dr. Grega have hosted more than a dozen virtual LMIGs and have covered essential topics, including nutrition, exercise, sleep, and behavior change.

A scholarship is available to medical and healthcare professional students who are striving to create and sustain an LMIG at their medical school. It is the Donald A. Pegg Award. This award was created in 2016. It is available through ACLM. Applications are typically due around April 1 each year, and a panel of judges selects four medical students. All information about past recipients and the award's history is available at www.lifestylemedicine.org. The students win money to use for lectures and lunches. In addition, they receive complimentary registration to ACLM's annual meeting, a copy of the *Lifestyle Medicine Handbook*, and financial assistance with travel to and from the meeting. The funds provided by this award have been used in many different capacities, including "hiring local chefs to demonstrate unique healthy recipes, hosting LMIG-sponsored plant-based cooking sessions, facilitating body weight–based exercise programs, and teaching mindfulness methodologies through presentations and hands-on exercises" (2). The LMIGs participate in a wide variety of activities. Over the years, the "LMIG activities have included students presenting research at national conferences, initiating a chapter of the national organization Walk with a Doc, hosting educational lectures on LM principles, sponsoring plant-based cooking sessions, facilitating stress management workshops, and hosting a national-level LM congress in Europe" (3). The benefits of the Pegg Award are far-reaching. "The fruits of the Pegg Award extend beyond individual recognition: between seed funding, conference scholarships, and travel support, the Pegg Award constitutes a foundational source of momentum for LMIGs at awardee institutions, catalyzing student engagement by facilitating invaluable connections with mentors, access to research opportunities, and broader community support within the esteemed ACLM network" (4).

LMIGs have grown steadily over the years. By the end of 2024, there were almost 190 total, including medical schools, bachelor's programs, master's/doctoral programs, and health systems (5). A decade earlier, there were only a handful of schools with LMIGs. According to an analysis of LMIGs performed by ACLM members and staff, titled "Lifestyle Medicine Interest Group Event Analysis," published in the *American Journal of Lifestyle Medicine*, most LMIG events focused on the pillars of nutrition (36.4%) and physical activity (22.2%) (5). The next most common pillars were stress management (10.1%), social connection (5.1%), sleep (3%), and avoidance of risky substances (1%). An additional 22.2% of events fell into an other category. In the article, there was an "other" category, and

22.2% of events fell into that category. The article also categorized LMIG events by format, including lectures, group physical activity, board meetings, webinars, cooking demonstrations, community service, fundraisers, and documentary screenings. Among these, lectures were the most common at 25.8%, followed by group physical activity (15.3%), board meetings (11.3%), webinars (9.1%), cooking demonstrations (8.8%), and community service (8.7%); fundraisers (1.8%) and documentary screenings (1.5%) were the least common, and 17.8% of events fell into an other category (5). The focus of the LMIG is often dictated by the interests of the students involved that year.

Building on the interest and passion of the lifestyle medicine faculty and student leaders in the LMIG at the medical school, the next step in integrating lifestyle medicine into the curriculum is to meet with other medical school faculty who teach in the core curriculum. There are many ways to provide lifestyle medicine learning opportunities to medical students, including developing a lifestyle medicine case study focused on a specific organ system, such as cardiovascular, renal, endocrine, musculoskeletal, or neurologic. By approaching faculty who teach in the core curriculum and offering to share a case, a faculty member can create opportunities to incorporate lifestyle medicine into various courses. Another option is to meet with the faculty involved in the core courses and describe the benefits to students of incorporating evidence-based information on a specific pillar, such as nutrition when teaching ketolysis and ketogenesis in biochemistry, or exercise when teaching cellular respiration in the mitochondria and mitogenesis. Connecting with the faculty members who oversee the curriculum committee is an essential step toward formally integrating lifestyle medicine into medical education.

Creating a curricular theme or thread on lifestyle medicine over the four years of medical school allows faculty to maintain their current course design and curricular structure without time-consuming disruption. Time is often a barrier to change, and this is no different when considering changes to the medical school curriculum. In fact, the most frequently cited barrier to incorporating lifestyle medicine into the curriculum is that the curriculum is already full. There is no room for additional courses or material. Adding a lifestyle medicine theme does not add extra time to the course load. It requires adding information on the six pillars of lifestyle medicine to existing courses. No change in curricular structure is needed.

Creating a thread or theme involves connection and collaboration with course faculty members. Educating faculty members about the science and research underpinning the six pillars helps them understand the importance of integrating lifestyle medicine into the four years of medical school. It can help them map out how the theme can be successfully integrated. A theme indicates that the topic is a focus of the curriculum and is addressed in a longitudinal, cross-cutting manner. The theme is addressed in the first, second, third, and fourth years and appears across many courses and learning opportunities, both preclinical and clinical. When a school adopts a lifestyle medicine theme, it also means there is a curriculum lead faculty member working with other faculty members to ensure the topic is included and to support the integration. Without a faculty member or group overseeing the integration of the theme, redundancies and missed opportunities may arise. A few medical schools have adopted a lifestyle medicine theme. Harvard, Northwestern, and the University of North Carolina are just three examples.

19.1 ELECTIVES

In general, electives provide faculty with the opportunity to share their expertise with medical students. Lifestyle medicine electives have been implemented at numerous medical schools across the country, including Harvard Medical School, Brown University Medical School, Loma Linda Medical School, the University of Central Florida Medical College, Stanford University School of Medicine, Yale Medical School, UT Southwestern, and many others. Electives typically range from one to four weeks. There are also opportunities for longitudinal electives at some schools. Harvard Medical School offers an elective titled Medical Exploratory Longitudinal Elective (ELO 700), which some students have taken, with a focus on lifestyle medicine education. Creating an elective requires time and commitment, as well as approval from the curriculum committee.

There are many examples of electives in lifestyle medicine that faculty can use as templates. An article on electives in medical school published in the American Journal of Lifestyle Medicine is available online as open access (6). It is titled, "Lifestyle Medicine Electives: Options for Creating Curricula Within Medical School Training." The article identifies different resources used by Loma Linda, University of Central Florida, Brown University, and the University of California-Irvine medical schools and shares the experience of creating an elective in lifestyle medicine. As noted in the article, medical schools use various resources to teach electives, including the LM 101 Curriculum and the Culinary Medicine Curriculum, available for free and downloadable via the ACLM website, as well as the Foundations of Lifestyle Medicine resources, which are also free and downloadable via the website http://www.lifestylemedicinecurriculum.org.

The Lifestyle Medicine 101 Curriculum (LM 101 Curriculum) is an excellent resource for medical school faculty (7). It was originally designed for both master's- and bachelor's-level learners, making it ideal for first-year medical students as well as second-, third-, and fourth-year students. Most medical students lack exposure to lifestyle medicine in college when they were premeds. So, this curriculum provides an appropriate level of content for an introduction to the six pillars of lifestyle medicine and coaching/motivational interviewing basics. As the curriculum is also used for master's level students, it can be directed to medical students in the second, third, and fourth years by incorporating additional research articles on the science of each pillar and clinical trials using lifestyle medicine to treat specific conditions. Additionally, the course level can be adjusted by incorporating varied in-class application activities and modifying assignments, with more clinical reasoning and decision-making for more experienced medical students.

The LM 101 is a free, full curriculum available for download from the American College of Lifestyle Medicine's website (7). Faculty simply need to complete a form to obtain access. The course curriculum comprises a syllabus, 13 PowerPoint slide decks, and a teacher's guide. It follows along with a textbook, the *Lifestyle Medicine Handbook* (8), all proceeds from which go to the American College of Lifestyle Medicine. The 13 PowerPoint decks in this curriculum correspond to the 13 chapters in the *Lifestyle Medicine Handbook.* Each PowerPoint deck has 150–200 slides. All six pillars of lifestyle medicine are covered. There are two chapters on behavior change, one chapter on positive psychology, and another chapter on how to implement this into the life of physicians and other healthcare professionals. This curriculum has been successfully employed in the United States and countries around the globe, such as Romania and South Korea. It is often used in medical school electives in lifestyle medicine and has also been employed by faculty for medical student presentations and classes. The LM 101 Curriculum provides 26 hours of material. It has been updated twice, and there are plans to make sure it is updated every two to three years.

Foundations of Lifestyle Medicine is a modular curriculum designed for flexible use across a range of teaching needs (9). Faculty may adopt it for an entire elective or integrate selected modules into just a few hours of instruction. The curriculum covers each of the six pillars, with a special emphasis on behavior change, and introduces the concept of integrating lifestyle factors in the treatment and prevention of cardiovascular disease, type 2 diabetes, and cancer. Each module includes activities and discussion questions to support faculty facilitation and to promote experiential learning for students. In addition to the core curriculum, educators are provided with a sample elective schedule and a spreadsheet summarizing the cited literature. This curriculum from Foundations of Lifestyle Medicine specifies what to do each day of a two- or four-week elective.

Another option for an elective is to offer the ACLM Foundations in Lifestyle Medicine CME course, which can be used as a self-paced learning elective. Collaborating with ACLM and coordinating logistics is recommended for each school or student. There are additional CME courses available at ACLM that can be purchased and used. These courses cover different topics, such as Food Is Medicine and Reversing Diabetes.

Additionally, faculty members can visit the LMEd website (10). The website hosts slide decks, case studies, videos, and recorded webinars on lifestyle medicine. The Ardmore Institute of Health generously funded the Lifestyle Medicine Education Collaborative starting in 2014 and continuing for a number of years. Some of the topics in the slide decks include lifestyle medicine and cancer, respiratory health, immune system, GI health, hematopoiesis, brain health, musculoskeletal health, and renal health. Case studies include cancer, immune system, bone health, psych-neuro, and skeletal muscle. These PowerPoints and case studies are from faculty at the University of South Carolina at Greenville.

19.2 FULL INTEGRATION INTO MEDICAL SCHOOL CURRICULA

ACLM is working to promote the full integration of lifestyle medicine into medical schools. One of its efforts in 2021 was to create an ACLM Curriculum Certification Committee and a process with different levels or tiers. This effort was also funded by the Ardmore Institute of Health (AIH). For certification, medical schools must apply for consideration and grading. There is a fee associated with the application process. AIH generously donated funds to support ten medical schools in using the program. ACLM education staff review the institution's curriculum and mapping work. They then evaluate it based on total training hours, the percentage of competencies covered, and the availability of enrichment opportunities for in-depth learning. This enrichment is noted by a plus in the certification level designation. There are platinum, gold, silver, and bronze levels of certification. The first publication sharing this curriculum certification opportunity was published in the American Journal of Lifestyle Medicine in 2021 (11). The ACLM Education Department staff and LMEd have partnered to provide recommendations to applicants to strengthen their LM offerings.

In the past five years, nine schools have completed the certification process with funding provided by AIH. The schools and their designation are as follows: Loma Linda (Platinum Plus), University of South Carolina-Greenville campus (Platinum Plus), Western University of Health Sciences College of Osteopathic Medicine of The Pacific (Gold), UT McGovern Medical School at Houston (Silver Plus), Touro University of California (Silver Plus), Oakland University William Beaumont School of Medicine (Bronze), University of Missouri-Kansas City School of Medicine (Bronze), Chicago Medical School (Bronze), and Ohio State University College of Medicine (Bronze).

The different levels indicate the number of hours spent on LM and the percentage of the LM competencies covered. All schools need to have a Lifestyle Medicine Interest Group as a baseline requirement. Platinum level means that 100 hours or more are spent on lifestyle medicine education, and 100% of the lifestyle medicine competencies are covered, and medical students across all four years receive LM education. Gold level means that 75–99 hours are spent on lifestyle medicine education, and 75% of the lifestyle medicine competencies are covered and all medical students receive LM education at some point in their four years. Silver level means that 50–74 hours are spent on lifestyle medicine education, and 50% of the lifestyle medicine competencies are covered, and all medical students receive LM education at some point in their four years. Bronze level means that 25-49 hours are spent on lifestyle medicine education, and 25% of the lifestyle medicine competencies are covered and all medical students receive LM education at some point in their four years. A plus designation indicates that the school has met the required hours and competency percentages by creating offerings in addition to the core curriculum, such as a Lifestyle Medicine Enrichment Track (e.g., a series of electives, in-depth education, and mentoring in LM) or an LM concentration at the school. As was shared in an article in the American Journal of Lifestyle Medicine titled The Evolution of Lifestyle Medicine Education: What, Why, How, Who, and What Now,

> Those schools that have been able to incorporate lifestyle medicine into the core curriculum for all 4 years and the follow-up of those students will be helpful for other older, more traditional medical schools to fully appreciate the value of such a comprehensive lifestyle medicine approach (12).

Only a small number of schools have participated in the ACLM curriculum certification, which may be because the science and research underlying the six pillars of lifestyle medicine have not yet been widely recognized or fully appreciated by leaders in academic medicine. Reaching leaders in academic medicine and sharing the rigorous research supporting the six pillars, as outlined in the first 17 chapters of this book, are critical steps toward integrating lifestyle medicine into the core curriculum in medical education (13). Regardless of whether a school chooses to pay and go through the ACLM certification process, mapping the school's curriculum to identify how many hours are dedicated to lifestyle medicine topics and what percentage of the LM competencies are covered is a worthwhile endeavor, as it provides insight into what topics are being taught and where there are opportunities to add more lifestyle medicine teaching (14).

19.3 SUMMARY

Seeds of change are being planted at many medical schools. More than 140 medical schools have established an LMIG, through which students can study the science of the six pillars of lifestyle medicine and the art of behavior change counseling in a parallel curriculum. A few schools have incorporated dedicated themes or threads in lifestyle medicine that focus efforts on integrating the pillars of lifestyle medicine across all four years of medical school, distributed across a variety of courses and learning opportunities. To date, only two schools have integrated 100 hours of lifestyle medicine, covering 100% of the LM competencies, into their course offerings. With each year, more LMIGs are created. With each year, more medical school faculty are board-certified in lifestyle medicine. Each year, faculty develop opportunities to share the science and research on the six pillars of lifestyle medicine with medical students. Progress has been made, but more work remains.

REFERENCES

1. Pojednic R, Frates E. A parallel curriculum in lifestyle medicine. *Clin Teach.* 2017;14(1):27–31. doi: 10.1111/tct.12475. Epub 2015 Dec 6. PMID: 26639320.
2. Stiegmann RA, Abreu A, Gardner JE, Hipple JM, Poling PE, Frates EP. Planting the seeds of change: growing lifestyle medicine interest groups with the Donald A. Pegg award. *Am J Lifestyle Med.* 2017;11(6):443–447. doi: 10.1177/1559827617714782. PMID: 30202369; PMCID: PMC6125011.
3. Jaini PA, Stiegmann RA, Barrera A, et al. Nurturing the seeds of change: strengthening the lifestyle medicine movement with the Donald A. Pegg student leadership award. *Am J Lifestyle Med.* 2018;12(6):476–478. doi: 10.1177/1559827618789354. PMID: 30783401; PMCID: PMC6367882.
4. Jacob Y, Srinivasan R, Ubbens E, Orme A, Shahinfar S, Frates B. Furthering lifestyle medicine through the Donald A. Pegg student leadership award: reflections from 2023 awardees. *Am J Lifestyle Med.* 2024;19(2):202–210. doi: 10.1177/15598276241274487. PMID: 39554955; PMCID: PMC11562118.
5. Vanderpool LE, Wong ML, Gama GO, et al. Lifestyle medicine interest group (LMIG) events analysis. *Am J Lifestyle Med.* 2025:15598276251337409.
6. Bansal S, Cramer S, Stump M, Wasserstrom S. Lifestyle medicine electives: options for creating curricula within medical school training. *Am J Lifestyle Med.* 2023;17(6):754–758. doi: 10.1177/15598276221147181. PMID: 38511111; PMCID: PMC10948920.
7. Lifestyle Medicine (LM) 101 Curriculum. American College of Lifestyle Medicine. Connect Platform. https://learning.lifestylemedicine.org/content/lifestyle-medicine-101-curriculum. Accessed December 22, 2025.
8. Frates B, Bonnet J, Joseph R, and Peterson J. *The Lifestyle Medicine Handbook* (2nd ed). Monterey, CA: Healthy Learning, 2021.
9. Foundations of Lifestyle Medicine. https://www.lifestylemedicinecurriculum.org/. Accessed December 22, 2025.
10. LMEd. https://lifestylemedicineeducation.org/. Accessed December 22, 2025.
11. Trilk JL, Worthman S, Shetty P, et al. Undergraduate medical education: lifestyle medicine curriculum implementation standards. *Am J Lifestyle Med.* 2021;15(5):526–530.
12. Frates B. The evolution of lifestyle medicine education: what, why, how, who, and what now. *Am J Lifestyle Med.* 2025:15598276251359562. doi: 10.1177/15598276251359562.
13. Rippe JM, Frates B. Academic lifestyle medicine and physician education. *Am J Lifestyle Med.* 2025:15598276251355163. doi: 10.1177/15598276251355163. Epub ahead of print.
14. Essa-Hadad J, Rudolf MC, Mani N, Malatskey L. Mapping lifestyle medicine in undergraduate medical education: a lever for enhancing the curriculum. *BMC Med Educ.* 2022;22(1):886.

20 Examples of Lifestyle Medicine in Medical Schools

This chapter presents examples of medical schools that are already incorporating lifestyle medicine (LM) education into their curricula. A wide variety of experiences are detailed in this chapter. Many more schools include lifestyle medicine in their curricula than are listed here. These are only a sampling.

20.1 UNIVERSITY OF MASSACHUSETTS SCHOOL OF MEDICINE—JAMES RIPPE, MD

Dr. Rippe was recruited to join the faculty at University of Massachusetts Chan Medical School (UMMC) in 2019 with the mandate to establish a robust, academically oriented lifestyle medicine program at a major academic medical school. Since that time, multiple achievements and parameters have been completed or are in progress.

The initial groundwork to launch lifestyle medicine at UMMC involved establishing a culture within the academic medical center that recognized that lifestyle medicine occupies a central role in evidence-based medicine. This foundation was essential in order to build among skeptical academicians the strong evidence base that supports lifestyle medicine.

Early efforts to establish this foundation and culture involved building a strong relationship with Terry Flotte, MD, Provost and Executive Deputy Chancellor, UMass Chan Medical School; Dean, Celia and Isaac Haidak Professor; and Professor of Pediatrics, T.H. Chan School of Medicine. In addition, Dr. Rippe built a strong supportive relationship with David D. McManus, MD ScM, Richard M. Haidack Professor; Chair, Department of Medicine, UMass Chan Medical School/UMass Memorial Health. Dr. Rippe's position as Professor of Medicine (Cardiology) lent further credibility to this effort.

In the past six years, Dr. Rippe has developed multiple other components of this initiative to begin to spread the word and credibility of lifestyle medicine amongst both undergraduate medical students and graduate interns and residents. With this goal in mind, he has given multiple lectures in the area of lifestyle medicine and health to the Primary Care Residents as well as the Categorical Residents (all the other Internal Medicine Residents). In addition, he has begun work with the key members of the committee that established the new VISTA Curriculum for undergraduate medical students at UMass Chan Medical School.

In 2024, Dr. Rippe applied for and received a grant from the Ardmore Institute of Health to establish a "High Level Medically Oriented Lifestyle Medicine Curriculum." The goal was to link the robust scientific evidence behind lifestyle medicine with a "hands-on" curriculum that academic physicians could utilize.

In order to continue to build on the academic underpinnings of lifestyle medicine, Dr. Rippe has launched an aggressive publication program. This includes the publication of his multi-authored, academic *Lifestyle Medicine* textbook (published in 2024). This publication has 325 co-authors, with Dr. Rippe serving as the editor-in-chief. In addition, he has developed a six-component CME lecture series and is working with the UMass Chan CME team to determine exactly the best way of delivering these six lectures. There is one lecture for each pillar of lifestyle medicine.

In addition to the above references, Dr. Rippe also serves as the editor-in-chief of the *Lifestyle Medicine Series* and has personally written for academic textbooks in this area over the past

DOI: 10.1201/9781003630043-20

five years including one in physical activity, a manual of lifestyle medicine, a book showing how lifestyle medicine fits into cardiovascular disease treatment and prevention, a book on obesity prevention and management, and a book on healthy nutrition (plant-based) for physicians. Dr. Rippe has also established relationships to publish additional books in the academic lifestyle medicine area.

Dr. Rippe continues to serve as editor-in-chief of the *American Journal of Lifestyle Medicine* (AJLM) and has written multiple state-of-the-art reviews in AJLM in areas related to academic LM, including a review of LM and cardiovascular disease, an overall review of LM and health, as well as a specific article (along with Dr. Beth Frates) on academic LM and physician education. References to the books published in academic LM, as well as some of the articles that Dr. Rippe has written, may be found in Appendix C. In addition, Dr. Rippe and Dr. Frates have written a book entitled *Academic Lifestyle Medicine: A Curriculum for Medical Educators,* which will be published in 2026.

During Dr. Rippe's service as editor-in-chief of the AJLM over the last five years, AJLM has grown to over 30,000 subscribers and, in 2024, had over 340,000 downloads of articles in the area of lifestyle medicine. AJLM also publishes academic abstracts that have been accepted at the American College of Lifestyle Medicine (ACLM). In 2025, AJLM published over 200 academic abstracts.

Having established a firm academic basis for lifestyle medicine, the next level of this initiative will be to integrate this robust information into various levels of education at UMass Chan Medical School and Harvard Medical School. Following this, the goal that Dr. Rippe and Dr. Frates have established is to offer this type of evidence-based, academic lifestyle medicine to other medical schools around the country. With this in mind, they have reached out to and received strong support from high-level academicians at UMass Chan Medical School, Harvard Medical School, Tufts Medical School, BU School of Medicine, Stanford University School of Medicine, and Johns Hopkins School of Medicine. The team has received an additional grant from the Ardmore Institute of Health to support the academic lifestyle medicine efforts.

20.2 HARVARD MEDICAL SCHOOL—BETH FRATES, MD

Harvard University is actively involved in lifestyle medicine from pre-med to medical school to CME. Harvard Medical School (HMS) started the first Lifestyle Medicine Interest Group (LMIG) in the 2008–2009 academic year (1). This parallel curriculum provides medical students with opportunities to learn about the six pillars of lifestyle medicine while enjoying a nutritious and delicious meal. There are at least six presentations a year, drawing on the expertise of HMS and the Harvard T.H. Chan School of Public Health faculty across the pillars of lifestyle medicine. Each year, the medical student leaders determine the activities they will undertake. Over the years, these have included a 5K to benefit the Massachusetts General Hospital (MGH) Revere Food Pantry, a kickball game, walk-and-talk lectures, cooking demonstrations, a panel of Harvard faculty practicing lifestyle medicine from different specialties, and journal clubs. The students from the LMIG at HMS have also helped faculty map nutrition and lifestyle medicine in the curriculum. A Nutrition Interest Group was later formed, and the two groups co-sponsor events.

In 2015, HMS adopted the theme of nutrition and lifestyle medicine in the core curriculum. Several HMS faculty are involved. With this theme in place, there have been opportunities to revise case studies and to incorporate more nutrition and lifestyle medicine into core courses and professional development week courses.

Dr. Beth Frates has routinely offered a workshop on well-being and lifestyle medicine during HMS professional development weeks for over a decade and continues to do so. Lifestyle medicine has also been included in the core curriculum before students' transition to the wards for clinical experience, with four lectures covering heart disease and stroke, diabetes, obesity, and frailty. In addition, faculty in the lifestyle medicine theme group delivered workshops on motivational interviewing for second-year students. More recently, HMS students were required to complete an online nutrition module, and faculty in the lifestyle medicine group provided comments to each student on the online platform. When students arrive at HMS, they take a course titled Introduction to the Professions (ITP) and HMS has included nutrition, sleep, and stress resiliency in this core curriculum course.

Over the years, several HMS students have focused on lifestyle medicine in their scholarly projects, producing work including a plant-based cookbook, the Lifestyle Medicine Pocket Guide, and a lifestyle medicine program in well-being spanning all four years, as described in an article published in the AJLM (2). The HMS graduates Case Brabham, MD, and Andre Dempsey, MD, used the *Lifestyle Medicine Handbook* by Frates, Bonnet, Joseph, and Peterson (3) and the LM 101 Curriculum available for free from the ACLM website to help them co-author the *Lifestyle Medicine Pocket Guide* (4), along with Dr. Beth Frates, their faculty advisor for their scholarly project. At HMS, some electives encourage students to partner with faculty on academic projects, such as an elective in medical education, and some students have chosen to focus on lifestyle medicine topics.

In 2024, the Harvard Medical School LMIG sought to bring lifestyle medicine to adolescents in underserved areas of Boston. HMS student Vivian Wang partnered with Dr. Beth Frates to co-create a lifestyle medicine curriculum based on the Teen Lifestyle Medicine Curriculum available for free from the ACLM. Dr. Frates and Vivian Wang recruited students from HMS and Harvard College pre-med/pre-healthcare professional students to join the LIVELY Team in the summer of 2024. LIVELY stands for "**L**ifestyle **I**nter**v**entions Through **E**mpowerment and **L**eadership in **Y**outh." The Office for Community Centered Medical Education at HMS helped sponsor and support this work (https://occme.hms.harvard.edu/news/lively-approach-mental-health). Dr. Frates and Vivian Wang partnered with the Boys and Girls Clubs of Boston to implement the program, which was highly successful and won the 2024 Best Program Award from the organization. The following summer, in 2025, the program was repeated and included pre-medical students from Boston University. One of the Harvard pre-med students, Noah Janfaza, won a fellowship to bring LIVELY to the Boys and Girls Clubs of Puerto Rico for the 2025–2026 academic year. With programs like this, HMS is working to teach medical students and Harvard College pre-meds the science and art of lifestyle medicine, train them to teach, and share LM basics with teens in underserved areas.

HMS offers specific electives in nutrition and lifestyle medicine, including Nutrition, Metabolism, and Lifestyle Medicine, Pediatric Nutrition, Pediatric Gastroenterology/Nutrition, Nutrition and Rural Medicine in Latin America, and Culinary Medicine and Nutrition. Some HMS students have also opted to focus on lifestyle medicine in the Medical Exploratory Longitudinal Elective (ELO 700).

Faculty at HMS work toward innovation in implementing lifestyle medicine in the curriculum. During the first summer with an eight-week vacation for first-year medical students at HMS, Dr. Beth Frates led a summer pilot program in lifestyle medicine that included participation by medical students and faculty. The program was a flipped classroom, using video content from a CME course created by Dr. Beth Frates and provided by Mass General Brigham (MGB). There were seven hours of content covering the lifestyle medicine pillars, as well as topics such as finding a sense of purpose, goal setting, and energy management. There was a mix of students and attendings as learners. For eight weeks, the learners met for an hour every Monday evening from 7 to 8 pm to discuss the topic covered in the video and share Aha moments. In addition, the course instructor, Beth Frates, facilitated a coaching session for a volunteer learner who sought to work on behavior change and goal setting related to the week's topic. Post-program evaluations indicated that both medical students and faculty enjoyed the program, watched the videos, and learned about the six pillars of lifestyle medicine and the process of coaching for behavior change. This was evident in their performance on the content quiz at the end of the program. This pilot was a novel approach to teaching lifestyle medicine, employing summer weeks, holding live sessions with mixed-level learners, and using the flipped classroom model. It helped educate HMS students and faculty.

Several faculty members at HMS are Board Certified in Lifestyle Medicine through American Board of Lifestyle Medicine (ABLM)/International Board of Lifestyle Medicine (IBLM) and American College of Lifestyle Medicine (ACLM). These faculty members are involved in teaching in the clinical years at HMS and training residents and fellows throughout the HMS system. In 2022, HMS began offering the Lifestyle Medicine Residency Curriculum (LMRC) to residents in the Occupational Medicine Residency Program, with excellent feedback and evaluations from residents (5). That expanded to the Physical Medicine and Rehabilitation Residency at Spaulding Rehabilitation Hospital, the Psychiatry Residency at MGH, and the Primary Care Residency at Brigham and Women's Hospital. The pediatric residency at MGH is also currently working to incorporate lifestyle medicine into its rotations.

HMS offers many CMEs, including but not limited to lifestyle medicine lectures, including courses in Internal Medicine Board Review, Women's Leadership, Women's Health, Primary Care, Mind-Body Medicine, Lifestyle Medicine Tools for Promoting Healthy Change, Rehabilitation Medicine, Sports Medicine, Anesthesia, General Internal Medicine for Specialists, Women's Health and Menopause, and the Surgical Leadership Program, among others. In addition, the Harvard Medical School Department of External Education offers two popular online courses in lifestyle medicine: Health and Wellness: Designing a Sustainable Eating Pattern. From March 2023 to March 2026, 2,900 learners enrolled in this online course from the United States and a wide variety of countries across the world. Given the success of this online course, HMS launched a second course titled, Nutrition and Lifestyle Coaching. From its launch in September 2024 to March 2026, 2,600 students have enrolled. Both online courses have an over 90% completion rate and the course receives excellent reviews, above average markings for its product type. Due to the popularity of these courses, HMS decided to offer an in-person, on campus, immersion program in lifestyle medicine and coaching in April 2026. It was a huge success, and there are plans to offer this immersion program twice a year moving forward.

Harvard Extension School has offered lifestyle medicine courses at the college and master's level since 2014. There are three online courses offered each year, including Wellbeing from the Inside Out: Cell to Community, Lifestyle Medicine 101, and Empowering People to Change. All of the courses enroll approximately 65 students per semester (and have active waitlists), and they have been recognized by ACLM as part of the Academic Partial Pathways Programs. Over the past decade, over a dozen students at the Harvard Extension School have elected to focus their theses on lifestyle medicine-related topics and have selected Dr. Beth Frates as their thesis advisor for these projects. In addition, dozens of students at the school have opted to work with a lifestyle medicine expert, Dr. Beth Frates, as their faculty advisor. With regard to medical students, so far, two Harvard Medical students have served as teaching assistants for the fall-semester course titled Wellbeing from the Inside Out: From Cell to Community. The medical students led small group sections. In this way, medical students gained experience not only in the science and art of lifestyle medicine but also in effective teaching strategies. Teaching assistants are often an essential component of a successful classroom experience (6).

A handful of pre-medical students at Harvard College have selected a lifestyle medicine focus for their Global Health and Health Policy (GHHP-91) supervised reading and research course with Dr. Beth Frates serving as their faculty advisor.

Harvard University is an example of an institution that has integrated lifestyle medicine across all aspects of its teaching and learning, including its college, extension school, medical school, community-centered medical education, and external medical education efforts. Faculty at Harvard are teaching lifestyle medicine topics at the pre-med, medical school, Graduate Medical Education (GME), and Continuing Medical Education (CME) levels. Graduates of HMS have interacted with and learned from HMS faculty experts in lifestyle medicine and have gone on to become leaders in the field, including Michelle Hauser, MD, an HMS graduate and the 2024 ACLM President-Elect. Richard Joseph, MD, was a resident in the Brigham and Women's Primary Care residency and became a co-author of the first and second editions of the *Lifestyle Medicine Handbook* (3,7). He is now running his own private practice in lifestyle medicine. Jacob Mirsky, MD, another resident in the Brigham and Women's Primary Care residency, is actively involved with shared medical appointments in lifestyle medicine and works at the MGH Healthy Lifestyles program at MGH Revere. Harvard University has three LMIGs: HMS, Harvard Extension School, and Harvard College, which serve students from pre-medical through medical studies.

20.3 STANFORD UNIVERSITY SCHOOL OF MEDICINE—MICHAEL FREDERICSON, MD

The Stanford University Lifestyle Medicine Center offers two elective, ten-week courses that undergraduate or medical students can take for one or two graded units. As part of this, students also complete a formal course evaluation at the end of every quarter. Stanford averages 60 students per quarter for the introductory course and 30 per quarter for the advanced course. Stanford University School of Medicine also serves as a hub for the ACLM LMRC program, an undergraduate research program, and sponsors the National Teen Lifestyle Medicine program and a three-week intensive summer program for high school students.

20.4 LIFESTYLE MEDICINE IN THE MOREHOUSE SCHOOL OF MEDICINE CURRICULUM—JENNIFER ROOKE, MD

Morehouse School of Medicine (MSM) is a private, historically Black medical school located in Atlanta, Georgia. MSM focuses on training primary care physicians and addressing health disparities among underserved communities.

First-year medical students are introduced to lifestyle medicine in the Clinical Preceptorship Component (CPC) of the Fundamentals of Medicine 1 (FOM1) course. The CPC component is the first exposure to patient care in the curriculum. Students spend a half day in clinical settings of their choice. The lifestyle medicine clinic is one of the options, along with the traditional primary care options, internal medicine, pediatrics, family medicine, and gynecology. The decision process is often the first time that medical students become aware of clinical lifestyle medicine as a viable clinical practice option.

The Medical Student Summer Research and Public Health Experience is designed to increase interest in biomedical, public health, and clinical research via a focused mentor-directed summer experience. In 2019, two first-year medical students assisted in analyzing lifestyle medicine clinic outcomes data. A lifestyle medicine research project was planned for 2020, but was cancelled because of coronavirus disease 2019 (COVID-19).

First- and second-year medical students have annual Wellness Workshops for MD1 and MD2 students. These workshops are a series of 2-hour presentations on different personal "wellness" topics. These workshops provide the opportunity to introduce the basics of lifestyle medicine.

Fourth-year medical students have a Public Health and Preventive Medicine Elective. This is a four-week elective rotation for fourth-year medical students. Students learn about traditional public health and lifestyle medicine. Medical students complete four 1-hour lifestyle medicine lectures and spend two weeks in the lifestyle medicine clinic. The rotation deliverables are a presentation on a public health/preventive medicine topic and a presentation on their personal experience with behavior modification in one or more lifestyle medicine pillars.

Fourth-year medical students also have extracurricular lifestyle medicine activities. All medical students are invited to join the LMIG's Lifestyle Intervention Workshops, consist of a series of 12 workshops which are held three times each year for lifestyle medicine clinic patients, along with their friends, family, and community members. The workshops initially began as in-person cooking classes, and medical students at all levels participated. Since 2020, the workshops have been virtual. LMIG students have requested that in-person cooking classes resume.

20.5 OKLAHOMA UNIVERSITY CULINARY MEDICINE PROGRAM, UNIVERSITY OF OKLAHOMA SCHOOL OF COMMUNITY MEDICINE, TULSA, OKLAHOMA—MARIANNA WETHERILL, PHD, MPH, RDN/LD; LORI WHELAN, MD; AND CHEF VALARIE CARTER, MPH

After receiving a pilot project grant from the Ardmore Institute of Health, the University of Oklahoma School of Community Medicine (Tulsa, OK) launched an extracurricular culinary medicine program in January 2018 as an initial step toward addressing nutrition curriculum gaps in medical school education. In its first year, 100% of medical students chose to participate in culinary medicine classes, and that summer, the school's Physician Assistant Program became one of the first in the nation to require culinary medicine for its students as part of its degree program (8).

In 2019, the school launched two new lifestyle medicine courses for first- and second-year medical students, which were used to meet the competencies defined in the school's community medicine specialty track. In 2020, the Physician Assistant Program expanded its two-credit-hour Culinary Medicine course to a three-credit-hour Lifestyle Medicine course. Both the medical and the physician assistant courses align with the ACLM's recommended competencies for undergraduate medical education, described in a publication co-authored by two of the program's founders (9).

Beyond the delivery of its mandatory coursework, the Culinary Medicine Program has created an environment that has enabled extracurricular, research, and other applied-learning opportunities to thrive at the University of Oklahoma Tulsa campus, attracting nearly $6 million in extramural funding. In 2024, the program's teaching kitchen relocated from a nearby community Young Men's Christian Association (YMCA) teaching kitchen to an on-campus location after two classrooms were successfully renovated. The Oklahoma University Culinary Medicine Program is currently led by its co-founders, an emergency room physician, a registered dietitian, and a chef who also directs community-based research, education, and service projects that advance the school's mission, such as the Food First Pharmacy for uninsured patients at the school's student teaching clinic. The school's culinary medicine curriculum and its LM courses are often a deciding factor for students who choose to attend the school. In 2025, two medical students at the College of Medicine's main campus (Oklahoma City, OK) founded the MedChef student interest group, which will increase access to additional healthcare student learners in the state.

20.6 ROSALIND FRANKLIN UNIVERSITY OF MEDICINE AND SCIENCE—CHICAGO MEDICAL SCHOOL—MELISSA BERNSTEIN, PHD

The Chicago Medical School LM curriculum has been awarded Bronze certification by ACLM undergraduate medical education (UME) in the Undergraduate Medical Education Lifestyle Medicine Curriculum Certification process, meaning that all students receive a minimum of 25–49 hours of UME LM competencies covered in the core curriculum. This highlights the institution's dedication to equipping future healthcare providers with a comprehensive understanding of the critical role of lifestyle factors in patient health. Additionally, a number of different popular electives are offered in lifestyle medicine, culinary medicine, and nutrition.

Rosalind Franklin University of Medicine and Science also has a Distinction in Nutrition and Health Promotion, which is a highly selective program for students to have the opportunity to take a deep dive into lifestyle medicine by participating in an immersive and experiential longitudinal program during their M2–M4 years. The Distinction in Nutrition and Health Promotion culminates with the completion of a capstone project. This final project, focused on a specific issue or problem in the area of lifestyle medicine, is designed to showcase the additional knowledge and skills students gain by completing this program. Capstone projects are creative, rigorous, and have the potential to make a meaningful contribution to Chicago Medical School and the surrounding community.

20.7 BROWN UNIVERSITY SCHOOL OF MEDICINE—MARIAH STUMP, MD

The Warren Alpert Medical School of Brown University offers one pre-clinical elective in Lifestyle Medicine and Culinary Medicine called "Food is Health," which is a semester-long course, and one two-week clinical elective for third- and fourth-year students called "Introduction to Lifestyle Medicine."

"Food is Health" is an elective course offered during the first and second years of medical school. The course is taught in conjunction with the Culinary School in Providence, Rhode Island, Johnson and Wales University, and the students use its kitchen for cooking, and its chef is involved as a co-course instructor. Each year, the course is capped at 25 students to enable each student enough space at the kitchen stations. For the past few years, there has been a waitlist to get into the course, so it is offered in the fall and spring semesters. The course is evaluated through student feedback, and students evaluate the course through online evaluations. The course has been offered as pass/fail.

"Introduction to Lifestyle Medicine" is a two-week clinical elective offered for third- and fourth-year students. This course is intended to provide the clinical context for lifestyle medicine, and students work alongside faculty who are incorporating lifestyle medicine into their practices. Cumulatively, through the academic year, about 20–30 students sign up for this course, which is about 20%–30% of the fourth-year class. Students are evaluated through a PASS/FAIL grading system, which is determined by the completion of their clinical work and educational activities and modules. Students evaluate the course formally through their online evaluation platform, "OASIS," where they can evaluate the course as a whole.

Dr. Mariah Stump, of Brown Medicine and an Assistant Professor at the Warren Alpert Medical School of Brown University, has also received a Department of Medicine grant to help fund the implementation of a culinary medicine curriculum into the Internal Medicine residency. This initiative consists of alternating culinary sessions with didactic lectures. The intention after this grant is that the Internal Medicine department will offer a formalized track of study/focus within the Internal Medicine residency for Culinary and Lifestyle Medicine.

Brown also has an active Walk with a Doc chapter in Providence, which is growing and thriving, and has featured Brown medical students coming on walks several times per year and leading teaching sessions for the walkers.

20.8 UNIVERSITY OF PITTSBURGH MEDICAL CENTER—MICHELLE THOMPSON, DO

Lifestyle medicine has become an essential component of medical education within the University of Pittsburgh School of Medicine's Family Medicine curriculum. As part of the department's didactic structure, a dedicated monthly lifestyle medicine lecture is offered to all students learning the essentials of primary care. These sessions provide evidence-based guidance on nutrition, physical activity, sleep health, stress management, social connection, and reduction of risky substances—core pillars that support improved patient outcomes. By integrating these lectures into routine didactics, students gain consistent reinforcement of practical skills they can immediately apply once they enter clinical care.

In addition to the lecture series, the University of Pittsburgh School of Medicine offers immersive lifestyle medicine rotations for medical students. Third- and fourth-year students can participate in either a two- or four-week elective, depending on their clinical schedule and interests. These rotations expose learners to outpatient Lifestyle and Integrative Medicine practices, interdisciplinary team visits with dietitians and health coaches, group medical visits, culinary medicine experiences, and hands-on approaches to behavior change counseling. Students gain valuable training in both preventive and therapeutic lifestyle medicine strategies, preparing them to incorporate these competencies into any specialty they choose.

Together, the monthly didactic lectures and structured student electives strengthen the pipeline of future physicians trained to deliver whole-person, lifestyle-focused care. This comprehensive educational approach ensures that lifestyle medicine is not an isolated topic but a sustained, integrated element of medical training at the University of Pittsburgh School of Medicine.

20.9 UNIVERSITY OF TEXAS SOUTHWESTERN MEDICAL SCHOOL—JACLYN ALBIN, MD

The Building a Food Foundation elective at University of Texas (UT) Southwestern, launched in 2018, is a fully remote, four-week experience designed for fourth-year medical students to explore the intersection of nutrition, policy, research, and clinical care. Students engage with books, articles, documentaries, and web-based tools to critically evaluate media and public discourse around food, building the skills needed to respond thoughtfully to the same information their patients encounter. Weekly activities encourage diverse modes of engagement, such as writing blog posts, critiquing news articles, creating social media content, and conducting nutrition assessments. This approach allows students to apply what they learn both personally and professionally.

The course emphasizes awareness of food policy and its influence on individual choices, equips students to navigate inconsistent nutrition research, and fosters understanding of food insecurity and community food resources. Students also apply dietary frameworks (such as the DASH and Mediterranean diets) to clinical case studies across diverse patient populations. The activities encourage students to reflect on their own food choices, share practical tools with patients, and practice conversations that can translate directly to future clinical encounters. While designed for virtual completion, the elective design offers opportunities to integrate community engagement through service learning and patient-facing shared medical appointments in Culinary Medicine. With 25 elective spots offered annually, the elective remains highly popular, with full enrollment and a waiting list for every block, reflecting strong student interest in gaining additional nutrition education.

The Culinary Medicine Enrichment Elective (ENRH 148) at UT Southwestern, launched in 2017, is a hands-on, interprofessional course designed primarily for pre-clerkship medical students but also open to other health professional students. Now structured in the fall semester, the elective blends evidence-based nutrition with practical culinary skills, emphasizing the physician–dietitian partnership in patient care. Rooted in curriculum from The American College of Culinary Medicine's *Health Meets Food* courseware, students engage in interactive cooking modules that pair clinical applications with the art of food preparation. Each session explores high-impact nutrition topics, including managing hypertension and diabetes, navigating food trends, awareness of food insecurity, and strategies for realistic dietary counseling.

Classes are held in UT Southwestern (UTSW)'s teaching kitchen and center on active participation, with students cooking, tasting, and applying key takeaways in a collaborative environment. The elective is pass/fail and emphasizes engagement over assessment, requiring at least three of four modules for credit. With its focus on both culinary literacy and clinical application, the course equips learners to integrate nutrition into patient care and their own lives, while modeling interprofessional collaboration in a teaching kitchen setting. Designed to be immersive and practical, the elective offers a unique blend of clinical application and practical skills that enriches early medical training and sets the stage for engagement in community education and practice of clinical culinary medicine, including shared medical appointments.

20.10 YALE MEDICAL SCHOOL—NATE WOOD, MD

Training in lifestyle medicine at the Yale School of Medicine (YSM) is largely focused on the nutrition pillar. All first-year medical students receive a short lecture series (three hours) on nutrition during their Energy and Metabolism course. This is taught by MDs and dietitians. During their primary care clerkship, all medical students participate in a workshop on dietary counseling. In this workshop, they learn to use the 5 As' method, take a 24-hour dietary recall, and make SMART goals to assist their patients in goal-setting. Medical students are also invited every year to participate in a two-hour, hands-on "Food & Nutrition Insecurity and Culinary Medicine" session at the Irving and Alice Brown Teaching Kitchen at Yale New Haven Health. These sessions are co-taught by an MD-chef (Dr. Wood) and a dietitian-chef and are offered on an opt-in basis. In March 2025, the LMIG at YSM was officially founded. In June 2025, the Educational Policy and Curriculum Committee at YSM approved plans for the implementation of a longitudinal curricular nutrition "thread." This pilot will begin with the 2026–2027 academic year.

20.11 UNIVERSITY OF CENTRAL FLORIDA COLLEGE OF MEDICINE—SHARON WASSERSTROM, MD, DIPABLM, AND MAGDALENA PASARICA, MD, PHD

At University of Central Florida (UCF) College of Medicine, lifestyle medicine is included in both the pre-clinical and clinical years. An example of a pre-clinical opportunity is the topic of Social Determinants of Health, which is introduced to medical students in their first year of the Health Systems Science Curriculum. The first session, taught to all 120 first-year medical students, is an exercise where, upon completion, the students should be able to identify primary, secondary, and tertiary treatment approaches for a given condition: asthma, HTN, metabolic syndrome, or obesity. Also, first-year medical students receive a one-hour lecture on Introduction to Lifestyle Medicine during the Psychosocial Issues in Healthcare course. At the end of the second year of medical school, during the transition to the clerkship course, all students are required to complete an asynchronous Lifestyle Medicine Hypertension assignment. UCF has a board-certified lifestyle medicine primary care physician who serves as a preceptor for four of the first-year four-week rotations in Community of Practice and for a subset of 30–40 third-year students during a one-month continuity clinic for the Core Clerkship in Internal and Family Medicine.

Electives have been another method to offer lifestyle medicine education to UCF COM medical students. Third- and fourth-year medical students can choose to be exposed to two- to four-week electives called Lifestyle Modification Skills in Practice, which is open to one to two students per month. They are assigned to work side by side with a board-certified lifestyle medicine primary care physician in the clinic to assist with lifestyle assessments, motivational interviewing, and formulating lifestyle prescriptions. Students also have a didactic component through weekly lectures on each of the pillars of lifestyle medicine. In addition, students go to a community medically integrated fitness facility to partake in lifestyle medicine opportunities outside of the clinic. Lastly, fourth-year medical students can choose a fourth-week elective in culinary medicine once a year. The goal is to teach medical students how to effectively communicate with and counsel patients on healthy cooking and eating habits at home. The elective is taught by a triad consisting of a chef, a nutritionist, and physicians. Students learn culinary skills, recipes, and the application of recipes to certain disease processes, and they go to various community and health settings to share what they have learned.

Lifestyle medicine is integrated within an interprofessional education framework for health promotion, addressing *Lifestyle Medicine Competency B: The Role of the Practitioner's Personal Health and Community Advocacy,* emphasizing the importance of personal well-being and interprofessional teamwork in promoting health. This is a four-week longitudinal curriculum designed to foster collaboration among students in medicine, nursing, counseling, social work, and pharmacy. Throughout the course, students work together to explore ten evidence-based health promotion interventions identified with high or moderate-to-high certainty of effectiveness (based on the United States Preventive Services Task Force criteria). These include nutrition, sleep, yoga, physical activity, active rest, mindfulness/cognitive behavioral strategies, emotional freedom techniques, acceptance and commitment practices, emotional intelligence, and psychological detachment. The curriculum combines team-based learning with individual self-practice. Students collaborate to review and discuss the scientific evidence supporting each intervention, then select two interventions to implement personally. Guided reflection activities are conducted immediately after the course and again at three and six months to reinforce learning and promote sustained behavioral change. By engaging in this experience, students enhance their awareness of factors that contribute to stress and well-being, gain practical skills to support their own health, and develop confidence in advocating for health promotion within their future clinical and community settings. The course has demonstrated effectiveness across all four levels of the Kirkpatrick evaluation model (reaction, knowledge, behavior, and results), and as such could be used by other institutions looking for effective evidence-based educational interventions.

20.12 NORTHWESTERN UNIVERSITY FEINBERG SCHOOL OF MEDICINE, CHICAGO, IL—ROBERT KUSHNER, MD

Lifestyle medicine was established as one of five new focused threads when the curriculum was redesigned in 2012. Integrated both horizontally and vertically, the thread is woven throughout the organ-based modules over the first two years of school. Within the first three months of matriculation, students are immersed in ten hours of introductory curricular content addressing health, diet, physical activity, and behavior change by pairing didactic sessions with small-group discussions and a patient panel. The sessions culminate with each student conducting an eight-week personalized behavior change plan, where they learn and implement the skills and strategies needed to change health behaviors.

Thereafter, these content areas, and the other lifestyle medicine pillars (substance misuse, sleep, stress) are pedagogically embedded within the organ-based modules. For example, sleep is addressed in the Neurology and Psychiatry modules, tobacco in the Pulmonary and Oncology modules, and diet is emphasized in the Cardiovascular, Renal, Gastrointestinal, and Endocrinology modules. In this way, students learn to holistically integrate lifestyle medicine concepts and counseling practices that are aligned with other scientific disciplines and patient presentations. Diet and physical activity counseling are assessed with a targeted objective structured clinical exam (OSCE) during the first and second years, and lifestyle medicine pillars are reinforced in the education-centered medical home (ECMH), a four-year longitudinal primary care experience in which students collaborate to care for a panel of patients with chronic illness.

20.13 UNIVERSITY OF ROCHESTER MEDICAL SCHOOL—SUSAN FRIEDMAN, MD

In 2021, the University of Rochester launched a two-week interdisciplinary elective for third- and fourth-year medical students. The elective combines clinical and experiential learning with in-depth reading. It is bookended by the Rochester Lifestyle Medicine Institute's 15-day Jumpstart—an online program that provides education and support to enable participants to move to a whole-food plant-based diet. The benefits of participating in the Jumpstart program are fourfold: (a) students are able to experience making a significant lifestyle change themselves; (b) they are able to observe seasoned coaches leading a small group; (c) they are able to learn the science behind the benefits of a whole-food plant-based diet; and (d) they are able to gain the clinical experience of seeing the outcomes of other participants in the program.

At the start of the elective, students are asked to complete their own SMART goals for the elective, incorporating the ACLM-recognized pillars of lifestyle, namely physical activity, diet, toxin avoidance, sleep hygiene, stress management, and social connection. The goals are not shared with the preceptor and are meant to provide a framework for lifestyle changes, as well as to gain experience with developing useful SMART goals. In addition to shadowing LM clinicians in the clinic, students work with wellness counselors at the School of Nursing, and with a registered dietitian and certified personal trainer at the university's Center for Community Health and Prevention. They complete an in-depth review of three to five papers on a lifestyle pillar and target condition of their choice.

20.14 TOURO UNIVERSITY CALIFORNIA COLLEGE OF OSTEOPATHIC MEDICINE (TUCCOM)—SHIPRA BANSAL, MD

TUCCOM has a long-standing commitment to advancing the understanding of healthy metabolism through primary research, student-coach training, and numerous community-based projects that promote wellness. In fall 2024, TUCCOM earned certification from the ACLM for its educational offerings in lifestyle medicine. As part of this certification, TUCCOM provides more than 60 hours of core curriculum covering the six lifestyle pillars and training in behavior change.

To meet UME certification requirements by graduation, students complete a pre-clinical elective, a clinical distinction rotation, and lifestyle medicine-based patient care activities that go beyond the core curriculum.

Pre-Clinical Elective: This course introduces students to the field of lifestyle medicine and the six foundational pillars. Students engage in activities such as grocery store tours, patient education video creation, and simulated clinical encounters where they take a full lifestyle medicine history and practice motivational interviewing with a standardized patient. In its inaugural year, 37 students participated, each completing 18 hours of coursework. The course is graded on a pass/fail basis, requiring a minimum score of 85% on course activities. All assignments and live sessions are mandatory. Course evaluation is conducted through anonymous surveys and focus groups to ensure ongoing improvement.

Clinical Distinction in Lifestyle Medicine: During their third year, students may participate in a four-week rotation designed to deepen their understanding of the six pillars through highly experiential learning. Students engage in personal health behavior trials guided by faculty, refine their motivational interviewing skills, and apply lifestyle medicine principles in patient care discussions. Students deepen their understanding of nutrition by preparing medically tailored meals for specific clinical presentations. Each student completes an independent project that enhances their familiarity with lifestyle medicine literature or clinical practice. In the first year, 10 students enrolled, committing 60–80 hours depending on their project scope. Assessment includes a goal-setting contract at the start of the rotation, self-reflection upon completion, and a final pass/fail determination following a faculty meeting. As a new course, feedback has been collected individually from participants, and iterative improvements are underway.

Continuity Intervention Requirement: Students must also complete a continuity intervention, where they conduct full lifestyle medicine histories and develop patient-centered plans. Two pathways are available to fulfill this requirement. Students may either (a) assist in leading a four-week culinary group visit program, or (b) participate in a longitudinal care initiative for older adults with multiple comorbidities during their fourth year. Students involved in the culinary group visits are currently participating in a research study assessing their perspectives and interest in group-based care. The fourth-year longitudinal program will launch in the upcoming academic year.

As an osteopathic training institution, TUCCOM has a strong commitment to equipping students with skills to deliver whole-person care that optimizes health outcomes. As the lifestyle medicine program continues to be integrated into the core curriculum, it also offers robust learning opportunities throughout students' undergraduate medical education.

20.15 LOMA LINDA UNIVERSITY SCHOOL OF MEDICINE—SYLVIA CRAMER, MD, BRENDA RAE, MD, AND APRIL WILSON, MD

Loma Linda University School of Medicine (LLUSM) has become a national leader in embedding lifestyle medicine into medical education (10,11), building on its long-standing heritage of health promotion and the Adventist Health Studies that demonstrated lifestyle's impact on longevity and chronic disease (12). In response to the American Medical Association's call for lifestyle medicine in physician training and the ACLM's core competency framework (9), LLUSM undertook a structured six-year effort to integrate over 100 hours of lifestyle medicine content across all four years of the curriculum. Lifestyle medicine is incorporated into all of the preclinical systems blocks, with dedicated sessions, threaded content, and experiential components such as culinary medicine, motivational interviewing, and Personal Improvement Projects that encourage students to apply lifestyle medicine principles in their own lives. Clinical training reinforces these foundations through Family Medicine clerkship workshops, integration weeks with lifestyle medicine specialists, the Preventive Medicine and Population Health clerkship, and the Whole Person Care clerkship.

Beyond the core curriculum, LLUSM established a Lifestyle Medicine Certificate Track (13), providing an additional 240 hours of advanced training. Graduate medical education opportunities, including an ACGME-accredited Preventive Medicine Fellowship and a Lifestyle Medicine Intensivist Fellowship (10,14), extend LLU's influence, as does its leadership in disseminating the national lifestyle medicine Residency Curriculum (11). Clinical services, including one of the nation's first inpatient lifestyle medicine consultation programs (15,16) and outpatient lifestyle medicine clinics (17), provide hands-on training and patient care experience. Through this comprehensive and longitudinal approach, LLUSM achieved ACLM's highest recognition—the Platinum Plus Tier designation —reflecting the breadth of lifestyle medicine exposure for all students, the depth of specialized training opportunities, and enabling all graduates to pursue board certification.

20.16 UNIVERSITY OF SOUTH CAROLINA SCHOOL OF MEDICINE AT GREENVILLE—JENNIFER TRILK, PHD

The University of South Carolina School of Medicine Greenville (SOMG) opened its doors with the principle that medical students would be comprehensively trained in lifestyle medicine to prevent and treat the nation's top chronic diseases. As a requirement, every medical student receives over 100 hours of all six pillars of LM content that is threaded into every year and throughout all organ systems. SOMG students are trained in an evidence-based, root-cause, classroom-clinic-community model. Medical students are also trained in behavior change, as well as medical student self-care and resilience for doctor readiness and reduction of physician burnout. SOMG's curriculum meets all lifestyle medicine competencies, earning the medical school a Platinum Plus certification from the ACLM. The training of SOMG future doctors in lifestyle medicine is a key aspect of community and population health.

20.17 SUMMARY

Currently, many medical schools are working to incorporate lifestyle medicine into their curricula. Faculty from each school are working to create opportunities and deliver high-impact learning experiences for medical students in the preclinical and clinical years. One institution, Harvard, has programs that span the spectrum from pre-med to CME. Most medical schools have an LMIG. Many are providing culinary medicine. Most are working toward delivering valuable hands-on activities for students. Most are providing some lifestyle medicine lectures and presentations in core coursework at some level. Many are offering elective courses. Only two schools, Loma Linda and SOMG, offer 100 hours of lifestyle medicine education and meet all the lifestyle medicine competencies.

This chapter presents a range of approaches to incorporating the six pillars of lifestyle medicine and behavior change into medical school curricula. There has been significant progress over the past two decades, but there is much more work to be done. With the support of deans and faculty involved in the core curriculum, lifestyle medicine efforts are more likely to succeed.

REFERENCES

1. Pojednic R, Frates E. A parallel curriculum in lifestyle medicine. *Clin Teach.* 2017;14(1):27–31.
2. Smith A, Barnett E, Frates B. WholeheartedMD: medical students embracing vulnerability and finding fulfillment. *Am J Lifestyle Med.* 2022;16(1):51–56.
3. Frates B, Bonnet J, Joseph R, Peterson J. *The Lifestyle Medicine Handbook* (2nd ed). Monterey CA: Healthy Learning, 2021.
4. Dempsey AM, Brabham CE. Medical education column, creating a high-yield guide to lifestyle medicine for medical students and healthcare professionals. *Am J Lifestyle Med.* 2023;18(3):332–334.
5. Lutchman K, Wan M, Lan FY, Kales SN, Frates EP. Integrating the lifestyle medicine residency curriculum into an occupational medicine training program. *J Occup Environ Med.* 2024;66(4):e143–e144.
6. Frates B, Kusnadi K, McCargo T. Teaching assistants: essential members of the teaching team. *Am J Lifestyle Med.* 2025;19(6):842–845. doi: 10.1177/15598276251328635.
7. Frates B, Bonnet J, Joseph R, Peterson J. *The Lifestyle Medicine Handbook* (1st ed). Monterey CA: Healthy Learning, 2018.
8. Wetherill MS, Davis GC, Kezbers K, et al. Development and evaluation of a nutrition-centered lifestyle medicine curriculum for physician assistant students. *Med Sci Educ.* 2018;29(1):163–172.
9. Trilk JL, Worthman S, Shetty P, et al. Undergraduate medical education: lifestyle medicine curriculum implementation standards. *Am J Lifestyle Med.* 2021;15(5):526–530.
10. Rea B, Holmes S, Bernstein M, et al. Cultivating the future: the intersection of education and lifestyle medicine. *Am J Lifestyle Med.* 2025:15598276251327925. doi: 10.1177/15598276251327925.
11. Rea B, Worthman S, Shetty P, Alexander M, Trilk JL. Medical education transformation: lifestyle medicine in undergraduate and graduate medical education, fellowship, and continuing medical education. *Am J Lifestyle Med.* 2021;15(5):514–525. doi: 10.1177/15598276211006629.
12. Fraser GE, Shavlik DJ. Ten years of life: Is it a matter of choice? *Arch Intern Med.* 2001;161(13):1645–1652. doi: 10.1001/archinte.161.13.1645.
13. Bansal S, Cramer S, Stump M, Wasserstrom S. Lifestyle medicine electives: options for creating curricula within medical school training. *Am J Lifestyle Med.* 2023;17(6):754–758. doi: 10.1177/15598276221147181.
14. Rea B, Wilson A. Creating a lifestyle medicine specialist fellowship: a replicable and sustainable model. *Am J Lifestyle Med.* 2020;14(3):278–281. doi: 10.1177/1559827620907552.
15. Cramer T, Wilson A, Rea B. Lifestyle medicine inpatient consultation services at Loma Linda University Health: a novel approach in a tertiary care center. *Am J Lifestyle Med.* 2018;12(3):227–229. doi: 10.1177/1559827618754860.
16. Annam R, Florian R, Johnson S, Mondala M, Wilson A, Rea B. Expanding the lifestyle medicine inpatient consultation services at Loma Linda University Health: a transformative tool for chronic diseases management in tertiary care settings. *Am J Lifestyle Med.* 2023;17(5):686–689. doi: 10.1177/15598276231172172.
17. Cramer T, Rea B. The lifestyle medicine outpatient clinic at Loma Linda University Health. *Am J Lifestyle Med.* 2018;12(5):425–427. doi: 10.1177/1559827618766487.

21 Teaching Strategies for Lifestyle Medicine Education

21.1 TEACHING VERSUS TALKING

"Tell me, and I forget. Teach me, and I remember. Involve me, and I learn." This quote often attributed to Benjamin Franklin helps make the point that students want more than having facts spewed at them by a faculty member in front of a chalkboard. Telling is different than teaching. Telling is a one-way road, as noted in Figure 21.1. Teaching is a two-way road that involves talking and listening, as noted in Figure 21.2.

Another way to think about this difference is that telling involves only talking, and teaching involves talking, asking questions, listening, and responding. When you are trying to enlighten people with fascinating facts, science, patient stories, research, and biochemistry, which way will work best? Telling students all the information, not checking in to gauge comprehension, and forging forward regardless of engagement may be rewarding and easy for a teacher, but that

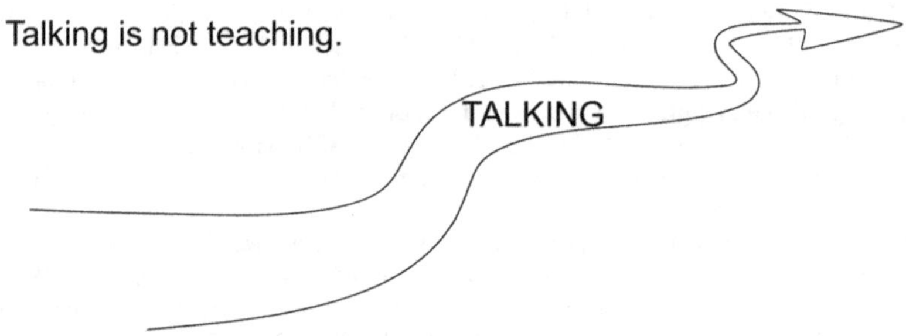

FIGURE 21.1 Talking is not teaching.

Modified from Shutterstock ID: 2459919087

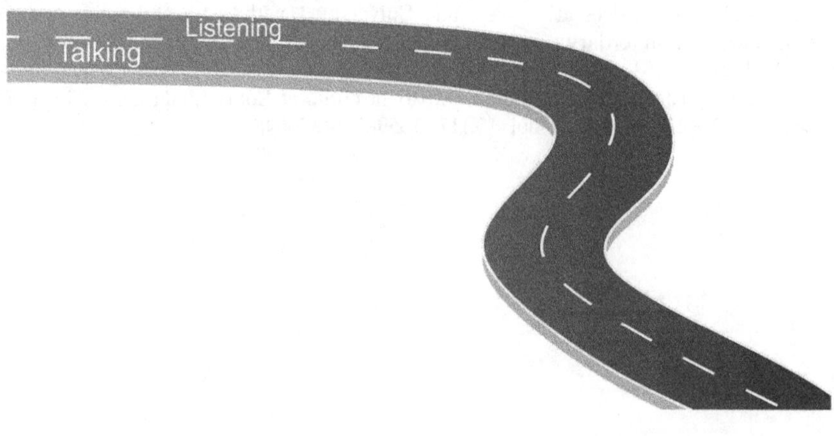

FIGURE 21.2 Teaching is a two-way road.

Modified from Shutterstock ID 2616774417

DOI: 10.1201/9781003630043-21

is not teaching. Teaching requires a give-and-take. It takes time, patience, and understanding to teach effectively. Asking students questions and addressing their specific queries along the way is essential.

If the goal is for students to learn the material, the teacher needs to pay attention to students and their responses. Responses indicate their comprehension, interest, mastery, confusion, their ability to relate the material to real-life scenarios, and their ability to build on their previous knowledge (whatever level that may be) and to consolidate the information presented. Thus, teachers use effective strategies to accomplish these goals.

Most importantly, the teacher must demonstrate they care—they care about the topic, and they care about the students. Listening to someone is a form of demonstrating caring and respect. It is good to be reminded of this quote from Theodore Roosevelt: "People don't care how much you know until they know how much you care."

21.2 MEDICAL STUDENTS AS ADULT LEARNERS

According to self-determination theory, individuals have three basic needs for sustained motivation: relatedness, competence, and autonomy (1). To keep adult learners motivated, these three needs must be considered.

Medical students are adult learners, and, as such, faculty in medical schools structure their lesson plans to motivate, inspire, and engage these adults. 'Malcolm Knowles' (Malcolm S. Knowles) shares his insights on teaching and learning in the learning theory known as andragogy—adult learning (2).

Here is a summary of the six principles of Knowles' Theory of Andragogy from the article Andragogy in Practice: Applying a Theoretical Framework to Team Science Training in Biomedical Research (3).

1. *Self-Concept*: Adults are self-directed and desire independence.
2. *Role of Experience*: Adults have years of experience that teachers can use in lesson plans.
3. *Readiness to Learn*: Adults are eager to learn more to help them in their current life roles.
4. *Orientation to Learning*: Adults take a problem-based approach to learning.
5. *Need to Know Why*: Adult learners want to know how the material being taught will impact their lives.
6. *Intrinsic Motivation*: Adult learners are motivated by internal factors like wanting to improve their quality of life, their self-esteem, or job satisfaction.

Medical school faculty serve more as facilitators than as lecturers. The days of long didactic lessons with students quietly sitting in their chairs, taking notes with pen and paper or on a computer, are no longer the norm. Today, medical school faculty spend significant time on how to engage medical students in the learning process. There is an emphasis on using activities to help students apply the concepts they are learning to their future professional endeavors. These application activities are as important as the slides and lectures that the faculty prepare.

Application activities help students with Knowles' principle 5 of the need to know why. Why is this material important to me? Additionally, these learning sessions incorporate problem-solving, a method known as problem-based learning (PBL). This addresses Knowles' principle 4. PBL in medical school can take the form of medical cases that describe patient experiences. Asking students to reflect on and discuss with fellow medical students how they would manage a particular patient case facilitates group discussion, peer-to-peer teaching, collaboration, and the development of social connections among classmates.

Taking into account Knowles' principle 2, medical educators can encourage students to share their prior research, insights from undergraduate or master's courses, and personal experiences to enrich and broaden the case. By using patient cases, students can see how learning this information will help them in their future roles as physicians, which aligns with Knowles' principle 3.

As Knowles' principle 6 points out, adult learners are motivated by a desire to improve their quality of life, self-esteem, and job satisfaction. Empowering students to reflect on what they learned in a teaching session or workshop, to identify their own knowledge gaps, or to explore and research new areas of medicine is one way to give medical students some autonomy, which aligns with Knowles' principle 1. This type of interactive and engaging instruction, grounded in the six principles of Knowles' andragogy, fosters autonomy, self-regulation, and critical thinking (4–8). All are key for the successful practice of medicine.

Educators are also "educational diagnosticians" for medical students, meaning they are responsible for knowing the students and understanding their learning styles. Some students are visual learners, others auditory, and still others tactile. For visual learners, the slides teachers use, the images in video clips they select, and the graphics they share will be critical for comprehension. For auditory learners, words spoken by the teacher or presented in a video will be absorbed more deeply. For tactile learners, simulation and hands-on workshops will be useful. Medical school educators can tailor instruction to students' learning styles and individual needs to the extent possible (6,9).

Understanding learners helps medical educators design activities, learning sessions, and interactive classroom experiences that engage and retain students' attention. It is essential to discuss the importance of active learning techniques with students so that they can better understand why they are used and how to participate confidently and comfortably. It is the medical educator's responsibility to create an environment conducive to active learning (10). Setting up this type of learning experience requires intentional design. Table 21.1 reviews strategies for medical educators to consider when facilitating courses and outlines how to apply the lens of lifestyle medicine to each strategy.

TABLE 21.1
Overview of Effective Teaching Strategies for Comprehension and a Strong Foundation

Strategy	Description	Lifestyle Medicine Focus
Case-based learning (CBL) (11,12)	A patient case is summarized with ID, chief complaint, PMH, medications, SH, SDOH, physical examination, labs, and tests. Students create differential diagnoses and explain their rationale for their choices. This can take many forms. In some cases, the patient tells their story to the students live or via a video recording.	Include information about the patient's exercise, nutrition, sleep, stress, social connection, and risky substance use (often already covered in social history). Include questionnaires on the six pillars and the validated Lifestyle Behavior Health Survey (13), which covers all six pillars in one short survey.
Problem-based learning (PBL) (11,14)	A patient with an ill-defined problem is presented. Students use group discussions, research in the medical literature, and clinical reasoning to develop a differential diagnosis. Students take the lead in determining what they need to know and learn to solve the problem.	Include discussions on how exercise, nutrition, sleep, stress, social connection, and risky substances could be part of the problem and the solution. Review the literature and identify rigorous studies to evaluate and bring them into the discussion.
Simulation-based learning (SBL) (11,15)	In safe and controlled environments that mirror real-life clinical settings, students work to manage specific patient scenarios, honing both procedural and counseling skills in a safe environment mimicking real-life situations. The debriefing after simulation exercises is an important part of the learning process.	During consultations for heart disease, diabetes, high blood pressure, and other chronic conditions, include counseling strategies like the 5 As, the COACH Approach, motivational interviewing, appreciative inquiry, and positive psychology to encourage students to practice and hone these skills.

(*Continued*)

TABLE 21.1 (*Continued*)
Overview of Effective Teaching Strategies for Comprehension and a Strong Foundation

Strategy	Description	Lifestyle Medicine Focus
Flipped classroom (16–19)	Students listen to videos or podcasts and read chapters in textbooks or journal articles outside class/lecture hours to gain knowledge. Usually, the material is assigned as homework. When they arrive at the classroom, students use that knowledge to solve problems, participate in discussions and debates, and then determine what they want to explore further to increase their knowledge and skills.	Use evidence-based pre-recorded lectures such as those provided by the American College of Lifestyle Medicine in the Virtual Lifestyle Medicine Interest Group series. Use PowerPoints from LMEd available for free. Use the LM 101 Curriculum available for free at the American College of Lifestyle Medicine. Use chapters or sections with specific page numbers in the Lifestyle Medicine Textbook, other books in the Rippe series, the Lifestyle Medicine Handbook, the Lifestyle Medicine Pocket Guide, and Lifestyle Medicine by Kales and Sidossis as pre-reading for class.
Peer teaching (20–22)	Students take ownership of certain topics or clinical cases and deliver brief presentations to each other. This helps learners master the material, practice teaching, and gain a new perspective on learning. It is peer to peer. To teach, one needs to have confidence in one's knowledge of the material.	Encourage students to consider how exercise, nutrition, sleep, stress, social connection or loneliness, and the use of risky substances could be impacting the patient and playing a role in chronic conditions like diabetes, obesity, heart disease, high blood pressure, stroke, cancer, and metabolic disease.
Self-explanation/ self-elaboration (23,24)	Students stop to reflect on a case or problem and to explain to themselves, out loud or in writing, the pathology, physiology, or biochemistry involved with the patient scenario being presented. Students may explain their own reasoning for a differential diagnosis, recommending a medication or procedure, or for ordering a specific diagnostic radiologic exam or laboratory blood test.	Encourage students to elaborate on the impact of the six pillars of lifestyle medicine as they relate to the case or problem. Recommend exploration of how the six pillars may be impacting the biochemistry, histology, and pathology of the condition being discussed.
Elaborative discussion (24)	In small groups, students debate concepts and elaborate on their own clinical reasoning, understanding of relevant biological mechanisms and pathways, and the importance of specific aspects of the case presentation in deep discussions with peers and faculty. They share their thinking, knowledge, and clinical reasoning in a space that allows for extensive elaboration.	Include topics on the six pillars of lifestyle medicine and debate how much of an impact exercise, nutrition, sleep, stress, social connection or loneliness, and the use of risky substances could have on the clinical scenario being discussed. Weigh the evidence from clinical trials.
Concept mapping (23,25)	Students work to connect concepts on a piece of paper, an index card, a chalkboard, a whiteboard, an electronic board, or a poster board. They map concepts from a central topic, such as the heart, using lines to connect them hierarchically, with subconcepts and interconnected lines revealing relevant relationships with organ systems, disease pathology, and treatment options.	Include topics of the six pillars of lifestyle medicine. For example, consider how exercise is impacting PGC-1-alpha levels and thus the number and health of the mitochondria, or if low fiber consumption is playing a role in the concept being mapped, then consider the impact on short-chain fatty acids like acetate, propionate, and butyrate.

(*Continued*)

TABLE 21.1 (*Continued*)
Overview of Effective Teaching Strategies for Comprehension and a Strong Foundation

Strategy	Description	Lifestyle Medicine Focus
Cognitive apprenticeship (26–28)	A medical educator or practicing clinician serves as the mentor and expert. The mentor shares their deductive reasoning, problem-solving strategies, clinical experience, and methodology for further exploration in the form of original research or review of the applicable medical literature. A quarter of the way into the 21st century, gaining exposure to the academic use of Artificial Intelligence (AI) will also serve the students well. This type of teaching involves modeling, coaching, scaffolding, articulation, reflection, and exploration.	Include faculty who have expertise and experience in lifestyle medicine. Consider inviting clinicians who are board-certified by the American Board of Lifestyle Medicine or the International Board of Lifestyle Medicine to be mentors. Including other healthcare professionals such as registered dietitians, physical therapists, and social workers in the mentoring team can also help medical students better understand their roles and thus work collaboratively with them in teams.
Chalk talk (29–31)	The medical educator captivates the learners by drawing a diagram, pathway, or cycle on the board, a piece of paper, or an index card in real time. The educator can ask the learners, "What's the next step? What do you think? Why?" This type of chalk talk is interactive and encourages interaction. It is well-suited to visual learners.	The medical educator can draw the five-step cycle of collaboration (32) and ask for input at each step to engage students in learning about behavior change. Another chalk talk could be on plant proteins, and students could list different plants with protein and then order them from most protein to least on the board.
Think-pair-share (33–38)	A medical educator can pose a question. Then, ask the students to think about the answer on their own. After a few minutes, the educator pairs up students, and they discuss their thoughts. After 10–15 minutes of discussion, the pair of students shares their takeaway points and Aha moments with the larger group. This ensures participation by all students and engages them in the learning process while opening their minds to different ideas and perspectives shared by classmates. This strategy encourages peer teaching and learning. It also encourages social connection and collaboration between students.	In lifestyle medicine, there are thought-provoking questions for each pillar. This exercise could be performed after the medical educator describes a recent research paper and asks, "What are the limitations of this study?" Alternatively, a piece of information from influencers or the media could be the topic of discussion, with the educator asking the question, "How can you verify or deny/reject this information?"

Medical educators need to consider how they facilitate and conduct teaching sessions, with particular attention to how they elicit factual responses from students, present material, build on prior information, and reinforce facts through repetition. Considering the techniques they use to enhance learners' memory will help medical students succeed on exams and in clinical practice. Some effective learning and teaching techniques to improve memory are summarized in Table 21.2.

There are several important learning theories to consider when creating courses. One has already been covered in this chapter. That is andragogy. Others include constructivism, cognitive load theory, and situated learning. Summaries of these are provided in Table 21.3.

During clinical years, medical educators need a different lens on learning, which will require additional teaching strategies to empower medical students to become clinicians. There is a focus

TABLE 21.2
Overview of Effective Learning and Teaching Techniques for Enhancing Memory

Learning Technique	Description
Active recall or practice testing (39)	Learning involves actively remembering information by taking a short quiz that could be fill-in-the-blank, multiple choice, matching, or short answer, which is graded or not graded. This could be pen and paper, online, verbal, or part of a class session with the questions on a PowerPoint slide or embedded in an anonymous polling system. The goal is to check recall of facts from memory, meaning without looking at notes or study guides. This is not open-book. Breaking up lectures and asking specific factual questions, taking a poll with a show of hands, or using a true/false question format can be another way to use this technique during class time. Students often use this learning technique themselves to study with flashcards or to quiz each other verbally when studying in pairs or groups.
Spaced repetition (39–41)	Students often use this learning technique when studying for exams with flashcards, either online, or on paper. Lecturers can use this in class by teaching a concept more than once and providing opportunities for students to test themselves on the material at different times. When teaching, referring back to concepts and facts from previous lectures or chapters covered helps learners consolidate information and store it in long-term memory. This type of verbal and written repetition of important facts during different lectures throughout a course is useful for long-term retention of facts and concepts.
Successive reinforcing/ successive relearning (39)	Repeating material strategically over the course of a class or curriculum so that the material is introduced at a basic level. Then, with each successive mention, the level is deeper and more complex. This allows students to build on a solid foundation of knowledge. An example of successive relearning is providing a quiz that students can take multiple times until they get all the questions correct.
Distributed practice (24,39)	Creating opportunities for learners to revisit material and test their memories as well as their understanding of concepts, multiple times distributed throughout the course with assignments, quizzes, and discussion prompts that ask about material covered previously, is considered distributed practice. Asking learners to connect new material to previously learned material is another way to use distributed practice. Spaced repetition and distributed practice are often used interchangeably.
Retrieval practice (24,42)	Providing opportunities for learners to retrieve information from their memories of concepts, facts, mechanisms, cycles, or procedures provided in lectures, research papers, book chapters, or other materials covered in a course is a strategy used repeatedly over time. This practice uses active recall.
Interleaving (24,43)	This is the opposite of blocking or studying only one subject at a time in a block of time. Instead, with interleaving, subjects are interwoven together. With this method, faculty discuss different topics during the same teaching session rather than focusing on one topic. Students can plan to do this themselves for their own self-study or group study sessions. For example, discuss the histology and the pathology of the same tissue, mixing both histology and pathology. Review EKGs revealing a variety of abnormalities, rather than teaching just one EKG pattern per session; students can do this with their own study sessions. For clinical cases, this can be accomplished by having students consider the case through the lens of different medical specialties. How would the cardiologist view this case? The endocrinologist? The primary care doctor? The lifestyle medicine expert?

on clinical reasoning and on developing the skills to care for patients. In the clinical setting, new surroundings for medical students open various avenues for teaching. The learning is inherently case-based and problem-based, as each patient presents a unique history, specific symptoms, and a range of differential diagnoses to consider. The clinic or hospital setting can be busy and chaotic. Thus, it is best to establish a routine for teaching sessions and for developing clinical reasoning skills.

TABLE 21.3
Summary of Four Important Learning Theories for Medical Education

Adult learning theory-andragogy (2,3)	Adult learners are self-directed, have life experience, desire relevance, take a problem-based approach, and have intrinsic motivation. (Discussed further in the text.)
Constructivism (44,45)	Learners construct their knowledge by adding to their previous experiences, using their own frameworks to understand new concepts, participating in hands-on activities, and engaging with the material through discussions, case-based learning, collaborative problem-solving, and other interactive activities. Constructing a building takes time and the use of many different materials. Constructing knowledge takes working with material from different angles and with new perspectives while building on past information.
Cognitive load theory (45,46)	There are three aspects of cognitive load: intrinsic, extrinsic, and germane. The intrinsic load is something that usually cannot be changed, in that it is related to the complexity and difficulty of the material itself, like the pathophysiology of cardiovascular disease. The extrinsic load is something that teaching strategies can impact and lessen. This is the load put upon the learner to decipher and follow the lesson plan set out to teach the concepts. Disorganization, distractions, contradictions, unclear images, murky explanations, and confusing diagrams will add to the extrinsic load. The germane load is the amount of energy and time the learner can use to actively process the new information and connect it to previous knowledge, creating novel schema, pathways, and frameworks for better understanding. Teachers can encourage germane load by using strategies that involve the learner, like asking questions, using self-explanation, providing practice problems, and using case-based or problem-based learning. As a general rule, teachers work to reduce extrinsic load and increase the germane load. The intrinsic load is inherent in the material itself.
Situated learning theory (47)	Learners who are in the actual situation of a clinic or hospital setting can actively engage with real-life scenarios and learn from them. Students can be assigned simple tasks within their skill level. They can learn about clinical reasoning and decision-making by shadowing a mentor. Case-based learning using patient scenarios that mimic real-life situations and simulated learning opportunities helps pre-clinical students gain experience in a clinic-like setting before clerkships.

The skills and strategies medical educators use in the preclinical years remain relevant in the clinical years, particularly when they take time to teach biochemical pathways, pharmacology, and pathology relevant to the patient case. Spending time with students and making it clear that there are specific learning and teaching sessions in the clerkship underscores their importance and relevance. It is recommended that the medical educator identify the session clearly by stating, "This is going to be a teaching session now." Sometimes students complete their clerkships and report in their evaluations that there was little or no teaching.

Case presentations provide an excellent opportunity for medical students to develop their clinical reasoning skills. They are often stressful for the medical student, but they do not have to be. Training students in the SNAPPS methodology for case presentation can alleviate some of the stress. The protocol gives the students structure. It is collaborative and invites self-reflection. The six steps of the SNAPPS approach are (48–51):

1. **Summarize** succinctly the history and findings.
2. **Narrow** the differential diagnosis to two to three possibilities.
3. **Analyze** the differential diagnoses by comparing and contrasting these possibilities.
4. **Probe** the preceptor by asking questions about uncertainties, difficulties, or alternative approaches.
5. **Plan** management for the patient's problem list and medical issues.
6. **Select** a case-related issue for self-directed learning.

Reviewing the protocol for the six steps of SNAPPS with the students, providing examples, and sharing a journal article on the topic can help medical students become familiar and comfortable with the process. By streamlining the case presentation and encouraging the student to ask questions of the medical educator (preceptor), some of the pressure and stress is removed from the student. Yet, the importance of learning is highlighted, especially with the last step, select. The student selects the topic that he or she is most curious about. This gives the student autonomy. This puts the self-determination theory into practice. For sustained motivation, people including medical students need autonomy, relatedness, and competence. The six SNAPPS steps can foster an environment that encompasses all three components of this theory: the autonomy to choose what the student will study: the relatedness and connection to the preceptor and team; and, lastly, competence, because they have a framework with which to work to feel successful in their clinical case presentations.

Another teaching strategy for the clinical years in medical school is the One Minute Preceptor. There are five steps to this teaching strategy for use with medical students during their clinical rotations after patient encounters. The five steps in the One Minute Preceptor process include (48,50–53):

1. *Get a Commitment*: Ask the learner to commit to a diagnosis or next step.
2. *Probe for Supporting Evidence*: Ask the learner to explain their reasoning.
3. *Teach General Rules*: Provide concise, high-yield teaching points relevant to the case.
4. *Reinforce What Was Done Well*: Give specific positive feedback.
5. *Correct Mistakes*: Offer constructive feedback on areas for improvement.

When presenting a patient case, the medical student can focus on identifying the most likely diagnosis based on their assessment. That is step 1. The second step uses self-explanation, in which the preceptor probes for supporting evidence for the selected diagnosis. The preceptor asks the medical student to explain their reasoning. At this point, their clinical reasoning is on display. By listening to the student in the clinic or on the wards, the preceptor can identify a few high-yield teaching points associated explicitly with the specific patient case presented by the medical student. That is step 3. In a busy outpatient clinic or hospital setting, the preceptor should not only teach general rules that the medical student can apply to the current case and future cases but also highlight specific aspects of the medical student's presentation that were particularly well executed. Reinforcing what was done well is step 4. This step also helps medical students gain confidence and feel competent. Steps 4 and 5 constitute feedback, which will be reviewed in an upcoming chapter. When providing feedback to medical students, it is recommended that the preceptor signal that the session is a feedback session by stating, "Now, I would like to provide you with some useful feedback. How does that sound?" Asking permission gives the student autonomy. Not only will the preceptor point out areas of strength, but they will also need to correct any errors, inaccuracies, or misinformation during the feedback session. Correcting mistakes is step 5 and is critical for the medical student's future and that of their future patients.

To facilitate recall of the steps in the One Minute Preceptor, the acronym DEFT was created (53). Deft means skillful. The acronym stands for **D**iagnosis, **E**vidence, **F**eedback, and **T**eaching. In the five-step model, teaching precedes feedback; however, in this acronym, feedback is first. Use the acronym if it helps. DETF is more challenging to remember, as it does not create a word. Consider a new acronym for this. DEAF could be the acronym. In this case, replace the term "teaching" with "advising." Preceptors could use the acronym DEAF to avoid appearing deaf to the student. Instead, they are eagerly listening and actively educating. Regardless of which acronym is used, the key is to support the medical student's clinical reasoning by focusing on identifying the diagnosis and providing evidence for its selection, thereby revealing the student's decision-making process and knowledge. Then, the preceptor needs to do their job by teaching (advising) and providing feedback.

This One Minute Preceptor is intended to enhance interactions between medical school faculty members and students. It helps faculty focus their clinical teaching sessions, work on clinical reasoning skills, provide just-in-time information by sharing clinical pearls related to the patient case, and help students develop and grow by giving concrete, constructive feedback.

Chalk talks, included in the chart on teaching strategies, are an old-school way of teaching that still works in medical education (54). The title of a medical education journal article on the topic speaks volumes: "Not yet a dinosaur: the chalk talk" (30). When people hear "chalk talk," many envision a sports coach with the team huddled around a chalkboard. The coach takes time out of practice to visually demonstrate new plays to the team. Instead of only using words, the coach draws in real time on the chalkboard. This is a compelling way to explain a new play, and it is also easier to follow than verbal instructions alone. There is often time for questions and answers in these scenarios, and players are invited to respond to the visual diagrams. Seeing the moves on the board also helps players remember them, especially visual learners. In medicine, the medical educator serves as the coach, and the players are members of the clinical team, including medical students, residents, nurses, and other healthcare professionals. The discussion is not about on-field maneuvers but about clinical decisions facing particular patients on the wards.

Although chalkboards are rarely, if ever, used in clerkships, having a planned, prepared, interactive, visually oriented talk ready when the appropriate teaching moment arises is helpful for medical school faculty teaching on the wards. Over time, faculty may collect several chalk talks to use at appropriate times. The talks may take place on a whiteboard rather than a chalkboard. They may even occur huddled around a piece of paper at the bedside or on an index card. Some faculty use a Rolodex-type index card system for their chalk talks.

Whenever and wherever these chalk talks occur, they are interactive and learner-centered. The name of this teaching technique is misleading, as it contains the word "talk." However, the medical educator is not just talking to the medical student. That is a one-way street, with information flowing only from the teacher to the learner. These chalk talks are intended to be two-way streets, with data flowing from the teacher to the learner and from the learner to the teacher. Students are encouraged to brainstorm during the chalk talk and help create a visual framework for specific concepts related to patient care, including clinical reasoning, diagnostic algorithms, and decision trees. Concept mapping could also be part of a chalk talk. The goal of the chalk talks is to promote conceptual understanding, review clinical reasoning, and inspire further exploration of pertinent medical concepts, using real-life patient cases to bring the material to life. The ideas shared are directly relevant to patients in clinical or hospital settings. This teaching aid often involves drawing and creating pathways. It is invaluable for visual learners.

21.3 SUMMARY

There are well-established teaching strategies that medical school faculty can utilize during the preclinical and clinical years. These strategies benefit both students and faculty. The most important lesson is to remember that medical students are adults with their own desires for autonomy, relatedness, and competence, as discussed in the self-determination theory covered at the beginning of this chapter. Simply providing information in a lecture-style format is neither ideal nor complete. Teaching is a two-way street, with the medical educator talking and listening. Asking learners questions engages them and helps assess their understanding. Being intentional in teaching strategies enables educators and students to use their time more effectively. It may seem time-efficient to simply tell students what they need to know. However, this methodology lacks feedback and will not check whether students understand the concepts taught, connect those concepts to patient care, value the information as beneficial for their future selves and careers, or engage in the learning process through problem-solving. This straight lecture style of teaching takes the learner out of the learning loop. To bring learners into the learning loop, medical educators should use case-based learning, problem-based learning, simulation-based learning, peer teaching, self-elaboration, and active teaching strategies such as concept mapping. Helping medical students comprehend vast amounts of knowledge also requires strategic teaching, which entails active recall, spaced repetition, successive reinforcement, distributed practice, retrieval practice, and interleaving. Understanding adult learning theory (andragogy), constructivism, cognitive load theory, and situated learning theory helps medical educators design courses and educational experiences that enhance students' medical school experience. Three specific strategies that can be helpful in clerkship experiences are SNAPPS (Summarize, Narrow, Analyze, Probe, Plan, Select), the One-Minute Preceptor, and Chalk Talks. Working to be intentional about instructional design for teaching sessions, whether a single lecture or an entire course, is the main takeaway of this chapter. Just sharing a PowerPoint lecture with medical students is not enough.

REFERENCES

1. Ryan RM, Deci EL. Self-determination theory and the facilitation of intrinsic motivation, social development, and well-being. *Am Psychol.* 2000;55(1):68–78.
2. Knowles M, Elwood F. Holton III, Swanson R. *The Adult Learner: The Definitive Classic in Adult Education and Human Resource Development.* Burlington, MA: Elsevier, 2005 and Knowles MS. *The Modern Practice of Adult Education: From Pedagogy to Andragogy.* Englewood Cliffs, NJ: Cambria Press, 1980.
3. Knapke JM, Hildreth L, Molano JR, et al. Andragogy in practice: applying a theoretical framework to team science training in biomedical research. *Br J Biomed Sci.* 2024;81:12651. doi: 10.3389/bjbs.2024.12651. PMID: 38605981; PMCID: PMC11008574.
4. Taylor DC, Hamdy H. Adult learning theories: implications for learning and teaching in medical education: AMEE guide No. 83. *Med Teach.* 2013;35(11):e1561–e1572. doi: 10.3109/0142159X.2013.828153. *Epub* 2013 Sep 4. PMID: 24004029.
5. Stagnaro-Green A. Applying adult learning principles to medical education in the United States. *Med Teach.* 2004;26(1):79–85. doi: 10.1080/01421590310001642957. PMID: 14744700.
6. Collins J. Education techniques for lifelong learning: principles of adult learning. *Radiographics.* 2004;24(5):1483–1489. doi: 10.1148/rg.245045020. PMID: 15371622.
7. Rashid P. Surgical education and adult learning: Integrating theory into practice. *F1000Res.* 2017;6:143. doi: 10.12688/f1000research.10870.1. PMID: 28357046; PMCID: PMC5345767.
8. Aulakh J, Wahab H, Richards C, Bidaisee S, Ramdass PVAK. Self-directed learning versus traditional didactic learning in undergraduate medical education: a systemic review and meta-analysis. *BMC Med Educ.* 2025;25(1):70. doi: 10.1186/s12909-024-06449-0. PMID: 39815233; PMCID: PMC11737201.
9. Schwartzstein RM, Dienstag JL, King RW, et al. The Harvard Medical School pathways curriculum: reimagining developmentally appropriate medical education for contemporary learners. *Acad Med.* 2020;95(11):1687–1695. doi: 10.1097/ACM.0000000000003270. PMID: 32134787.
10. Heng W, Ho MH, Mah XH, et al. Exploring pre-clinical medical students' perception of and participation in active learning: a mixed-methods transnational study. *Med Educ.* 2025;59(6):615–629. doi: 10.1111/medu.15611.
11. Zhang SL, Ren SJ, Zhu DM, et al. Which novel teaching strategy is most recommended in medical education? A systematic review and network meta-analysis. *BMC Med Educ.* 2024;24(1):1342. doi: 10.1186/s12909-024-06291-4.
12. Bowe CM, Voss J, Thomas Aretz H. Case method teaching: an effective approach to integrate the basic and clinical sciences in the preclinical medical curriculum. *Med Teach.* 2009;31(9):834–841.
13. Pangalangan J, Puma J, Tollefson M, Frates B. Development and psychometric evaluation of the lifestyle medicine health behavior scale. *Am J Lifestyle Med.* 2024:15598276241280207. doi: 10.1177/15598276241280207. Epub ahead of print. PMID: 39540170; PMCID: PMC11556621.
14. Lim WK. Problem based learning in medical education: handling objections and sustainable implementation. *Adv Med Educ Pract.* 2023;14:1453–1460.
15. Elendu C, Amaechi DC, Okatta AU, Amaechi EC, Elendu TC, Ezeh CP, Elendu ID. The impact of simulation-based training in medical education: a review. *Medicine.* 2024;103(27):e38813. doi: 10.1097/MD.0000000000038813. PMID: 38968472; PMCID: PMC11224887.
16. Phillips J, Wiesbauer F. The flipped classroom in medical education: a new standard in teaching. *Trends Anaesth Crit Care.* 2022;42:4–8.
17. Hurtubise L, Hall E, Sheridan L, Han H. The flipped classroom in medical education: engaging students to build competency. *J Med Educ Curric Dev.* 2015;2:JMECD.S23895.

18. Mengesha AK, Ayele HS, Misker MF, Beyna AT. Assessing the effectiveness of flipped classroom teaching-learning method among undergraduate medical students at Gondar university, College of Medicine and Health Sciences: an interventional study. *BMC Med Educ.* 2024;24(1):1108. doi: 10.1186/s12909-024-06105-7. PMID: 39375705; PMCID: PMC11460021.
19. Ang KCS, Afzal F, Crawford LH. Transitioning from passive to active learning: preparing future project leaders. *PLAS.* 2021;2:100016.
20. Yu TC, Wilson NC, Singh PP, Lemanu DP, Hawken SJ, Hill AG. Medical students-as-teachers: a systematic review of peer-assisted teaching during medical school. *Adv Med Educ Pract.* 2011;2:157–172.
21. Avonts M, Bombeke K, Michels NR, et al. How can peer teaching influence the development of medical students? a descriptive, longitudinal interview study. *BMC Med Educ.* 2023;23:861. doi: 10.1186/s12909-023-04801-4.
22. House JB, Choe CH, Wourman HL, Berg KM, Fischer JP, Santen SA. Efficient and effective use of peer teaching for medical student simulation. *West J Emerg Med.* 2017;18(1):137–141.
23. Torre D, Chamberland M, Mamede S. Implementation of three knowledge-oriented instructional strategies to teach clinical reasoning: self-explanation, a concept mapping exercise, and deliberate reflection: AMEE guide No. 150. *Med Teach.* 2023;45(7):676–684. doi: 10.1080/0142159X.2022.2105200. Epub 2022 Aug 7. PMID: 35938204.
24. Schmidt HG, Mamede S. How cognitive psychology changed the face of medical education research. *Adv Health Sci Educ Theory Pract.* 2020;25(5):1025–1043.
25. Torre D, German D, Daley B, Taylor D. Concept mapping: an aid to teaching and learning: AMEE guide No. 157. *Med Teach.* 2023;45(5):455–463. doi: 10.1080/0142159X.2023.2182176. Epub 2023 Mar 2. PMID: 36862077.
26. Collins A, Brown JS, Newman SE. Cognitive apprenticeship: teaching the crafts of reading, writing, and mathematics. In Resnick LB (ed.) *Knowing, Learning, and Instruction: Essays in Honor of Robert Glaser.* Hillsdale, NJ: Lawrence Erlbaum Associates, Inc., 1989, pp. 453–494.
27. Stalmeijer RE, Dolmans DH, Wolfhagen IH, Scherpbier AJ. Cognitive apprenticeship in clinical practice: can it stimulate learning in the opinion of students? *Adv Health Sci Educ Theory Pract.* 2009;14(4):535–546. doi: 10.1007/s10459-008-9136-0.
28. Salajegheh M. Application of cognitive apprenticeship model in clinical education: a scoping review. *J Med Educ Devel.* 2023;61(49):68–78.
29. Armour C, Schneid SD, Brandl K. Writing on the board as students' preferred teaching modality in a physiology course. *Adv Physiol Educ.* 2016;40(2):229–233. doi: 10.1152/advan.00130.2015. PMID: 27105742.
30. Singh N, Phoon CKL. Not yet a dinosaur: the chalk talk. *Adv Physiol Educ.* 2021;45(1):61–66. doi: 10.1152/advan.00126.2020. PMID: 33502289.
31. Brooks ES, Cho NL. How I do it: improving resident led medical student education with premade chalk talks. *J Surg Educ.* 2025;82(8):103551. doi: 10.1016/j.jsurg.2025.103551. Epub 2025 May 24. PMID: 40414178.
32. Frates EP, Moore MA, Lopez CN, McMahon GT. Coaching for behavior change in physiatry. *Am J Phys Med Rehabil.* 2011;90(12):1074–1082. doi: 10.1097/PHM.0b013e31822dea9a. PMID: 22019966.
33. D'Antoni AV, Mtui EP, Loukas M, Tubbs RS, Zipp GP, Dunlosky J. An evidence-based approach to learning clinical anatomy: a guide for medical students, educators, and administrators. *Clin Anat.* 2019;32(1):156–163.
34. Guenther AR, Abbott CM. Think-pair-share: promoting equitable participation and in-depth discussion. *PRiMER.* 2024;8:7. doi: 10.22454/PRiMER.2024.444143. PMID: 38406233; PMCID: PMC10887392.
35. Rao SP, DiCarlo SE. Peer instruction improves performance on quizzes. *Adv Physiol Educ.* 2000;24(1):51–55. doi: 10.1152/advances.2000.24.1.51. PMID: 11209565.
36. Arasappa Vishwanath V, Raghuramaiah S, Rasalkar K. Exploring peer learning module vs. conventional tutorials: effects on engagement and learning outcomes among first-year medical students. *BMC Med Educ.* 2025;25(1):101. doi: 10.1186/s12909-024-06549-x. PMID: 39838387; PMCID: PMC11753065.
37. Fakoya AOJ, Ndrio M, McCarthy KJ. Facilitating active collaborative learning in medical education; a literature review of peer instruction method. *Adv Med Educ Pract.* 2023;14:1087–1099. doi: 10.2147/AMEP.S421400. PMID: 37810958; PMCID: PMC10559896.
38. Lyman F. The responsive classroom discussion. In Anderson AS (ed.) *Mainstreaming Digest.* College Park, MD: University of Maryland, College of Education, 1981, pp. 109–113.
39. Price DW, Wang T, O'Neill TR, et al. The effect of spaced repetition on learning and knowledge transfer in a large cohort of practicing physicians. *Acad Med.* 2025;100(1):94–102.

40. Burel J, Trost O, Demeyere M, et al. Spaced repetition and other key factors influencing medical school entrance exam success: insights from a French survey. *BMC Med Educ.* 2025;25:1036. doi: 10.1186/s12909-025-07605-w.
41. Upegui A, Awan OA. Spaced repetition in medical education: its importance and applications. *Acad Radiol.* 2024;31(12):5339–5340.
42. Serra MJ, Kaminske AN, Nebel C, Coppola KM. The use of retrieval practice in the health professions: a state-of-the-art review. *Behav Sci.* 2025;15(7):974. doi: 10.3390/bs15070974. PMID: 40723757; PMCID: PMC12292765.
43. Van Hoof TJ, Sumeracki MA, Madan CR. Science of learning strategy series: article 3, interleaving. *J Contin Educ Health Prof.* 2022;42(4):265–268. doi: 10.1097/CEH.0000000000000418. Epub 2022 Feb 17. PMID: 35170479.
44. Richardson V. Constructivist pedagogy. *Teach Coll Rec.* 2003;105(9):1623–1640.
45. Dong H, Lio J, Sherer R, Jiang I. Some learning theories for medical educators. *Med Sci Educ.* 2021;31(3):1157–1172.
46. Young JQ, Van Merrienboer J, Durning S, Ten Cate O. Cognitive load theory: implications for medical education: AMEE guide No. 86. *Med Teach.* 2014;36(5):371–384.
47. Mann KV. Theoretical perspectives in medical education: past experience and future possibilities. *Med Educ.* 2011;45(1):60–68.
48. Pierce C, Corral J, Aagaard E, Harnke B, Irby DM, Stickrath C. A BEME realist synthesis review of the effectiveness of teaching strategies used in the clinical setting on the development of clinical skills among health professionals: BEME guide No. 61. Med Teach. 2020;42(6):604–615.
49. Wolpaw TM, Wolpaw DR, Papp KK. SNAPPS: a learner-centered model for outpatient education. *Acad Med.* 2003;78(9):893–898.
50. Pascoe JM, Nixon J, Lang VJ. Maximizing teaching on the wards: review and application of the one-minute preceptor and SNAPPS models. *J Hosp Med.* 2015;10(2):125–130.
51. Teixeira Ferraz Grünewald S, Grünewald T, Ezequiel OS, Lucchetti ALG, Lucchetti G. One-minute preceptor and SNAPPS for clinical reasoning: a systematic review and meta-analysis. *Intern Med J.* 2023;53(5):680–689. doi: 10.1111/imj.16005. Epub 2023 May 5. PMID: 36625402.
52. Lockspeiser TM, Kaul P. Applying the one minute preceptor model to pediatric and adolescent gynecology education. *J Pediatr Adolesc Gynecol.* 2015;28(2):74–77. doi: 10.1016/j.jpag.2014.07.014. Epub 2014 Aug 1. PMID: 25850586.
53. Savaria MC, Min S, Aghagoli G, Tunkel AR, Hirsh DA, Michelow IC. Enhancing the one-minute preceptor method for clinical teaching with a DEFT approach. *Int J Infect Dis.* 2022;115:149–153. doi: 10.1016/j.ijid.2021.12.314. Epub 2021 Dec 7. PMID: 34883233; PMCID: PMC8805221.
54. Orlander JD. Twelve tips for use of a white board in clinical teaching: reviving the chalk talk. *Med Teach.* 2007;29(2–3):89–92. doi: 10.1080/01421590701287913. PMID: 17701616.

22 Assessment and Feedback in Lifestyle Medicine Education

This book emphasizes the development of courses and the teaching of lifestyle medicine topics in medical school. Without assessing students and providing feedback, there is no way to evaluate the impact of these courses or to share that impact with students. Without assessment and feedback strategies, a course is a one-way road, much like a straight lecture that provides only information by talking at students. For a course to be effective, it must have an impact on the learner and teach materials and skills. The only way to determine whether the course was successful is to assess the learner's knowledge and skills. In this way, the course speaks back to the educator, providing information on the effectiveness of the teaching strategies employed. Assessments reflect how well students learned the material and how well the medical educator taught it.

In medical school, courses are designed to develop the competencies required to become a practicing physician who is competent and compassionate. Assessments can evaluate competencies. Medical schools are moving toward competency-based education systems. Competencies need to be set. Courses need to target these competencies. Then, competencies need to be checked. Assessments check them.

Feedback helps learners understand how the course or educational experience has influenced their growth and development as physicians, including knowledge acquisition, comprehension of key medical information, and clinical reasoning skills. Feedback from a teacher to a student can have a lasting impact. The manner in which a medical educator provides feedback to a student is vital to consider. On the one hand, feedback is necessary to course-correct if a student is on the wrong track. On the other hand, it is essential to encourage and uplift students as they make progress. The journey through medical school and training is long and often arduous.

Feedback is like the centerboard of a sailboat, improving the boat's stability in heavy winds. Medical students are under significant pressure, like a sailboat in heavy winds. The medical system propels them forward, like strong winds propel a boat. In a storm, the wind can get tricky, and a ship can become unstable. In medical school, academic pressure can be high, and family or life stressors can exacerbate these challenges, creating waves, and difficult situations for students. Faculty feedback can help stabilize students and reduce pressure, guiding those who are struggling to find a safe way forward with less turbulence. It is important to remember that one of the primary roles of feedback is to support and empower students.

22.1 ASSESSMENTS

Competency in lifestyle medicine can be evaluated through various mechanisms, including written or oral assignments, tests, or simulation exercises. Assessment should be formative and summative. Table 22.1 reveals the difference between formative and summative assessments. Formative assessment helps students build and solidify their knowledge, while summative assessment helps students understand how they performed at the end of a course, workshop, or program. It is a summary of their knowledge acquisition and skill level. Notably, Table 22.1 illustrates interleaving, a teaching strategy discussed in Chapter 21.

The assessments for lifestyle medicine ideally center on foundational knowledge of the science of the six pillars, the art of prescribing the pillars with **F**requency, **I**ntensity, **T**ime, and **T**ype of behavior (**FITT** prescription for each pillar), and counseling on behavior change. Formative assessments

DOI: 10.1201/9781003630043-22

TABLE 22.1
The Difference Between Formative and Summative Assessments Using Five Indicators

Indicator	Formative (1–4)	Summative (5,6)
Purpose	Motivate students, monitor learning, provide early and ongoing feedback, help with mastery and retention of material and skills, identify strengths and weaknesses, and discover areas of confusion and of comprehension. Aligned with the course objectives.	Evaluate overall learning and determine competency for knowledge and skill sets. Identify if remedial work is necessary. Used to determine if students have met the required benchmarks or competencies. Essential for professional accountability, licensing, and board certification.
Timing	Repeated. Performed throughout the course: early, midway, and toward the end of the course. Completed in person during class time or after as a homework-style assignment.	One time. This is a summary of knowledge acquired and skills mastered, so it is completed at the end of the course, workshop, or instructional period.
Feedback	Delivered immediately or as soon as possible. It is specific and as detailed as possible to guide future learning and studying. Feedback is meant to inspire learners to work on areas of weakness and to acknowledge areas of strength. Feedback is meant to be part of the continued learning process as students continue to form their knowledge and skills throughout the course or class.	Often minimal, used primarily for grading purposes, as in a final exam, project, or paper. Ideally, feedback is delivered soon after the assessment is completed. Detailed information on performance should be shared so that the student actually learns from taking the assessment. Students should also be encouraged to provide their own feedback on their overall course or class performance as they understand and experience it. Areas of future exploration and focus should be identified. If there are areas of deficiency, a plan to bolster those areas needs to be determined and agreed upon by the student.
Examples	Quizzes, rough draft or second draft submissions, in-class activities to check on comprehension, class discussions inviting self-explanation, polls in class that test facts covered, discussion posts online that require reflection and self-explanation, one-minute summaries or reflections, sharing AHA moments, and case presentations.	End-of-term or class test/exam, in-class final essay, standardized exams, licensing exams, end-of-term paper, capstone project, scholarly project, or thesis.
Impact on learning and teaching	Guides instructional design for teachers/educators. Guides review and study sessions for the learners. Helps students self-regulate, reflect, plan, and direct their own learning. Helps give learners autonomy over their studying by demonstrating areas of strength and weakness before the final or summative assessment.	Provides a measure of student learning outcomes. Grades students. It can be used to rank students. It demonstrates the level of effectiveness of the teaching methodology. It can be used to determine the level of competency in knowledge and skills for the learners.

could be short polls administered before class, completed via an app (e.g., Poll Everywhere) to maintain anonymity, or administered in a Zoom meeting if the class is delivered online. Examples of knowledge-based questions to assess understanding of the reading material are shared below. These questions are from the *Lifestyle Medicine Handbook* (7), published by Healthy Learning and co-authored by Drs. Beth Frates, Jon Bonnet, Richard Joseph, and James Peterson. Medical school faculty can ask these questions before and/or after a learning session to serve as a knowledge check. These questions can be used by students themselves when reading through the *Lifestyle Medicine Handbook*. This type of formative assessment is low-stakes and designed to keep learners engaged and motivated to learn more. In addition, faculty could use the questions before and after a class

TABLE 22.2
The FIT and ABLE Mnemonic for Feedback

F-Frequent
I-Interactive
T-Timely

A-Appropriate for learner level
B-Behavior-specific and balanced
L-Labeled
E-Empathetic

to check recall when using the LM 101 Curriculum from ACLM (8). The questions are divided to cover each chapter of the *Lifestyle Medicine Handbook* separately. The handbook chapters correspond to modules in the LM 101 Curriculum. Thus, the questions can be presented to learners once per week if the course covers one chapter or module per week. In this way, the questions can be used as a formative assessment. In addition, the questions can be used as a final exam or as a summative assessment.

Below are examples of questions that are fact-checking. They do not test clinical reasoning. These questions demonstrate ways to use questions as a formative assessment of knowledge throughout the course, or all the questions can be used at the end of a class as a final summative assessment of learning for an introductory lifestyle medicine course in the first or second year of medical school.

Examples of Assessment Questions for an Introduction to Lifestyle Medicine Course.

Lifestyle Medicine Handbook Quiz

Chapter 1: Understanding Lifestyle Medicine

1. According to Mokdad and colleagues' JAMA article published in 2004, the actual causes of death in order of most prevalent to least prevalent were:
   a. Firearms, microbial agents, tobacco, poor diet/physical inactivity
   b. **Tobacco, poor diet/physical inactivity, alcohol consumption, microbial agents**
   c. Tobacco, illicit drug use, firearms, and alcohol consumption
   d. Poor diet/physical inactivity, motor vehicles, microbial agents, tobacco
   (page 21 Edition 2)
2. According to Chapter 1 of the *Lifestyle Medicine Handbook*, heart disease causes approximately how many deaths in the United States each year,
   a. One out of every 10 deaths
   b. One out of every 15 deaths
   c. **One out of every 4 deaths**
   d. One out of every 2 deaths
   (page 22 Edition 2)
3. According to Chapter 1 of the *Lifestyle Medicine Handbook*, heart disease and stroke cost the United States how much money in health care expenditures and lost productivity, approximately?
   a. $300 million
   b. $500 million
   c. $3 billion
   d. **$300 billion**
   (page 22 Edition 2)

4. According to Chapter 1 of the *Lifestyle Medicine Handbook*, the average life expectancy in the United States is
   a. 85.9 years old
   b. 63.9 years old
   c. **77.9 years old**
   d. 81.9 years old
   (page 20, Edition 2)
5. Inventions that changed society norms included the three big Ts, according to Chapter 1 of the *Lifestyle Medicine Handbook*. What are the three big Ts?
   a. Telemedicine, Trains, Transcription
   b. **Transportation, Television, Technology**
   c. Transportation, Time clocks, Telemarketing
   d. Trains, Time clocks, Technology
   (page 19 Edition 2)

Chapter 2: Empowering People to Change

1. Hettler's Six Dimensions of Wellness include emotional, physical, and social. What are the other three?
   a. **Spiritual, intellectual, occupational**
   b. Financial, family, sleep
   c. Spiritual, financial, and educational
   d. Occupational, family, nature
   (Page 47, Edition 2)
2. An Expert-Like Approach includes the following
   a. Helping patients to help themselves
   b. Focusing on what is working well
   c. Building motivation, confidence, and engagement
   d. **Striving to have all the answers**
   (page 51 Edition 2)
3. A Coach-Like Approach includes the following
   a. **Collaborates**
   b. Advises
   c. Focuses on the problem
   d. Relies on their skills and knowledge as an expert
   (page 51 Edition 2)
4. In the Frates COACH acronym, the two Cs stand for
   a. Compassion and caring
   b. **Curiosity and compassion**
   c. Calm and curious
   d. Caring and cumulative
   (page 52 Edition 2)
5. In a coach approach, the coach does more listening than talking.
   a. **True**
   b. False
   (page 61 Edition 2)
6. Health coaching is a relatively new concept, and there are no randomized controlled studies yet published in the medical literature.
   a. True
   b. **False**
   (page 69 Edition 2)

7. There are five stages in the Transtheoretical Model of Change, including Pre-Contemplation, Contemplation, Preparation, Action, and
   a. Completion
   b. Relapse
   c. **Maintenance**
   d. Acceptance
   (page 75 Edition 2)
8. When patients who smoke are in pre-contemplation, it is advised that the healthcare providers
   a. Insist that the patient commit to changing by providing a quit date right then and there
   b. Tell the patient to quit and set up an appointment in one week for a check-up
   c. **Ask if the patient wants to hear a story of someone who successfully quit smoking after multiple attempts**
   d. Sign the patient up for a smoking cessation support group
   (page 76 Edition 2)
9. When patients are in the Maintenance stage of the Transtheoretical Model of Change with regard to exercise, the healthcare provider
   a. Does not need to discuss exercise with the patient
   b. **Is encouraged to check in with the patient to see how things are going with the exercise**
   c. Is encouraged to ensure the patient is logging their exercise minutes or steps
   d. Does not need to check blood pressure
   (page 81 Edition 2)
10. In the contemplation stage of change, according to the Transtheoretical model of change,
   a. A person is already planning to change
   b. A person is refusing to change
   c. A person is not interested in change
   d. **A person is considering a change**
   (page 77 Edition 2)

Chapter 3: Collaborating, Motivating, Goal-Setting, and Tracking

1. Motivational interviewing focuses on encouraging the patient to
   a. **Engage in change talk**
   b. Engage in sustain talk
   c. Engage in real talk
   d. Engage in lifestyle talk
   (page 91 Edition 2)
2. The R in the RULE mnemonic in Motivational Interviewing stands for
   a. **Resist the righting reflex**
   b. Right the wrong
   c. Reflection
   d. Range of emotions
   (page 93 Edition 2)
3. The U in the RULE mnemonic in Motivational Interviewing stands for
   a. **Understand the patient's motivation**
   b. Understand your own emotions
   c. Understand the disease
   d. Understand the damage
   (page 93 Edition 2)

4. The L in the RULE mnemonic in Motivational Interviewing stands for
   a. Love
   b. Loyalty
   c. Language
   d. **Listen**
   (page 93 Edition 2)
5. The E in the RULE mnemonic in Motivational Interviewing stands for
   a. Energize the patient
   b. Empathize with the patient
   c. Express kindness to the patient
   d. **Empower your patient**
   (page 93 Edition 2)
6. The 5 D model of Appreciative Inquiry includes
   a. **Define, discover, dream, design, deliver**
   b. Dig, do, deliver, design, destiny
   c. Dump, drain, destroy, delight, dream
   d. Danger, drama, dream, define, discover
   (Page 98–99 Edition 2)
7. The sociological model of change includes
   a. **Individual, relationship, community, societal**
   b. People, places, parties, patronage
   c. Single, family, pets, plants
   d. Personality, attitudes, mindsets, judgments
   (page 100 Edition 2)
8. The 5 Step Coaching Model for Creating a Collaborative Coach-Client Relationship involves
   a. Be energetic, be appreciative, be compassionate, be responsible, be trustworthy
   b. Be authentic, be honest, be respectful, be kind, be accountable
   c. **Be empathic, align motivation, build confidence, set SMART goals, and set accountability**
   d. Be energized, create connection, set SMART goals, internalize motivation, and report back
   (Page 101 Edition 2)
9. Self-efficacy is
   a. Belief that one is better than they were before
   b. Treating mistakes like opportunities to learn and grow
   c. **Confidence that a person can complete a task**
   d. Knowing one's strengths and using them to find flow
   (page 91 Edition 2)
10. An example of an intrinsic motivator is
   a. **Feeling energized and creative after a run**
   b. Treating yourself with a cookie after a run
   c. Rewarding yourself with a movie after a run
   d. Running so that you can lose weight and receive a gift certificate after you lose 10 pounds
   (page 90 and 106 Edition 2)

Chapter 4: Improving Health Through Exercise

1. Muscular strength is:
   a. the ability of a muscle or a muscle group to carry heavy weight
   b. **the ability of a muscle or a muscle group to exert a short-term maximum force**

   c. the ability of a muscle or a muscle group to exert submaximal force for an extended period of time
   d. the ability of a muscle or a muscle group to exert minimal force for an extended period of time

   (Page 134, Edition 2)

2. Muscular endurance is:
   a. the ability of a muscle or a muscle group to carry heavy weight
   b. the ability of a muscle or a muscle group to exert a short-term maximum force
   c. **the ability of a muscle or a muscle group to exert submaximal force for an extended period of time**
   d. the ability of a muscle or a muscle group to exert minimal force for an extended period of time

   (Page 134, Edition 2)
3. The Frates **MOSS** method used in coaching patients in lifestyle change stands for:
   a. Motivation, overcoming, strategies, stability
   b. Movement, obstacles, strategies, strengths
   c. Movement, overcoming, stability, strengths
   d. **Motivation, obstacles, strategies, strengths**

   (Page 154, Edition 2)
4. What are the four basic health-related components of total fitness?
   a. **Cardiorespiratory fitness, muscular fitness, flexibility, and body composition**
   b. Cardiorespiratory fitness, movement, flexibility, and cognitive strength
   c. Cognitive strength, medicine, body composition, and capability
   d. Muscle mass, flexibility, VO2max, and body composition

   (Page 132, Edition 2)
5. What is the most widely accepted measure for aerobic fitness?
   a. Body composition
   b. **VO2max**
   c. The sing test
   d. Waist measurements

   (Page 133, Edition 2)
6. What is hydrostatic weighing?
   a. Using an at-home scale to measure body weight
   b. Field test of a person's body fat distribution pattern
   c. **Underwater weighing**
   d. Quick and painless procedure to measure bone density

   (Page 139, Edition 2)
7. What does NEAT stand for?
   a. **Non-exercise activity thermogenesis**
   b. New energy and thermogenesis
   c. Nesting, eating, and talking
   d. Nourish, exercise, activity, tighten

   (Page 120, Edition 2)
8. How does exercise impact the dermatologic system?
   a. Promotes healthy digestion at rest
   b. Can result in muscle strength
   c. Raises HDL cholesterol
   d. **Helps cool the body by enabling heat to cool the pores**

   (Page 122, Edition 2)

9. What is released during exercise that helps the development of new brain cells?
   a. Hemoglobin
   b. **Brain-derived neurotrophic factor**
   c. Ferritin
   d. Secretin
   (Page 124, Edition 2)
10. Dopamine levels, which are elevated after exercise, are associated with:
   a. Control of eating, appetite, and regulation of pain
   b. Sexual arousal, memory, and regulation of pain
   c. Fight-or-flight response and mood
   d. **Reward, motivation, and pleasure**
   (Page 126, Edition 2)

Chapter 5: The Nutrition-Health Connection

1. What are the six essential nutrients?
   a. Macronutrients, micronutrients, fiber, minerals, water, and vitamins
   b. Macronutrients, micronutrients, fiber, minerals, vitamins, and alcohol
   c. **Water, vitamins, minerals, protein, carbohydrates, and fat**
   d. Alcohol, vitamins, minerals, protein, carbohydrates, and fat
   (Page 177, Edition 2)
2. What is the primary site of digestion and absorption of nutrients in the body?
   a. The esophagus
   b. The stomach
   c. **The small intestine**
   d. The large intestine
   (Page 178, Edition 2)
3. According to the CDC's *Morbidity and Mortality Weekly Report*, how many adults meet the federal fruit or vegetable consumption recommendations?
   a. 0 in 10 adults
   b. **1 in 10 adults**
   c. 3 in 10 adults
   d. 7 in 10 adults
   (Page 179, Edition 2)
4. Which nutrient is associated with protecting eye health?
   a. Vitamin D
   b. Folate
   c. Cobalamin
   d. **Vitamin A**
   (Page 180, Edition 2)
5. Which nutrient is associated with building bones?
   a. Vitamin A
   b. Folate
   c. **Calcium**
   d. Iodine
   (Page 181, Edition 2)
6. The MIND diet is a hybrid of which two dietary patterns?
   a. Paleo and Mediterranean
   b. Paleo and DASH

c. **DASH and Mediterranean**
d. DASH and Keto
(Page 200, Edition 2)

7. According to the Harvard Healthy Eating Plate, how much of the plate should be fruit and vegetables?
   a. ⅕
   b. ¼
   c. ½
   d. ¾
   (Page 205, Edition 2)
8. Which molecules protect the body's cells from free radicals?
   a. Carbon
   b. **Antioxidants**
   c. Dietary Fiber
   d. Water
   (Page 284, Edition 2)
9. What is ACLM's dietary "North Star"?
   a. Vegan
   b. Paleo
   c. **Whole Foods, plant-based**
   d. High Fiber Low Fat
   (Page 207, Edition 2)
10. What does the FITT prescription for nutrition stand for?
    a. Food, Intensity, Testing, Tolerance
    b. Fiber, Iron, Tryptophan, Tapioca
    c. Frequency, Iron, Timing, Tolerance
    d. **Frequency, Intensity, Time, Type**
    (Page 212, Edition 2)

Chapter 6: Weight Management

1. What is energy balance?
   a. Calories consumed
   b. Macronutrients + Micronutrients
   c. **Energy inputs – energy outputs**
   d. Energy outputs + energy inputs
   (Page 252, Edition 2
2. RMR or resting metabolic rate represents how much daily expenditure?
   a. 20%–30%
   b. 50%
   c. **60%–75%**
   d. 85%
   (Page 233, Edition 2)
3. EEPA or energy expenditure due to physical activity represents how much energy is expended?
   a. 5%–10%
   b. **15%–30%**
   c. 30%–45%
   d. 40%–60%
   (Page 233, Edition 2)

4. According to the *Lifestyle Medicine Handbook*, what is the best exercise for weight loss?
   a. **Aerobic conditioning and strength training**
   b. Only low-impact aerobic training
   c. Only strength training
   d. HIIT cardio
   (Page 241, Edition 2)
5. Which two hormones play a role in appetite regulation?
   a. Ghrelin and cortisol
   b. Growth hormone and oxytocin
   c. Growth hormone and calcitonin
   d. **Ghrelin and leptin**
   (Page 247, Edition 2)
6. Why do low-calorie, nutrient-dense foods tend to be filling?
   a. Due to carbohydrate content
   b. **Due to the fiber and water content**
   c. Due to the protein and carbohydrate content
   d. Due to high sodium content
   (Page 235, Edition 2)
7. Which hormone acts to increase satiety?
   a. Ghrelin
   b. Oxytocin
   c. Cortisol
   d. **Leptin**
   (Page 247, Edition 2)
8. When gauging portion sizes using your hands, what does your thumb represent?
   a. 1 cup
   b. 3 oz.
   c. **1 oz.**
   d. 1 teaspoon
   (Page 249, Edition 2)
9. According to the *Lifestyle Medicine Handbook*, a child with one obese parent has what chance of being obese?
   a. 25%
   b. **50%**
   c. 80%
   d. 95%
   (Page 238, Edition 2)
10. According to the *Lifestyle Medicine Handbook*, a child with both obese parents has what chance of being obese?
   a. 25%
   b. 50%
   c. **80%**
   d. 95%
   (Page 238, Edition 2)

Chapter 7: Sleep Matters

1. According to the *Lifestyle Medicine Handbook*, which stage of sleep comprises 40%–50% of sleep time over the course of the night?
   a. Stage N1
   b. **Stage N2**

c. Stage N3
d. Stage REM
(Page 266, Edition 2)

2. According to the *Lifestyle Medicine Handbook*, which stage of sleep occurs in increasingly long episodes across the night between 1.5 and 2 hours?
    a. Stage N1
    b. Stage N2
    c. Stage N3
    d. **Stage REM**
    (Page 267, Edition 2)
3. According to the National Sleep Foundation, what is the recommended number of hours of sleep for adults?
    a. 9.5–11 hours
    b. 9–11 hours
    c. 7.5–10 hours
    d. **7–9 hours**
    (Page 269, Edition 2)
4. Sleeping less than six to eight hours a night increases the risk of early death by how much?
    a. 10%
    b. **12%**
    c. 25%
    d. 37%
    (Page 270, Edition 2)
5. What is the most common sleep disorder?
    a. **Insomnia**
    b. Restless leg syndrome
    c. Sleep apnea
    d. Narcolepsy
    (Page 275, Edition 2)
6. How does poor sleep impact the cardiovascular system?
    a. **Decreases a person's heart rate variability**
    b. Increases a person's muscular endurance
    c. Decreases respiratory rate
    d. Increases digestion rate
    (Page 271, Edition 2)
7. How does poor sleep impact the digestive system?
    a. Increases blood pressure
    b. Decreases blood pressure
    c. **Increases ghrelin**
    d. Decreases ghrelin
    (Page 271, Edition 2)
8. According to the CDC, how many Americans suffer from sleep deprivation?
    a. 100,000
    b. 1,000,000
    c. 25–50 million
    d. **50–70 million**
    (Page 275, Edition 2)
9. What is sleep apnea?
    a. A condition characterized by an irresistible urge to move the legs, particularly in the evenings

b. **A sleep disorder in which breathing repeatedly stops and starts**
c. The inability to fall asleep
d. Excessive daytime sleepiness
(Page 277, Edition 2)

10. What is narcolepsy?
a. **A chronic sleep disorder that causes overwhelming drowsiness in the daytime**
b. A condition characterized by an irresistible urge to move the legs, particularly in the evenings
c. The inability to fall asleep
d. Disturbed sleep from severe nighttime terrors
(Page 278, Edition 2)

Chapter 8: Stress and Resilience

1. Who was the first to coin the term "stress" in 1936?
a. Dr. Mihaly Csikszentmihalyi
b. Drs. Robert M. Yerkes
c. Dr. John Dodson
d. **Dr. Hans Selye**
(Page 296, Edition 2)
2. According to information in Chapter 8 of the *Lifestyle Medicine Handbook*, how many of doctors' visits are stress-related ailments?
a. 10%
b. 25%
c. 50%
d. **75%**
(Page 296, Edition 2)
3. What is eustress?
a. The stress of pain, sorrow, or suffering
b. **Good stress, which motivates you**
c. Bad stress, which can be harmful and draining
d. The body's resistance to stress
(Page 297, Edition 2)
4. What does the Yerke's Dodson law depict the relationship of?
a. Sleep and stress/arousal
b. **Performance and stress/arousal**
c. Energy and stress/arousal
d. Nutrition and stress/arousal
(Page 297, Edition 2)
5. How does stress impact the respiratory system?
a. It can exacerbate inflammatory bowel disease
b. It can decrease the regulation of blood pressure
c. It can cause an upset stomach
d. **It can make it more difficult to breathe**
(Page 306, Edition 2)
6. Unchecked chronic stress can lead to an excess of which hormone?
a. Epinephrine
b. Oxytocin
c. Dopamine
d. **Cortisol**
(Page 302, Edition 2)

7. How does chronic stress impact the skeletal system?
   a. Depresses the production of testosterone
   b. Increases the production of testosterone
   c. **Decreases the level of bone density**
   d. Increases the level of bone density
   (Page 306, Edition 2)
8. What is the parasympathetic nervous system (PNS) responsible for?
   a. Irritating the gastrointestinal tract
   b. Controlling the muscles
   c. **The state of rest and digestion**
   d. The state of fight-or-flight
   (Page 306, Edition 2)
9. What is the sympathetic nervous system (SNS) responsible for?
   a. Irritating the gastrointestinal tract
   b. Controlling the muscles
   c. The state of rest and digestion
   d. **The state of fight-or-flight**
   (Page 306, Edition 2)
10. What is an example of an internal risk factor for chronic stress?
   a. Family-related issues
   b. **Excessive caffeine**
   c. Excessive exercise
   d. An all-or-nothing attitude
   (Page 308, Edition 2)

Chapter 9: Peace of Mind with Meditation, Mindfulness, and Relaxation

1. According to the Merriam-Webster Online Dictionary, what is meditation?
   a. **An act or process of spending time in quiet thought**
   b. The act of increasing blood flow to the brain
   c. A program developed by Dr. Jon Kabat-Zinn for health and well-being
   d. Tensing the body, followed by relaxing it
   (Page 320, Edition 2)
2. What is focused attention meditation?
   a. Remaining open to any and all aspects of the present experience
   b. Engaging in a repetitive activity, such as walking or practicing yoga
   c. **Focusing attention on a single object, such as a candle, sound, mantra, or internal object**
   d. Focusing on nothing but one's thoughts
   (Page 323, Edition 2)
3. What is the impact of meditation on the circulatory system?
   a. Stimulates digestion
   b. Facilitates restful sleep patterns
   c. Increases the rate of breathing
   d. **Decreases blood pressure**
   (Page 326, Edition 2)
4. What is considered an impact of meditation?
   a. Increases blood pressure
   b. Reduces digestion
   c. **Reduces markers of inflammation**
   d. Increases markers of inflammation
   (Page 326, Edition 2)

5. What are the four areas of the brain that may be affected by meditation
   a. Prefrontal cortex, occipital lobe, frontal cortex, insula
   b. Prefrontal cortex, occipital lobe, amygdala, hippocampus
   c. **Prefrontal cortex, insula, amygdala, hippocampus**
   d. Occipital lobe, amygdala, insula, hippocampus
   (Page 329, Edition 2)
6. People who practice mindfulness-based stress reduction (MBSR) strive to be able to
   a. Draw pictures mindfully to relax and breathe rhythmically
   b. **Respond consciously to circumstances by pausing and breathing before reacting**
   c. Sit in silence for over an hour to calm down and hold thoughtful conversations
   d. Walk to clear one's head to make a conscious decision while deep breathing
   (Page 333, Edition 2)
7. What is exercise-induced ischemia?
   a. Chest pain at rest
   b. Irregular heartbeat from decreased exercise
   c. Irregular heartbeat from excessive exercise
   d. **Lack of oxygen to the heart muscle with exercise**
   (Page 338, Edition 2)
8. What does the insula do?
   a. Dictates complex behavior, executive functioning
   b. **Modulates self-awareness, perception, and cognitive functioning**
   c. Regulates emotional control
   d. Helps modulate cortical arousal and responsiveness
   (Page 329, Edition 2)
9. What do the amygdala do?
   a. Dictates complex behavior, executive functioning
   b. Modulates self-awareness, perception, and cognitive functioning
   c. **Regulates emotional control**
   d. Helps modulate cortical arousal and responsiveness
   (Page 329, Edition 2)
10. What is open monitoring meditation?
    a. **Remaining open to any and all aspects of the present experience**
    b. Engaging in a repetitive activity, such as walking or practicing yoga
    c. Focusing attention on a single object such as a candle, sound, mantra, or internal object
    d. Focusing on nothing but one's thoughts
    (Page 324, Edition 2)

Chapter 10: The Power of Connection

1. Which hormone is also called "the love hormone"?
   a. Ghrelin
   b. Leptin
   c. Norepinephrine
   d. **Oxytocin**
   (Page 351, Edition 2)
2. What is the difference between loneliness and social isolation?
   a. Loneliness is when someone is alone due to introversion; social isolation is the voluntary state of choosing not to connect with others
   b. Loneliness is a physical state of not being with people; social isolation is an emotional state of someone not connecting with others
   c. **Loneliness is an emotional state of feeling disconnected from others; social isolation is a physical state of the lack of available relationships**

   d. Loneliness is when someone is alone due to introversion; social isolation is isolation due to a physical lack of relationships
   (Page 356, Edition 2)
3. What is included in Maslow's Hierarchy of Needs?
   a. Physiological, Safety, Love/Belonging, Esteem, Self-Actualization
   b. Physiological, Safety, Love/Belonging, Physical, Awareness
   c. Love/Belonging, Physical, Esteem, Awareness, Self-Actualization
   d. **Physiological, Safety, Love/Belonging, Esteem, Self-Actualization**
   (Page 350, Edition 2)
4. Who is known for doing extensive work in creating high-quality connections?
   a. **Dr. Jane Dutton**
   b. Dr. Beth Frates
   c. Nathan Pritikin
   d. Dr. Walter Willett
   (Page 358, Edition 2)
5. What does a FITT prescription stand for?
   a. Fundamentals, Intensity, Time, Training
   b. **Frequency, Intensity, Time, Type**
   c. Fundamentals, Increments, Type, Training
   d. Frequency, Increments, Time, Type
   (Page 362, Edition 2)
6. In a landmark study conducted in 1979, which researchers studied the relationship between social and community ties and mortality?
   a. Dr. Walter Willett and Dr. Jane Dutton
   b. **Lisa F. Berkman and S. Leonard Syme**
   c. Dr. Nicholas Christakis and Dr. Jane Dutton
   d. Lisa F. Berkman and Dr. Walter Willett
   (Page 356, Edition 2)
7. What did research by Dr. Nicholas Christakis show?
   a. Individuals who are socially isolated have disrupted sleep patterns
   b. Stress levels increase hunger
   c. The most effective way to lose weight is through a combination of strength training and cardio
   d. **Health behaviors are spread among members who are not only geographically close, but also socially close**
   (Page 357, Edition 2)
8. What is an adverse health effect of social isolation?
   a. Low resting heart rate
   b. Low C-Reactive Protein
   c. **High blood pressure**
   d. High levels of immunity
   (Page 356, Edition 2)
9. What is a barrier to social connection?
   a. An increased sense of community
   b. High blood pressure
   c. **Lack of self-confidence**
   d. Having a large family
   (Page 355, Edition 2)
10. According to the *Lifestyle Medicine Handbook*, when does the "default network" of the brain come on?
   a. When someone is exercising

b. **When someone is resting**
c. When someone is connecting with others
d. When someone is eating
(Page 353, Edition 2)

Chapter 11: Positively Positive

1. According to information in chapter 11 of the *Lifestyle Medicine Handbook*, what is positive psychology?
   a. A way of thinking or feeling about something
   b. A mental or emotional state of well-being
   c. The desire to change one's mood after an altering life event
   d. **The scientific study of optimal human functioning**
   (Page 372, Edition 2)
2. According to the *Lifestyle Medicine Handbook*, what is gratitude?
   a. A way of thinking or feeling about something
   b. **The quality of being thankful**
   c. A feeling of expectation and desire for a certain thing to occur
   d. The scientific study of optimal human functioning
   (Page 372, Edition 2)
3. What is Dr. Carol Dweck most known for?
   a. **Characterizing the "growth mindset"**
   b. Nutritional Epidemiology research
   c. Applying lifestyle medicine approaches in underserved populations
   d. Studying the benefits of relaxation
   (Page 374, Edition 2)
4. According to the *Lifestyle Medicine Handbook*, what is a benefit optimistic people experience?
   a. Reduced sleep quality
   b. Increased breathing patterns
   c. **Lower likelihood of suffering from depression**
   d. Slower cognitive processing
   (Page 373, Edition 2)
5. When Dr. Kokoro Shirai and colleagues looked at the association between perceived level of enjoyment and risk of cardiovascular disease incidence and mortality in 90,000 Japanese men and women, what did they find?
   a. Those who spent more time moving during the day were less likely to develop cardiovascular disease
   b. There was no difference between those who engaged in positive psychology practices versus those who did not, and the risk of developing cardiovascular disease
   c. **There is a protective role of positive psychological conditions against cardiovascular disease**
   d. Extremely high levels of enjoyment were associated with increased risk of cardiovascular disease
   (Page 373, Edition 2)
6. What did Dr. Jason S. Moser and colleagues find in a study regarding growth mindset?
   a. **Individuals who believed they could learn from their mistakes performed better after making a mistake**
   b. Individuals with a fixed mindset could learn from mistakes just as much as those with a growth mindset

   c. People are born intrinsically with a fixed or growth mindset
   d. Individuals with a fixed mindset could learn from their mistakes more than those without
   (Page 374, Edition 2)
7. What did studies from Dr. Ruby Nadler and colleagues show?
   a. Increased levels of sleep were connected to positive psychology
   b. **Positive moods allow for increased cognitive flexibility**
   c. Having a fixed mindset versus a growth mindset does not determine levels of success
   d. Positive moods have no effect on cognitive flexibility
   (Page 374, Edition 2)
8. Which feel-good hormones are associated with smiling?
   a. Ghrelin and leptin
   b. Oxytocin and ghrelin
   c. Endorphins and testosterone
   d. **Endorphins and serotonin**
   (Page 376, Edition 2)
9. What does Dr. Barbara Frederickson's research suggest?
   a. Increased levels of sleep were connected to positive psychology
   b. Having a fixed mindset versus a growth mindset does not determine levels of success
   c. **Positive emotions lead to novel, exploratory, and creative behaviors**
   d. Creative behaviors are innate and cannot be malleable
   (Page 377, Edition 2)
10. Who is considered the father of the field of positive psychology?
   a. **Dr. Martin Seligman**
   b. Dr. Walter Willett
   c. Dr. Egil Martinsen
   d. Dean Ornish
   (Page 379, Edition 2)

Chapter 12: Substance Use Disorder

1. According to the information in chapter 12 of the *Lifestyle Medicine Handbook*, what is addiction?
   a. **A compulsive use of a habit-forming substance despite negative consequences**
   b. The body's physical need for a specific substance, as evidenced by withdrawal
   c. When the body receives a level of drugs that it cannot tolerate
   d. Specific signs and symptoms occurring after discontinuing the given substance
   (Page 398, Edition 2)
2. According to information from chapter 12 in the *Lifestyle Medicine Handbook*, what is withdrawal?
   a. A compulsive use of a habit-forming substance despite negative consequences
   b. The body's physical need for a specific substance, as evidenced by withdrawal
   c. When the body receives a level of drugs that it cannot tolerate
   d. **Specific signs and symptoms occurring after discontinuing the given substance**
   (Page 398, Edition 2)
3. Which part of the brain establishes associations between environmental cues and whether or not that particular experience is rewarding or aversive?
   a. Nucleus accumbens
   b. Hippocampus
   c. Prefrontal cortex
   d. **Amygdala**
   (Page 399, Edition 2)

4. What does the ASAM acronym "ABCDE" stand for in helping diagnose a person who suffers from addiction?
   a. Abstain, behavior control, craving, diminished recognition, enable activity
   b. **Abstain, behavior control, craving, diminished recognition, emotional response**
   c. Addiction, behavior control, cardiovascular disease, detrimental activity, emotional response
   d. Addiction, behavior control, cardiovascular disease, diminished recognition, enable activity
   (Page 400, Edition 2)
5. What are the most common substance use disorders in the United States?
   a. Heroin, cannabis, alcohol use disorder, Narcan, PCP
   b. Sedatives, PCP, LSD, cannabis, anxiolytics
   c. **Alcohol use disorder, tobacco use disorder, cannabis use disorder, stimulant use disorder, opioid use disorder**
   d. Sedatives, Narcan, PCP, cannabis use disorder, melatonin
   (Page 400, Edition 2)
6. According to the AHA guidelines for alcohol use, what is the recommended number of drinks per day for men?
   a. 0
   b. **≤2 drinks per day**
   c. 2 or 3 drinks per day
   d. 5–7 drinks per day
   (Page 403, Edition 2)
7. According to the AHA guidelines for alcohol use, what is the recommended number of drinks per day for women?
   a. 0
   b. **≤1 drink per day**
   c. ≤2 drinks per day
   d. 3–5 drinks per day
   (Page 403, Edition 2)
8. According to the information in the *Lifestyle Medicine Handbook*, how many people in the United States struggle with alcohol use disorder (AUD)?
   a. 10,000
   b. 10 million
   c. **16 million**
   d. 22 million
   (Page 403, Edition 2)
9. According to the AHA guidelines for alcohol use, what is considered binge drinking for women?
   a. ≥4 drinks in 30 minutes
   b. **≥4 drinks in about 2 hours**
   c. ≥8 drinks in 1 hour
   d. ≥10 drinks in 2 hours
   (Page 403, Edition 2)
10. What is one impact of alcohol on heart health?
    a. High blood pressure
    b. Low blood pressure
    c. Fibrosis
    d. Pancreatitis
    (Page 405, Edition 2)

Chapter 13: Staying the Course

1. According to the *Lifestyle Medicine Handbook*, what is burnout?
   a. **Physical or mental collapse resulting from overwork or stress**
   b. The quality of being dedicated to a cause
   c. Any activity undertaken by a person to take care of other people
   d. The ability to do something effectively and efficiently
   (Page 432, Edition 2)
2. According to the information in Chapter 13 of the *Lifestyle Medicine Handbook*, what is competence?
   a. Physical or mental collapse resulting from overwork or stress
   b. The quality of being dedicated to a cause
   c. Any activity undertaken by a person to take care of other people
   d. **The ability to do something effectively and efficiently**
   (Page 432, Edition 2)
3. What is an example of an emotional reaction of an individual not active in practicing self-care?
   a. Festuge
   b. Sleep disturbances
   c. Mind wandering
   d. **Feeling inadequate**
   (Page 435, Edition 2)
4. What is an example of a cognitive reaction of an individual not active in practicing self-care?
   a. Consuming a calorie-dense diet
   b. Fatigue
   c. Headaches
   d. **Decreased level of concentration**
   (Page 436, Edition 2)
5. What is the common barrier to engaging in self-care?
   a. Disturbed sleep
   b. Disrupted hormone levels
   c. Lack of money
   d. **Lack of time**
   (Page 444, Edition 2)
6. According to Dr. John Travis' Illness-Wellness Continuum, how does lifestyle medicine differ from traditional medicine?
   a. **Traditional medicine focuses on slowing the progression of disease and death; lifestyle medicine reverses this trajectory and moves people toward wellness and optimal functioning**
   b. Lifestyle medicine focuses on slowing the progression of disease and death; traditional medicine reverses this trajectory and moves people toward wellness and optimal functioning
   c. Traditional medicine focuses on the prognosis and treatment of disease; lifestyle medicine only focuses on the treatment of disease
   d. Lifestyle medicine focuses on the prognosis and treatment of disease; traditional medicine only focuses on the treatment of disease
   (Page 451, Edition 2)
7. What are four core attributes that lifestyle medicine practitioners who want to stay the course should strive to have?

a. Strive to achieve seven to eight hours of sleep each night, always eat only plant-based foods, always be learning, always be a difference-maker
b. Strive to achieve seven to eight hours of sleep each night, always practice what they preach, always be learning, always be a difference-maker
c. **Strive to practice what they preach, always be learning, always be values-oriented, always be a difference-maker**
d. Strive to practice what they preach, always eat only plant-based, always be learning, always be values-oriented
(Page 432, Edition 2)

8. According to the *Lifestyle Medicine Handbook*, what factors does self-care encompass?
a. Hygiene, meditation, HIIT workouts, screentime, gardening, playtime
b. Meditation, environment, lifestyle, screentime, playtime, nutrition
c. **Hygiene, nutrition, lifestyle, environment, socioeconomic circumstances, self-medication**
d. Mediation, nutrition, lifestyle, screentime, socioeconomic circumstances, self-medication
(Page 433, Edition 2)

9. According to the *Lifestyle Medicine Handbook*, what causes job burnout?
a. Early mornings or shifts
b. **Work-life imbalance**
c. Eating throughout the day
d. Only medical professionals experience job burnout
(Page 441, Edition 2)

10. According to the *Lifestyle Medicine Handbook*, how is health optimization defined?
a. Giving healthcare and health outcomes the same priority as other life events
b. Minimizing the priority of overall health
c. **Maximizing an individual's well-being, functioning, and quality of life**
d. Viewing nutrition as the most important aspect of one's better health
(Page 453, Edition 2)

Other examples of formative assessment resources for lifestyle medicine include the lifestyle medicine question bank available through the American College of Lifestyle Medicine's website at www.lifestylemedicine.org. A 2021 book titled *Lifestyle Medicine: Essential MCQs for Certification in Lifestyle Medicine* contains 531 multiple-choice questions in lifestyle medicine. There are 25 questions on the introduction to the field, including definitions, distinctions between lifestyle medicine and other fields, and physicians' competencies in the practice of lifestyle medicine. There are 62 questions on health behavior change; 88 on nutrition science, assessment, and prescription, including food labels and prescribing nutrition; and 47 on key clinical processes in lifestyle medicine, including the classification of lifestyle-related illnesses, measures of fitness, and fitness testing options. These questions could be used in medical school courses as part of formative or summative assessments.

There is a focus on formative assessments in medical education. A recent article titled Formative assessment and feedback in medical education: A practical guide: AMEE Guide No. 189 authored by Anastasiya A. Lipnevich, Krista Mattern, and Christopher Feddock from the National Board of Medical Examiners, highlights essential practice points for formative assessments as follows (1):

(*AMEE stands for Association for Medical Education in Europe, and the organization is referred to as the International Association for Health Professions. More information is available on its website https://amee.org/)

1. Continuous and regular assessment
   a. Schedule frequent, low-stakes assessments to monitor progress.
   b. Use a variety of assessment methods to capture diverse learning outcomes.
2. Alignment with learning objectives
   a. Ensure assessments directly measure the intended learning goals.
   b. Use rubrics or criteria that reflect the objectives.
3. Inclusivity and fairness
   a. Design assessments that are accessible to all learners.
   b. Avoid biases by using clear, objective criteria.
4. Evidence of validity and efficacy
   a. Regularly review assessment tools to ensure they measure what they intend to and are resulting in the intended learner outcomes.
   b. Collect feedback from students and instructors to refine assessments.

With the move toward competency-based medical education rather than time-based medical education, the importance of formative assessments becomes even greater. Medical students must become proficient in specific competencies to support their learning, development, and proficiency. It is important that they track their progress. Formative assessments can help them accomplish this and meet competency expectations. With frequent formative assessments, feedback is also frequent. This enables students to identify areas in which they may be failing to progress and enables teachers to identify students who require more focused work in specific areas. Formative assessments help students and teachers take a more individualized approach to medical education, fostering openness to addressing areas of weakness and identifying students who are struggling earlier rather than later (1–4). In fact, according to a small study of students at a Chinese medical school, the use of formative assessments improved students' performance on summative assessments, particularly for those struggling in the course. In addition, the results of this study indicated that students' satisfaction with the course increased over time in the formative assessment group (9).

Using formative assessments for clinical skills can also be a powerful tool for medical educators in lifestyle medicine. One standard method of assessing competency in medical school is the observed structured clinical examination (OSCE) using standardized patients, which could be used to evaluate lifestyle medicine core competencies. Direct observation of peer-to-peer work, simulated patient interactions, or in-clinic interactions could be part of the assessment strategies. This would be well suited to counseling skills necessary for behavior change, such as motivational interviewing. In lifestyle medicine, OSCEs can be used to assess students' understanding of the six pillars of lifestyle medicine through the history taking process with identification of the patient, chief complaint, history of the present illness, past medical/surgical history, medications/supplements, allergies, family history, and social history with a focus on living environment, occupation, physical activity, nutrition, sleep, stress resilience, social connection, and risky substance use. Asking about food insecurity, loneliness, and social determinants of health would be important to include in this section. Review of systems and physical exam follows. The social history section provides the opportunity to include lifestyle medicine questions. Watching and listening to a student acquire information on the patient's social history during an OSCE is one form of lifestyle medicine assessment. Assessing a visit and determining if it was consistent with motivational interviewing is another way to evaluate lifestyle medicine skills.

Experiential assessments, such as self-monitoring of lifestyle behaviors and reflective assignments on goal setting and behavior change, are also practical for evaluating students' ability to apply lifestyle medicine principles (10,11). In this case, students apply the principles to themselves. The validated tool, the Lifestyle Behavior Health Survey (12), could be utilized as a pre- and post-assignment for medical students in a course.

22.2 FEEDBACK FOR LEARNERS

Another aspect of teaching is providing meaningful feedback. Feedback is listed as an indicator in Table 22.1, and reviewing formative and summative assessments is essential. With every assessment, it is helpful to give feedback to the student on their performance. Every assessment is an opportunity to teach. That teaching takes the form of feedback after the assessment and a careful, comprehensive review and evaluation of the student's performance.

Feedback is often overlooked, ignored, or given cursory attention. In some situations, a faculty member may provide the student with feedback, but if it is not formally designated as a feedback session, students may not realize that the session serves this purpose. Stating to the learner, "This is a feedback session," is helpful. It is advisable to ask the student whether this is a good time for a meeting to discuss feedback. If the student declines, the next step is to identify an appropriate day and time in the near future.

Asking for input on the feedback process once it is complete is another chance to remind the student that the session was a formal part of their educational journey. Toward the end of the feedback session, the medical educator can ask the student, "What do you think about this feedback session?" To elicit further information from the student, the final question might be: "What feedback do you have for me on this feedback session?" Given the numerous references to the word "feedback" in this conversation, the student is likely to recognize the session as a feedback session. The fact that the medical educator is open to feedback for themselves also provides a powerful example of lifelong learning, with a focus on continued growth, development, and improvement, while honoring and respecting the student's views and perspectives and recognizing them as an adult learner (drawing on andragogy discussed in Chapter 21).

22.3 POSITIVITY RATIO

Students are often sensitive to negative comments or constructive criticism, also called useful or helpful feedback. As Barbara Frederickson, PhD, reported in her book titled *Positivity: Top-Notch Research Reveals the 3:1 Ratio That Will Change Your Life*, it is recommended to provide three positive comments for every negative comment (13). This exact ratio was called into question when Dr. Frederickson's statisticians' work was scrutinized. However, the notion that students require more positive than negative feedback remains. The exact number is debatable.

22.4 THE SANDWICH TECHNIQUE

Starting with a positive reflection on a student's performance, placing constructive criticism in the middle, and concluding with a positive comment can help the student remain positive and motivated in their learning. This is known as the sandwich technique. It gained significant traction when it was first shared in the 2010s. More recently, medical educators have observed that medical students are aware of the sandwich technique and therefore simply wait for the middle and focus on it, which creates tension (14). Some educators continue to use it or a variation of it.

Explaining that constructive criticism is vital for pushing oneself to learn more and improve helps frame the feedback session. Asking students to provide their own feedback on their assessment results or work to date is an interesting and informative endeavor. Often their impressions are quite accurate. Asking students what they believe they need to work on and what they want to work on can motivate them. In many cases, the student-identified areas align with those identified by the faculty as areas for growth. Even if the student's feedback does not align precisely with that of the educator, the process underscores the need for development in medical practice and that professional growth is lifelong.

22.5 GROWTH MINDSET

Using Carol Dweck's growth mindset in teaching helps students view mishaps and mistakes as opportunities for learning and growth (15). With a growth mindset, people believe that they can improve; with practice and attention to the information or skill, they can learn more and get better. This is an essential mindset for medical students and faculty alike. Learning this early in their medical careers will empower medical students to keep striving and making progress. Realizing that they do not have to be perfect and that medicine is a process of lifelong learning is a valuable lesson for medical students. It is expected that people will make mistakes, fail at times, and then learn and grow from any mishap. Morbidity and mortality conferences are meant to demonstrate a growth mindset.

22.6 THE FIT AND ABLE METHOD

The mnemonic FIT and ABLE (16) can help medical educators remember the importance of feedback for their learners. It stands for frequent, interactive, timely, appropriate to the learner level, behavior-specific, balanced, labeled, and empathetic, as noted in Table 22.2.

Many aspects of the FIT and ABLE mnemonic have been covered in this chapter already. An essential part of the feedback emphasized in the mnemonic, as the last point but certainly not the least valuable, is empathy. Just as it is crucial to schedule time for feedback and ensure it is acceptable to the student, it is equally essential that the time is suitable for the medical educator. Specifically, the medical educator needs to have the time, focus, and energy to give the feedback session their full attention. Additionally, the medical educator needs to carefully formulate the content of the feedback session, taking into account the learner's level and the behavior to be addressed or corrected, and ensuring that it is balanced by highlighting positive behaviors and identifying areas for growth.

Behaviors and actions are the focus of feedback sessions. It is important not to criticize or provide feedback on personality traits or personal characteristics. This can feel like an attack on a person and their identity. Actions and behaviors are the focus of feedback sessions, and these can be addressed, changed, and improved. This refocuses the medical educator's attention on empathy. No one wants to feel attacked. If someone feels attacked, they become defensive. Then, the session loses its power as a teaching tool and becomes an exercise in making excuses.

The medical educator needs to remember what it was like to receive feedback when they were an impressionable young medical student. Careful attention to word choice, tone, and body language is recommended. Speaking to the student the way the medical educator would have wanted to be spoken to when they were a student is a good guideline to follow. In the past, feedback sessions were often not part of the educational process, and when they were, they may have been harsh and public. Remembering that the medical educator is the preceptor, mentor, ally, and teacher for the student, the student's success reflects on the educator, and their failure does, too. In some cases, the student will require remedial support or mental health counseling; in all cases, the teacher needs to be empathetic and attuned to what is occurring with the student at school and, if applicable, at home, if the student is facing challenges. Medical educators need to realize that outside influences could be impacting a student's performance and behaviors.

22.7 PENDLETON'S MODEL

One commonly used protocol for providing feedback is Pendleton's Model. There are five steps in this model (17,18).

1. The feedback provider asks the feedback recipient to mention two or three points that are going well.

2. The feedback provider shares two or three points that are going well.
3. The feedback provider asks the feedback recipient to mention two or three points that can be improved.
4. The feedback provider shares two or three points for improvement and discusses strategies based on the input for closing the gap.
5. The feedback provider or the feedback recipient summarizes the key points from the conversation.

This model has been used for decades and encourages conversation and collaboration between the educator and the student. Using a model such as Pendleton's provides structure for the feedback session and facilitates reflection (19). Some educators observe that learners are aware of looming negatives even when discussing two to three points that are going well, which can create tension, similar to how the sandwich model can. Thus, another model can be used if the educator chooses not to employ Pendleton's Model.

22.8 THE ALOBA MODEL—AGENDA-LED OUTCOME-BASED ANALYSIS

Another model that educators find helpful is the ALOBA Model. ALOBA stands for Agenda-Led Outcome-Based Analysis. There are five steps to this process (14).

1. Learner is asked to reflect and identify their learning needs, objectives, and agenda for the feedback encounter.
2. Educator encourages the learner to self-assess, reflect on their situation, and problem-solve.
3. Educator reinforces theory-practice links and delivers descriptive and balanced feedback.
4. Educator and learner discuss suggestions and alternatives to reach the objectives and learning needs.
5. Educator checks feedback acceptance, provides a summary, and they agree on the action plan.

In this model, the learner sets the agenda. The learner provides a self-assessment, reflects on their situation, and does the problem-solving. The educator plays a role in discussing the theory-practice links and also offers descriptive and balanced feedback. There is a conversation and discussion between the learner and the educator. This way, together, they work to make progress toward the objectives and learning needs. In the end, the educator checks in with the learner and provides a summary of the session. Finally, the learner and educator agree on an action plan. This is a conversational model in which the learner leads.

22.8.1 "Ask-Tell-Ask" Approach

Sometimes, feedback is warranted in response to a specific situation that is alarming or concerning. This is usually something negative. In these situations, there is a three-step method that can be used, called "ask-tell-ask" (20). With "ask-tell-ask," the flow is clear. The educator initiates the first "ask" by asking the learner for a self-assessment of the specific situation. After the learner shares, it is the educator's turn to share, or "tell," the learner what they observed and what their assessment is. Finally, the educator performs a second "ask" and asks the learner if they have any questions. After the learner's questions are answered, the educator concludes the session by asking (not telling) the learner what the action plan is to address the issue raised. This is also meant to be a collaborative conversation seeking solutions and ways forward toward improvement.

22.8.2 Advocacy-Inquiry Technique

Another methodology for addressing concerning situations involving learners is the "Advocacy-Inquiry Technique" (21). This may be necessary if, for example, a medical student or resident recommends a beta-blocker for a patient with a blood pressure of 130/80 at their annual exam, without checking the records to determine their previous blood pressures and without repeating the blood pressure measurement. If the learner did not inquire about dietary salt intake or dietary patterns, this would also be cause for concern. With the "Advocacy-Inquiry Technique," the first step is to point out the problem or discrepancy with non-judgmental language and factual observations, such as "I noticed that you recommended a beta blocker for Patient X after measuring his blood pressure and getting one reading of 130/80." This first statement, the advocacy statement, is intended to be self-reflective and self-oriented, using phrases such as "I noted," "I saw," "I observed," or "I noticed." Then comes the inquiry. The inquiry requires an open-ended, nonjudgmental question such as "Can you tell me more about your decision process?" or "Can you help me understand your thinking?"

After the first two steps of inquiry and advocacy (the name of the feedback technique), there are two additional steps: identify and teach. For the identification step, listening is the skill to focus on. After asking an open-ended question to elicit clarification, listen carefully and quietly to determine where the decision-making, clinical reasoning, or thought process went awry. You must listen to identify.

Although it is tempting to tell the student what is wrong and why, and to talk the whole time, this will not likely help the student learn. Thus, the Advocacy-Inquiry Method is recommended. It is important to listen, not talk, during the identify step. The final step is to teach, and this is where talking comes back in.

After sharing observations, requesting an explanation of the rationale for the actions, and listening carefully to the response, the faculty member should formulate concrete teaching points in a nonjudgmental manner. The goal is to address the clinical or framework error to prevent recurrence and to ensure that the learner is confident that they can handle the situation differently next time. Providing an alternative, evidence-based method for handling the problem helps the learner understand how to work with another patient in a similar situation. Sharing articles, guidelines, or a chalk talk on the subject may be useful, depending on the situation. Focusing on a growth mindset where each mishap is an opportunity to learn and grow is key when there are concerning situations to address.

22.9 THE COACH APPROACH FOR FEEDBACK

In lifestyle medicine, clinicians are trained to collaborate and negotiate with patients to support behavior change across the six pillars of lifestyle medicine. Patients are often struggling with their exercise routine, eating patterns, sleep, stress management, social connections, or use of risky substances, and lifestyle medicine physicians use the COACH approach to hold conversations with patients. COACH is a mnemonic for curiosity, openness (nonjudgmental, without shame, blame, or guilt), appreciation (of any movement in a positive direction), compassion, and honesty. In some respects, the physician is providing feedback to the patient regarding their lifestyle. They often have the patient complete an assessment, such as the Lifestyle Behavior Health Scale, and then provide feedback on the results. This is an opportunity for a conversation, not a lecture.

The lifestyle medicine clinician expresses empathy, aligns motivation, builds confidence, sets SMART goals, and establishes accountability to empower the patient to change. This process is similar to the feedback methods recommended for faculty use with students. In lifestyle medicine, this is called the five-step collaboration cycle, as depicted in Figure 22.1 (22,23). The same five-step collaboration cycle can be used during feedback sessions for learners. As you can see, it aligns with many of the recommended frameworks published in the medical education literature.

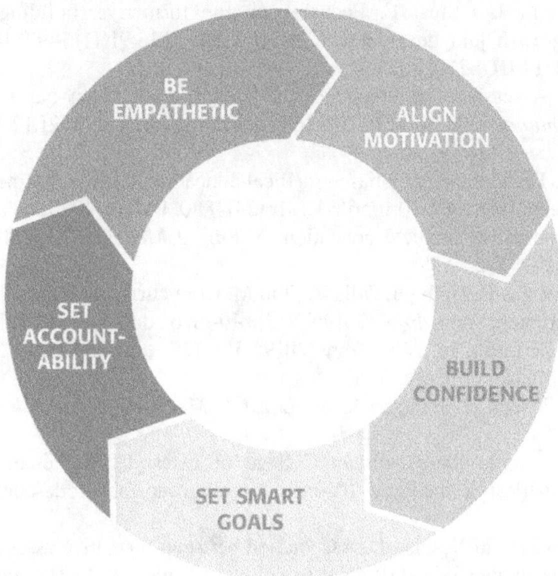

FIGURE 22.1 The five-step collaboration cycle for behavior change. (Used with permission from: Frates B, Bonnet JP, Joseph R, Peterson JA. *Lifestyle Medicine Handbook: An Introduction to the Power of Healthy Habits* (2nd ed). Monterey, CA: Healthy Learning, 2021.)

22.10 SUMMARY

Assessments are an integral part of education. Assessing learners is critical for successful teaching and learning. For medical students to become competent physicians, they must pass several summative assessments throughout their medical education. Using formative assessments is recommended, as these can help learners identify areas of strength and weakness, thereby enabling them to focus their attention on specific subjects or skills for improvement. Summative assessments are necessary for professional credentialing and standardization. Medical educators in medical schools and training programs can focus on formative assessments aligned with course objectives, as discussed in the next chapter. Formative assessments should be administered frequently and accompanied by specific, timely feedback.

Feedback is an essential part of medical education. It is often overlooked, but this does a disservice to students. To make the process of providing feedback easier for faculty, many educators have developed structures and frameworks to guide these important sessions. Examples of frameworks include the Sandwich Technique, the FIT and ABLE Model, the Pendleton Model, the ALOBA Model, the "Ask-Tell-Ask" Method, and the Advocacy-Inquiry Technique. Learning these models and practicing with them will help faculty select the framework that best suits their style. It takes time and practice to adopt behavior change as an educator.

In lifestyle medicine, behavior change and the COACH Approach are critical components of patient counseling. Using curiosity, openness (without judgment, shame, blame, or guilt), appreciation, compassion, and honesty, which are key elements of the COACH way of being, will also serve faculty well when delivering feedback to students. The same type of collaboration and conversation is necessary for a partnership to develop, based on trust and understanding, when counseling patients on behavior change and when counseling students on behavior change during feedback sessions.

REFERENCES

1. Lipnevich AA, Mattern K, Feddock C. Formative assessment and feedback in medical education: a practical guide: AMEE guide No. 189. *Med Teach.* 2025:1–20. doi: 10.1080/0142159X.2025.2569623. Epub ahead of print. PMID: 41134874.

2. Konopasek L, Norcini J, Krupat E. Focusing on the formative: building an assessment system aimed at student growth and development. *Acad Med.* 2016;91(11):1492–1497. doi: 10.1097/ACM.0000000000001171. PMID: 27028028.
3. Lee GB, Chiu AM. Assessment and feedback methods in competency-based medical education. *Ann Allergy Asthma Immunol.* 2022;128(3):256–262. doi: 10.1016/j.anai.2021.12.010. Epub 2021 Dec 17. PMID: 34929390.
4. Cooper D, Holmboe ES. Competency-based medical education at the front lines of patient care. *N Engl J Med.* 2025;393(4):376–388. doi: 10.1056/NEJMra2411880. PMID: 40700689.
5. Epstein RM. Assessment in medical education. *N Engl J Med.* 2007;356(4):387–396. doi: 10.1056/NEJMra054784. PMID: 17251535.
6. Safdieh JE, Govindarajan R, Gelb DJ, Odia Y, Soni M. Core curriculum guidelines for a required clinical neurology experience. *Neurology.* 2019;92(13):619–626. doi: 10.1212/WNL.0000000000007187. Epub 2019 Feb 22. Erratum in: *Neurology.* 2019;93(3):135. doi: 10.1212/WNL.0000000000007481. PMID: 30796141; PMCID: PMC6453766.
7. Frates B, Bonnet J, Joseph R, Peterson J. *The Lifestyle Medicine Handbook* (2nd ed). Monterey, CA: Healthy Learning, 2021.
8. LM 101 Curriculum from the American College of Lifestyle Medicine. https://learning.lifestylemedicine.org/content/lifestyle-medicine-101-curriculum#group-tabs-node-course-default3. Accessed November 8, 2025.
9. Zhu T, Liang J, Mao M, Liu X, Qian D. Association between formative assessment and academic performance for undergraduate medical students in a chinese clinical skills training course. *Med Sci Monit.* 2021;27:e929068. doi: 10.12659/MSM.929068. PMID: 33484506; PMCID: PMC7839276.
10. McGrady A, Badenhop D, Lynch D. Effects of a lifestyle medicine elective on self-care behaviors in preclinical medical students. *Appl Psychophysiol Biofeedback.* 2019;44(2):143–149.
11. Barss P, Grivna M, Al-Maskari F, Kershaw G. Strengthening public health medicine training for medical students: development and evaluation of a lifestyle curriculum. *Med Teach.* 2008;30(9–10): e196–e218. doi: 10.1080/01421590802334267. PMID: 19117217.
12. Pangalangan J, Puma J, Tollefson M, Frates B. Development and psychometric evaluation of the lifestyle medicine health behavior scale. *Am J Lifestyle Med.* 2024:15598276241280207
13. Frederickson BL. *Positivity: Top-Notch Research Reveals the 3-to-1-Ratio That Will Change Your Life.* New York: Three Rivers Press, 2009.
14. Orsini C, Rodrigues V, Tricio J, Rosel M. Common models and approaches for the clinical educator to plan effective feedback encounters. *J Educ Eval Health Prof.* 2022;19:35. doi: 10.3352/jeehp.2022.19.35. Epub 2022 Dec 19. PMID: 36537186; PMCID: PMC9842479.
15. Dweck CS. *Mindset: The New Psychology of Success—How We Can Learn to Fulfill Our Potential* (Updated ed). New York: Ballantine Books, 2016.
16. Beckman TJ, Lee MC. Proposal for a collaborative approach to clinical teaching. *Mayo Clin Proc.* 2009;84(4):339–344.
17. van de Ridder JMM. Pendleton's rules: a mini review of a feedback method. *Am J Biomed Sci Res.* 2023;19(1):19–21. doi: 10.34297/AJBSR.2023.19.002542.
18. Pendleton D, Schofield T, Tate P, Havelock P. *The New Consultation: Developing Doctor-Patient Communication.* Oxford: Oxford University Press, 2003.
19. Burgess A, van Diggele C, Roberts C, Mellis C. Feedback in the clinical setting. *BMC Med Educ.* 2020;20(Suppl 2):460. doi: 10.1186/s12909-020-02280-5. PMID: 33272265; PMCID: PMC7712594.
20. Lee GB, Chiu AM. Assessment and feedback methods in competency-based medical education. *Ann Allergy Asthma Immunol.* 2022;128(3):256–262. doi: 10.1016/j.anai.2021.12.010. Epub 2021 Dec 17. PMID: 34929390.
21. Castillo AY, Chan JD, Lynch JB, Bryson-Cahn C. How to disagree better: utilizing advocacy-inquiry techniques to improve communication and spur behavior change. *Antimicrob Steward Healthc Epidemiol.* 2023;3(1):e201. doi: 10.1017/ash.2023.457. PMID: 38028895; PMCID: PMC10654947.
22. Frates EP, Bonnet J. Collaboration and negotiation: the key to therapeutic lifestyle change. *Am J Lifestyle Med.* 2016;10(5):302–312. doi: 10.1177/1559827616638013. PMID: 30202286; PMCID: PMC6125074.
23. Frates EP, Moore MA, Lopez CN, McMahon GT. Coaching for behavior change in physiatry. *Am J Phys Med Rehabil.* 2011;90(12):1074–1082. doi: 10.1097/PHM.0b013e31822dea9a. PMID: 22019966.

23 Developing and Designing Lifestyle Medicine Courses with Objectives and Goals

23.1 DEVELOPING AND DESIGNING COURSES

Depending on the medical school, the process of course development, proposal submission, proposal acceptance, and course delivery can take months to a year or longer. The curriculum committee has many responsibilities. Reviewing proposals for new core curriculum courses or electives is only one of their responsibilities. In addition, they review course content, manage course feedback, oversee assessments, promote the integration of basic science, clinical skills, and professionalism, and ensure compliance with accreditation standards and requirements set by governing bodies, including the Liaison Committee on Medical Education (LCME). For example, if a school has a lifestyle medicine theme or thread and is integrating lifestyle medicine into the curriculum, the curriculum committee oversees this process. Lastly, they need to work on continual improvements and adjustments in response to students, standards, and science. The medical school's curriculum committee is busy. When a faculty member is considering a proposal for a new course, it is essential to carefully consider the process in order to avoid wasting time: the curriculum committee's time or the faculty member's time. Time is our most precious commodity.

To use time wisely, medical faculty should familiarize themselves with the course proposal process. In general, there are eight steps with specific focal points: identifying a clear need for the course; proposal preparation; stakeholder support; submission and review; the revision process; launch preparation; student assessments and course evaluation; and, lastly, iterative improvements year after year.

1. *Identify the Gap and Need*: Map the current curriculum to determine the time currently allocated to the proposed subject. Ensure the proposed topic aligns with the school's educational goals and competencies by explicitly mapping the course content to the school's priorities and competencies. Demonstrate the gap in the current curriculum and clearly state its importance. Connect the gap to a need or needs. Make the case that the school and the students need the proposed course information using medical education research or statistics. Connect the course topic to the institutional priorities and to the LCME's requirements and expectations. The students' voices carry weight. A focus group of students can provide important perspectives for the committee to consider.
2. *Prepare a Proposal Draft*: Prepare a detailed proposal that includes all the necessary elements, including course title and description; objectives and learning outcomes (to be reviewed in this chapter) in alignment with core competencies (to be examined in this chapter) and priorities of the institution; content overview and course syllabus; teaching method description (reviewed in Chapter 21); materials and resources required; assessments for the students (reviewed in Chapter 22); evaluation of the course (to be examined in this chapter); and a plan for redesign or revisions.
3. *Obtain Stakeholder Support*: Share a draft of the proposal with relevant department faculty members, curriculum committee members, and student leaders for initial review and feedback. Speaking with faculty and students and gathering their feedback will support the

DOI: 10.1201/9781003630043-23

proposal process and help publicize the possibility of offering this new course in the near future. This can increase interest in the material and topic of focus.

4. *Submission of the Proposal and Review by the Curriculum Committee or a Subcommittee, Such as the Subcommittee on Electives*: Once complete, the faculty member formally submits the final draft of the proposal. Then, members of the curriculum committee, subcommittee, and/or academic councils carefully evaluate the proposal. They assess the proposal's educational value and rigor, feasibility, alignment with core competencies, and importance with regard to institutional and national needs. These committees usually meet at a cadence of about once a month, which can extend the proposal process to several months, given the back-and-forth often required.
5. *Revision Process*: Based on feedback, faculty may need to revise the proposal. The curriculum committee may have questions, require explanations, and request specific revisions for subsequent reviews. A proposal may undergo multiple resubmissions and revisions. The curriculum committee may evaluate the proposal several times before final approval. Some proposals do not reach the stage of final approval. In that case, the only option is to reconsider the strategy by considering a new course title, different content, a fresh design with varied teaching methods, and returning to step one to ensure the course meets a high value need.
6. *Final Approval and Launch Preparation*: If the course is approved, it is added to the official curriculum, and implementation is planned, including scheduling, faculty assignment, and resource allocation. Some faculty forget to advocate for compensation for their time in preparing and delivering the course. This is critical to consider if the course is going to be sustainable over time. People need compensation for their work, including medical educators. If the course is an elective, the faculty member should help market the course by speaking with medical students they know through school activities, research projects, other courses, or interest groups such as the lifestyle medicine interest group. Just because an elective is approved does not mean that students will enroll in it. It is critical to market the new elective. Faculty can also connect with colleagues who teach in the core curriculum or other electives to determine whether they are willing to make announcements about the new course, particularly if the elective's topic aligns with the current course. If the course is required, no marketing or extra effort is needed.
7. *Evaluation with Assessments and Feedback*: Collect data to inform ongoing improvements. The proposal included a description of assessment strategies for measuring student success, learning, and growth in the course. Assessments are formative and summative, as discussed in Chapter 22. Selecting or crafting the assessment tools to make sure they align with course objectives and student development is key. Without formal assessments, it is difficult to track the student's progress or the value of the course. Giving feedback to the students is critical and was covered in Chapter 22. Getting feedback on the course from the students—their evaluation of the course—is an integral part of course delivery, as it forms the next iteration of the course, if it is approved to run again. This type of evaluation is discussed later in the current chapter. Evaluation of the course also informs medical education research and advances the field.
8. *Revisions and Updates*: Each year, the teaching faculty should review the objectives and reevaluate their alignment with core competencies. They should make any adjustments that reflect updated research findings and the latest science. If the institution's priorities have changed, they need to take them into account. For example, in 2025, many medical schools began discussions about when and how to incorporate Artificial Intelligence (AI) into healthcare. Course faculty may need to add an objective on AI in future iterations, particularly if students request this information in their evaluations.

When developing a course, it is recommended that faculty discuss their ideas with a seasoned faculty member who has already undergone the process at the same institution. The steps covered are general steps and not specific to any institution. Each institution will have its own standardized, formal process. Meeting with a member of the curriculum committee before preparing a course proposal is ideal; the sooner, the better. Faculty want to provide excellent courses for their students. This is why there is a formalized, lengthy proposal review process for new courses in the core curriculum or as electives. The course developer and the curriculum committee share the same goal: educating the next generation of physicians to be outstanding clinicians, educators, and researchers.

Prior to developing a course proposal, reviewing various models of course development will be beneficial. In this chapter, Kern's Six-Step Approach, the Tyler Model, and Backward Design are highlighted.

23.2 KERN'S SIX-STEP APPROACH FOR DEVELOPING COURSES AND CURRICULA IN MEDICAL EDUCATION

Kern's Six-Step Approach for developing courses and curricula in medical education was first published in 1998 (1). Over a quarter of a century later, Kern's Six-Step Approach is still utilized successfully in medical school curricula in a variety of areas, including online medical school curricula (2), integrating health systems science into medical school curricula (3), and implementing basic science in a cardiology clerkship (4). The six steps are outlined in Table 23.1. They are similar to the eight steps for proposing a new course at a medical school presented earlier in this chapter.

Understanding Kern's Six-Step Approach and working through each step will help medical school faculty be successful in their educational efforts at all stages of training. A review of the steps as they may apply to a lifestyle medicine course follows.

This book highlights the lack of emphasis on lifestyle medicine in medical school curricula. That is step 1 in Kern's approach: problem identification and general needs assessment. Each medical school must conduct its own targeted needs assessment, as discussed earlier in this chapter in the section on course proposals. That's step 2 in Kern's six-step approach: perform a targeted needs assessment. There is no one-size-fits-all approach for curricula. Each school, each residency, and each institution will need its own needs assessment. Mapping lifestyle medicine to the school's curriculum will identify which of the six pillars and behavior change topics are covered and in which courses they are covered, thereby informing a needs assessment for lifestyle medicine courses.

Creating course objectives and goals is one of the most crucial steps in developing and designing curricula, courses, classes, workshops, presentations, or lectures. That is Step 3, and it will be addressed in greater detail in the next section of this chapter. Bloom's Taxonomy and the SMART goal framework will be helpful to faculty in crafting objectives and goals, both of which are required for any CME talk. Most educators give CME talks and are familiar with this task. Rather than dreading it, this task can be viewed as the key step toward a successful talk. This can happen if the faculty member has a framework to work with and an understanding of the power of objectives.

Step 4 in Kern's Six-Step Approach is identifying which educational strategies to employ in the course. Examples of educational strategies were reviewed in Chapter 21, "Teaching Strategies

TABLE 23.1
Kern's Six-Step Approach for Developing Courses and Curricula in Medical Education

1. Problem identification and general needs assessment
2. Targeted needs assessment
3. Goals and objectives
4. Educational strategies
5. Implementation
6. Evaluation and feedback

for Lifestyle Medicine Education." One of the most important concepts to keep in mind during this step is that engagement is the primary goal. Relaying information is not the primary goal, although many faculty members were trained and attended medical school when instruction was passive—essentially a transfer of information from faculty to students. Teaching is so much more than that.

Step 5 is often the most intimidating but can also be the most rewarding. It is the implementation step. Chapter 20 presents numerous examples of implementing lifestyle medicine education in medical schools, drawn from programs across the country and including input from a wide range of faculty members. Step 5 will also be discussed in this chapter using a different example: a lifestyle medicine master's and bachelor's course at Harvard Extension School.

The final step in Kern's Six-Step Approach addresses evaluation and feedback. This topic is discussed in greater detail later in this chapter, with an emphasis on the Kirkpatrick levels for evaluating medical school courses. This book is designed to help readers successfully follow each of these six steps.

23.3 TYLER'S BASIC PRINCIPLES OF CURRICULUM AND INSTRUCTION

Kern's Six-Step Approach is not the only curriculum methodology that medical educators consider when creating courses, nor is it the oldest. There is also the work of Ralph W. Tyler, who wrote the book *Basic Principles of Curriculum and Instruction* in 1949 (5).

Here are the four guiding questions that Tyler proposed (6).

1. What educational purposes should the school seek to attain?
2. What educational experiences can be provided that are likely to attain these purposes?
3. How can these educational experiences be effectively organized?
4. How can we determine whether these purposes are being attained?

This methodology asks the medical educator to consider what educational purposes the school should seek. This is a broad overview of education. This question asks the faculty member to consider the school's purpose. For medical schools, the overarching purpose is to train medical students to become competent, compassionate physicians in the 21st century. This is the time to reflect on how the purpose of medical education has remained constant over the years and how it has shifted to meet the needs of the current generation and the current disease burden of the patient population. There may be multiple purposes guiding a school, not just one.

Purpose can also be understood as goals, although they are not identical. Merriam-Webster online dictionary defines purpose as "the reason something is done or used" (https://www.merriam-webster.com/dictionary/purpose). It defines a goal as "the end toward which effort is directed" (https://www.merriam-webster.com/dictionary/goal). You need to know the reason why something is going to be done. As with a needs assessment, one seeks to determine the gap or need that a program or course addresses. What does the world of medical education need? Then, the goals align with this need and purpose. What are the medical school's intended outcomes?

The second question the Tyler Method asks is: What educational experiences will the school provide to students to attain this purpose or these purposes? This is akin to identifying teaching strategies to achieve a course's objectives. Will the course be a hands-on workshop, a flipped classroom with application activities planned for the in-person session, a debate-based session, or a role-playing session? Will simulation be utilized? Will the class revolve around a patient case? Will a patient join the live class? The aim is to make the educational experiences engaging and interactive for medical school students, as described in Chapter 21.

Once brainstorming a list of possible educational experiences is complete, the next step is to organize it. This is question 3 in the Tyler Method. An organization or strategy is required to create and deliver successful, impactful educational experiences. It is not enough to list several engaging educational experiences. The experiences need to be planned and organized to achieve the purpose of building the course in the first place (question 1). In what order will the educational experiences flow? Will the first week focus on the flipped classroom material, with debates and discussions to enhance interaction and engagement? Whether motivational interviewing works in the hospital setting with acute care is a debatable question, and students would need to consult the medical literature to identify research supporting or refuting this claim.

Once a baseline level of knowledge on the topic, such as motivational interviewing, is established, role-playing may be a strategic educational experience to employ with medical students. After role-playing, a simulation lab could be used with actors who have chronic conditions and are working to change their lifestyles. When would be an appropriate time for a real patient to share their experience of behavior change, with a focus on their conversations with a physician who used motivational interviewing? All of this takes careful planning and organization. This example demonstrates that sequencing educational experiences and identifying the flow of interactive activities are crucial to course design.

Lastly, in Tyler's four-step methodology, the fourth step is to determine whether the purposes were successfully achieved or the goals were attained. This is similar to the evaluation and assessment step in Kern's Six-Step Approach. Identifying which surveys students will complete before and after class, or which skills assessment will be employed using an OSCE or another methodology, is the focus of this final step. Which level of Kirkpatrick's model is being assessed: students' reactions to the material; their learning of facts, skills, or concepts; their behavior—personally or professionally—using the skills and knowledge gained in the clinical setting; or results, such as patient outcomes? Did the course affect how students care for patients and, in turn, patients' outcomes? As mentioned earlier, the Kirkpatrick model is reviewed in detail later in this chapter.

Over the years, there has been some criticism of Tyler's Model (7). In 2024, in the World Journal of Arts, Education, and Literature, the authors wrote, "While recognizing Tyler's vital contributions, the article criticizes the limitations of the model, particularly its descriptive nature, which can limit creativity, adaptability, and inclusion of diverse student needs" (7). Tyler's model, like many models created 75 years ago, has limitations. It is vital to evaluate current world events and adapt models to the needs of diverse student bodies, with creativity and an open-minded approach. As the article acknowledges, global interconnectedness, technological advances such as artificial intelligence, and an emphasis on critical thinking skills must be considered when developing new courses; many existing frameworks were not designed to address these areas (7). Some aspects of the Tyler Model still hold, including "the importance of clear objectives, systematic design, and measurable outcomes in program planning" (7).

23.4 BACKWARD DESIGN

To begin, educators are advised to start at the end. This is backward design, not backward thinking. It is actually forward-thinking. As Kern's Six-Step Approach suggests, after identifying the need, medical educators jump to goals and objectives. Tyler's Method also begins by questioning the purpose or goal the school seeks to achieve. Educators should begin by considering the end goals. As Stephen R. Covey says, "Begin with the end in mind." This is his second habit for highly effective people, as outlined in *The 7 Habits of Highly Effective People: Powerful Lessons in Personal Change* (8).

Backward design has been on the minds of educators since 1998, with the publication of Understanding by Design by Grant Wiggins and Jay McTighe, published by the Association for Supervision and Curriculum Development (9). This book was updated into its second edition in 2005 (10). The concept of backward design was introduced in the book *Understanding by Design*. This concept has been described in the medical education literature as early as 2006 with the article,

"Backward course design: making the end the beginning" (11). The steps for backward design were described in that article as:

1. Identify the desired results
2. Determine the acceptable evidence
3. Plan learning experiences and instruction

In this model, outcomes come first by identifying the desired results. The next step is similar to showing competency or determining how to assess proof that the desired result was achieved. After those two steps, the educator can begin building their instructional plan and determining the teaching strategies to use, the third and final step in backward design.

Many educators begin with only the beginning in mind. They rush to create a PowerPoint on a topic to share their information, experience, and wisdom, without clearly identifying the course objectives and how the slides will align with them. They may invite colleagues to present on specific topics, but neglect to share the course's overall goals with that guest speaker and to instruct the faculty on the main purpose of inviting them to lecture in the course. In addition, faculty are often excited to bring a patient to class to share their story because students love interacting with patients. However, faculty may fail to consider how the session fits within the course's overall objectives and, in some cases, may not even plan any goals or objectives for the session when the patient is sharing his or her story.

There are various frameworks for implementing backward design in course development. One example of such a framework is Understanding by Design (UbD). Newell and colleagues shared 12 tips for using Understanding by Design in an article published in Medical Teacher (12). Their twelve tips are shared here as a direct quote. These are good to keep in mind.

"1. **Conceptualize 'understanding' in the UbD context.**
   ('Understandings' are demonstrations of outcomes, not regurgitations of facts.)
2. **Start with big ideas to identify and prioritize key understandings.**
3. **Differentiate between outcomes and objectives and identify the need for your context.**
   (Formulate measurable learner outcomes. Think of objectives as course goals and outcomes as goals for the learner, specifically.)
4. **Invest in the process and give yourself time to develop quality outcomes.**
5. **Keep outcomes in mind as you prepare for assessment development.**
   (Think of assessments as tools for learning and focus on progress toward competencies.)
6. **Think beyond standard approaches when designing assessments.**
7. **Embrace active and learner-centered approaches at the right time in the planning process.**
   (Instead of jumping to determine which engaging teaching strategies, like role playing, an instructor wants to use, it's best to figure out the learner outcomes and assessments first, and then focus on the active and learner-centered approaches.)
8. **Understand your educational culture and prepare for resistance.**
9. **Select appropriate stakeholders to optimize buy-in.**
   (Including students early in the process is helpful, and representation from a variety of faculty at different stages of their careers is also useful.)
10. **Create a safe environment for experimentation and setbacks.**
   (Feedback from peers and learners is important in the development of courses, and in order for people to give and receive constructive criticism, there must be a sense of trust and non-judgment in the group.)
11. **Effective UbD implementation requires educator development.**
12. **Foster a Continuous Quality Improvement (CQI) mindset.**"

Two other educational frameworks that will help medical educators develop compelling, well-designed courses in lifestyle medicine include the Four-Dimensional Curriculum Framework (4DF) and the 3P-6C toolkit (13). Educational frameworks are helpful as they provide guidance and step-by-step instruction for faculty, new and experienced, to adapt curricula and integrate new topics.

The Four-Dimensional Curriculum Framework (4DF) is particularly useful for lifestyle medicine, as it accounts for instruction for a variety of healthcare professional learners, not just physicians. Lifestyle medicine is practiced by physicians, nurses, registered dietitians, physical therapists, mental health therapists, and advanced practice practitioners/providers. Education efforts in lifestyle medicine need to take this into account (14). Because a variety of healthcare professionals are involved in the practice of lifestyle medicine, it is often described as a "team sport." This may impact how curricula are developed in some schools. Thus, the 4DF is a framework that lifestyle medicine educators need to be familiar with (15). As outlined in an article by Steketee and colleagues, the four dimensions are: Dimension 1 is a focus on the future of healthcare and the clinical practice of medicine; Dimension 2 has a focus on professionalism, including professional values, attitudes, and standards, as well as the acquisition of knowledge and skills necessary for the practice of medicine; Dimension 3 considers the competencies and capabilities required to practice medicine successfully as healthcare evolves and patient needs shift successfully; and Dimension 4 takes into account the larger systems involved with education, including organizational governance and administrative processes required for course development and delivery (15).

The 3P-6C framework is useful for lifestyle medicine faculty at medical schools. As the authors of the paper point out, "A substantial shift in thinking is therefore required from conceiving of a curriculum as a single mechanical entity that can be 'fixed' by attending to individual elements toward understanding the ecology of how various intersecting and interrelating curricular components impact a learner's trajectory from *being* an individual student to *becoming* a member of a community of practice" (16). The 3P-6C framework is about becoming a member of a community of practice, which is essential for all healthcare professionals. The 3Ps are personal, program, and practice. There are 6Cs for the program piece and 3Cs for the personal and practice piece: the 6Cs for the program are commands, contextualization, coordination, collections, collations, and connections; the 3Cs for personal are content, cognition, and confirmation; and the 3Cs for practice are calibration, collaboration, and continuous development (16).

For medical school educators, regardless of the course design framework employed, developing objectives, outcomes, and goals is a critical component of the process. Spending time on course objectives is time well spent. This is the topic of the next section of the chapter.

23.5 IMPORTANCE OF COURSE OBJECTIVES USING BLOOM'S TAXONOMY

23.5.1 Bloom's Taxonomy Is an Excellent Tool to Use for Determining Course Objectives

In 1956, Benjamin Bloom and colleagues, including Max Engelhart, Edward Furst, Walter Hill, and David Krathwohl (a name that will come up again shortly), published the original Bloom's Taxonomy in a book titled *Taxonomy of Educational Objectives: Handbook I* (17), Cognitive Domain. This original pyramid was helpful for educators in crafting course objectives using the hierarchy of six cognitive domains: knowledge, comprehension, application, analysis, synthesis, and evaluation. The levels were labeled with nouns. Each level had corresponding verbs for crafting course objectives, and this approach was applied across all levels, K-12 and college.

There are cognitive domains, psychomotor domains, and affective domains in Bloom's Taxonomy, as noted in Figure 23.1. Most people only mention the cognitive domain.

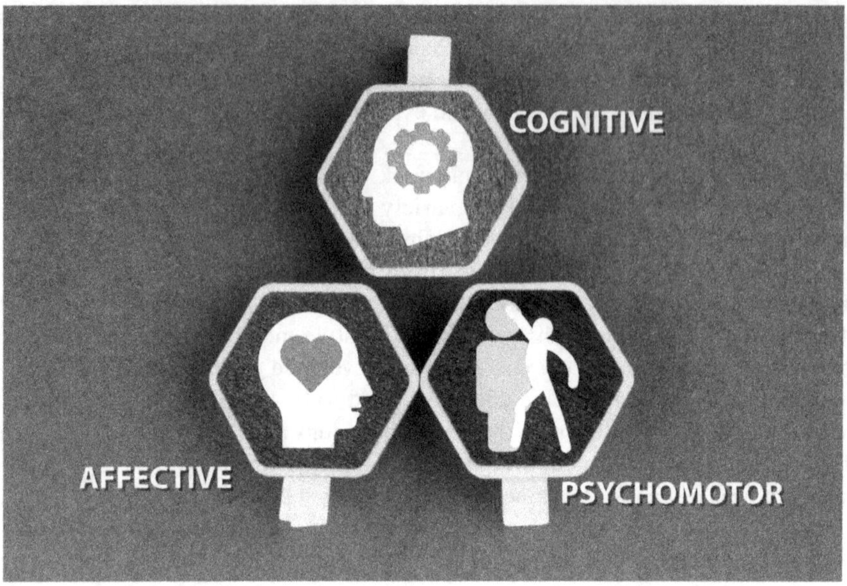

FIGURE 23.1 The three domains described in Bloom's Taxonomy.

Shutterstock Asset ID; 2521738159

Cognitive objectives are the main focus in many academic programs. Considering the psychomotor and affective domains in medical education is useful. For example, courses focused on surgical skills (18) and emergency medicine skills (19) can draw on Bloom's Taxonomy in the Psychomotor and Cognitive Domains. Physical exam skills and other procedures may also fall into the psychomotor domain. Figure 23.2 shares a depiction of a pyramid for Bloom's Taxonomy in the psychomotor domain.

The pyramid starts from the most basic and progresses to the more complex. Descriptions of each level of the pyramid are provided below (20):

1. *Perception*: Having a basic sensory awareness, using sensory cues to guide movements.
2. *Set*: Being ready to act physically and mentally.
3. *Guided Response*: An early stage of learning a skill or procedure, progressing through initial performance with guidance.
4. *Mechanism*: Progressing in skill development, increasing proficiency, intermediate stage of learning a skill or procedure, able to follow a series of predetermined steps independently.
5. *Complex Overt Response*: The skilled and coordinated performance of complex maneuvers independently.
6. *Adaptation*: The ability to modify and adapt steps of a procedure or skill to respond to real-time situations, and unforeseen complexities.
7. *Origination*: Creating new procedures or maneuvers independently, using highly developed skills to address a specific situation.

Concerning the Affective Domain in Bloom's Taxonomy, Figure 23.3 depicts the different levels. The affective domain is often used to address students' attitudes, values, and beliefs, as well as the actions and behaviors that stem from them.

For courses focused on professionalism and topics such as expressing empathy or reducing bias and stigma (21), the affective domain is helpful. For example, in lifestyle medicine, courses that

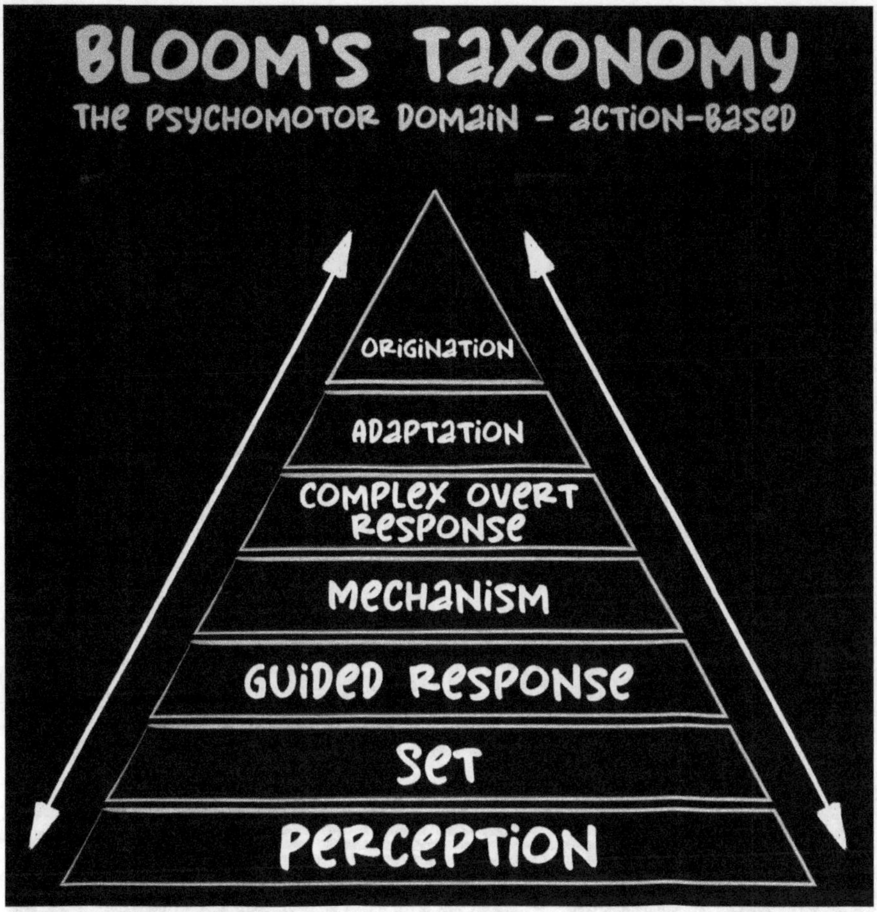

FIGURE 23.2 Bloom's Taxonomy and the psychomotor domain.

Shutterstock Asset ID: 2379801373

teach the COACH Approach and counsel patients on behavior change may include objectives from Bloom's Taxonomy's Affective Domain. The different levels are described below (22,23):

1. *Receiving*: Being open to new experiences and receiving novel information and stimuli.
2. *Responding*: Actively participating and reacting to information and experiences by naming responses and emotions and reflecting in a journal or discussion.
3. *Valuing*: Evaluating and attaching worth or value to a particular concept, behavior, or approach that was recently learned.
4. *Organization*: Adopting, comparing, integrating, organizing, and prioritizing new values, allowing for the synthesis of a new perspective.
5. *Characterization*: Internalizing values to the extent that they influence behavior and decision-making and become part of a person's character.

The Cognitive Domain is the one most commonly used in medical education. In 2001, Bloom's Taxonomy Cognitive Domain was updated by one of the original authors and collaborators of Benjamin Bloom, David Krathwohl (24). David Krathwohl worked with Lorin Anderson to revise the 1956 version of Bloom's Taxonomy. They labeled the levels with verbs rather than nouns and reordered the levels, specifically switching synthesis and evaluation so that synthesis was at the top, considered the highest order. They also changed the term synthesis, not to the verb synthesizing but

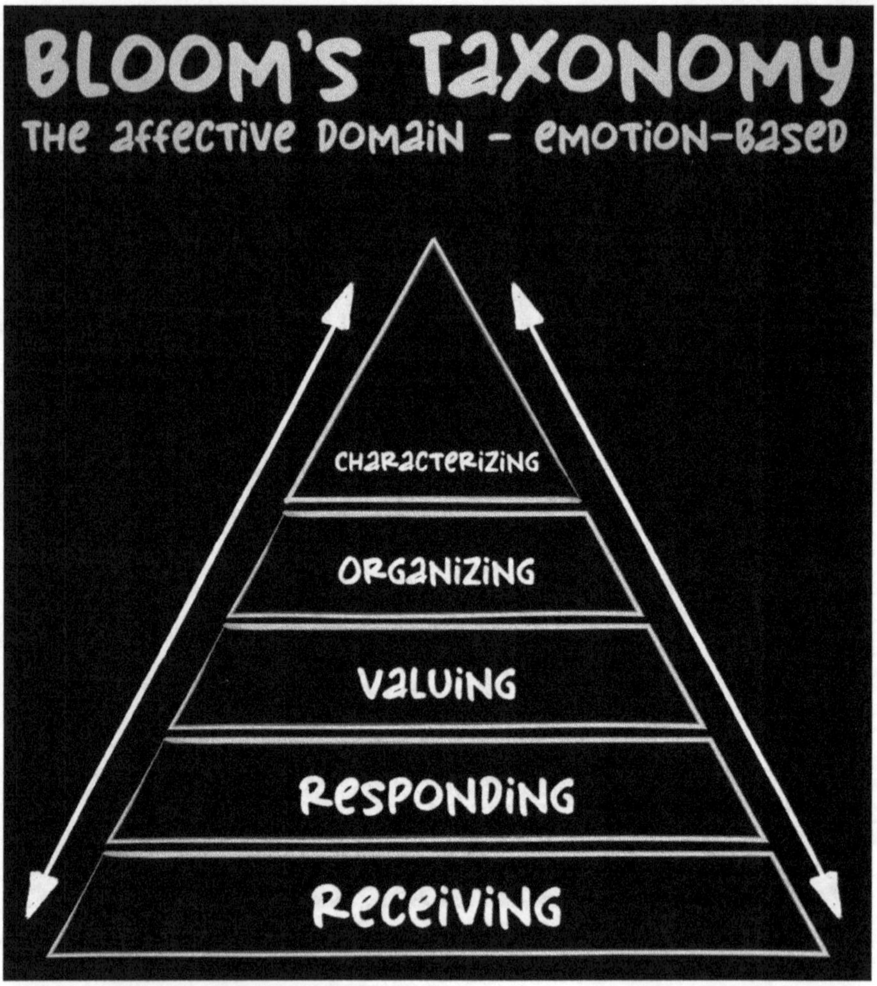

FIGURE 23.3 Bloom's Taxonomy and the affective domain.
Shutterstock Asset ID: 2379453519

to the verb creating. With the new verb nomenclature, evaluating is one step lower than creating, which is the highest order. This is shown in Figure 23.4.

Using the 2001 version of the original taxonomy created by Benjamin Bloom in 1956 can help faculty better plan their goals for the course and what they want learners to know, how they want them to learn, and what application activities they will incorporate to help learners reach the higher-order learning objectives, like applying, analyzing, evaluating, and creating (Figure 23.5) (25–27).

Recall of facts is covered under the first level of Bloom's Taxonomy. The verbs used at the first level of Bloom's Taxonomy to create learning objectives include list, memorize, define, duplicate, repeat, and state. There are many facts that a medical student must memorize to become a competent physician and to pass the United States Medical Licensing Examination (USMLE) exams for licensure. Identifying essential facts that students need to know is a vital role for faculty. Memorizing everything is neither possible nor helpful.

In the age of online information and artificial intelligence, one could argue that a physician no longer needs to memorize all these facts. But that is not entirely accurate. There are specific facts that physicians need to know off the top of their heads, especially in emergencies when time is of the essence. For example, knowing the causes of shortness of breath that are deadly, such as heart attack, heart failure, pneumothorax, airway obstruction, respiratory failure, acute trauma, or

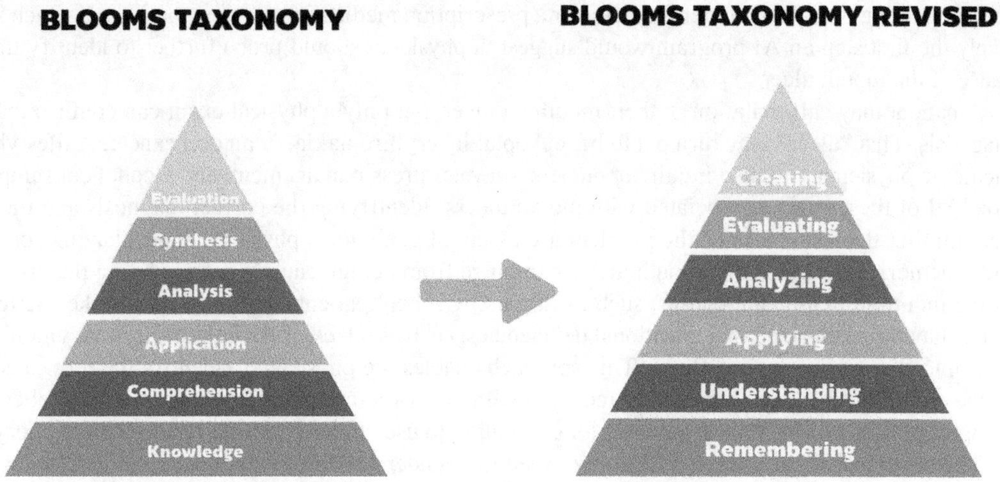

FIGURE 23.4 The original Bloom's Taxonomy compared to the updated 2001 version.

Shutterstock Asset ID: 2122194074

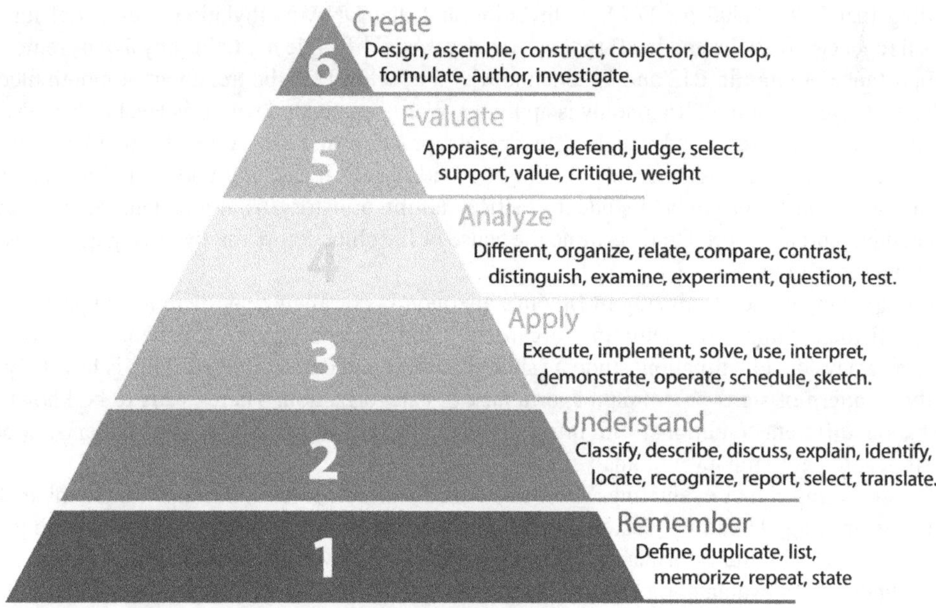

FIGURE 23.5 Verbs associated with the different levels of Bloom's Taxonomy.

Shutterstock Asset ID: 2401212047

overdoses of medications or risky substances, is information that all practicing physicians need to know because by the time someone puts a potentially deadly case scenario into an artificial intelligence site, the patient may take their last breath. The sooner the physician determines the cause of the shortness of breath, the better.

In lifestyle medicine, knowing that someone is vegan and reports mouth ulcers will prompt probing questions, such as, "Are you taking a multivitamin with B12, using nutritional yeast in your food or paying attention to how much vitamin B12 you are consuming from fortified foods like plant-based milks, cereals, and soy products?" Recalling that certain foods are sources of B12 and recognizing that someone who recently adopted a vegan diet may be at risk of B12 deficiency will be helpful when listening to the patient's chief complaint of mouth ulcers. Instead of merely recommending over-the-counter medicine or a prescription medication for the mouth sore, which is likely the first step an AI program would suggest, a physician should probe further to identify the cause of the mouth ulcer.

A patient may call irritation in their mouth an ulcer, but only a physical exam can confirm that diagnosis. That "ulcer" may turn out to be leukoplakia, erythroplakia, or an oral cancer. A lifestyle medicine physician will also inquire about stress levels, stress management, and alcohol consumption. All of these can be associated with mouth ulcers. Identifying the correct diagnosis and then determining the root cause of the problem are essential goals for a physician. Thus, having some facts memorized, such as that mouth ulcers can range from benign causes, such as biting the inside of the mouth, to malignant causes, such as tumors, will help patients and physicians alike. Better still is having memorized that nutritional deficiencies, such as a lack of B vitamins, iron, or vitamin C, can lead to benign mouth ulcers. This approach enables the physician to identify the root cause of the mouth ulcer rather than merely recommending over-the-counter gels or ointments to relieve symptoms. This is one of the arguments for continuing to use objectives in the recall-facts category.

The next level of the Bloom Taxonomy pyramid is understanding. Words used in this category include describe, discuss, explain, paraphrase, identify, recognize, translate, and summarize. For example, describe why vitamin B12 is a factor contributing to mouth ulcers, especially those that will not heal. In research, a drop in B12 has been correlated with a drop in DNA methylation (28). A lack of DNA methylation has been associated with reduced oral mucosal regeneration (29). Recalling that B12 is vital for DNA methylation and that DNA methylation is essential for oral mucosal regeneration helps medical students, residents, and lifestyle medicine physicians remember the importance of vitamin B12 and understand why it is helpful for the treatment of mouth ulcers.

The next level in Bloom's Taxonomy is applying. Words associated with this level of the pyramid include implement, execute, solve, calculate, operate, practice, and use. At this level of learning and teaching, the student and teacher are working beyond instant recall and understanding. They are working on "doing." For apply, a student practices taking a history from a patient (actor, peer, or simulated patient) and works to determine the cause of the chief complaint by asking questions and examining the patient.

After applying comes analyzing in Bloom's Taxonomy. For analyzing, there is comparing, contrasting, distinguishing, differentiating, organizing, and categorizing. In a patient case, after the history and physical examination, students should analyze the data collected. This is how they can identify a pattern of signs or symptoms, or a lack of categorization. There needs to be knowledge stored about different conditions, with information on the typical presentations by patients, in order for a student to get to the level of analyzing.

After analyzing comes evaluating. Verbs associated with this level in Bloom's Taxonomy include appraising, arguing, defending, debating, judging, selecting, valuing, critiquing, and weighing. The student sorts through the information from the history and physical exam, analyzes the data, and then evaluates it. To evaluate, the student assesses all possibilities, weighs the pros and cons of different interventions, appraises the options, makes judgment calls, and selects specific medications, procedures, and lifestyle medicine pillars as treatments for the chronic conditions. This evaluation requires extensive knowledge, experience, and understanding of the human body and pathology.

The last level of Bloom's Taxonomy is creating. The verbs at this level include constructing, formulating, investigating, inventing, generating, authoring, composing, assembling, developing, and designing. In medicine, this can involve building a treatment plan for a cancer patient in collaboration with the medical team and the patient, using shared decision-making, or creating a research study or a new protocol for the management of a disease. It could be writing a review article on a topic of interest or generating a new model or framework for patient communication and collaboration. Creating requires proficiency in a specific area and expertise, enabling the formulation and implementation of novel ideas. To get to creating, one must have already been through remembering, understanding, applying, analyzing, and evaluating. Creating is at the top of the pyramid. Note that the order was changed in 2001, and creating moved to above evaluating in the hierarchy.

Classes, lessons, and workshops can be designed to address different levels of Bloom's Taxonomy. In many respects, they build on one another. You need to recall facts (remembering), comprehend pathological pathways (understanding), implement frameworks for diagnosis (applying), carefully compare data points with previous ones or reference-range values (analyzing), then make a judgment call as to the correct diagnosis (evaluating), and finally generate a plan for treatment (creating).

A lesson plan for first-year medical students or master's-level students might include reviewing the guidelines for physical activity at the level of remembering. Then, describing why those guidelines exist would be the next level of understanding. Applying this would involve using a case study and a target heart rate calculator (220-age) × 0.70 to determine the recommended heart rate for moderate-intensity exercise. The analysis would involve reviewing research and comparing blood pressures pre- and post-12-week exercise program, along with hemoglobin A1c, high-sensitivity CRP, and HDL levels, to determine the impact of the exercise program on patient health. Evaluating would entail critiquing the research, the exercise routine employed, and the results to determine whether the program was effective and how it should be enhanced or modified. Creating would include writing up an exercise protocol for a specific patient based on all the information gathered, analyzed, and evaluated.

Learners can use Bloom's Taxonomy to help them appreciate the level at which they are studying. If they are memorizing definitions and muscle insertions, they are at the level of remembering. This is important, but it is not sufficient to pass an exam or score highly on an OSCE. After the student gains confidence with the facts, they can move on to understanding and looking for ways to make sense of the material they have memorized. Identifying connections between ideas and concepts and mapping them using a concept map can improve understanding. Solving clinical problems and reading cases while pausing to ask questions can help apply and implement the frameworks learned for remembering and understanding. Then, for analyzing, comparing the signs and symptoms of the patient in the case with other clinical vignettes already covered and studied will help with contrasting, organizing the data, and categorizing it. For evaluating and making a judgment about the clinical case, the student needs confidence and courage to take a stand and commit to a diagnosis. To create a treatment plan, the student must have enough knowledge to design or generate a safe and effective protocol for the patient.

When faculty design courses and consider which objectives to use, Bloom's Taxonomy helps identify the targeted level of learning. The words associated with each level can be used as the verbs that start each objective. Ensuring that objectives extend beyond the remember and understand domains is critical to developing medical students' critical-thinking skills. Critical thinking does not factor into Bloom's Taxonomy until the analyze level. Everything above the applying level requires critical thinking skills.

Using the SMART goal framework when crafting course objectives and goals can be helpful. In lifestyle medicine, healthcare professionals assist patients in creating SMART goals. A SMART goal is specific, measurable, attainable, relevant, and time-bound (Figure 23.6).

Bloom's Taxonomy helps identify verbs suited to the level and type of learning. The SMART goal framework helps frame the goal so that it is targeted to a specific type of learner and relevant to that learner. This is a learner-centric process. If the objective is a four-week course, it must be realistically attainable within that period. If the aim is a two-hour workshop, it must be modified to be achievable within a short timeframe. The measurable piece is often neglected when creating objectives. How will the educator determine whether the learner has met the objective? How can it be measured? Table 23.2 presents examples of vague objectives that do not conform to the SMART framework and compares them with similar objectives modified to conform to the SMART framework.

The objectives must be well thought out. Connecting objectives to the medical school's core competencies, and specifically to lifestyle medicine's core competencies, helps faculty ensure they cover all essential material. This section on course objectives emphasizes the importance of carefully

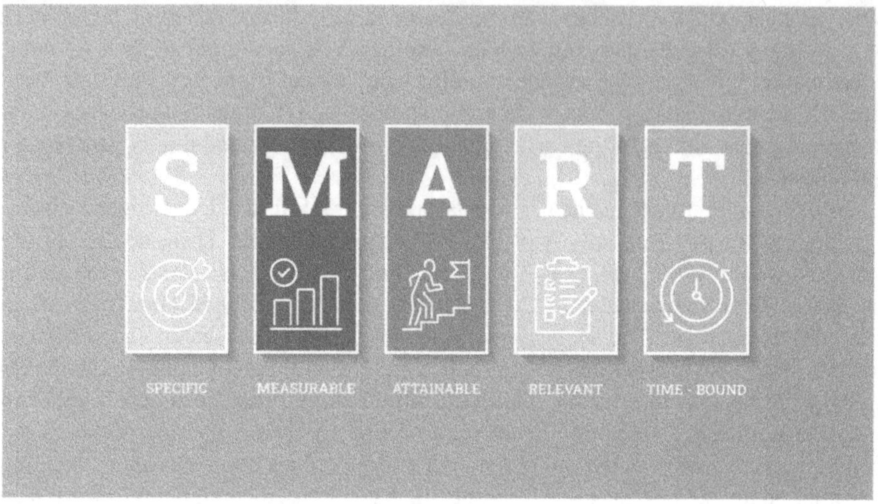

FIGURE 23.6 The SMART mnemonic.

TABLE 23.2
Vague Objectives Compared to SMART Objectives

Vague Objective	SMART Objective
Students will learn about the benefits of exercise.	By the end of the two-hour session, students will be able to list at least three health benefits of regular aerobic exercise, as demonstrated by correctly answering at least 80% of questions on the topic.
Students will understand the importance of sleep.	By the end of the 45-minute workshop, students will collaboratively create a concept map that links at least five key aspects of sleep physiology to its health impacts.
Students will learn about stress and its effects on health.	By the end of the semester, students will be able to identify and explain at least five physiological and psychological responses to stress, as demonstrated in their three-page paper assignment on stress.
Physicians will learn about various aspects of nutrition relevant to clinical practice.	By the end of the hour-long lecture, participating physicians will be able to list at least three evidence-based dietary recommendations for managing diabetes.

planning course content and development. It is not sufficient to identify the topic and materials a faculty member intends to teach. That is only the very beginning. Crafting course objectives is one of the most critical early steps in course creation.

23.6 SUMMARY

Developing courses in lifestyle medicine and proposing them to medical school curriculum committees are major goals for several physicians who are lifestyle medicine experts. Kern's Six-Step Approach is a valuable framework for creating courses. The steps are (a) Problem Identification and General Needs Assessment, (b) Targeted Needs Assessment, (c) Goals and Objectives, (d) Educational Strategies, (e) Implementation, and (f) Evaluation and Feedback. Each step needs to be considered carefully. Using backward design strategies and keeping the end goal in mind first will help medical educators craft powerful courses that meet their objectives.

Objectives direct the course design, content, and teaching strategies. Bloom's Taxonomy is a key framework for crafting meaningful objectives. The objectives of a course in lifestyle medicine should align with the medical school's core competencies and the lifestyle medicine core competencies for medical education. As indicated in the sixth step of Kern's Six-Step Approach for course creation, a concrete plan for evaluation and feedback is vital. How will medical educators determine whether they have met their goals? This careful consideration of each step in the creation, proposal, implementation, and evaluation of a course is the goal for all educators in the field of lifestyle medicine.

REFERENCES

1. Kern DE, Thomas PA, Howard DM. *Curriculum Development for Medical Education: A Six-Step Approach.* Baltimore, MD: Johns Hopkins University Press, 1998.
2. Chen BY, Kern DE, Kearns RM, Thomas PA, Hughes MT, Tackett S. From modules to MOOCs: application of the six-step approach to online curriculum development for medical education. *Acad Med.* 2019;94(5):678–685. doi: 10.1097/ACM.0000000000002580. PMID: 30681454.
3. Singh MK, Gullett HL, Thomas PA. Using Kern's 6-step approach to integrate health systems science curricula into medical education. *Acad Med.* 2021;96(9):1282–1290. doi: 10.1097/ACM.0000000000004141. PMID: 33951679.
4. Hashmi S, Riaz Q, Qaiser H, Bukhari S. Integrating basic sciences into clerkship rotation utilizing Kern's six-step model of instructional design: lessons learned. *BMC Med Educ.* 2024;24(1):68. doi: 10.1186/s12909-024-05030-z. PMID: 38233860; PMCID: PMC10795218.
5. Tyler RW. *Basic Principles of Curriculum and Instruction.* Chicago, IL: University of Chicago Press, 1949.
6. Prideaux D. ABC of learning and teaching in medicine. Curriculum design. *BMJ.* 2003;326(7383):268–270. doi: 10.1136/bmj.326.7383.268. PMID: 12560283; PMCID: PMC1125124.
7. Sata SK. A critical analysis of Ralph Tyler's principles: their role in shaping historical and foundational curriculum theories and contemporary educational practices. *World J Arts Educ Lit.* 2024;1(3):1–8.
8. Covey SR. *The 7 Habits of Highly Effective People: Powerful Lessons in Personal Change.* New York: Free Press, 2004.
9. Wiggins G, McTighe J. *Understanding by Design.* Alexandria, VA: Association for Supervision and Curriculum Development, 1998.
10. Wiggins G, McTighe J. *Understanding by Design.* Alexandria, VA: Association for Supervision and Curriculum Development, 2005.
11. Daugherty KK. Backward course design: making the end the beginning. *Am J Pharm Educ.* 2006; 70(6):135. doi: 10.5688/aj7006135. PMID: 17332861; PMCID: PMC1803709.
12. Newell AD, Foldes CA, Haddock AJ, Ismail N, Moreno NP. Twelve tips for using the understanding by design® curriculum planning framework. *Med Teach.* 2024;46(1):34–39. doi: 10.1080/0142159X.2023.2224498. *Epub* 2023 Jun 19. PMID: 37334694; PMCID: PMC10728343.
13. Godfrey EM, Kim ES, Frates B. Lifestyle medicine: the case for using educational frameworks and instructional approaches that meet adult learning needs. *Am J Lifestyle Med.* 2025:15598276251393587. doi: 10.1177/15598276251393587.
14. Clarke CA, Frates J, Pegg Frates E. Optimizing lifestyle medicine health care delivery through enhanced interdisciplinary education. *Am J Lifestyle Med.* 2016;10(6):401–405. doi: 10.1177/1559827616661694. PMID: 30202301; PMCID: PMC6124981.
15. Steketee C, Moran M, Brewer M, Rogers GD. The four-dimensional curriculum framework: 10 years on. *FoHPE.* 2024;25(2):98–109.
16. Khanna P, Roberts C, Lane AS. Designing health professional education curricula using systems thinking perspectives. *BMC Med Educ.* 2021;21(1):20. doi: 10.1186/s12909-020-02442-5. PMID: 33407403; PMCID: PMC7789213.
17. Bloom BS, Engelhart MD, Furst EJ, WALTER H. Hill, Krathwohl DR. *Taxonomy of Educational Objectives: The Classification of Educational Goals.* London: Longmans Green and Co Ltd, 1956. https://eclass.uoa.gr/modules/document/file.php/PPP242/Benjamin%20S.%20Bloom%20-%20Taxonomy%20of%20Educational%20Objectives%2C%20Handbook%201_%20Cognitive%20Domain-Addison%20Wesley%20Publishing%20Company%20%281956%29.pdf. Accessed November 9, 2025.
18. Tuma F, Nassar AK. Applying Bloom's taxonomy in clinical surgery: practical examples. *Ann Med Surg.* 2021;69:102656. doi: 10.1016/j.amsu.2021.102656. PMID: 34429945; PMCID: PMC8371225.

19. Kovacs G. Procedural skills in medicine: linking theory to practice. *J Emerg Med.* 1997;15(3):387–391. doi: 10.1016/s0736–4679(97)00019-x. PMID: 9258796.
20. White CB, Ross PT, Haftel HM. Assessing the assessment: are senior summative OSCEs measuring advanced knowledge, skills, and attitudes? *Acad Med.* 2008;83(12):1191–1195. doi: 10.1097/ACM.0b013e31818c6f6a. PMID: 19202499.
21. Muzyk AJ, Lentz K, Green C, Fuller S, May DB, Roukema L. Emphasizing Bloom's affective domain to reduce pharmacy students' stigmatizing attitudes. *Am J Pharm Educ.* 2017;81(2):35. doi: 10.5688/ajpe81235. PMID: 28381895; PMCID: PMC5374924.
22. Rogers GD, Mey A, Chan PC. Development of a phenomenologically derived method to assess affective learning in student journals following impactive educational experiences. *Med Teach.* 2017;39(12):1250–1260. doi: 10.1080/0142159X.2017.1372566. Epub 2017 Sep 21. PMID: 28933577.
23. Krathwohl DR, Bloom BS, Masia BB. *Handbook II: Affective Domain.* New York: David McKay, 1964.
24. Anderson LW, Krathwohl DR (eds.). *A Taxonomy for Learning, Teaching, and Assessing: A Revision of Bloom's Taxonomy of Educational Objectives.* New York: Longman, 2001.
25. Adams NE. Bloom's taxonomy of cognitive learning objectives. *J Med Libr Assoc.* 2015;103(3):152–153. doi: 10.3163/1536–5050.103.3.010. PMID: 26213509; PMCID: PMC4511057.
26. Larsen TM, Endo BH, Yee AT, Do T, Lo SM. Probing internal assumptions of the revised Bloom's taxonomy. *CBE Life Sci Educ.* 2022;21(4):ar66. doi: 10.1187/cbe.20–08–0170. PMID: 36112622; PMCID: PMC9727608.
27. Phillips AW, Smith SG, Straus CM. Driving deeper learning by assessment: an adaptation of the revised Bloom's taxonomy for medical imaging in gross anatomy. *Acad Radiol.* 2013;20(6):784–789. doi: 10.1016/j.acra.2013.02.001. PMID: 23664405.
28. Fernàndez-Roig S, Lai SC, Murphy MM et al. Vitamin B_{12} deficiency in the brain leads to DNA hypomethylation in the TCblR/CD320 knockout mouse. *Nutr Metab.* 2012;9:41. doi: 10.1186/1743-7075-9-41.
29. Akiyama N, Yamamoto-Fukuda T, Yoshikawa M, Kojima H. Regulation of DNA methylation levels in the process of oral mucosal regeneration in a rat oral ulcer model. *Histol Histopathol.* 2020;35(3):247–256. doi: 10.14670/HH-18–147. Epub 2019 Jul 9. PMID: 31286466.

24 Core Competencies in Medical Education and Lifestyle Medicine

24.1 CORE COMPETENCIES

Given that medical educators design courses with the end in mind, it is unsurprising that focusing on core competencies at every stage of medical education is crucial. For medical educators, the primary goal is to work with students over the years to help them become competent and compassionate physicians. Medical school students must be deemed qualified to graduate from medical school and residency. Hence, competencies and the alignment of course objectives with core competencies are key.

A core competency is an essential skill required for success in a job or profession. The focus on competencies starts in college with pre-medical students. The Association of American Medical Colleges (AAMC) has listed 17 core competencies, divided into three sections—professional, science, and critical thinking—for pre-medical students entering medical school. They are as follows (1):

Professional Competencies:

1. Commitment to Learning and Growth
2. Cultural Awareness
3. Cultural Humility
4. Empathy and Compassion
5. Ethical Responsibility to Self and Others
6. Interpersonal Skills
7. Oral Communication
8. Reliability and Dependability
9. Resilience and Adaptability
10. Service Orientation
11. Teamwork and Collaboration

Science Competencies:

12. Human Behavior
13. Living Systems

Thinking and Reasoning Competencies:

14. Critical Thinking
15. Quantitative Reasoning
16. Scientific Inquiry
17. Written Communication

In medical school, students must meet core competencies and complete numerous requirements to graduate. The exact requirements vary by school, but all schools require students to complete

DOI: 10.1201/9781003630043-24

specific courses and clerkships and achieve a satisfactory grade or assessment. Passing the United States Medical Licensing Examination (USMLE) Steps 1 and 2 is also required for graduation. There are additional requirements regarding professionalism, technical standards, health and immunization requirements, Health Insurance Portability and Accountability Act (HIPAA) training, basic research training, and safety training. The requirements from Stanford University School of Medicine, as listed on the school's website, are provided below (2).

"2.2: Specification of Requirements for Graduation

The requirements for the MD degree are established by the Stanford School of Medicine Faculty Senate and allow no exceptions. Those requirements are as follows:

1. *Satisfaction of Academic Requirements*: To graduate, students must satisfy all academic requirements, as outlined here (http://med.stanford.edu/md/mdhandbook/section-4–discovery-curriculum-overview/4-3–academic-requirements-for-graduation.html).
2. *United States Medical Licensing Examination*: To graduate, students must achieve overall passes on the USMLE Step 1 and Step 2 CK (Clinical Knowledge) examinations, as outlined here (http://med.stanford.edu/md/mdhandbook/section-3-md-requirements-procedures/section-3-22-united-states-medical-licensing-examinations-requirements.html).
3. *Satisfaction of Professionalism Requirement*: To graduate, students must meet the standards of professionalism set forth in the *School of Medicine Professionalism Principles* (http://med.stanford.edu/md/mdhandbook/section-2-general-standards/section-2-4-school-of-medicine-professional-principles.html).
4. *Satisfaction of Technical Standards*: To graduate, students must meet the requirements set forth in the *School of Medicine Technical, Non-Academic Standards* (http://med.stanford.edu/md/mdhandbook/section-2-general-standards/section-2-3-school-of-medicine-technical-non-academic-standards.html).
5. *Residency Requirement*: To graduate, students must enroll in and be assessed for 12-quarters of full "Med-MD" tuition. MD degree candidates must be registered for the quarter during which the degree is conferred. Students must apply for conferral of a degree by submitting an 'Application to Graduate' in Axess. Students may graduate in any quarter by completing their degree requirements and submitting the 'Application to Graduate' by the application to graduate deadline date for that quarter.
6. *Medical Health Requirements and Immunizations* (http://med.stanford.edu/md/mdhandbook/section-3-md-requirements-procedures/section-3-11-medical-health-requirements-and-mmunizations.html): MD degree candidates must be in compliance with medical health requirements at all times. Entering medical students must complete certain health-related forms, immunizations, and tests before beginning studies at Stanford and, for some of these, annually thereafter.
7. *Data Security and Privacy (HIPAA) Training*: MD degree candidates must be in compliance with Stanford's *Data Security and Privacy (HIPAA) Training* (https://med.stanford.edu/md/mdhandbook/section-3-md-requirements-procedures/section-3-3-data-security-and-privacy-hipaa-training.html).
8. *Safety Training*: MD degree candidates must be in compliance with Bloodborne Pathogens, Hospital-Acquired Infections training, Safety and Emergency Preparedness training requirements and N95 Respirator training and fitting.
9. *Ethical Conduct of Biomedical Research*: MD degree candidates must be in compliance with the *CITI training requirement* (http://med.stanford.edu/md/mdhandbook/section-3-md-requirements-procedures/section-3-6-ethical-conduct-of-biomedical-research.html)."

https://med.stanford.edu/md/mdhandbook/section-2-general-standards/section-2-2-specification-requirements-for-graduation-with-md-degree.html

There are no specific requirements for medical schools to teach nutrition or the other lifestyle medicine pillars. Most schools do not teach enough in these vital areas. For many large, traditional medical schools, the curriculum is set and full. The faculty have been teaching their subjects for years, and they are masters at their craft. According to a paper in Mayo Clinic Proceedings: Innovations, Quality, and

Outcomes, titled "Lifestyle Medicine in Medical Education: Maximizing Impact," very little attention is currently given to the six pillars of lifestyle medicine (exercise, nutrition, sleep, stress resilience, social connection, and avoidance of risky substances) in medical education (3). The paper revealed that of the pillars, most medical schools spent the most time on nutrition (14.3 hours), then physical activity (8 hours), and then sleep (less than 2.5 hours). There was insufficient data to quantify the number of hours spent on stress resilience and social connection. Most medical schools do cover risky substances such as cigarettes and alcohol. This may change soon, as the current Secretary of the United States Health and Human Services Department, Robert F. Kennedy Jr., and his team made a proclamation on August 27, 2025, that all medical schools need to include nutrition in their education (4).

Lifestyle medicine core competencies for medical students were published in the *American Journal of Lifestyle Medicine* in 2021 (5). They have been mapped to the Entrustable Professional Activities (EPAs) from the AAMC (6). EPAs are activities that medical students must be able to perform before entering residency. The 13 EPAs are listed below.

EPA 1: Gather a History and Perform a Physical Examination
EPA 2: Prioritize a Differential Diagnosis Following a Clinical Encounter
EPA 3: Recommend and Interpret Common Diagnostic and Screening Tests
EPA 4: Enter and Discuss Orders and Prescriptions
EPA 5: Document a Clinical Encounter in the Patient Record
EPA 6: Provide an Oral Presentation of a Clinical Encounter
EPA 7: Form Clinical Questions and Retrieve Evidence to Advance Patient Care
EPA 8: Give or Receive a Patient Handover to Transition Care Responsibility
EPA 9: Collaborate as a Member of an Interprofessional Team
EPA 10: Recognize a Patient Requiring Urgent or Emergent Care and Initiate Evaluation and Management
EPA 11: Obtain Informed Consent for Tests and/or Procedures
EPA 12: Perform General Procedures of a Physician
EPA 13: Identify System Failures and Contribute to a Culture of Safety and Improvement

The Entrustable Professional Activities can be found on the AAMC website at https://www.aamc.org/media/20211/download

https://www.aamc.org/about-us/mission-areas/medical-education/cbme/core-epas

The AAMC provides many resources for faculty, including:

- *Core Entrustable Professional Activities for Entering Residency*: Curriculum Developers' Guide (https://store.aamc.org/downloadable/download/sample/sample_id/63/)
- *Core Entrustable Professional Activities for Entering Residency*: Faculty and Learners' Guide (https://store.aamc.org/downloadable/download/sample/sample_id/66/)
- CoreEPA Toolkits (https://www.aamc.org/what-we-do/mission-areas/medical-education/cbme/core-epas/publications)
- *Core Entrustable Professional Activities for Entering Residency*: Summary of the 10-School Pilot, 2014–2021 (https://store.aamc.org/core-entrustable-professional-activities-for-entering-residency-summary-of-the-10-school-pilot-2014-2021.html)
- Annotated Bibliography for Core EPAs for Entering Residency Pilot Project (https://www.aamc.org/media/62326/download?attachment) (Updated through July 31, 2022)

The Lifestyle Medicine core competencies have been mapped to the 13 EPAs listed in Table 24.1. The EPAs in bold, italics, and underlined are ones added for this book, and the others are those shared in the original article published in AJLM 2021 (5).

There were 31 lifestyle medicine core competencies for medical students, as listed above. In September 2024, a JAMA Network Open article on the proposed nutrition competencies for medical students and

TABLE 24.1
Lifestyle Medicine Competencies for Medical Students Mapped to EPAs

- I. Patient care and procedural skills
  1. Conduct a comprehensive, lifestyle-focused history, and physical examination, including appropriate screenings, to assess the six pillars of lifestyle medicine (EPA 1). **Added EPA10**
  2. Apply evidence-based lifestyle medicine guidelines for the development of a comprehensive lifestyle medicine assessment and plan for chronic disease prevention, treatment, and reversal, including lifestyle medicine prescriptions (EPA 7). **Added EPA2, EPA3, EPA4, EPA5, EPA6**
  3. Effectively apply clinical reasoning skills when ordering and interpreting appropriate tests to screen, diagnose, and guide the prevention, treatment, and reversal of common lifestyle-related chronic diseases (EPA 3, 7). **Added EPA2**
  4. Utilize evidence-based models of health behavior change to assess patients' readiness and ability to make lifestyle changes (EPA 7). **Added EPA 2**
  5. Utilize evidence-based behavior change counseling to support patients in lifestyle changes (EPA 7).
  6. Collaborate in a patient-centered approach with patients and their families to develop evidence-based, achievable, specific, written action plans such as lifestyle prescriptions (EPA 9).
  7. Apply pharmaceutical knowledge to adjust medication doses as patients adopt a healthier lifestyle (EPA 4, 5).
  8. Compare effective dosing of lifestyle medicine strategies based on progression and severity of disease (EPA 4).
- II. Medical knowledge
  1. Discuss the pathophysiology of lifestyle-related chronic diseases.
  2. Evaluate and discuss the scientific evidence and physiological mechanisms by which lifestyle changes can treat and reverse lifestyle-related chronic disease (EPA 7).
  3. Discuss how lifestyle-related chronic disease treatment and reversal is dependent on disease severity and lifestyle medicine intervention dose. **Added EPA4**
  4. Discuss the six pillars of lifestyle medicine and the expected disease prevention, treatment, and reversal outcomes when lifestyle medicine is utilized. **Added EPA 7, EPA9**
  5. Demonstrate how the six pillars of lifestyle medicine fit into a comprehensive treatment framework, including pharmaceuticals and surgery (EPA 9, 10, 11).
- III. Practice-based learning and improvement
  1. Critically evaluate national guidelines for alignment with the six pillars of lifestyle medicine (EPA 7).
  2. Utilize resources to locate, interpret, and apply evidence from scientific studies regarding lifestyle medicine to prevent, treat, and reverse lifestyle-related chronic disease (EPA 7).
  3. Work collaboratively within an interprofessional team dedicated to multifactorial lifestyle change (EPA 9).
  4. Utilize information technology to optimize the delivery of lifestyle interventions and track changes over time (EPA 5).
- IV. Interpersonal and communication skills
  1. Collaborate with patients and their family members utilizing effective patient-centered relationship skills and shared decision-making to cultivate confidence and readiness for action (EPA 1, 11).
  2. Communicate and effectively lead an interprofessional health care team related to LM treatment plans and goals (EPA 8, 9).
  3. Educate patients, students, residents, and other health professionals on the appropriate use of LM as a sustainable approach for prevention, treatment, and reversal of lifestyle-related chronic disease. **Added EPA 9**
  4. Tailor lifestyle education based on the health literacy and learning needs of the patient (EPA 1, 2).
- V. Professionalism
  1. Describe how a physician's personal LM engagement can benefit patients' health behaviors.
  2. Demonstrate compassion, respect, and autonomy for patients, regardless of their readiness or ability to engage in lifestyle change. **Added EPA 1**
  3. Model an authentic journey of healthful lifestyle choices.
  4. Demonstrate the ability to perform LM counseling in a culturally competent manner. **Added EPA 1**
- VI. Systems-based practice
  1. Describe the role of LM within the health care system framework (EPA 9, 13).
  2. Advocate for policies that support treating the root cause of chronic disease through LM (EPA 13). **Added EPA 9**
  3. Describe practice systems that support and optimize LM-focused interventions (EPA 13).

(*Continued*)

TABLE 24.1 (*Continued*)
Lifestyle Medicine Competencies for Medical Students Mapped to EPAs

4. Describe costs of common lifestyle-related chronic diseases at the individual, health care system, and community levels and the impact of LM interventions on cost containment (EPA 13).
5. Integrate appropriate LM referrals to community organizations and health care professionals into patient treatment plans (EPA 8, 9).
6. Describe how lifestyle medicine can decrease health inequities among populations experiencing higher burdens of chronic disease, including adaptation strategies for patients and populations with limited resources (EPA 13).

residents was published (7). For nutrition alone, 33 proposed competencies are identified. These proposed competencies are organized into four groups in Table 24.2, including social determinants of health, nutrition knowledge, assessment and consultation skills, and teamwork and collaboration.

Proposed core competencies in nutrition can also be used to map how textbooks or courses fulfill them. For example, the textbook *Essentials of Clinical Nutrition in Healthcare*, published by McGraw-Hill (8), fulfills the proposed core competencies, as noted in Table 24.3.

Faculty with intimate familiarity with the book and the core competencies can complete this exercise of mapping the proposed competencies across different textbooks. This type of mapping can help faculty determine which book best suits their nutrition course. These proposed nutrition competencies (7) can also be used to develop a curriculum for medical school education.

The lifestyle medicine core competencies for medical students, as outlined in an article published in the American Journal of Lifestyle Medicine in 2021 (5) and listed earlier in this chapter, can be used to develop pre-medical school, master's-level, PhD-level courses, and medical school courses on lifestyle medicine. For the ACLM Academic Pathway program, faculty teaching lifestyle medicine courses are asked to map their courses to the ACLM core competencies. After completing the mapping and submitting the paperwork for evaluation by the Education Department at ACLM, the course is approved for the Academic Pathway program, in whole or in part. In this way, the course can be recognized as aligning with the ACLM's core competencies. An example of that is available for review in Table 24.4 with one of the courses at Harvard Extension School created and taught by Past President of ACLM, Dr. Beth Frates, Associate Professor, Part-Time at Harvard Medical School in the Department of Physical Medicine and Rehabilitation. This example can help other faculty members appreciate the power of mapping and recognize that it is not difficult. In fact, some faculty even find it enjoyable.

The Introduction to Lifestyle Medicine (Lifestyle Medicine 101) Course, first delivered in 2014 at the Harvard Extension School and subsequently modified and updated, is a 12-week, full-semester, college- and master's-level course with 24 hours of instruction. Table 24.5 presents the titles of all 12 lectures in the full-semester course, along with brief outlines for each lecture in the Lifestyle Medicine 101 curriculum.

Table 24.6 presents the Introduction to Lifestyle Medicine course objectives and teaching strategies and identifies the Bloom's Taxonomy level for each. A version of this was also shared in the book, *Lifestyle Medicine: Closing Research, Practice, and Knowledge Gaps,* which was co-edited by Mechanick and Kushner (9). As was described in Chapter 23, Bloom's Taxonomy has three domains: cognitive, psychomotor, and affective. Two of the objectives from the Introduction to Lifestyle Medicine course do not neatly fit within Bloom's Taxonomy Cognitive Domain. The verb utilize is used. In the recommendations for Bloom's Taxonomy, the verb use is listed, not utilize. This is a reminder that the verbs for Bloom's Taxonomy are tools to aid medical educators. They are not the only verbs one can use or utilize. There is some flexibility in the use of the verbs. The second word that does not fit into the commonly used Bloom's Taxonomy for the Cognitive Domain is the verb commit. This verb is used for the final project. There are cognitive and affective aspects to this

TABLE 24.2
Nutrition Competencies as listed in the *JAMA Network Open* article titled Proposed Nutrition Competencies for Medical Students and Physician Trainees: A Consensus Statement

Category	Competency
Social determinants of health	• Provides evidence-based, culturally sensitive nutrition and food recommendations to the patient for the prevention and treatment of disease. • Screens for food insecurity and nutrition insecurity and makes appropriate referrals for those identified at risk. • Demonstrates sensitivity to the social, cultural, emotional, economic, educational, and psychological factors that may affect an individual's nutrition behavior, food choices, and health status. • Identifies community-based nutrition resources for patients experiencing food and nutrition insecurity. • Communicates diet, food, and nutrition information to patients using their preferred language, via interpretive services if needed, based on education and health literacy levels. • Identifies factors that affect their personal health and nutrition status.
Nutrition knowledge	• Identifies pathophysiological and/or socioeconomic circumstances that may lead to metabolic syndrome or malnutrition. • Demonstrates knowledge of the nutritional content of foods, including the major dietary sources of macronutrients and micronutrients. • Demonstrates knowledge of public health nutrition, including the social determinants of health, and how it can reduce the burden of disease and improve access to adequate, healthy food. • Demonstrates knowledge of pathological states that can affect the absorption of macronutrients, micronutrients, and other food-based compounds. • Demonstrates knowledge of the difference between food allergies and food intolerance. • Demonstrates knowledge of how energy and nutrient requirements in health and disease states differ across the lifespan. • Demonstrates knowledge of possible drug-nutrient interactions between certain foods, beverages, and medications. • Demonstrates knowledge of nutritional differences between unprocessed, minimally processed, and ultra-processed foods. • Demonstrates knowledge of the environmental impact of food production and how food choices can promote or diminish both personal and planetary health. • Demonstrates knowledge of breastfeeding, chestfeeding, and complementary feeding practices. • Demonstrates knowledge of the functions of essential nutrients. • Demonstrates knowledge of the principles of a healthy, balanced diet, in accordance with national nutritional guidelines.
Assessment and consultation skills	• Assesses the nutritional status of a patient with a brief diet and food history or questionnaire, anthropometric measurements, and appropriate laboratory tests. • Integrates evidence-based nutrition information from national nutrition guidelines, scientific publications, and other sources into patient care. • Identifies nutrient deficiencies and recommends foods and/or supplements as needed. • Demonstrates empathy and sensitivity when counseling patients with obesity and eating disorders. • Assesses diet and food intake and performs a comprehensive nutrition-focused physical examination to identify factors affecting a patient's health status. • Utilizes evidence-based models of behavior change to assess patients' readiness in order to effectively counsel patients on how to modify their diet and food choices to improve health.

(*Continued*)

TABLE 24.2 (*Continued*)
Nutrition Competencies as listed in the *JAMA Network Open* article titled Proposed Nutrition Competencies for Medical Students and Physician Trainees: A Consensus Statement

Category	Competency
	• Guides patients with regard to food choices in establishing lifelong dietary patterns to promote healthy weight and prevent or address chronic disease. • Interprets physical examination data and biomarkers against reference ranges to identify patients at risk of malnutrition. • Listens carefully, compassionately, and nonjudgmentally while taking a nutrition history. • Demonstrates awareness of one's own biases about food, food choices, obesity, and "healthy eating." • Provides brief counseling interventions to help patients decrease visceral adiposity or reduce the risk of metabolic syndrome. • Interprets information on nutrition facts panels, nutrition labels, and menus to make appropriate recommendations to support patients' individual needs and food choices. • Demonstrates knowledge of how to create a culinary nutrition SMART goal for personal use and for patient use. • Describe indications, administration, and complications of clinically assisted nutrition and hydration support (oral, enteral, and parenteral).
Teamwork and collaboration	• Works with other health professionals to deliver a multidisciplinary approach to nutrition care. • Identifies and refers patients for eating disorders and psychosocial problems, including emotional eating and binge eating. • Makes appropriate referrals to a range of professionals to support the patient in achieving their health goals.

Source: Eisenberg et al. (7).

TABLE 24.3
Mapping the Nutrition Core Competencies from the *JAMA Network Open* article, Proposed Nutrition Competencies for Medical Students and Physician Trainees: A Consensus Statement, with the nutrition textbook *Essentials of Clinical Nutrition in Healthcare*

Competency	Chapter in the Textbook
1. Provides evidence-based, culturally sensitive nutrition and food recommendations to the patient for the prevention and treatment of disease.	Chapter 29. Culinary Medicine Chapter 30. Nutrition Counseling with Group Visits
2. Screens for food insecurity and nutrition insecurity and makes appropriate referrals for those identified at risk.	Chapter 4. Food Insecurity
3. Works with other health professionals to deliver a multidisciplinary approach to nutrition care.	Chapter 28. A Multidisciplinary Approach for Nutrition Counseling
4. Identifies pathophysiological and/or socioeconomic circumstances which may lead to metabolic syndrome or malnutrition.	Chapter 13. Severe Malnutrition and Refeeding Syndrome Chapter 17. Overweight and Obesity Chapter 18. Diabetes Mellitus Chapter 19. Stroke and Hypertension Chapter 20. Cardiovascular Disease

(*Continued*)

TABLE 24.3 (*Continued*)
Mapping the Nutrition Core Competencies from the *JAMA Network Open* article, Proposed Nutrition Competencies for Medical Students and Physician Trainees: A Consensus Statement, with the nutrition textbook *Essentials of Clinical Nutrition in Healthcare*

Competency	Chapter in the Textbook
5. Assesses the nutritional status of a patient with a brief diet and food history or questionnaire, anthropometric measurements, and appropriate laboratory tests.	Chapter 3. Nutritional Assessment
6. Starts a sensitive, nonjudgmental conversation about food and lifestyle in a brief consultation within a primary or secondary care setting.	Chapter 26. Introduction to Behavior Change Chapter 27. Sustaining Change-Challenging Cases
7. Demonstrates knowledge of the nutritional content of foods, including the major dietary sources of macronutrients and micronutrients.	Chapter 1. Macronutrient Metabolism Chapter 2. Micronutrient Metabolism
8. Integrates evidence-based nutrition information from national nutrition guidelines, scientific publications, and other sources into patient care.	Chapter 5. Nutrition Through the Life Span
9. Demonstrates knowledge of public health nutrition, including the social determinants of health, and how it can reduce the burden of disease and improve access to adequate, healthy food.	Chapter 9. Healthy and Sustainable Diets Chapter 26. Introduction to Behavior Change Chapter 31. The Six Pillars of Lifestyle Medicine and Nutrition Chapter 32. The Physician as Nutrition Change Agent
10. Demonstrates sensitivity to the social, cultural, emotional, economic, educational, and psychological factors that may affect an individual's nutrition behavior, food choices and health status.	Chapter 26. Introduction to Behavior Change
11. Demonstrates knowledge of the pathological states that can affect the absorption of macronutrients, micronutrients, and other food-based compounds.	Chapter 1. Macronutrient Metabolism Chapter 2. Micronutrient Metabolism
12. Identifies nutrient deficiencies and recommends foods and/or supplements as needed.	Chapter 1. Macronutrient Metabolism Chapter 2. Micronutrient Metabolism Chapter 3. Nutrition Assessment Chapter 7. Herbs and Supplements
13. Demonstrates empathy and sensitivity when counseling patients with obesity and eating disorders.	Chapter 17. Overweight and Obesity Chapter 25. Eating Disorders Chapter 26. Introduction to Behavior Change Chapter 27. Sustaining Change—Challenging Cases
14. Assesses diet and food intake and performs a comprehensive nutrition-focused physical examination to identify factors affecting a patient's health status.	Chapter 3. Nutritional Assessment
15. Utilizes evidence-based models of behavior change to assess patients' readiness in order to effectively counsel patients for how to modify their diet and food choices to improve health.	Chapter 26. Introduction to Behavior Change Chapter 27. Sustaining Change—Challenging Cases Chapter 30. Nutrition Counseling with Group Visits
16. Guides patients with regard to food choices in establishing lifelong dietary patterns to promote healthy weight and prevent or address chronic disease.	Chapter 17. Overweight and Obesity Chapter 26. Introduction to Behavior Change Chapter 27. Sustaining Change—Challenging Cases Chapter 31. The Six Pillars of Lifestyle Medicine and Nutrition

(*Continued*)

TABLE 24.3 (*Continued*)
Mapping the Nutrition Core Competencies from the *JAMA Network Open* article, Proposed Nutrition Competencies for Medical Students and Physician Trainees: A Consensus Statement, with the nutrition textbook *Essentials of Clinical Nutrition in Healthcare*

Competency	Chapter in the Textbook
17. Identifies community-based nutrition resources for patients experiencing food and nutrition insecurity.	Chapter 26. Introduction to Behavior Change Chapter 28. A Multidisciplinary Approach to Nutrition Counseling Chapter 31. The Six Pillars of Lifestyle Medicine and Nutrition
18. Communicates diet, food, and nutrition information to patients using their preferred language, via interpretative services if needed, based on education and health literacy levels.	Chapter 26. Introduction to Behavior Change Chapter 31. The Six Pillars of Lifestyle Medicine and Nutrition
19. Listens carefully, compassionately, and nonjudgmentally while taking a nutrition history.	Chapter 26. Introduction to Behavior Change Chapter 28. A Multidisciplinary Approach to Nutrition Counseling Chapter 31. The Six Pillars of Lifestyle Medicine and Nutrition
20. Demonstrates knowledge of the difference between food allergies and food intolerance.	Chapter 16. Diseases of the Gastrointestinal Tract
21. Interprets physical examination data and biomarkers against reference ranges to identify patients at risk of malnutrition.	Chapter 3. Nutrition Assessment
22. Demonstrates awareness of one's own biases about food, food choices, obesity, and "healthy eating."	Chapter 17. Overweight and Obesity
23. Provides brief counseling interventions to help patients decrease visceral adiposity or reduce the risk of metabolic syndrome.	Chapter 17. Overweight and Obesity Chapter 26. Introduction to Behavior Change
24. Demonstrates knowledge of how energy and nutrient requirements in health and disease states differ across the lifespan.	Chapter 5. Nutrition Through the Lifespan
25. Demonstrates knowledge of possible drug-nutrient interactions between certain foods, beverages, and medications.	Chapter 18. Diabetes Mellitus Chapter 19. Stroke and Hypertension
26. Demonstrates knowledge of nutritional differences between unprocessed, minimally processed, and ultra-processed foods.	Chapter 6. Popular Diets Chapter 9. Healthy and Sustainable Diets Chapter 29. Culinary Medicine
27. Interprets information on nutrition facts panels, nutrition labels, and menus to make appropriate recommendations to support patients' individual needs and food choices.	Chapter 26. Introduction to Behavior Change Chapter 27. Sustaining Change—Challenging Cases Chapter 29. Culinary Medicine
28. Identifies factors that affect their personal health and nutritional status.	Chapter 26. Introduction to Behavior Change Chapter 31. The Six Pillars of Lifestyle Medicine and Nutrition
29. Demonstrates knowledge of the environmental impact of food production and how food choices can promote or diminish both personal and planetary health.	Chapter 9. Healthy and Sustainable Diets
30. Demonstrates knowledge of how to create a culinary nutrition SMART goal for personal use and for patient use.	Chapter 26. Introduction to Behavior Change Chapter 29. Culinary Medicine.

(*Continued*)

TABLE 24.3 (*Continued*)
Mapping the Nutrition Core Competencies from the *JAMA Network Open* article, Proposed Nutrition Competencies for Medical Students and Physician Trainees: A Consensus Statement, with the nutrition textbook *Essentials of Clinical Nutrition in Healthcare*

Competency	Chapter in the Textbook
31. Identifies and refers patients for eating disorders and psychosocial problems, including emotional eating and binge eating.	Chapter 24. Depression and Anxiety Chapter 25. Disordered Eating
32. Makes appropriate referrals to a range of professionals to support the patient in achieving their health goals.	Chapter 28. Multidisciplinary Approach to Nutrition Counseling
33. Describe indications, administration, and complications of clinically assisted nutrition and hydration support (oral, enteral, and parenteral).	Chapter 10. Specialized Nutrition Therapies Chapter 12. Critical Illness Chapter 13. Severe Malnutrition and Refeeding Syndrome

TABLE 24.4
Mapping of the Harvard Extension School Course, Lifestyle Medicine 101, with the Lifestyle Medicine Core Competencies for Medical School by the ACLM

Competency Domain	Competency	Y	N	Method of Instruction/ Assessment of Learning	Comments
Introduction to Lifestyle Medicine	Discuss lifestyle medicine and its unique role in healthcare practice.	X		L, R, D	
	Describe the lifestyle medicine core competencies as identified by a national consensus panel.	X		L, R, D	
	Compare and contrast lifestyle medicine with other fields of health and medicine.	X		L, R, D	
	Summarize the scientific evidence that shows health behaviors are associated with key health outcomes.	X		L, R, D	
	Describe the evidence showing that lifestyle interventions effectively impact disease pathophysiology.	X		L, R, D	
	Describe the priority of lifestyle medicine in the spectrum of treatment algorithms for chronic, lifestyle-related diseases across the lifespan.	X		L, R, D	
	Discuss the prevalence and associated cost burden of lifestyle-related diseases, such as hyperlipidemia, cardiovascular disease, pre-diabetes, diabetes, hypertension, obesity, and cancer.	X		L, R	
	Explain the impact of lifestyle choices on planetary health and sustainable living.		X		Can add reading assignments

(*Continued*)

TABLE 24.4 (*Continued*)
Mapping of the Harvard Extension School Course, Lifestyle Medicine 101, with the Lifestyle Medicine Core Competencies for Medical School by the ACLM

Competency Domain	Competency	Y	N	Method of Instruction/ Assessment of Learning	Comments
The Role of the Practitioner's Personal Health and Community Advocacy	Examine scientific evidence indicating that clinicians who maintain healthy lifestyles are more likely to provide counseling, serve as role models, and improve patient outcomes.	X		L, R, D	
	Develop a culture of leadership by modeling personal health behaviors.				
	Describe strategies for incorporating personal wellness for practitioners into clinics, medical offices, or other healthcare settings, including wellness programs.	X		L, R, D, O-case study	
	Examine essential practitioner characteristics and practices that increase the capacity and impact of the therapeutic alliance.	X		L, R, D, O-case study	
	Integrate personal readiness assessments and lifestyle action plans into sustainable life patterns for clinicians.	X		L, R, D, Q, O-case study	
	Explore the role of lifestyle medicine in promoting personal practitioner resiliency and reducing burnout.		X		Can add extra reading.
	Advocate for lifestyle medicine directly with patients and their families, as well as policy and decision makers within the community.	X		L, R, D	
Nutrition Science, Assessment, and Prescription	Analyze the importance and limitations of global food-based dietary guidelines.	X		L, R, D	
	Assess food intake patterns and nutrient deficiencies and excesses.	X		L, R, D, Q	
	Summarize the health impact of prominent dietary patterns, including plant-predominant and non–plant–predominant patterns.	X		L, R, D	
	Describe how the level of processing in a food affects health and discuss the evidence base for these effects.		X		Can add extra reading.
	Describe the practice of culinary medicine and its role in sustainable, healthy eating behavior.		X		Can add extra reading.
	Demonstrate the ability to write evidence-based nutrition prescriptions.	X		L, R, D	
	Apply the science behind nutrition prescriptions to address the pathophysiology of most chronic diseases, including inflammation, oxidation, glycosylation, epigenetic expression, as well as food and its effects on the microbiome.	X		L, R, D	Can add extra reading.

(*Continued*)

TABLE 24.4 (*Continued*)
Mapping of the Harvard Extension School Course, Lifestyle Medicine 101, with the Lifestyle Medicine Core Competencies for Medical School by the ACLM

Competency Domain	Competency	Y	N	Method of Instruction/ Assessment of Learning	Comments
	Summarize the major studies of nutrition in the prevention, treatment, and reversal of hyperlipidemia, cardiovascular disease, pre-diabetes, diabetes, hypertension, obesity, and cancer.	X		L, R, D	
	Analyze food labels for the health impacts of ingredients.		X		Can add extra reading.
	Describe indications for referral to a lifestyle medicine-trained registered dietitian to translate and further personalize nutrition prescriptions.		X	This comes up in discussion, but is not covered thoroughly in the lecture or book to date. It will be updated.	
Physical Activity Science, Assessment, and Prescription	Discuss the aerobic, strength, flexibility, and balance components of physical activity.	X		L, R, D	
	Examine the evidence and pathophysiology between physical activity components and health outcomes.	X		L, R, D	
	Describe the benefits of physical activity in preventing or treating disease in special populations, such as healthy older adults, pregnant women, children and adolescents, persons with obesity or disability, cardiovascular disease, diabetes, cancer, disability, and stroke.	X		L, R, D	Can add reading materials for specific populations
	Summarize the role of physical activity guidelines.	X		L, R, D	
	Integrate key physical activity assessment tools into clinical practice.	X		L, R, D	
	Define fitness terminology relevant to writing exercise prescriptions.	X		L, R, D, Q	
	Integrate evidence from relevant physical activity literature into treatment protocols for management, remission, or reversal in patients with diabetes, cancer, cardiovascular, and cerebrovascular disease.	X		L, R, D	
	Describe indications for referral to health fitness professionals.		X	Discusses this but does not cover in enough detail. Will include in update.	Can add extra reading.
	Develop physical activity prescriptions appropriately modified for special populations, such as healthy older adults, pregnant women, children and adolescents, persons with obesity or disability, cardiovascular disease, diabetes, cancer, disability, and stroke.		X		Can add extra reading.

(*Continued*)

TABLE 24.4 *(Continued)*
Mapping of the Harvard Extension School Course, Lifestyle Medicine 101, with the Lifestyle Medicine Core Competencies for Medical School by the ACLM

Competency Domain	Competency	Y	N	Method of Instruction/ Assessment of Learning	Comments
Sleep Health Science and Interventions	Describe sleep's role in health and chronic disease pathophysiology.	X		L, R, D	
	Perform sleep assessments to identify patients with insufficient or poor-quality sleep.	X		L, R, D	
	Summarize lifestyle-based interventions that can improve sleep health.	X		L, R, D	
	Assess the risk for common sleep disturbances, such as obstructive sleep apnea, chronic insomnia, and restless legs syndrome, and refer to sleep specialists when applicable.	X		L, R, D	
	Describe indications for referral to a program or specialist in cognitive behavioral therapy for insomnia.		X		Can add extra reading.
	Describe the indications for referral to a sleep specialist or for a sleep study to assess for sleep apnea.		X	L, R, D	Can add extra reading. Mentions this with\sleep apnea and snoring but needs to be more specific and thorough.
Treating Tobacco Use Disorder and Managing Other Toxic Exposures (Including Vaping, Alcohol Use, and Other Illicit Substances)	Describe the health effects of tobacco, alcohol, and other frequently used substances, and the benefits of cessation.	X		L, R, D	
	Apply patient screening tools for substance use.	X		L, R, D	
	Create patient-centered substance use treatment plans using practice guidelines and behavioral interventions.	X		L, R, D	
	Summarize the diagnostic criteria for common substance use disorders.	X		L, R, D, Q	
	Integrate behavioral therapy with pharmacotherapy for tobacco and other substance use disorder plans, and refer to a substance use disorder specialist when indicated.	X		R, D	Can add reading materials
	Apply the United States Preventive Services Task Force guidelines for patients with tobacco use disorder.	X		L, R, D	Cover the five As in behavior change counseling, coaching.

(Continued)

TABLE 24.4 (*Continued*)
Mapping of the Harvard Extension School Course, Lifestyle Medicine 101, with the Lifestyle Medicine Core Competencies for Medical School by the ACLM

Competency Domain	Competency	Y	N	Method of Instruction/ Assessment of Learning	Comments
Key Clinical Processes in Lifestyle Medicine	Integrate lifestyle vital signs into components of the patient history and physical exam.	X		L, R, D	Assessment tools are shared in the Appendix of the Lifestyle Medicine Handbook
	Analyze and implement evidence-based clinical practice guidelines relevant to lifestyle medicine for prevention, treatment, and reversal of chronic diseases.	X		L, R, D	
	Describe the treatment of disease with the lifestyle medicine pillars as compared with medication.	X		L, R, D (One of the class break-out sessions is to see how many medications it would take to replicate the impact of exercise)	
	Demonstrate how to screen, diagnose, treat, and monitor a lifestyle-related disease and provide lifestyle medicine–focused anticipatory guidance.	X		L, R, D	
	Discuss strategies for a clinical practice to access and implement the use of local, national, and global resources.		X		Can add lists of resources with websites.
	Describe the key strategies for leveraging inter-professional teams to enhance health behavior change interventions.	X		L, R, D	
	Examine how group visits and telehealth can optimize lifestyle medicine treatment encounters.		X		Can add extra reading.
	Create and utilize data from office systems, such as electronic health records with lifestyle medicine guidance, in clinical decisions and care, including tracking screening frequency, test results, referrals, and recommended follow-up.		X		Can add extra reading.
	Analyze the evidence for collaborative and chronic care models on improved lifestyle outcomes.		X		Can add extra reading and discussion questions
	Discuss successful primary care and office-based models for lifestyle modification.		X		Can add extra reading and discussion questions
	Design a quality improvement project for lifestyle medicine clinical practice, using tools such as Plan-Do-Study-Act (PDSA) cycles.		X		Can add as an experiential exercise

(*Continued*)

TABLE 24.4 (*Continued*)
Mapping of the Harvard Extension School Course, Lifestyle Medicine 101, with the Lifestyle Medicine Core Competencies for Medical School by the ACLM

Competency Domain	Competency	Y	N	Method of Instruction/ Assessment of Learning	Comments
	Explain principles of evidence-based medicine and their application to lifestyle medicine.	X		L, R, D	
	Describe methods of assessing the effectiveness of interventions, such as patient activation measures and therapeutic alliance measures.	X		L, R, D	
Fundamentals of Health Behavior Change	Summarize health behavior change theories, such as the health belief model, the social learning theory, and the transtheoretical model (TTM), and their application to lifestyle medicine practice.	X		L, R, D, O=case study homework	
	Demonstrate key elements of conducting a patient assessment within the TTM and collaborate to develop stage-matched responses.	X		L, R, D, Q, O=case study homework	
	Apply the process of building effective and therapeutic alliances with patients that foster their personal growth.	X		L, R, D, O=case study homework	
	Explain how to collaborate with your patients to promote health behavior changes.	X		L, R, D, Q, O=case study homework	
	Apply motivational interviewing, cognitive behavioral, health coaching, and positive psychology techniques.	X		L, R, D, Q, O=case study homework	
	Summarize the evidence to support the use of behavior change techniques in clinical practice.	X		L, R, D, O=case study homework	
	Use the skills of open inquiry, reflection, and empathy to develop and maintain a therapeutic alliance.	X		L, R, D, Q, O=case study homework	
	Describe the impact of positive emotions on the success of health behavior change.	X		L, R, D, O=case study homework	
	Develop patient-centered, written action plans based on the appropriate stage of change of the TTM.	X		L, R, D, Q, O=case study homework	
	Summarize the process of follow-up for ongoing lifestyle change progress, including building patient self-efficacy and relapse prevention.	X		L, R, D, Q, O=case study homework	
	Describe the factors that support sustained behavior change.	X		L, R, D, Q, O=case study homework	
	Explain the role of family and other support in initiating and maintaining health behavior change.	X		L, R, D, O=case study homework	
	Manage disruptions to the therapeutic alliance.	X		L, R, D, O=case study homework	

(*Continued*)

TABLE 24.4 (*Continued*)
Mapping of the Harvard Extension School Course, Lifestyle Medicine 101, with the Lifestyle Medicine Core Competencies for Medical School by the ACLM

Competency Domain	Competency	Y	N	Method of Instruction/ Assessment of Learning	Comments
	Identify patient resources for sustainable behavior change in relation to the pillars of lifestyle medicine.	X		L, R, D, O=case study homework	
Emotional and Mental Health Assessment and Interventions	Apply screening tools for stress, depression, and anxiety in clinical practice.		X		Can add surveys as an additional reference for reading.
	Explain the relationship and pathophysiology between emotional and physical health.	X		L, R, D	
	Summarize the nature of stress, the role of stressors, such as adverse childhood experiences, and identify manageable elements of pathogenic stress reactions.		X		Can add reading.
	Describe and utilize evidence-based and patient-centered mental and emotional health interventions, including self-management and resilience-building techniques.	X		L, R, D, Q	
	Analyze the clinical relevance and evidence base for mindfulness-based stress reduction (MBSR) and related stress management strategies.	X		L, R, D	
	Manage treatment plans for lifestyle-related mental health diseases, such as depression and anxiety.		X		Can add reading.
	Describe indications for referral to mental health professionals (versus when clinically indicated).		X		Can add reading and a discussion question for this
	Apply mindfulness skills to enable presence, clarity, and curiosity in the clinical encounter.	X		L, R, D, Q	
The Role of Connectedness and Positive Psychology	Apply positive psychology in health behavior change counseling.	X		L, R, D, Q	
	Describe how positive psychology strategies support achieving and sustaining healthy behaviors.	X		L, R, D	
	Compare and contrast eudaimonia and hedonia, and explain their effect on physical health, including longevity.	X		L, R, D	
	Describe how social connectedness and social networks affect emotional well-being, physical health, and longevity.	X		L, R, D	

(*Continued*)

TABLE 24.4 (*Continued*)
Mapping of the Harvard Extension School Course, Lifestyle Medicine 101, with the Lifestyle Medicine Core Competencies for Medical School by the ACLM

Competency Domain	Competency	Y	N	Method of Instruction/ Assessment of Learning	Comments
	Summarize the deleterious and positive effects social media has on emotional well-being and flourishing.	X		L, R, D	Can add more in reading.
	Explain the relationship among the lifestyle pillars, positive emotions, and flourishing.	X		L, R, D	
	Describe positive psychology activities that can boost emotional well-being and flourishing.	X		L, R, D, Q	

Key—Y for Yes this competency is included in the course.
N for No this competency is not included in this course.
L = Lecture
R = Required Reading
D = Discussion
E = Experiential
G = Group Project
P = Paper
Q = Quiz, Test
O = Other

TABLE 24.5
Lecture Topics, Required Reading, and Summary for the Week for Each Lecture in the Introduction to Lifestyle Medicine Curriculum

Week #	Lecture Topics	Required Reading	Summary for Week
1	Introduction and Overview of Lifestyle Medicine	*Lifestyle Medicine Handbook*—Chapter 1 *Recent Research article sharing results of a lifestyle medicine intervention	• Define Lifestyle Medicine and name the six pillars of lifestyle medicine. • Contrast Lifestyle Medicine to usual medical care • Create a framework for the six pillars of lifestyle medicine and a skeleton on which to attach information as the weeks proceed. • Identify the pioneers in lifestyle medicine, starting with Hippocrates. • Critique key statistics and landmark research studies. • Explore student perspectives on lifestyle medicine • Debate the impact of the lifestyle medicine intervention in the required research article.
2	How to Evoke Behavior Change for Self and Those You Care For Personally and Professionally	*Lifestyle Medicine Handbook*—Chapter 2 *Research article on the impact of a Motivational Interviewing intervention	• Differentiate between the COACH Approach ™ and the Expert Approach. • Identify the five elements in the COACH Approach ™ way of being. • Describe how to use the Transtheoretical Model of Change, Appreciative Inquiry, Motivational Interviewing, Socio-Ecological Model of Change, and the five As when counseling patients on behavior change.

(*Continued*)

TABLE 24.5 (*Continued*)
Lecture Topics, Required Reading, and Summary for the Week for Each Lecture in the Introduction to Lifestyle Medicine Curriculum

Week #	Lecture Topics	Required Reading	Summary for Week
			• Explore students' experiences with behavior change. • Analyze the results of the required research article.
3	Goal Setting, Accountability, and Tracking for Lifestyle Medicine	*Lifestyle Medicine Handbook*-Chapter 3 *Research article on the topic of goal setting for behavior change	• Explain Goal Setting Theory and demonstrate how to set SMART goals. • Describe the Five-Step Collaboration Cycle and weigh the importance of each step. • Demonstrate how to create goals that are connected to people's vision, values, purpose, and priorities. • Interpret the findings of the research study from the required reading.
4	Physical Activity Guidelines and Prescription	*Lifestyle Medicine Handbook*- Chapter 4 *Research article on an exercise intervention	• Compare physical activity recommendations over the years. • Identify benefits of aerobic exercise, strength training, balance exercises, and flexibility routines. • Describe the mechanisms by which exercise impacts health. • Demonstrate how to personalize exercise recommendations using the FITT prescription. • Analyze the results of the research article from the required reading.
5	Nutrition Guidelines and Prescription	*Lifestyle Medicine Handbook*-Chapter 5 *Research article on a whole food plant predominant study	• Contrast nutrition recommendations from the 1950s to today. • Describe different dietary patterns. • Explain the benefits of eating a whole-food, plant-predominant diet rich in vegetables, fruit, whole grains, nuts, seeds, and legumes. • Recognize the importance of macronutrients and micronutrients. • Demonstrate how to write a personalized nutrition prescription. • Evaluate the research article provided for the week.
6	Sleep and Its Effect on Health and Well-Being	*Lifestyle Medicine Handbook*-Chapter 7 *Research article on sleep and its impact on chronic conditions	• Identify the National Sleep Foundation's Sleep guidelines. • Define sleep hygiene and identify sleep strategies for restorative sleep. • Examine how insufficient sleep impacts the body and brain. • Describe the homeostatic and circadian sleep drives. • Demonstrate how to write a sleep prescription and when to refer to a sleep specialist. • Debate the value of sleep interventions after reading the research article.
7	Stress Resilience	*Lifestyle Medicine Handbook*-Chapter 8 *Research article on the impact of stress on the immune system	• Debate whether all stress is bad for your health. • Explain how stress impacts different organs of the body. • Explore the concept of stress resilience and identify ways to counsel toward this goal. • Analyze guidelines and recommendations for stress reduction. • Evaluate the results of the research study on stress.

(*Continued*)

TABLE 24.5 (*Continued*)
Lecture Topics, Required Reading, and Summary for the Week for Each Lecture in the Introduction to Lifestyle Medicine Curriculum

Week #	Lecture Topics	Required Reading	Summary for Week
8	Relaxation, Mindfulness, and Meditation	*Lifestyle Medicine Handbook*-Chapter 9 *Research article on mind-body interventions to reduce stress	• Define relaxation, mindfulness, and meditation. • Compare different mind-body techniques. • Describe the evidence-based benefits of participating in mind-body exercises. • Practice a variety of mind-body techniques during class. • Explain ways to counsel patients on adopting mind-body practices. • Debate the results of the research study on mind-body interventions.
9	The Connection Prescription	*Lifestyle Medicine Handbook*-Chapter 10 *Research article on social connection and its impact on chronic conditions	• Define social connection. • Identify the 12 Vital Ties described by Dr. Ned Hallowell. • Describe a high-quality connection as defined by Dr. Jane Dutton. • Explain the connection between social connections and chronic conditions. • Recognize the landmark studies on the power of social connection. • Practice writing a prescription for social connection. • Debate the importance of social connection for health based on the research article of the week.
10	Positive Emotions: Laughter, Optimism, and Gratitude	*Lifestyle Medicine Handbook*-Chapter 11 *Research article on gratitude and health outcomes	• Explore the evidence connecting positive emotions to physical and mental health. • Describe ways to counsel patients about adopting positive mindsets. • Practice writing a personalized prescription for increasing positive emotions. • Analyze the results of the research study in the weekly reading.
11	Avoidance of Risky Substances	*Lifestyle Medicine Handbook*-Chapter 12 *Research on interventions to reduce the use of risky substances	• Identify the DSM-5 criteria for substance use disorder for tobacco, alcohol, opioids, and other substances. • Describe the health risks of using tobacco, alcohol, and other risky substances. • Explore counseling strategies that are effective when helping people who are struggling with the use of risky substances. • Debate the risks of using alcohol compared to the possible benefits.
12	Review of Lifestyle Medicine	*Students identify research articles of interest	• Identify the benefits of the six pillars of lifestyle medicine with regard to preventing, treating, and putting chronic conditions into remission. • Explore students' Aha moments and lessons learned. • Describe how the material in this course can be used in the future. • Explain how to use this course to help identify misinformation. • Develop a plan to continue learning about lifestyle medicine.

TABLE 24.6
Course Objectives, Teaching Strategies, and Bloom's Taxonomy Level for the Introduction to Lifestyle Medicine Course

Course Objectives	Teaching Strategies	Bloom's Taxonomy Level
Define lifestyle medicine, identify the six pillars, and describe the difference between lifestyle medicine and usual care in traditional medicine.	Lectures with PowerPoint, required reading, quizzes for homework, questions in class, polls in class, discussion posts for homework, sharing Aha moments, and opportunities for elaborative discussions.	Remember and understand
Recognize and describe the impact that the six pillars of lifestyle medicine have on the development and progression of chronic conditions, and evaluate their importance based on analysis of research studies.	Lectures with PowerPoint, required readings, research studies, quizzes for homework, discussion posts for homework, in-class polls, questions in class, breakout sessions with peer-to-peer teaching, and opportunities for elaborative discussions.	Remember, understand, analyze, and evaluate
List the current guidelines for exercise, nutrition, sleep, and avoidance of risky substances, and discuss the recommendations for stress resilience and social connectedness.	Lectures with PowerPoint, required readings, and quizzes for homework.	Remember and understand
Define the COACH™ Approach and the EXPERT Approach, describe the main components of each, contrast the two approaches, and analyze when the COACH™ Approach can be most effective.	Lectures with PowerPoint, sections with Teaching Assistants, required readings, quizzes for homework, case studies, class demonstrations, role playing, and opportunities for elaborative discussions.	Remember, understand, analyze, and evaluate
Utilize evidence-based coaching techniques to empower people to adopt and sustain behavior change.	Sections with Teaching Assistants, Case Studies, and Course Project.	Apply, evaluate, and create
Analyze how the six pillars of lifestyle medicine and positive emotions can impact physical and mental health.	Lectures with PowerPoint, Sections with Teaching Assistants, discussion posts for homework, breakout sessions with peer-to-peer teaching, and opportunities for elaborative discussions.	Apply, analyze, and evaluate
Commit to improvements in personal healthy lifestyle behaviors, evaluate options, create SMART goals, apply lessons learned in class, readings, research articles, and discussions, and analyze the results.	Course project involving selecting a behavior to change throughout the course, creating SMART goals, tracking the behavior, and journaling about the change process, including struggles, surprises, and successes.	Apply, analyze, evaluate, and create

objective. The word commit aligns more closely with the affective domain in Bloom's Taxonomy, specifically with the valuing and organizing levels. The objective is "Commit to improvements in personal healthy lifestyle behaviors to best serve as role models." Lifestyle Medicine courses may include objectives from Bloom's Taxonomy Affective and Psychomotor Domains in addition to the Cognitive Domain.

This Introduction to Lifestyle Medicine course, taught at the Harvard Extension School since 2014, has been updated and enhanced each year. Following best practices in education as described earlier, the faculty and teaching assistants work to improve the lectures, experiential learning, discussion posts, assignments, and final projects. More recently, the faculty added assignments that allow for flexibility and creativity for learners who are less adept at verbal and written expression and who excel with out-of-the-box thinking expressed in the form of art such as drawing, photography, poetry, music, dance, video creation, explanatory images with vectors, or diagrams and flow charts. Providing exercises that engage and excite the learners is the key.

The importance of the teaching team needs to be emphasized. Teaching assistants and course administrators are critical to a course's success (10). Providing medical students with the opportunity to serve as teaching assistants enables them to deepen their understanding of the material and develop their teaching skills. If a student is tasked with teaching material, they have an added incentive to master it fully. For students interested in teaching, offering electives such as Harvard Medical School's Exploratory Longitudinal Elective (ELO) elective is an excellent way to foster their interest. To improve medical education and teaching, medical schools must prioritize the development of critical teaching skills. Including medical students in curriculum discussions is another way to garner interest in education. Medical students can be helpful in many ways, including mapping the hours spent on lifestyle medicine topics over their four years of medical school. Often, the students involved with the Lifestyle Medicine Interest Groups (LMIGs), introduced in Chapter 18, are interested in and eager to participate in this way.

Mapping the curriculum to determine how much time is devoted to lifestyle medicine topics and which topics are covered is an academic exercise that faculty can use to assess their current progress in teaching the core competencies of lifestyle medicine and their future direction. Results such as these were collected by Bar-Ilan University in 2017, which found that the school offered 58 hours of lifestyle medicine teaching, 49 hours of pre-clinical training, and 9 hours of clinical training. Of the 58 hours, 42 covered theoretical knowledge, and 16 focused on practical skills related to lifestyle behavior change (11). After a school determines its baseline for lifestyle medicine offerings, faculty can plan future efforts to expand them. There can be a five-year long-term plan, a two-year short-term plan, and an immediate plan for the following year.

24.2 MOVE TOWARD COMPETENCY-BASED CURRICULUM

Mapping curricula often involves identifying the time spent on subjects, specifically hours. Many medical education articles reviewing lifestyle medicine and the incorporation of the six pillars report the hours spent on each pillar. However, with the shift to competency-based medical education, it is essential to focus on the competencies taught in a given course. And just because something is taught does not mean it is learned, memorized, or instilled in the student's clinical reasoning or decision-making. Identifying competencies is one aspect of medical education, and assessing competency is another. Faculty members in a school can teach all the competencies, but do the students demonstrate competency? That is an important question. Moving away from a focus on hours taught to competencies taught and then ultimately to checking on competency demonstration by students is the future of medical education–competency-based medical education.

The AAMC defines competency-based medical education (CBME) as follows:

> CBME is an outcomes-based approach to the design, implementation, and evaluation of education programs and to the assessment of learners across the continuum that uses competencies or observable abilities. The goal of CBME is to ensure that all learners achieve the desired patient-centered outcomes during their training (12).

An article in the *New England Journal of Medicine* by Cooper and Holmboe in 2025, titled "Competencies-Based Medical Education at the Front Lines of Patient Care," describes the differences between the models (13). Competency-based medical education strives to meet the quintuple aim: improved population health, health equity, better patient care, better support for healthcare professionals, and cost reduction (13). In addition, there is a focus on the learner-faculty-patient triad, rather than on the two dyads of learner-faculty and learner-patient (13).

One of the main differences between competency-based medical education and the traditional model of medical education is that, in the latter, students exit the system at a fixed time (graduation), based on years in school, time spent in rotations, and passing critical summative assessments (13). In contrast, in the competency-based medical education model, students would exit when competency was met. In competency-based medical education, time is not a requirement but rather a resource for reaching competence. Assessments are formative and used to help students meet competency.

Schools are publishing their core competencies online. For example, Harvard Medical School shares its updated core competencies on its website (14).

Competencies and Program Objectives from the Harvard Medical School (HMS) Handbook are available on its public website, last updated 8/1/24 (14). The seven competencies, which are bolded, italicized, and underlined, are those that lifestyle medicine courses can uniquely address, thereby helping to achieve the quintuple aim.

By the time of graduation, all HMS students are expected to:

Medical Knowledge:

1. Explain the foundational principles that underlie the medical sciences and integrate this knowledge across disciplines.
2. Apply their understanding of established knowledge in medical sciences to problems in clinical medicine and the care of individuals and populations.
3. Apply their understanding of how the scientific method works and how it advances the medical sciences.
4. Identify and integrate evolving information in medical sciences, and apply this knowledge to clinical problem solving.

Patient Care:

1. Provide compassionate, inclusive, trauma-informed, and affirming patient-centered care in order to promote and improve health.
2. Obtain and collect information from patients, including a complete and accurate medical history and physical examination, and other sources relevant to the diagnosis, treatment, and prevention of common and urgent conditions, including the performance of diagnostic procedures.
3. Efficiently interpret, analyze, assess, and prioritize relevant data from patient sources as well as from the medical literature to establish a diagnosis and management plan, including the initiation of clinically reasoned interventions.
4. Work collaboratively as part of an interprofessional team to ensure safe, appropriate care for a service of patients.

Interpersonal and Communication Skills:

1. Form collaborative and trusting relationships with patients, caregivers, and all members of the healthcare team.
2. Effectively communicate with patients, caregivers, and all members of the healthcare team, using all available resources, to promote informed consent and shared decision-making.
3. Effectively communicate medical information in oral, written, and electronic form to advance patient care.
4. Demonstrate the interpersonal and communication skills required to be an effective member of a health care team.

Critical and Informed Thinking, Adaptive Expertise, and Scientific Inquiry:

1. Evaluate, analyze, and apply new and existing knowledge with advances and discoveries in biomedical, clinical, social, behavioral, and population and data sciences.
2. Identify and describe gaps in their knowledge and skills, while managing uncertainty, to continually advance their professional development.
3. Apply the skills necessary for self-reflection, self-assessment, self-directed learning, and lifelong learning.
4. Recognize and explain cognitive biases and how they impact decision-making and patient care.
5. Identify gaps in the literature and engage in scholarly inquiry and innovation with the goal of advancing knowledge in the service of the mission of medicine and exceptional patient care.

Professionalism:

1. Exemplify the professional values of medicine, including compassion, integrity, social responsibility, and respect for all persons and identities.
2. Demonstrate the responsible behaviors expected of physicians, including accountability, patient confidentiality and safety, punctuality, and the prioritizing of the needs of others while maintaining appropriate self-care.
3. Demonstrate and embody ethical standards, principles, and moral reasoning in all professional interactions with patients, caregivers, colleagues, and society at large.
4. Apply the skills and incorporate the attitudes needed to maintain and promote personal well-being while ensuring patient safety.

Health Equity and the Structural and Social Determinants of Health:

1. Demonstrate the ability to operate effectively within health systems and to improve access, safety, quality, equity, and value of those systems.
2. Provide care with cultural humility and appreciation of the needs of diverse populations.
3. Demonstrate the skills needed to advocate in partnership with patients and communities to improve health outcomes at the individual, organizational, and societal levels.
4. Demonstrate through actions and reflections an understanding of and sensitivity to the social determinants of health and opportunities to address health inequities.

Medical schools have a variety of core competencies, primarily falling into four of the six ACGME categories: medical knowledge, patient care, professionalism, and interpersonal and communication skills. When proposing lifestyle medicine courses, faculty members need to review their medical school's specific focus and determine how the medical school elective or core course will help the school fulfill its mission and help students achieve competency by graduation.

24.3 SUMMARY

Core competencies drive curriculum creation in many ways. The knowledge, skills, and attitudes required to practice medicine are articulated in the core competencies for pre-medical students and the Entrustable Professional Activities (EPAs) defined by the Association of American Medical Colleges (AAMC) (6). The American College of Lifestyle Medicine (ACLM) has core competencies that map to the EPAs (5) and help guide curriculum development in medical schools. As interest in nutrition education in medical school grows, the core competencies for lifestyle medicine (5) and the proposed core competencies for nutrition (7) will be critical resources for medical school deans and faculty on curriculum committees.

The move toward a competency-based curriculum will benefit students and faculty alike. It will shift the focus from the hours spent on a subject to the learners themselves. Progress toward achieving competency and mastering EPA will take center stage in medical schools. Time spent on a topic does not translate to competency. Focused attention, practice, study, individualized formative feedback, and tracking progress with competency levels lead to mastery. This underscores the importance of competency milestones, which will be discussed in the next chapter.

REFERENCES

1. Association of American Medical Colleges. https://students-residents.aamc.org/real-stories-demonstrating-premed-competencies/premed-competencies-entering-medical-students. Accessed November 10, 2025.
2. Stanford University School of Medicine Graduation Requirements. https://med.stanford.edu/md/mdhandbook/section-2-general-standards/section-2-2-specification-requirements-for-graduation-with-md-degree.html. Accessed November 9, 2025.
3. Frates B, Ortega HA, Freeman K, et al. Lifestyle medicine in medical education: maximizing impact. *Mayo Clin Proc Innov Qual Outcomes*. 2024;8(5):451–474.
4. Secretaries Kennedy, McMahon Demand Comprehensive Nutrition Education Reforms, United States Health and Human Services Department. https://www.hhs.gov/press-room/hhs-education-nutrition-medical-training-reforms.html. Accessed November 10, 2025.
5. Trilk JL, Worthman S, Shetty P, et al. Undergraduate medical education: lifestyle medicine curriculum implementation standards. *Am J Lifestyle Med*. 2021;15(5):526–530.
6. The Entrustable Professional Activities. AAMC. https://www.aamc.org/media/20211/download and https://www.aamc.org/about-us/mission-areas/medical-education/cbme/core-epas.
7. Eisenberg DM, Cole A, Maile EJ, et al. Proposed nutrition competencies for medical students and physician trainees: a consensus statement. *JAMA Netw Open*. 2024;7(9):e2435425.
8. Frates B, Hivert MF, Christopher Duggan. *Essentials of Nutrition in Healthcare*. New York: McGraw Hill, 2024.
9. Mechanick JI, Kushner RF (eds.). *Lifestyle Medicine: Closing Research, Practice, and Knowledge Gaps*. New York: Springer, 2025.
10. Frates B, Kusnadi K, McCargo T. Teaching assistants: essential members of the teaching team. *Am J Lifestyle Med*. 2025;19(6):842–845. doi: 10.1177/15598276251328635.
11. Essa-Hadad J, Rudolf MC, Mani N, Malatskey L. Mapping lifestyle medicine in undergraduate medical education: a lever for enhancing the curriculum. *BMC Med Educ*. 2022;22(1):886.
12. Competency-Based Medical Education from the Association of American Medical Colleges (AAMC). https://www.aamc.org/about-us/mission-areas/medical-education/cbme. Accessed December 20, 2025.
13. Cooper D, Holmboe ES. Competency-based medical education at the front lines of patient care. *N Engl J Med*. 2025;393(4):376–388. doi: 10.1056/NEJMra2411880.
14. The Harvard Medical School Student Handbook Online. 1.08 MD Program Objectives. https://medstudenthandbook.hms.harvard.edu/md-program-objectives. Accessed December 20, 2025.

25 Evaluations and Assessments for Lifestyle Medicine Courses

25.1 STUDENT EVALUATIONS OF THE COURSE

Medical school faculty members spend a significant amount of time developing and delivering courses with engaging and compelling teaching strategies. They work diligently to craft objectives with Bloom's Taxonomy and align them with the core competencies. There's also the student assessment and feedback part of teaching courses. All of this work will be of limited value if there is no assessment or feedback on the course itself. The only way to know if a course was successful is to measure outcomes. As was discussed in Chapter 23 on developing and designing courses, medical educators begin with the end in mind. The end results are the course outcomes. This shifts the focus of assessments and student feedback from students to medical educators.

One crucial component of teaching and learning experiences is the assessment of the teacher, teaching team, teaching strategies, and course materials. Sometimes, teachers create the course assessment instruments. In addition, the medical school or university always provides standardized course evaluation surveys for each course. In some cases, the university allows faculty to add questions relevant to their course or course material. Clearly, this is different from an assessment used to check a student's knowledge. This is an assessment of the course itself: how organized it was, if the course assignments were too challenging or easy, if the reading and homework were at the right level, if the assessments were reflective of the material covered in class, and if the course met student expectations. There are also questions specifically about individual faculty members, lecturers, teaching assistants, and others involved in delivering the course material. There are Likert-scale and open-ended questions. The Likert questions may include general items such as how you would rate the course overall, the course material, and the professor, all on a 1–5 scale. Open-ended questions may include suggestions for how faculty could improve this course. Other questions could include: What were the most effective parts of the course? What were the least effective parts of the course? And why?

The results of the survey are usually sent directly to the faculty. Often, charts indicate where the course rates relative to university or medical school averages. In general, faculty read their own survey responses and respond accordingly. It is essential to encourage students to fill out these survey instruments. It is this type of evaluation and feedback that enables faculty to improve their teaching techniques and strategies as well as the overall design of their courses each year.

To follow the Plan-Do-Study-Act methodology for improving courses, faculty need the "study" phase of the process (1,2). In this context, the word "study" means to evaluate. Faculty want to have an impact. They want the time and energy they put into creating the course to be worthwhile for the students, themselves, and the teaching team. A team at Baylor, in the Department of Internal Medicine, Division of Infectious Diseases, used the Plan-Do-Study-Act model to work with students on an antibiotic utilization curriculum (3). The authors reported that the Plan-Do-Study-Act method they employed from February 2017 to July 2019 allowed them to enhance their course guided by feedback from their students, ultimately achieving more positive ratings for the active learning format of the course, and improvements in understanding antibiotic medications and their clinical applications when compared to scores before the Plan-Do-Study-Act intervention. What did they change? Based on student feedback, educators addressed the timing of their sessions, the content of their handouts, and the organization of the gaming component of their class (3). This example demonstrates that students in a course can be the most effective guides for future improvements.

DOI: 10.1201/9781003630043-25

It is helpful if faculty conduct their own mid-year assessment of their courses so that they can course-correct midway. By administering an anonymous online survey, faculty can gain insight into how the course is progressing before it concludes. In addition, soliciting student feedback after individual lessons can be beneficial, particularly when faculty are implementing new approaches. A faculty member could ask, "How did you enjoy the breakout sessions today?" or "What did you enjoy about class today?" The one-minute reflections, during which students summarize an "Aha moment" or a meaningful moment in the session, can also help guide faculty. If students repeatedly mention the richness of discussions about clinical cases, this indicates that the class is gaining valuable insight during those activities. In this way, faculty can receive feedback well before the formal, official student input at the end of the course.

25.2 TRACKING RESULTS OF MEDICAL EDUCATION PROGRAMS AND COURSES

The Donald Kirkpatrick Model helps to analyze the impact of training programs. It was originally focused on businesses, but it has been used in health information management courses (4), in healthcare staff teaching and learning workshops (5), and in medical school education (6). The model demonstrates that there are different levels of impact a program can have.

The four Kirkpatrick levels for medical education are (6):

- *Level 1: Reaction*: This includes learner satisfaction, engagement, and relevance.
- *Level 2: Learning*: This includes changes in knowledge, skills, attitudes, confidence, and commitment.
- *Level 3: Behavior*: This includes the application of what was learned and a change in learner behavior.
- *Level 4: Results*: This includes achieving outcomes and indicators of progress toward those outcomes. Figure 25.1 demonstrates the four levels of the Kirkpatrick model.

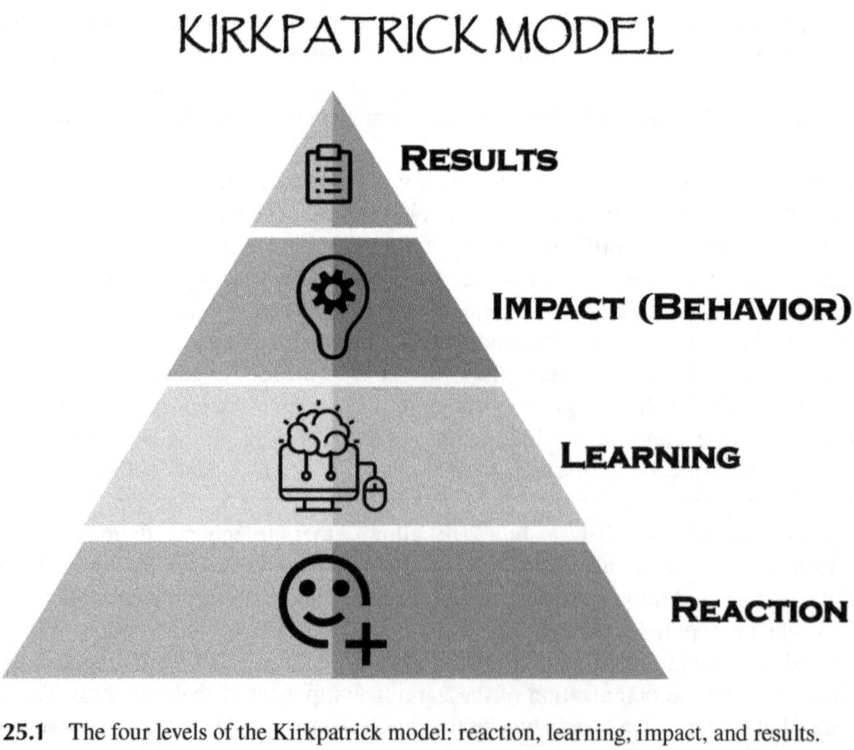

FIGURE 25.1 The four levels of the Kirkpatrick model: reaction, learning, impact, and results.

Asset ID: 2143753285

Level 1 is the reaction to the program or course. This is the level of engagement, relevance, and satisfaction. Then, there is level 2. In this level, learning is assessed. Knowledge, skills, attitudes, confidence, and commitment are evaluated and measured. Level 3 refers to the behavioral level. Has behavior changed? If so, how? Level 4 is the results level. At this level, the initiative or course outcomes are reviewed, and the organizational outcomes or medical school outcomes are evaluated.

In medical school courses, level 1 is typically assessed through a school- or course-administered survey administered at the end of the course, with questions such as "How satisfied were you with this course?" Engagement can be assessed by attendance, survey response rates, and student participation in class discussions and assignments.

One of the early medical education efforts to integrate lifestyle medicine into the four-year curriculum was delivered by Dr. Erica Frank and her colleagues at Emory University School of Medicine in the early 2000s. She provides level 1 feedback per Kirkpatrick's model, which can be helpful 25 years later. Dr. Frank and her colleagues implemented a comprehensive "Healthy Doc-Healthy Patient" intervention spanning all four years of medical school for the Class of 2003, incorporating extracurricular components, and intending to promote healthy lifestyles among the students. They compared the Class of 2003 with the Class of 2002. Here is a list of the interventions from their article in MedGenMed (7). Reviewing this article can generate ideas for faculty interested in incorporating lifestyle medicine into the medical school curriculum. Highlights from the article are included below, including lists of curricular interventions targeted to the whole class and interventions that were not lecture-based, as shown below.

LIST 1 HD CURRICULAR INTERVENTIONS: LECTURES TO WHOLE CLASS (ONLY IN PRE-CLINICAL YEARS)

First year

- Orientation: half-hour Principal Investigator (PI) lecture with questions and answers on scientific basis for HD

Sophomore year

- Behavioral science: physician panel of former substance users (also done in previous years, with a new [minor] emphasis on normativeness of healthful behaviors)
- Behavioral science: 1-hour talk on alcohol and tobacco use habits of physicians, US medical students, and Emory 2003 medical students by PI
- Nutrition course: plant-based diet lecture (given yearly by the PI and her physician-husband) with new emphasis on personal dietary practice
- Pathophysiology: mention made of need for students to have healthful drinking habits themselves in lecture on alcoholic liver disease by regular pathophysiology lecturer

LIST 2 HD CURRICULAR INTERVENTIONS: NON-LECTURE FORMAT

First year

- Anatomy: booklet on strengthening particular muscles, given by anatomists
- Medical decision-making: used their own data to learn statistics, with homework assignment (from dean/professor) and in-class discussion (from dean/professor and PI)
- Patient-doctor small groups: pairs of students presented papers they chose to write on physician/medical student health (averaging 1 such paper in half the small groups)
- Problem-based-learning small groups: unit on a substance-abusing physician (also done in prior years), with accompanying email from PI on physicians' substance use rates

Sophomore year

- Clinical methods: an afternoon on exercise with mixed lectures and demonstrations, moderated by the PI with guest lecturers

Junior year

- Dermatology: letter on the importance of skin cancer prevention for themselves and their patients, a review article on skin cancer-prevention strategies, and a container of sunscreen for their own use, all from clerkship director
- Ethics/medicine: completed advanced directives and living wills for themselves
- Ethics/psychiatry: completed a Beck Depression Inventory and an alcohol (CAGE) screening questionnaire on themselves
- Family/internal medicine orientation: instead of role-playing being patients, students practiced patient counseling with their own personal health practices (with 2 follow-ups in family medicine, all with PI, for a total of 1–3 hours)
- Family/internal medicine orientation: 30 minutes of instruction and practice with health-risk appraisals (HRAs), reviewing results of their HRAs on their own and with a classmate
- Family medicine: students (and occasional preceptors) kept 1-week logs of daily number of fruits/vegetables and exercise amount/type, and submitted them to the clerkship director
- Family medicine: wrote a description of their ideal lifestyle a decade hence
- Ob/Gyn: articles assigned on women physicians' characteristics during pregnancy, sexual abuse/domestic violence rates, and depression/suicide rates in preparation for lectures by Ob/Gyn faculty on these topics
- Ob/Gyn: students given American Cancer Society breast self-exam shower card
- Ob/Gyn: students given condoms and emergency contraception, offered as requested (also offered occasionally in prior years)

Senior year

- Medicine sub-internship: Under the PI's (and, later in the year, other preventionists') supervision, students practiced taking histories, performing physical exams, and developing assessments and plans on each other, with an emphasis on reviewing their personal health practices for 1–2 hours
- Medicine sub-internship: All ward attendings and supervising physical exam faculty were sent a 1-page email message explaining HD prior to beginning a month supervising the seniors, asking them to reinforce HD concepts; students did not receive the intervention."

Here is a list of extracurricular activities included in the intervention from their article.

LIST 3 EXTRACURRICULAR ACTIVITIES INCLUDED IN THE INTERVENTION

First year

- Saturday visit to PI's mountain house (10 students)
- One-hour healthy, quick-cooking class by PI and a nutritionist (10)
- One-hour lunchtime (with free healthy lunch) panel (including PI and her husband) on living a well-balanced life (30, SI)
- Personal health prescriptions provided to students subsequent to lifestyle review with PI (5)

- Afternoon hike and healthy dinner with PI (4)
- Emailed message inviting M1s to submit projects that they would like done for HD intervention (all)
- Emailed note to students encouraging a healthful and pleasant summer vacation (all)
- Students worked full-time with the PI over the summer on new interventions for their class (3, SI)

Sophomore year

- "Health Heads Up" – monthly emailed summary of a half-dozen prevention-related studies, written by a classmate (all, SI)
- Lunchtime massage "hands-on" seminar with data on the physiological effects of massage (free healthy lunch provided) (30, SI)
- Lunchtime yoga/meditation seminar by a visiting MD on the health and psychological effects of yoga and meditation (free healthy lunch provided) (50, SI)
- A piece of fruit and a "have a healthy/happy holiday" note put into students' boxes the day before pre-winter holiday exams, and a similar note posted to their emails (all)
- Personal health prescriptions provided to students subsequent to lifestyle review with the PI (5)
- Lunchtime talk (free healthy lunch provided) on the pathophysiology of stress and what can be done about it by Emory PhD counselor (30)
- Emailed message that HD was featured on the back cover (and on page 8) of *Emory Medicine* magazine (message read by 104 students)
- Two wine-tasting seminars (attended by about 30 students each time, SI) to teach about using alcohol for purposes other than inebriation at the PI's house
- Monthly walks/runs (1–10, SI)
- Weekly yoga classes (1–6, SI)
- Sponsored entrance fees for races (5, SI)
- Healthy breakfasts prior to joint exams (all, SI)
- Healthy Quick Asian Cooking class, proposed by and cosponsored with Asian student group (30, all)
- PI presented HD at a plenary for the Student National Medical Association meeting in Atlanta (10 Emory students and 200 other medical students, SI)

Junior year

- Validation study for HD food-frequency screener, including 5 in-person 24-hour recalls; 2 HD food-frequency questionnaires; personal analysis of fat and fruit and vegetable intake; and $100 for participants (20)

Senior year

- Students given toothpaste and a travel toothbrush imprinted with "Well, at least my teeth are healthy" (all)
- PI attended Match Day and graduation activities and attended the senior banquet, giving students champagne and flutes (engraved with ""EUSM Class of 2003 – To your health!"), and toasted/thanked them." (6)

The authors used focus groups to gather data on the impact of their intervention. This list of themes is from their article and provides essential and relevant information to this day.

LIST 4 MAJOR THEMES FROM THE FOCUS GROUPS

- Listen to the students early and often; respond to them substantively; and make sure that they know that you're listening and responding.
- Have this be a multipronged effort, incorporating many faculty, the administration, and peer role modeling.
- Integrate the curricular activities thoroughly into the curriculum.
- Provide a strong, science-based, pragmatic prevention curriculum, giving them many practical strategies for helping patients.
- Don't just use lectures to teach.
- Offer plentiful, nonrequired, fun extracurriculars.
- Don't nag or induce guilt.
- Have interventions and recommendations seem achievable to the students.
- Provide collective data, but don't overexpose the students to it, and don't assume that collective data apply to every student, especially if it's unpleasant news.
- Provide personalized data when possible.
- Uncouple evaluations from the intervention, and keep evaluations brief" (6).

Test results are an indicator for level 2 in the Kirkpatrick Model. Did the students pass the quizzes, tests, and other assessments? Did their knowledge increase? Questions on a questionnaire that ask about confidence level, such as "How confident are you in your ability to counsel a person with diabetes on lifestyle factors on a scale of 1–5?" are examples of level 2 questions. Another level 2 question is "How important do you believe lifestyle medicine counseling is for patient management and prevention of disease?" Skills in lifestyle medicine are often evaluated through Objective Structured Clinical Examination (OSCE) assessments and through role-play exercises in class.

Another example of a level 2 outcome in the Kirkpatrick Model is a lifestyle medicine education program offered at Harvard Medical School, a small research study in which medical students were asked about their confidence in counseling on lifestyle medicine pillars and tested on counseling strategies pre- and post a one-hour lecture on behavior change (8). This small study demonstrated that, following a one-hour presentation, first-year medical students' knowledge and confidence regarding counseling and behavior change increased. Bar-Ilan University, a school in Israel, assessed students' confidence levels following an internal medicine rotation. They found that students were relatively confident in providing general LM counseling but less confident in specific topics such as exercise, nutrition, stress, and sleep (9).

Level 3 in the Kirkpatrick Model includes an assessment of behavior. Do students who are exposed to lifestyle medicine in the first and second years spend more time counseling patients on the six pillars of lifestyle medicine when they enter their clinical rotations? A level 3 outcome could be the answer to the question, "Do students who take courses in lifestyle medicine counsel patients on the six pillars when they enter internship?" or "Do medical students graduating from schools that have 100+ hours of lifestyle medicine education incorporated into their four-year curriculum counsel more on the six pillars of lifestyle medicine compared to students at schools that offer less than 25 hours of lifestyle medicine education in the four years of medical school?" These are research questions that remain unanswered.

Level 3 results can include personal behavior and lifestyle practices. The University of Toledo Medical Center reported its findings on medical students' self-care behaviors following a lifestyle medicine elective (10). In the fall of 2015, their study began. It ended in the spring of 2017. Sixty-one students participated in the study. The faculty offered a lifestyle medicine elective to first- and second-year medical students, comprising four sessions.

Session One: The faculty provided information on the effects of lifestyle behaviors on physical and mental health. During the same session, the students completed self-report surveys on their physical activity and nutrition levels, as well as questionnaires assessing anxiety and depression.

Session Two: Students' scores were shared, and they then selected one of three areas of focus for the remainder of the session (physical activity, nutrition, or stress management).

Sessions Three and Four: The faculty reviewed patient cases.

At the end of the four sessions of this elective, the students filled out the same self-report measures (10).

The results demonstrated that, as a group, the students in the elective reported statistically significant improvements in nutrition, depression, and anxiety. Regarding the specific focus groups, the students who chose the stress management group reported lower scores on anxiety levels after the elective. Students who selected the nutrition focus reported lower fat intake and higher fruit and vegetable intake after the elective. Interestingly, the students who chose the physical activity group did not significantly increase their daily physical activity by the end of the elective. This elective demonstrated that the students who participated in the nutrition focus group changed their own personal eating behaviors (10). This is an example of a Kirkpatrick level 3 result.

Level 4 outcomes would include behavior change at the system level or medical school level. The goal is for physicians to counsel patients on the six pillars of lifestyle medicine, with patients benefiting by preventing or controlling chronic conditions with fewer medications and fewer procedures than when physicians do not counsel on the six pillars. Does providing 100+ hours of lifestyle medicine education produce practicing physicians who can successfully manage patients with chronic conditions with more prescriptions for the pillars and fewer prescriptions for pills and procedures, and do their patients better control their blood pressure, cholesterol, and hemoglobin A1C? These research questions remain unanswered. To date, there are no Kirkpatrick level 4 research results for lifestyle medicine medical education courses (11). Lifestyle medicine has come a long way as a field and specialty with board certification and medical schools, including Lifestyle Medicine Interest Groups (LMIGs), as well as offering elective courses on lifestyle medicine and more schools using lifestyle medicine themes/threads, but the research on lifestyle medicine education needs to grow (12). This book will hopefully support the development of more lifestyle medicine courses and research on those courses.

As noted at the beginning of the section, Kirkpatrick's model was originally developed for business training but is readily applicable to medical school education. The descriptions of each level are shown in Figure 25.2. Level 1 represents the students' reaction level. Level 2 represents the success

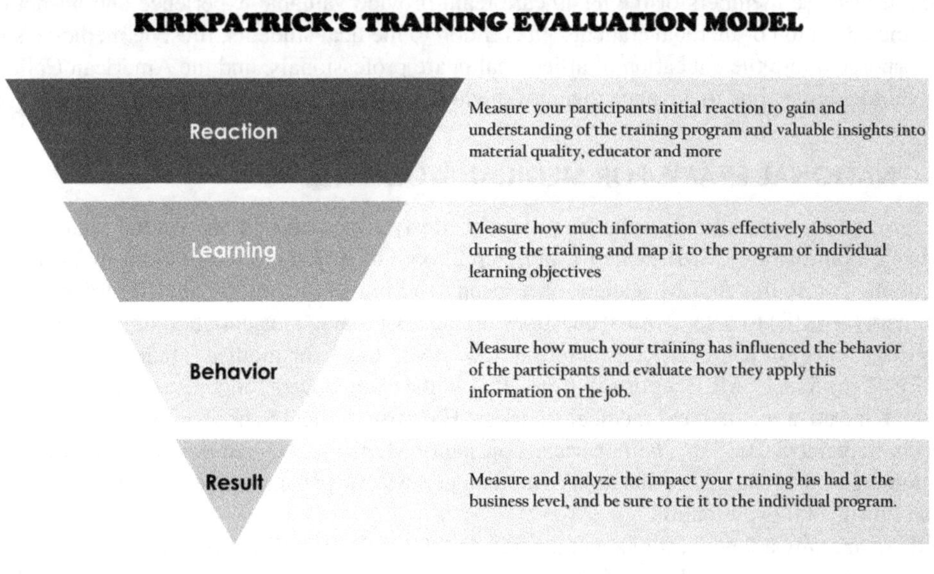

FIGURE 25.2 Kirkpatrick's training evaluation model with descriptions.

the students achieved through their learning opportunities in courses, classes, or workshops. Level 3 assesses how their learning has impacted their personal and professional behavior, including how they treat and counsel patients. Level 4 represents the impact that the students' learning had on the healthcare system and the patients they treat. Did the patients experience benefits, such as lower hemoglobin A1C, lower blood pressure, and ultimately improved longevity and quality of life?

25.3 IMPLEMENTATION CHALLENGES TO INCORPORATING LIFESTYLE MEDICINE INTO MEDICAL SCHOOLS

The main implementation challenges in incorporating lifestyle medicine fall into three categories: faculty expertise, curriculum overload, and national exams.

In terms of faculty expertise, the field of lifestyle medicine is only two decades old, and the first board certification was in 2017. There are thousands of physicians and other healthcare professionals trained and certified in lifestyle medicine worldwide, but the majority of medical school faculty are not. To teach lifestyle medicine, it helps if the faculty member is an expert in at least one of the six pillars of lifestyle medicine, such as exercise physiology, nutrition science, sleep medicine, stress management, social connection, or avoidance of risky substances. However, endocrinologists, cardiologists, family medicine physicians, pediatricians, obstetricians and gynecologists, primary care physicians, nephrologists, rheumatologists, and other specialists who manage patients with chronic conditions know a great deal about these diseases, their pathology and pathophysiology, and their treatments. A board-certified specialist in these areas, in addition to lifestyle medicine, would be an ideal faculty member to teach lifestyle medicine to medical students.

Faculty members can collaborate with colleagues to leverage their own strengths and areas of expertise, combining them with those of colleagues who have different training, knowledge, and skills in lifestyle medicine. In addition, including other healthcare professionals in the teaching helps medical students better understand the value of teamwork. By learning from nurses, registered dietitians, physical therapists, exercise physiologists, and health coaches, medical students better appreciate these members of the healthcare team and the expertise they bring.

Lifestyle medicine is a team-based specialty (13,14). Collaborating with physical therapists, social workers, registered dietitians, community health workers, and mental health professionals enables physicians to help patients address social determinants of health and mental health conditions. All of these members of the healthcare team provide valuable experience and wisdom that add to the education of medical students. In addition to medical students, lifestyle medicine should be incorporated into the education of allied healthcare professionals, and the American College of Lifestyle Medicine aims to advance this movement through the Academic Pathways system (15).

25.4 NATIONAL EXAMS FOR MEDICAL STUDENTS

There are very few questions on the six pillars of lifestyle medicine on the United States Medical Licensing Examination USMLE Step 1 and Step 2, both of which are required for medical school graduation. For years, ACLM leaders have been working with the National Board of Medical Examiners (NBME) to help identify questions on the six pillars. This collaboration is key.

To date, nutrition has been considered a "low yield" topic for medical students preparing for USMLE 1 (16). The USMLE reports that 5%–15% of the exam covers "Biochemistry and Nutrition." As John Kincaid, a second-year medical student at Harvard Medical School, wrote in an article published in September 2025 in The American Journal of Medicine, "Given the high level of national attention focused on nutrition education in medicine, it was surprising to see scant mention of nutrition on this pivotal examination."

If there are only a few questions on nutrition and the other five pillars of lifestyle medicine, students may not feel motivated to study these topics, and medical schools may not feel compelled to devote time to teaching them, especially given the material they already need to cover. Most faculty involved in curriculum development struggle to find time for essential topics that medical students must master to become competent physicians. High-yield USMLE subjects are necessary for medical students to master and, therefore, must be included in the core curriculum. It is a difficult task to revamp and update medical school curricula that provide foundational knowledge across all organ systems, the latest scientific and research findings on disease pathophysiology, and treatment options. The art of medicine, professionalism, and whole-person compassionate care also need to be taught.

Until the NBME includes questions on the six pillars of lifestyle medicine in a noticeable manner for test takers, medical students will continue to ignore the "low yield" subjects and focus on the "high yield" ones. In turn, medical school curriculum development teams often focus on USMLE content to ensure that their students pass these exams and graduate from their schools. The USMLE Step 1 changed from a score-based to a pass/fail format in January 2022. This relieves some of the pressure on medical students, which is beneficial for stress resilience. Adding questions on stress, nutrition, exercise, sleep, social connection, and avoidance of risky substances will be a groundbreaking advancement for the USMLE Step 1 and will impact medical education. Teaching to the test is a well-known strategy employed by educators at all levels.

When national exams include material in the questions, schools ensure that the material is included in the curriculum. Incorporating questions on exercise, nutrition, sleep, stress resilience, social connection, and avoidance of risky substances into the USMLE Step 1, 2, and 3 exams would encourage schools to include this material in the core curriculum. As mentioned in Chapter 24, in 2025, Robert F. Kennedy JR., Secretary of the United States Department of Health and Human Services, and Linda McMahon, Secretary of the United States Department of Education, issued a recommendation that medical schools include nutrition in their curricula (17). At that time, there was mention of withholding funding from schools that did not teach nutrition. This is a step in the right direction. Time will tell if medical schools comply with the recommendations and what will happen if they do not.

25.5 SUMMARY

A concrete plan for evaluating and providing feedback on a medical school course is vital. How will medical educators determine whether they have met their goals? Kirkpatrick's Model for determining the results of a medical education study is useful. Level 1 covers the students' reactions to the course. Level 2 covers the students' learning. Level 3 addresses students' behavior change in their own practice and in their clinical practice, including how they treat patients. Level 4 covers the impact on patient outcomes and the healthcare system. Lifestyle medicine education requires more level 4 research evidence. The first step is to implement successful lifestyle medicine courses that are carefully designed with clear objectives and goals, employ effective, engaging teaching techniques, assess students and provide feedback, and evaluate the course and receive student feedback. Assessment and feedback are the means by which lifestyle medicine courses can demonstrate their impact. Level 4 impact in the Kirkpatrick model is the goal. This is a call to action for medical educators in lifestyle medicine. There is work to be done, and this book will help accomplish it.

REFERENCES

1. Bradham TS, Sponsler KC, Watkins SC, Ehrenfeld JM. Creating a quality improvement course for undergraduate medical education: practice what you teach. *Acad Med.* 2018;93(10):1491–1496. doi: 10.1097/ACM.0000000000002253. PMID: 29727320.
2. Mills G, Kelly S, Crittendon DR, Cunningham A, Arenson C. Evaluation of a quality improvement experience for family medicine clerkship students. *Fam Med.* 2021;53(10):882–885. doi: 10.22454/FamMed.2021.702090. PMID: 34780656.

3. Rose S, Hamill R, Caruso A, et al. Applying the plan-do-study-act cycle in medical education to refine an antibiotics therapy active learning session. *BMC Med Educ.* 2021;21:459. doi: 10.1186/s12909-021-02886-3.
4. Rouse DN. Employing Kirkpatrick's evaluation framework to determine the effectiveness of health information management courses and programs. *Perspect Health Inf Manag.* 2011;8(Spring):1c.
5. Heydari MR, Taghva F, Amini M, et al. Using Kirkpatrick's model to measure the effect of a new teaching and learning methods workshop for health care staff. *BMC Res Notes.* 2019;12:388. doi: 10.1186/s13104-019-4421-y.
6. Ragsdale JW, Berry A, Gibson JW, Herber-Valdez CR, Germain LJ, Engle DL. Evaluating the effectiveness of undergraduate clinical education programs. *Med Educ Online.* 2020;25(1). doi: 10.1080/10872981.2020.1757883.
7. Frank E, Smith D, Fitzmaurice D. A description and qualitative assessment of a 4-year intervention to improve patient counseling by improving medical student health. *MedGenMed.* 2005;7(2):4. PMID: 16369383; PMCID: PMC1681578.
8. Frates EP, Xiao RC, Simeon K, McCargo T, Guo M, Stern TA. Increasing knowledge and confidence in behavioral change: a pilot study. *Prim Care Companion CNS Disord.* 2016;18(6). doi: 10.4088/PCC.16m01962. PMID: 27922227.
9. Essa-Hadad J, Rudolf MC, Mani N, Malatskey L. Mapping lifestyle medicine in undergraduate medical education: a lever for enhancing the curriculum. *BMC Med Educ.* 2022;22(1):886. doi: 10.1186/s12909-022-03929-z. PMID: 36539724; PMCID: PMC9769064.
10. McGrady A, Badenhop D, Lynch D. Effects of a lifestyle medicine elective on self-care behaviors in preclinical medical students. *Appl Psychophysiol Biofeedback.* 2019;44(2):143–149. doi: 10.1007/s10484-019-09431-5. PMID: 30826911.
11. Pasarica M, Boring M, Lessans S. Current practices in the instruction of lifestyle medicine in medical curricula. *Patient Educ Couns.* 2022;105(2):339–345. doi: 10.1016/j.pec.2021.05.042. Epub 2021 Jun 2. PMID: 34116891.
12. Frates B. The evolution of lifestyle medicine education: what, why, how, who, and what now. *Am J Lifestyle Med.* 2025:15598276251359562. doi: 10.1177/15598276251359562. Epub ahead of print. PMID: 40692611; PMCID: PMC12276203.
13. Kent K, Johnson JD, Simeon K, Frates EP. Case series in lifestyle medicine: a team approach to behavior changes. *Am J Lifestyle Med.* 2016;10(6):388–397. doi: 10.1177/1559827616638288. PMID: 30202299; PMCID: PMC6124983.
14. Millstein RA, Winters L, Sullivan C, Eisenstat S, Sorg E, Comander A. Implementing a multidisciplinary lifestyle medicine clinic for cancer survivorship. *Oncology.* 2024;38(11):421–425. doi: 10.46883/2024.25921030. PMID: 39570709.
15. Brown Z, Freeman K, Räisänen AM. Integrating lifestyle medicine content into health professions programs. *Am J Lifestyle Med.* 2025:15598276251321418. doi: 10.1177/15598276251321418. Epub ahead of print. PMID: 39991019; PMCID: PMC11840824.
16. Kincaid JWR, Devries S. Nutrition on the United States medical licensing step 1 exam: a 'low-yield' topic? *Am J Med.* 2025;138(9):1173–1174. doi: 10.1016/j.amjmed.2025.04.005. Epub 2025 Apr 12. PMID: 40228601.
17. Secretaries Kennedy, McMahon Demand Comprehensive Nutrition Education Reforms. United States Health and Human Services Department. https://www.hhs.gov/press-room/hhs-education-nutrition-medical-training-reforms.html. Accessed November 10, 2025.

26 Lifestyle Medicine in Graduate Medical Education (GME)

Board Certification, Core Competencies, Milestones, and Intensivist Designation

26.1 INTRODUCTION

Many medical students enter medical school seeking to cure disease, heal patients, and learn how lifestyle behaviors (nutrition, exercise, sleep, stress, social connection, and avoidance of risky substances) affect health and well-being. As noted in previous chapters, medical schools do not provide comprehensive coverage of all six pillars of lifestyle medicine. Thus, graduating medical students seek this type of knowledge during residency and graduate medical education (GME).

There is no standalone Accreditation Council for Graduate Medical Education (ACGME)-accredited residency in lifestyle medicine. To fill this gap, the American Board of Lifestyle Medicine developed a Lifestyle Medicine Residency Curriculum (LMRC), which can be purchased by any residency program site nationwide. There is a free introductory offer that residency programs can utilize. The LMRC provides a standardized curriculum in all six pillars. There is an online didactic component, required application activities, a necessary number of patient encounters related to lifestyle medicine, and required group and Intensive Therapeutic Lifestyle Change (ITLC) interventions. These align with the core competencies in lifestyle medicine, as detailed in this chapter.

For board certification in lifestyle medicine, the American Board of Lifestyle Medicine (ABLM) administers a board examination. A physician can be board-certified in lifestyle medicine only after passing the board examinations and obtaining certification from a recognized American Board of Medical Specialties (ABMS)- or American Osteopathic Association (AOA)-recognized specialty. In other words, a physician first needs ABMS or AOA board certification to be eligible for board certification in lifestyle medicine.

Medical students and residents can learn the principles, practices, skills, and knowledge of the six pillars of lifestyle medicine throughout their educational journey. Examples of medical school educational offerings and experiences have been described in previous chapters. This chapter will focus on graduate medical education (GME) options.

26.2 LIFE AFTER MEDICAL SCHOOL

Residency is a time of rapid growth and development for medical trainees. Suddenly, they graduate from medical school and are placed in a hospital setting as practicing physicians. After graduating from medical school, they earn the title of Medical Doctor (MD) and are referred to as doctor (Dr.) Being called doctor (Dr) for the first time can be intimidating for new interns. It is also a source of great pride, given the hard work and perseverance required to earn that title. By the time medical trainees are interns, they have passed the United States Medical Licensing Examination (USMLE) Step 1 and Step 2 CK (Clinical Knowledge). But there is more.

DOI: 10.1201/9781003630043-26

26.3 UNITED STATES MEDICAL LICENSING EXAMINATIONS (USMLE)

The journey to earn a medical license and become board-certified is a long one. It starts in medical school with the United States Medical Licensing Examination (USMLE). The USMLE Step 1 is a one-day examination lasting eight hours. It comprises seven blocks of 60-minute sessions, totaling 280 multiple-choice questions. It is graded pass or fail. The USMLE Step 2 CK is a one-day examination lasting nine hours. It comprises eight blocks of 60-minute sessions, totaling 318 items, some of which are multiple-choice questions. There is also a scientific abstract as well as items with audio and visual findings. This test is scored.

The USMLE Step 3 is required for a physician to obtain licensure to practice medicine. This third test occurs after the first year of residency, which is the internship, preliminary, or transitional year. This final examination in the USMLE series is a two-day examination. The first-day exam consists of multiple-choice questions focused on the foundations of independent clinical practice, and the second-day examination consists of multiple-choice questions and computer-based case simulations focused on advanced clinical medicine. This examination is scored.

There are interesting findings with regard to the lifestyle medicine pillars on the USMLE Content Outline PDF online (1).

Exercise: Only mentioned in the section on Human Development, Normal Age-Related Findings and Care of the Well Patient.

Nutrition: "This is a quote. For example, there has been an emphasis on new content developed assessing competencies related to geriatric medicine, nutrition, and prescription drug use." (1) Nutrition is mentioned in the section on Human Development, Normal Age-Related Findings and Care of the Well Patient, disorders of the small intestine and colon with malnutrition, under the biliary section with cholestasis with parenteral nutrition, under prenatal care with nutritional assessment for preconception counseling and care and supervision of normal pregnancy, and under multisystem processes and disorders, there is an entire nutrition section that covers "protein-calorie malnutrition (kwashiorkor, marasmus), vitamin deficiencies and/or toxicities including vitamin A; vitamin B; vitamin B1; thiamine (e.g., Wernicke–Korsakoff syndrome, beriberi); vitamin B3, niacin; vitamin B6, pyridoxine; vitamin B9, folic acid; vitamin B12, cobalamins (pernicious anemia); vitamin C (scurvy); vitamin D (rickets); vitamin E; vitamin K, mineral deficiencies and/or toxicities, obesity, and enteral/parenteral nutrition (TPN)" (1).

Sleep: Mentioned under neurology with sleep disorders, pulmonology with sleep apnea, patient safety with physician factors in the medical errors category, and under human development care of the well patient.

Stress: Mentioned in the section on Human Development, Normal Age-Related Findings and Care of the Well Patient, under the Behavioral Health Section, with anxiety disorders and psychosocial disorders/behavior.

Social Connection: Not mentioned.

Risky Substances: Under the section of behavioral health, there is a section on substance use disorders, including alcohol, tobacco, nicotine, and prescription drug use.

Thus, to pass all three USMLE examinations and become a licensed physician, a medical trainee requires minimal knowledge of the six pillars of lifestyle medicine. However, to become board-certified in lifestyle medicine after residency, a physician needs to know and understand a significant amount of medical knowledge in the six pillars of lifestyle medicine, be adept at communication skills for behavior change, master clinical processes needed to practice lifestyle medicine, work with interprofessional teams to help patients adopt and sustain healthy lifestyles, and practice with professionalism.

After residency, physicians must pass their specialty board examinations. Physicians are first board-certified in general internal medicine, pediatrics, or surgery, and then board-certified in a subspecialty such as cardiology, endocrinology, or nephrology. As a reminder, to be board-certified in lifestyle medicine, medical trainees must complete and graduate from an ACGME-accredited residency program, pass their primary board examination, and be board-certified in their primary specialty before being board-certified in lifestyle medicine. There are two different pathways to board certification in lifestyle medicine. However, they must first graduate from an ACGME-accredited residency program. That is the next focal point for this chapter.

26.4 ACCREDITATION COUNCIL FOR GRADUATE MEDICAL EDUCATION (ACGME)

Just passing USMLE Step 1, Step 2 CK, and Step 3 will not lead to residency graduation or board certification in a medical specialty, which requires its own examination process. The Accreditation Council for Graduate Medical Education (ACGME) oversees resident training in the United States. Resident training is a significant responsibility that affects the future of the healthcare system. Medical school faculty members help run graduate medical education departments at hospitals and academic institutions. Each residency has a residency program director and, likely, an associate or assistant residency program director. Many medical educators are involved with residents in training.

ACGME focuses on six core competencies, including:

1. Professionalism;
2. Patient care and procedural skills;
3. Medical knowledge;
4. Practice-based learning and improvement;
5. Interpersonal and communication skills;
6. Systems-based practice.

For all ACGME-accredited residencies, there are milestones associated with each of the six core competencies. These milestones are competency-based developmental outcomes (knowledge, skills, attitudes, performance) that are structured and progressive, helping residents learn and grow each year from novice (Level 1) to advanced beginner (Level 2), competent (Level 3), proficient (Level 4), and expert (Level 5). Milestones vary by specialty and are specific to the work physicians in that specialty perform. Milestones for a surgeon vary from milestones for a pediatrician, for example. The milestones are intended to help medical educators support residents on their journey toward proficiency and expertise. There are no specific requirements for graduation based on the milestones. The milestones are assessment and feedback tools for residents and faculty alike. The lifestyle medicine residency is not an ACGME-approved program, and it does not yet have official milestones from the ACGME or ACLM.

26.5 BOARD CERTIFICATION AND ELIGIBILITY

To graduate from residency, a resident must complete the required years of training (2–6), meet the specific requirements set by the residency program, demonstrate clinical competency, and receive satisfactory performance reviews throughout their rotations. The residency program director determines whether a resident can graduate. After completing residency, the resident is eligible for board certification in that specialty.

The use of the ACGME milestones by residency program directors helps residents improve, perform at a high level, and demonstrate clinical competency. In this way, milestones serve as tools that can assist residents in their journey toward expertise and their goal of graduating from residency. After residency, residents are eligible to sit for the board certification examination in their specialty. They are considered board-eligible by the American Board of Medical Specialties (ABMS) or the American Osteopathic Association (AOA). They are board-certified by ABMS or AOA in their specialty after successfully passing the board examination for their specific specialty. This often includes written and oral board examinations. It varies for each specialty.

26.6 BOARD CERTIFICATION IN LIFESTYLE MEDICINE

For lifestyle medicine, there are two pathways to board certification: experiential and educational. Both require board certification in a primary specialty by an ABMS or AOA board, as described above.

For the experiential pathway, a physician achieves board certification status through the ABMS or the AOA. They must complete two years of practice prior to applying for board certification in lifestyle medicine. The requirements are clearly stated on the American Board of Lifestyle Medicine's website (7). After two years, the physician needs to complete:

- 30 hours of online CME from an approved course
- 20 hours of event CME from an approved event or combination of approved events
- A case study outlining your personal experience with lifestyle medicine
  - Case study instructions from the template available on the ABLM website:
  - Please summarize the case of a patient (can be yourself) to whom you prescribed lifestyle change as the primary treatment for one or more chronic diseases. Provide:
  - a brief history or background about the patient and the assessment
  - the types, intensity (length), and frequency of interventions offered (counseling, group visits, digital apps, phone support, dietician visits, etc.)
  - lifestyle areas of focus (nutrition, movement, social connection, stress management/emotional well-being, or sleep)
  - lifestyle change results, such as level of increase in movement in frequency/minutes per week; frequency/amount of plant-based meals added; other dietary changes; increase in sleep; stress management activities added
  - health outcomes, such as decrease in hospitalizations, symptoms, improved vital signs and key labs, and decrease/change in medications
  - patient's view of changed/improved quality of life and life satisfaction
- Pass the examination, which consists of 150 multiple-choice questions written to NBME standards for physicians and 120 multiple-choice questions written to NBME standards for health care professionals with a master's degree or PhD in a health-related field. The test takers get four hours to complete the proctored examination. There is a registration fee for the examination.
- If all eligibility requirements are met and the physician or healthcare professional passes the examination, there is then a fee to become certified.

For the educational pathway, the Lifestyle Medicine Residency Curriculum (LMRC) is required. Faculty can learn alongside residents and participate in the LMRC, even if they are not residents, and scholarships are available. This is called the Faculty Learner LMRC or FLMRC. Here are the steps for the educational pathway to board certification in lifestyle medicine from the ABLM:

1. *Complete Residency*: Finish an ACGME-accredited residency program.
2. Complete the LMRC during the primary residency. Finish the 100-hour LMRC standardized curriculum. The LMRC is designed to be completed within one to three years. The LMRC includes 40 hours of online didactic instruction and 60 hours of application activities.
3. Or complete an ABLM-approved Lifestyle Medicine Educational Equivalency Pathway with 100% of all ABLM competencies covered, 100 hours of educational content (40 hours of didactics and 60 hours of application activities).

4. *Fulfill Practicum Requirements for LMRC and Equivalency Pathways*: Complete 400 patient encounters related to lifestyle medicine, 10 hours of Intensive Therapeutic Lifestyle Change (ITLC) interventions, and 10 hours of group facilitation.
5. *Take the ABLM Board Certification Examination*: After completing the requirements, you are eligible to sit for the ABLM certification examination. Passing the ABLM examination is a requirement to be board-certified in lifestyle medicine.
6. Certification will only be granted after successfully passing the primary board examination.
7. Submission of a letter of attestation from the program director is required to ensure completion of LMRC or equivalency residency program.

The board examination in lifestyle medicine is structured around the lifestyle medicine core competencies for physicians, which is the topic of the next section. The same examination is administered to international physicians, and the International Board of Lifestyle Medicine oversees their certification process. Healthcare professionals with a master's degree in a health-related field can be certified in lifestyle medicine through the American College of Lifestyle Medicine after meeting all eligibility requirements, writing up a case study, and passing the board certification examination (4).

26.7 LIFESTYLE MEDICINE CORE COMPETENCIES FOR RESIDENTS AND PRACTICING PHYSICIANS

To be board-certified in lifestyle medicine, a physician must know a significant amount of material in the six pillars. The field of lifestyle medicine has core competencies that guide the education, growth, and development of residents and practicing physicians to become competent in delivering lifestyle medicine to patients. The competencies are not broken up into the six pillars. There are different sections as noted below.

There are different sets of core competencies. Chapter 24 covered lifestyle medicine core competencies for medical school students. The Entrustable Professional Activities (EPAs) that all entering residents are expected to perform without supervision on day one of internship were also reviewed. The lifestyle medicine core competencies were mapped to these EPAs in Chapter 24. This chapter extends the core competencies to the resident and practicing physician levels.

There are ten lifestyle medicine core competencies, as identified and described in the original 2010 JAMA publication (2), the first to describe them. Twelve years later, in 2022, the updated core competencies were published in the *American Journal of Lifestyle Medicine* (3). The 2022 updated lifestyle medicine core competencies include ten areas of focus:

1. Introduction to lifestyle medicine;
2. The role of the practitioner's personal health and community advocacy;
3. Nutrition science, assessment, and prescription;
4. Physical activity science, assessment, and prescription;
5. Sleep health science and interventions;
6. Treating tobacco use disorder and managing other toxic exposures (including vaping, alcohol use, and other illicit substances);
7. Key clinical processes in lifestyle medicine;
8. Fundamentals of health behavior change;
9. Emotional and mental health assessment and interventions;
10. The role of connectedness and positive psychology.

Across the ten areas of focus, there are 6–14 specific core competencies, for a total of 88 core competencies in lifestyle medicine. These will be listed in the next section. The six pillars of lifestyle medicine are embedded in these ten core competencies, with five of them—including nutrition, physical activity, sleep, social connectedness, and avoidance of risky substances—holding their own competency titles. Stress resilience is covered in the competency for emotional and mental health assessment and interventions.

26.8 MAPPING THE 88 LIFESTYLE MEDICINE COMPETENCIES TO THE SIX ACGME CORE COMPETENCIES

The 88 core sub-competencies in lifestyle medicine are categorized into ten different focal areas listed earlier. These core competencies and subcompetencies had existed for 14 years before they were mapped to the ACGME core competencies. This is a crucial step because there is currently no ACGME-accredited residency in lifestyle medicine. For this reason, the medical education efforts proposed by lifestyle medicine experts must align with the ACGME's national standards. For the first time, the lifestyle medicine core competencies were mapped to the ACGME core competencies in Mayo Clinic Proceedings: Innovations, Quality, and Outcomes, Lifestyle Medicine in Medical Education: Maximizing Impact in 2024 (4). In some cases, the lifestyle medicine core competency was not specific to one ACGME core competency, and in those cases, two ACGME core competencies were identified. See the Mayo Clinic Proceedings article for the original breakdown.

At the time of writing this chapter, the sub-competencies were not yet categorized and listed under the six ACGME core competencies. But now they are. This is the initial attempt at breaking down the subcompetencies of lifestyle medicine in this manner. In cases where one lifestyle medicine subcompetency overlaps with two ACGME core competencies, the competency is listed twice.

1. *Professionalism*: Three subcompetencies
    1. Develop a culture of leadership by modeling personal health behaviors.
    2. Integrate personal readiness assessments and lifestyle action plans into sustainable life patterns for practitioners.
    3. Explore the role of lifestyle medicine in promoting personal practitioner resilience and reducing burnout
2. *Patient Care and Procedural Skills*: 24 subcompetencies
    1. Assess food intake patterns and nutrients of deficit and excess.
    2. Analyze food labels for the health impacts of ingredients.
    3. Apply nutrition prescriptions based on science that shows how nutrition can address the pathophysiology of most chronic diseases, including inflammation, oxidation, glycosylation, epigenetic expression, and the microbiome.
    4. Demonstrate the ability to write evidence-based nutrition prescriptions.
    5. Integrate key physical activity assessment tools into clinical practice.
    6. Integrate evidence from relevant physical activity literature into treatment protocols for management, remission, or reversal in patients with diabetes, cancer, cardiovascular, and cerebrovascular disease.
    7. Develop physical activity prescriptions appropriately modified for special populations, such as healthy older adults, pregnant women, children and adolescents, persons with obesity or disability, cardiovascular disease, diabetes, cancer, and stroke.
    8. Perform sleep assessments to identify patients with insufficient or poor-quality sleep.
    9. Assess the risk for common sleep disturbances, such as obstructive sleep apnea, chronic insomnia, and restless legs syndrome, and refer to sleep specialists when applicable.
    10. Apply patient screening tools for substance use (Patient Care and Procedural Skills).
    11. Create patient-centered substance use treatment plans using practice guidelines and behavioral interventions.
    12. Integrate behavior therapy with pharmacotherapy for tobacco and other substance use disorder plans and refer to a substance use disorder specialist when indicated.

13. Apply the United States Preventive Services Task Force guidelines for patients with tobacco use disorder.
14. Integrate lifestyle vital signs into components of the patient history and physical examination.
15. Analyze and implement evidence-based clinical practice guidelines relevant to lifestyle medicine for prevention, treatment, and reversal of chronic diseases.
16. Demonstrate how to screen, diagnose, treat, and monitor a lifestyle-related disease and provide lifestyle medicine-focused anticipatory guidance.
17. Demonstrate key elements of conducting a patient assessment within the TTM and collaborate to develop stage-matched responses.
18. Develop patient-centered, written action plans based on the appropriate stage of change of the TTM.
19. Summarize the process of follow-up for ongoing lifestyle change progress, including building patient self-efficacy and relapse prevention.
20. Apply screening tools for stress, depression, and anxiety in clinical practice.
21. Describe and use evidence-based and patient-centered mental and emotional health interventions, including self-management and resilience-building techniques.
22. Manage treatment plans for lifestyle-related mental health conditions, such as depression and anxiety.
23. Apply mindfulness skills to enable presence, clarity, and curiosity in the clinical encounter.
24. Apply positive psychology in health behavior change counseling.

3. *Medical Knowledge*: *fourteen* subcompetencies
   1. Discuss lifestyle medicine and its unique role in health care practice.
   2. Describe the lifestyle medicine core competencies as identified by a national consensus.
   3. Compare and contrast lifestyle medicine with other fields of health and medicine.
   4. Summarize the scientific evidence that shows health behaviors are associated with key health outcomes.
   5. Describe the evidence showing that lifestyle interventions effectively impact disease pathophysiology
   6. Describe the priority of lifestyle medicine in the spectrum of treatment algorithms for chronic, lifestyle-related diseases across the lifespan.
   7. Discuss the prevalence and associated cost burden of lifestyle-related diseases, such as hyperlipidemia, cardiovascular disease, pre-diabetes, diabetes, hypertension, obesity, and cancer.
   8. Explain the impact of lifestyle choices on planetary health and sustainable living.
   9. Examine scientific evidence that suggests practitioners who practice healthy lifestyles are more likely to offer counseling, serve as role models, and improve patient outcomes.
   10. Analyze food labels for the health impacts of ingredients.
   11. Discuss commonalities and key messages of global dietary guidelines.
   12. Summarize the health impact of prominent dietary patterns, including plant-predominant and non–plant-predominant patterns.
   13. Describe how the level of processing in a food affects health and discuss the evidence base for these effects.
   14. Describe the practice of culinary medicine and its role in sustainable healthy eating behavior.
   15. Summarize the major studies of nutrition in the prevention, treatment, and reversal of hyperlipidemia, cardiovascular disease, pre-diabetes, diabetes, hypertension, obesity, and cancer.
   16. Discuss the aerobic, strength, flexibility, and balance components of physical activity.

17. Examine the evidence and pathophysiology between physical activity components and health outcomes.
18. Describe the benefits of physical activity in preventing or treating disease in special populations, such as healthy older adults, pregnant women, children and adolescents, persons with obesity or disability, cardiovascular disease, diabetes, cancer, and stroke.
19. Summarize the role of physical activity guidelines.
20. Define fitness terminology relevant to writing exercise prescriptions.
21. Describe sleep's role in health and chronic disease pathophysiology.
22. Summarize lifestyle-based interventions that can improve sleep health.
23. Describe the health effects of tobacco, alcohol, and other frequently used substances and the benefits of cessation.
24. Describe the treatment of disease with the lifestyle medicine pillars compared with medication.
25. Explain principles of evidence-based medicine and their application to lifestyle medicine.
26. Describe methods of assessing effectiveness of interventions, such as patient activation measures and therapeutic alliance measures.
27. Summarize health behavior change theories, such as the health belief model, social learning theory, and the transtheoretical model (TTM), and their application to lifestyle medicine practice.
28. Explain how to collaborate with patients to promote health behavior changes.
29. Summarize the evidence to support the use of behavior change techniques in clinical practice.
30. Describe the impact of positive emotions on the success of health behavior change.
31. Summarize the process of follow-up for ongoing lifestyle change progress, including building patient self-efficacy and relapse prevention.
32. Describe the factors that support sustained behavior change.
33. Explain the role of family and other support in initiating and maintaining health behavior change.
34. Identify patient resources for sustainable behavior change in relation to the pillars of lifestyle medicine.
35. Explain the relationship and pathophysiology between emotional and physical health.
36. Summarize the nature of stress, the role of stressors such as adverse childhood experiences, and identify manageable elements of pathogenic stress reactions.
37. Describe how positive psychology strategies support achieving and sustaining healthy behaviors (Medical Knowledge).
38. Compare and contrast eudaimonia and hedonia and explain their effect on physical health, including longevity.
39. Describe how social connectedness and social networks affect emotional well-being, physical health, and longevity.
40. Summarize the deleterious and positive effects social media has on emotional well-being and flourishing.
41. Explain the relationship among the lifestyle pillars, positive emotions, and flourishing.
42. Describe positive psychology activities that can boost emotional well-being and flourishing.

4. *Practice-Based Learning and Improvement*: Nine subcompetencies
   1. Apply nutrition prescriptions based on science that shows how nutrition can address the pathophysiology of most chronic diseases, including inflammation, oxidation, glycosylation, epigenetic expression, and the microbiome.
   2. Integrate evidence from relevant physical activity literature into treatment protocols for management, remission, or reversal in patients with diabetes, cancer, cardiovascular, and cerebrovascular disease.

3. Analyze and implement evidence-based clinical practice guidelines relevant to lifestyle medicine for prevention, treatment, and reversal of chronic diseases.
4. Examine how group visits and telehealth can optimize lifestyle medicine treatment encounters.
5. Analyze the evidence for collaborative and chronic care models on improved lifestyle outcomes.
6. Design a quality improvement project for lifestyle medicine clinical practice using tools such as Plan-Do-Study-Act cycles.
7. Explain principles of evidence-based medicine and their application to lifestyle medicine.
8. Describe methods of assessing the effectiveness of interventions, such as patient activation measures and therapeutic alliance measures.
9. Analyze the clinical relevance and evidence base for mindfulness-based stress reduction and related stress management strategies.

5. *Interpersonal and Communication Skills*: Eight subcompetencies
   1. Examine essential practitioner characteristics and practices that increase the capacity and impact of the therapeutic alliance.
   2. Advocate for lifestyle medicine directly with patients and their families, as well as policy and decision makers within the community.
   3. Apply the process of building effective and therapeutic alliances with patients that foster their personal growth.
   4. Apply motivational interviewing, cognitive behavioral, health coaching, and positive psychology techniques.
   5. Use the skills of open inquiry, reflections, and empathy to develop and maintain a therapeutic alliance.
   6. Describe the factors that support sustained behavior change.
   7. Manage disruptions to the therapeutic alliance.
   8. Apply mindfulness skills to enable presence, clarity, and curiosity in the clinical encounter.
6. *Systems-Based Practice*: fourteen subcompetencies
   1. Discuss lifestyle medicine and its unique role in health care practice.
   2. Discuss the prevalence and associated cost burden of lifestyle-related diseases, such as hyperlipidemia, cardiovascular disease, prediabetes, diabetes, hypertension, obesity, and cancer.
   3. Explain the impact of lifestyle choices on planetary health and sustainable living.
   4. Describe strategies for incorporating personal wellness for practitioners into clinics, medical offices, or other health care settings, including wellness programs.
   5. Advocate for lifestyle medicine directly with patients and their families, as well as policy and decision makers within the community.
   6. Describe indications for referral to health fitness professionals.
   7. Describe the indications for referral to a sleep specialist or for a sleep study to assess for sleep apnea.
   8. Describe indications for referral to a program or specialist in cognitive behavioral therapy for insomnia.
   9. Integrate behavior therapy with pharmacotherapy for tobacco and other substance use disorder plans and refer to a substance use disorder specialist when indicated.
   10. Create and use data from office systems, such as electronic health records with lifestyle medicine guidance, in clinical decisions and care, including tracking screening frequency, test results, referrals, and recommended follow-up.
   11. Discuss successful primary care and office-based models for lifestyle modification.
   12. Discuss strategies for a clinical practice to access and implement use of local, national, and global resources.

13. Describe the key strategies for leveraging interprofessional teams to enhance health behavior change interventions.
14. Describe indications for referral to mental health professionals when clinically indicated.

The 88 competencies are distributed across the ACGME competencies and some are counted twice as they fall under two domains. So total there are 100 counts for the competencies matching to ACGME domains. There are 42 competencies in the medical knowledge category, 24 in patient care and procedural skills, 14 in systems-based practice, nine in practice-based learning and improvement, eight in interpersonal and communication skills, and three in professionalism.

The competencies were updated in November 2025 (5). One sub-competency under the Lifestyle Medicine Introduction section was added on social determinants of health. Sub-competency A9 is: "Apply LM interventions in the context of social determinants of health (SDOH) to improve health outcomes and health equity." This was not categorized within the six ACGME core competencies in the most recent article on the lifestyle medicine competencies update. Still, it would fit within patient care and procedural skills, systems-based practice, professionalism, and interpersonal skills categories. The other updates were modifications of existing subcompetencies. One was in the Lifestyle Medicine Introduction section: "Explain the impact of lifestyle choices on planetary health and sustainable living" was updated to "Examine the relationship between lifestyle medicine, planetary health, and sustainable living." The other modification was in the Nutrition Science, Assessment, and Prescription section. The 2022 sub-competency "Describe how the level of processing in a food affects health and discuss the evidence base for these effects" was modified in the 2025 update to "Appraise the evidence base related to how the level and type of food processing affects health outcomes." At the time of this writing, there are efforts to revamp the lifestyle medicine competencies, and the process is set to begin in early 2026.

With regard to the competencies and how they are weighted on the ABLM examination, the ABLM website reports the weighting for the ten main core competencies in lifestyle medicine as follows (6):

1. Introduction to Lifestyle Medicine —4%
2. Fundamentals of Health Behavior Change —10%
3. Key Clinical Processes in Lifestyle Medicine —8%
4. The Role of the Practitioner's Personal Health and Community Advocacy —4%
5. Nutrition Science, Assessment, and Prescription — 26%
6. Physical Activity Science and Prescription — 14%
7. Emotional Well-being, Assessments, and Interventions — 10%
8. Sleep Health Science and Interventions — 8%
9. Managing Tobacco Cessation and Other Toxic Exposures — 8%
10. The Role of Connectedness and Positive Psychology — 8%

When studying for the ABLM examination, it is useful to keep this breakdown in mind. The American College of Lifestyle Medicine (ACLM) has a Board Review Course that is recommended for those seeking certification in lifestyle medicine by the ABLM.

26.9 LIFESTYLE MEDICINE MILESTONES FOR RESIDENTS

Residents need to be evaluated and their progress tracked. As mentioned earlier in the chapter, ACGME provides milestones for medical educators and supervising physicians to use with residents every six months. These milestones serve as checkpoints to monitor knowledge acquisition, skill proficiency, clinical reasoning, and interpersonal communication skills. The specific milestones vary across residencies but center on the six core competencies of the ACGME: professionalism, patient care and procedural skills, medical knowledge, practice-based learning and improvement, interpersonal and communication skills, and systems-based practice. The milestones are broken down into five levels. These levels include:

Level 1 = Novice,
Level 2 = Advanced Beginner,
Level 3 = Competent,
Level 4 = Proficient,
Level 5 = Expert.

The milestones are intended to be formative assessments and to be continuous over time. At this time, Lifestyle Medicine does not have milestones that accompany its core competencies. However, working with the lifestyle medicine core competencies and identifying key aspects of each that can be monitored and measured will help residents understand what is expected of them and how to succeed. This is the first published list of milestones for lifestyle medicine. They will need to be modified and updated, requiring consensus building and collaboration with the ACGME, before they are accepted and official. There are 88 competencies which will likely be edited and shortened in future editions of the Lifestyle Medicine Core Competencies. However, these milestones represent the inaugural attempt to establish lifestyle medicine milestones based on the current core competencies. Going through the process of creating milestones is a useful exercise to help hone teaching objectives.

26.10 MILESTONE EXAMPLES FOR LIFESTYLE MEDICINE

26.10.1 Intro to Lifestyle Medicine

1. Discuss lifestyle medicine and its unique role in health care practice (Medical Knowledge and Systems-Based Practice).
   Novice: Defines lifestyle medicine (LM) and identifies the importance of each of the six pillars.
   Advanced Beginner: Describes lifestyle medicine's scope within healthcare.
   Competent: Explains lifestyle medicine's role in the prevention, treatment, and remission of chronic conditions
   Proficient: Integrates lifestyle medicine principles into clinical practice and health systems.
   Expert: Leads or develops lifestyle medicine initiatives at institutional or policy levels.
2. Describe the lifestyle medicine core competencies as identified by a national consensus panel (Medical Knowledge).
   Novice: Identifies the core competencies.
   Advanced Beginner: Summarizes the purpose of each competency and how it relates to the field of lifestyle medicine.
   Competent: Explains how the competencies interrelate and advance patient care and healthcare systems.
   Proficient: Applies these competencies in clinical and educational contexts.
   Expert: Contributes to updating current competencies or developing new competencies.
3. Compare and contrast lifestyle medicine with other fields of health and medicine (Medical Knowledge).
   Novice: Names related fields like preventive medicine, public health, family medicine, internal medicine, integrative medicine, and functional medicine.
   Advanced Beginner: Describes key differences in scope and approach among the different fields.
   Competent: Analyzes similarities and overlaps in terms of clinical care, research, and medical education, and distinguishes differences.

Proficient: Explains how lifestyle medicine works independently with teams of health-care professionals and how it integrates with other fields of medicine.

Expert: Develops interdisciplinary models that highlight lifestyle medicine for the prevention, treatment, and remission of chronic conditions, and integrates these models with other specialties.

4. Summarize the scientific evidence that shows health behaviors are associated with key health outcomes (Medical Knowledge).

   Novice: States foundational research findings linking lifestyle behaviors and health.

   Advanced Beginner: Describes rigorous research studies showing associations between the six pillars of lifestyle medicine and the prevention, treatment, and remission of chronic diseases.

   Competent: Explains mechanisms behind lifestyle behaviors' impact on health (physical and mental) and identifies the pathophysiological pathways contributing to the connection.

   Proficient: Uses evidence to inform clinical practice and/or health policy.

   Expert: Contributes to research, systematic reviews, or guidelines in the six pillars of lifestyle medicine, behavior change, and the clinical practice of lifestyle medicine.

5. Describe the evidence showing that lifestyle interventions effectively impact disease pathophysiology (Medical Knowledge).

   Novice: Identifies evidence-based lifestyle interventions.

   Advanced Beginner: Describes the effects of lifestyle medicine evidence-based interventions on specific disease mechanisms.

   Competent: Evaluates scientific evidence and research studies connecting evidence-based lifestyle medicine interventions to different chronic conditions.

   Proficient: Integrates basic science and current research on lifestyle medicine interventions into clinical practice, health systems, and medical education.

   Expert: Leads research (original clinical trials, systematic reviews, meta-analyses, or umbrella reviews) translating pathophysiological effects of unhealthy lifestyle behaviors into clinical practice.

6. Describe the priority of lifestyle medicine in the spectrum of treatment algorithms for chronic, lifestyle-related diseases across the lifespan (Medical Knowledge).

   Novice: Recognizes why lifestyle medicine is a vital component of the treatment spectrum.

   Advanced Beginner: Explains where lifestyle medicine fits within prevention, early intervention, and treatment of chronic conditions.

   Competent: Critiques evidence supporting lifestyle medicine as the core treatment for chronic conditions, their prevention, and, when possible, their remission.

   Proficient: Advocates for lifestyle medicine as first-line or adjunct therapy for chronic conditions with 1:1 visits and group interventions, such as Shared Medical Appointments.

   Expert: Develops models for integrating lifestyle medicine across care pathways for the treatment, prevention, and, when possible, remission of chronic conditions.

7. Discuss the prevalence and associated cost burden of lifestyle-related diseases (Medical Knowledge and Systems-Based Practice).

   Novice: Lists lifestyle-related diseases, identifies how common they are, and explains costs associated with them.

   Advanced Beginner: Describes epidemiologic trends and the economic impact of chronic conditions in the United States, discussing the current magnitude, trends, and trajectory.

   Competent: Analyzes the health system costs and resource utilization caused by chronic conditions, discussing the magnitude, trends, and trajectory.

   Proficient: Uses data to support lifestyle medicine implementation for cost savings in the treatment, prevention, and remission of chronic conditions.

Expert: Leads policy initiatives to reduce disease burden and costs by using evidence-based lifestyle medicine interventions, including 1:1 and group interventions such as Shared Medical Appointments.

8. Explain the impact of lifestyle choices on planetary health and sustainable living (Medical Knowledge and Systems-Based Practice).

   Novice: Illustrates how lifestyle behaviors impact the environment.

   Advanced Beginner: Describes connections between lifestyle behaviors and global sustainability.

   Competent: Explains how lifestyle interventions can promote planetary health at the individual, societal, and global levels.

   Proficient: Integrates sustainability principles into clinical and community practice, research, and education.

   Expert: Contributes to policies, education, or research promoting sustainable health behaviors.

26.10.2 The Role of the Practitioner's Personal Health and Community Advocacy

1. Examine scientific evidence that suggests healthcare professionals who practice healthy lifestyles are more likely to offer counseling, serve as role models, and improve patient outcomes (Medical Knowledge).

   Novice: Recognizes that healthy healthcare professionals may influence patient care.

   Advanced Beginner: Describes basic studies linking healthcare professionals' health with patient outcomes.

   Competent: Interprets research on the impact of healthcare professionals' behavior on counseling and role modeling.

   Proficient: Integrates evidence of the role of healthcare professionals' behaviors into practice and leadership roles.

   Expert: Contributes to research or advocacy regarding how healthcare professionals' lifestyle behaviors influence patients and public health.

2. Develop a culture of leadership by modeling personal health behaviors (Professionalism).

   Novice: Identifies the importance of personal health behaviors as a role model for patients.

   Advanced Beginner: Demonstrates putting effort into basic healthy lifestyle behaviors.

   Competent: Consistently puts effort into modeling healthy lifestyle behaviors that promote health among colleagues.

   Proficient: Leads initiatives promoting a healthy culture across medical organizations, medical schools, healthcare professional schools, and healthcare systems.

   Expert: Advocates for institutional change, mentors others, and leads health promotion policy.

3. Describe strategies for incorporating personal wellness for practitioners into clinics, medical offices, or other healthcare settings, including wellness programs (Systems-Based Practice).

   Novice: Recognizes different types of wellness/ wellbeing programs and resources.

   Advanced Beginner: Participates in wellness/wellbeing activities for self-care at work and at home.

   Competent: Implements wellness/wellbeing strategies within clinical practice and/or medical education.

   Proficient: Designs or promotes wellness/wellbeing initiatives at organizational levels in hospitals, clinics, medical schools, and other academic or clinical institutions.

   Expert: Leads systematic efforts to embed wellness/wellbeing into healthcare culture and policy, and/or medical education.

4. Examine essential practitioner characteristics and practices that increase the capacity and impact of the therapeutic alliance (Interpersonal and Communication Skills).

   Novice: Recognizes traits like empathy, deep listening, collaborating, and trust-building.

   Advanced Beginner: Demonstrates basic application of empathy, deep listening, collaborating, and building trust.

   Competent: Consistently employs key leadership characteristics, including but not limited to empathy, deep listening, collaborating, and building trust, to strengthen alliances.

   Proficient: Adapts relational skills to complex situations, difficult conversations, and diverse patient populations.

   Expert: Coaches others and champions relational skills as core to clinical practice, medical education and healthcare professions' education.
5. Integrate personal readiness assessments and lifestyle action plans into sustainable life patterns for practitioners (Professionalism).

   Novice: Recognizes own physical and mental health needs and goals.

   Advanced Beginner: Evaluates basic physical health with a primary care physician, mental health with a mental health professional as needed, and performs well-being self-assessments, with a focus on each of the six pillars of lifestyle medicine.

   Competent: Develops and implements personal physical and mental health plans aligned with professional life, home life, and a sense of purpose.

   Proficient: Uses self-assessment data to maintain long-term vitality and role modeling.

   Expert: Leads by example, mentors others, and advances institutional physical health models, mental health models, and wellbeing models.
6. Explore the role of lifestyle medicine in promoting personal practitioner resiliency and reducing burnout (Professionalism).

   Novice: Recognizes that lifestyle medicine evidence-based principles, including the science of the six pillars and the art of behavior change, can support resilience.

   Advanced Beginner: Practices self-care strategies related to the six pillars of lifestyle medicine.

   Competent: Integrates resilience-building practices into routine life at home and at work.

   Proficient: Uses lifestyle medicine knowledge to design programmatic burnout prevention, well-being optimization, and healthcare professionals' physical and mental health initiatives.

   Expert: Contributes to research, policy development, medical education, or organizational culture change on resilience, well-being, and burnout.
7. Advocate for lifestyle medicine directly with patients and their families, as well as policy and decision-makers within the community (Interpersonal and Communication Skills/Systems-Based Practice).

   Novice: Recalls basic advocacy principles.

   Advanced Beginner: Participates in advocacy efforts with support.

   Competent: Leads or independently advocates for lifestyle medicine in clinical practice, medical school, healthcare professional school, and/or community settings.

   Proficient: Engages stakeholders, develops campaigns, and influences policy at the local or national level.

   Expert: Shapes community health agendas, mentors others, and leads advocacy coalitions at the local, national, or international level.

26.10.3 Nutrition Science, Assessment, and Prescription

1. Assess food intake patterns and nutrients of deficit and excess (Patient Care and Procedural Skills).

   Novice: Identifies basic dietary assessment tools.

Advanced Beginner: Collects dietary histories with guidance.
Competent: Performs and interprets standard dietary assessments independently.
Proficient: Identifies specific nutrient deficits/excesses and relates them to health and disease.
Expert: Designs comprehensive, personalized nutrition assessments for complex cases.

2. Analyze food labels for the health impacts of ingredients (Medical Knowledge and Patient Care).
   Novice: Recognizes the importance of all food label components.
   Advanced Beginner: Explains the significance of macronutrients and additives on food labels.
   Competent: Critically evaluates food labels for health impacts.
   Proficient: Uses food label information to guide clinical recommendations.
   Expert: Teaches and develops strategies for food label literacy and policy advocacy.
3. Discuss commonalities and key messages of global dietary guidelines (Medical Knowledge).
   Novice: Recalls major dietary guidelines from key evidence-based sources.
   Advanced Beginner: Summarizes core messages of global evidence-based guidelines.
   Competent: Compares and contrasts different evidence-based guidelines.
   Proficient: Integrates evidence-based global dietary messages into patient counseling.
   Expert: Contributes to evidence-based guideline development or education initiatives.
4. Summarize the health impact of prominent dietary patterns, including plant-predominant and non–plant-predominant patterns (Medical Knowledge).
   Novice: Identifies common dietary patterns.
   Advanced Beginner: Describes basic health benefits/risks associated with these patterns.
   Competent: Analyzes evidence linking dietary patterns and health outcomes.
   Proficient: Applies knowledge to tailor evidence-based dietary recommendations.
   Expert: Engages in research or policy to shape evidence-based dietary guidance.
5. Describe how the level of processing in a food affects health and discuss the evidence base for these effects (Medical Knowledge).
   Novice: Identifies the difference between unprocessed, minimally, highly, ultra-processed foods.
   Advanced Beginner: Explains basic health effects of different processing levels.
   Competent: Analyzes scientific evidence on processing levels and disease.
   Proficient: Incorporates processing considerations into patient counseling.
   Expert: Contributes to research or policy on food processing and health impacts.
6. Describe the practice of culinary medicine and its role in sustainable healthy eating behavior (Medical Knowledge).
   Novice: Describes what culinary medicine involves.
   Advanced Beginner: Explains how culinary practices influence health.
   Competent: Integrates culinary skills and culinary medicine into patient education.
   Proficient: Develops or leads culinary medicine interventions 1:1 and group interventions or Shared Medical Appointments.
   Expert: Advances culinary medicine research or curricula.
7. Summarize the major studies of nutrition in prevention, treatment, and reversal of chronic diseases (Medical Knowledge).
   Novice: Names key studies related to nutrition and chronic disease.
   Advanced Beginner: Summarizes main findings of major studies.
   Competent: Critically appraises scientific evidence and its clinical implications.
   Proficient: Integrates scientific evidence into disease management plans.
   Expert: Contributes to nutrition research or evidence-based guideline development.
8. Apply nutrition prescriptions based on science addressing chronic disease pathophysiology (Practice-Based Learning and Patient Care).

Novice: Recognizes nutritional factors affecting biochemical pathways and disease mechanisms.

Advanced Beginner: Applies basic evidence-based nutrition principles to treatment plans.

Competent: Develops tailored evidence-based nutrition prescriptions addressing specific mechanisms (e.g., inflammation).

Proficient: Integrates complex scientific evidence into personalized nutrition prescription strategies.

Expert: Conducts or contributes to translational research influencing the practice of evidence-based nutrition prescription.

9. Demonstrate the ability to write evidence-based nutrition prescriptions (Patient Care and Procedural Skills).

   Novice: Drafts simple, sample nutrition recommendations.

   Advanced Beginner: Writes basic, evidence-based prescriptions with supervision.

   Competent: Independently formulates personalized, evidence-based prescriptions.

   Proficient: Adjusts prescriptions based on patient response and emerging scientific evidence.

   Expert: Educates others on writing complex evidence-based prescriptions and/or developing evidence-based protocols.

10. Describe indications for referral to a lifestyle medicine-trained registered dietitian to translate and further personalize nutrition prescriptions (Systems-Based Practice).

    Novice: Identifies the educational experience of different nutrition specialists, including a registered dietitian, and their roles in the healthcare team.

    Advanced Beginner: Describes common indications warranting referral to a nutrition specialist.

    Competent: Independently identifies when to refer patients for specialized nutrition counseling based on patients' chief complaints, past medical histories, physical examination, social history, and social determinants of health (SDOH).

    Proficient: Coordinates and advocates for referral to a nutrition specialist when personalized, comprehensive dietary interventions are needed, and works collaboratively with nutrition specialists.

    Expert: Leads development of institutional referral pathways, educates teams on when and how to refer, and participates in multidisciplinary evidence-based nutrition care models.

26.10.4 Physical Activity Science, Assessment, and Prescription

1. Discuss the aerobic, strength, flexibility, and balance components of physical activity (Medical Knowledge).

   Novice: Identifies basic definitions of aerobic, strength, flexibility, and balance exercises.

   Advanced Beginner: Describes the components of exercise programs and their general roles in fitness and health.

   Competent: Explains how each component of exercise affects health and fitness.

   Proficient: Integrates knowledge of components of exercise to advise on comprehensive activity programs.

   Expert: Conducts research and/or teaches advanced understanding of exercise program design.

2. Examine the evidence and pathophysiology between physical activity components and health outcomes (Medical Knowledge).

   Novice: Recognizes that physical activity/exercise impacts health outcomes.

   Advanced Beginner: Describes basic evidence linking physical activity/exercise components and common health outcomes.

Competent: Analyzes research evidence and underlying mechanisms for multiple health benefits of exercise and risks of sedentary behavior.

Proficient: Critically evaluates studies evaluating exercise and applies evidence to clinical practice with a variety of patient scenarios.

Expert: Contributes to research, synthesizing complex evidence and underlying pathophysiology.

3. Describe the benefits of physical activity in preventing or treating disease in special populations (Medical Knowledge).

Novice: Lists general benefits of physical activity/exercise for common patient populations categorized by age or disease.

Advanced Beginner: Describes specific benefits of physical activity/exercise for select patient populations.

Competent: Explains how physical activity/exercise impacts disease prevention/treatment in various patient populations.

Proficient: Integrates evidence to tailor evidence-based counseling for individual patient populations.

Expert: Develops advanced evidence-based guidelines and contributes to the literature on special populations with research (original studies, systematic reviews, meta-analyses, or umbrella articles).

4. Summarize the role of physical activity guidelines (Medical Knowledge).

Novice: Recites basic national or international guidelines in physical activity/exercise.

Advanced Beginner: Explains core physical activity/exercise recommendations and rationale.

Competent: Discusses how physical activity/exercise guidelines apply to different populations and clinical scenarios.

Proficient: Critically evaluates evidence-based guidelines and adapts recommendations accordingly.

Expert: Leads efforts to update or develop evidence-based guidelines and educates peers through national CME and other conferences/presentations national and/or international.

5. Integrate key physical activity assessment tools into clinical practice (Patient Care and Procedural Skills).

Novice: Identifies basic physical activity/exercise assessment tools such as self-report questionnaires, 12-minute walk/run test, 30-second sit-to-stand test, and YMCA 3-minute step test.

Advanced Beginner: Administers surveys and assessment physical activity/exercise tools with supervision.

Competent: Independently selects and interprets physical activity/assessment surveys and assessment results.

Proficient: Incorporates physical activity/exercise surveys and assessments into comprehensive patient evaluations.

Expert: Develops or modifies validated physical activity/exercise survey or assessment tools for specific populations or settings.

6. Define fitness terminology relevant to writing exercise prescriptions (Medical Knowledge).

Novice: Recalls basic fitness terms (e.g., aerobic, strength training, balance, and flexibility).

Advanced Beginner: Defines key terms like frequency, intensity (low, moderate, and vigorous), time, and type (FITT).

Competent: Explains terms in the context of exercise prescription writing.

Proficient: Uses terminology accurately when developing exercise prescriptions.

Expert: Educates others and advances the safe, and evidence-based use of exercise prescriptions.

7. Integrate evidence from relevant physical activity literature into treatment protocols (Practice-Based Learning and Patient Care).
   Novice: Recognizes that physical activity/exercise enhances the treatment of certain chronic diseases.
   Advanced Beginner: Summarizes key studies relevant to the impact of physical activity/exercise on treating common conditions.
   Competent: Incorporates scientific evidence and guidelines for physical activity/exercise into patient treatment plans.
   Proficient: Critically appraises physical activity/exercise research studies and personalizes physical activity/exercise prescriptions.
   Expert: Contributes to research in exercise prescription and develops new evidence-based exercise intervention models for the treatment of different conditions and diseases.
8. Describe indications for referral to health fitness professionals (Systems-Based Practice).
   Novice: Identifies indications for a referral to a health fitness professional.
   Advanced Beginner: Refers patients appropriately to a health fitness professional with guidance and supervision.
   Competent: Independently identifies indications for referral to a health fitness professional and completes the referral.
   Proficient: Coordinates care with fitness professionals to optimize outcomes for patients.
   Expert: Creates system-wide referral networks for patients to health fitness professionals.
9. Develop physical activity prescriptions modified for special populations (Patient Care and Procedural Skills).
   Novice: Identifies general considerations for physical activity/exercise in special populations.
   Advanced Beginner: Creates basic modifications to the exercise prescription with supervision for special populations.
   Competent: Independently develops individualized exercise prescriptions for special populations.
   Proficient: Tailors complex, multifactorial physical activity/exercise plans considering comorbidities for special populations.
   Expert: Innovates and educates on advanced, personalized exercise prescription strategies for special populations.

26.10.5 Sleep Health Science and Interventions

1. Describe sleep's role in health and chronic disease pathophysiology (Medical Knowledge).
   Novice: Recalls basic concepts of sleep physiology and its stages as well as sleep's connection to health.
   Advanced Beginner: Explains the general impact of sleep on chronic diseases such as diabetes, high blood pressure, dyslipidemias, and obesity.
   Competent: Describes the role of sleep in the pathophysiology of multiple chronic conditions.
   Proficient: Analyzes the complex relationships between sleep and chronic diseases.
   Expert: Integrates and teaches advanced knowledge about sleep physiology, pathophysiology, and disease mechanisms.
2. Perform sleep assessments to identify patients with insufficient or poor-quality sleep (Patient Care and Procedural Skills).
   Novice: Identifies validated sleep assessments.
   Advanced Beginner: Performs basic sleep assessments with patients suffering from insufficient sleep.

Competent: Analyzes sleep assessments for various conditions and makes recommendations.

Proficient: Interprets sleep assessments and nuances in sleep quality.

Expert: Trains others in sleep evaluations and develops innovative assessment tools.

3. Summarize lifestyle-based interventions that can improve sleep health (Medical Knowledge).

   Novice: Lists common lifestyle interventions for sleep improvement.

   Advanced Beginner: Summarizes evidence for lifestyle changes affecting sleep.

   Competent: Details evidence-based sleep interventions and their mechanisms of action.

   Proficient: Customizes and integrates evidence-based sleep interventions into whole-person care plans.

   Expert: Conducts research and disseminates advanced intervention strategies.

4. Assess the risk for common sleep disturbances, such as obstructive sleep apnea, chronic insomnia, and restless legs syndrome, and refer to sleep specialists when applicable (Patient Care and Procedural Skills).

   Novice: Recalls basic symptoms of common sleep disturbances.

   Advanced Beginner: Assesses the risk of common sleep disturbances and identifies basic referral protocols.

   Competent: Evaluates the risk of common sleep disturbances comprehensively and initiates appropriate referrals to sleep medicine experts.

   Proficient: Anticipates complex cases and coordinates interdisciplinary care.

   Expert: Innovates system-wide screening and referral practices for sleep disorders in a lifestyle medicine clinic or practice.

5. Describe the indications for referral to a sleep specialist or for a sleep study to assess for sleep apnea (Systems-Based Practice).

   Novice: Recognizes fundamental reasons for referrals to sleep medicine specialists.

   Advanced Beginner: Describes common scenarios requiring sleep studies.

   Competent: Identifies and accurately acts on indications for sleep medicine specialist referrals.

   Proficient: Optimizes referral processes and collaborates effectively with sleep medicine specialists.

   Expert: Leads initiatives to refine referral guidelines to sleep medicine specialists and educate peers.

6. Describe indications for referral to a program or specialist in cognitive behavior therapy for insomnia (Systems-Based Practice).

   Novice: Recognizes the benefits of cognitive behavior therapy as a treatment option for sleep disturbances and disorders.

   Advanced Beginner: Describes simple indications for referrals to CBT-I (Cognitive Behavioral Therapy-Insomnia).

   Competent: Identifies appropriate candidates and initiates referrals confidently to sleep medicine specialists.

   Proficient: Enhances sleep medicine referral networks and interdisciplinary cooperation.

   Expert: Develops and evaluates sleep medicine referral systems and provides education on CBT-I.

26.10.6 Treating Tobacco Use Disorder and Managing Other Toxic Exposures (Including Vaping, Alcohol Use, and Other Illicit Substances)

1. Describe the health effects of tobacco, alcohol, and other frequently used substances and the benefits of cessation (Medical Knowledge).

Novice: Lists the toxic effects of using risky substances and the benefits of quitting tobacco, alcohol, and opioids.

Advanced Beginner: Explains mechanisms and evidence linking risky substances to health outcomes.

Competent: Analyzes individual effects of risky substances in relation to a specific patient.

Proficient: Evaluates the risks of continued use of a risky substance in patient populations with complex medical conditions.

Expert: Leads or contributes to education/research on risky substance use effects and cessation benefits.

2. Apply patient screening tools for substance use (Patient Care and Procedural Skills).

   Novice: Identifies evidence-based screening tools (e.g., AUDIT, DAST).

   Advanced Beginner: Demonstrates basic administration of evidence-based survey tools under supervision.

   Competent: Independently uses evidence-based survey tools and interprets results.

   Proficient: Integrates evidence-based screening into routine practice and follow-up.

   Expert: Trains others to use evidence-based screening tools, researches the use of these tools, and/or works to develop new screening strategies.

3. Create patient-centered substance use treatment plans using practice guidelines and behavioral interventions (Patient Care and Procedural Skills).

   Novice: Outlines treatment components for patients using risky substances.

   Advanced Beginner: Drafts simple, evidence-based guideline plans for patients using risky substances.

   Competent: Creates tailored consultations 1:1 or in groups to address substance use and writes personalized prescriptions for reducing and stopping risky substances.

   Proficient: Modifies treatment plans and prescriptions for reducing and stopping risky substances for patients with complex medical conditions.

   Expert: Leads development of evidence-based protocols for discontinuing the use of risky substances and trains others.

4. Summarize the diagnostic criteria for common substance use disorders (Medical Knowledge).

   Novice: Recalls basic criteria for substance use disorders.

   Advanced Beginner: Explains key features of the criteria for substance use disorders.

   Competent: Uses criteria in the differential diagnosis of patients.

   Proficient: Applies diagnostic criteria when counseling patients with complex medical conditions.

   Expert: Contributes to diagnostic evidence-based guidelines or education.

5. Integrate behavior therapy with pharmacotherapy for substance use disorder plans and refer to specialists (Patient Care/Systems-Based Practice).

   Novice: Identifies combined treatment options using behavior therapy and pharmacotherapy for patients with substance use disorder and recognizes the need to refer to specialists.

   Advanced Beginner: Refers to addiction medicine specialists and/or implements combined therapy with supervision.

   Competent: Independently develops integrated plans for combined treatment for patients with substance use disorder or refers appropriate patients to addiction medicine specialists.

   Proficient: Coordinates multidisciplinary team care of patients with substance use disorder using combined therapy and/or appropriate referral to addiction medicine specialists.

   Expert: Leads system-wide integration and evidence-based education in the management of patients with substance use disorder using combined therapy and/or uses appropriate referral methods to addiction medicine specialists when needed.

6. Apply USPSTF guidelines for tobacco use disorder (Patient Care and Procedural Skills).

Novice: Recognizes USPSTF basic guidelines for tobacco use disorder.

Advanced Beginner: Explains routine evidence-based screening procedures for tobacco use disorder.

Competent: Routinely applies evidence-based guidelines for tobacco use disorder in practice.

Proficient: Uses tailored evidence-based screening and counseling for patients with tobacco use disorder.

Expert: Participates in policy or evidence-based guideline development for the management of patients with tobacco use disorder.

26.10.7 Key Clinical Processes in Lifestyle Medicine

1. Integrate lifestyle vital signs into components of the patient history and physical examination (Patient Care and Procedural Skills).

   Novice: Recognizes lifestyle factors and their relevance and identifies validated lifestyle medicine survey tools such as the Lifestyle Medicine Behavior Health Scale and the Lifestyle Medicine Assessment.

   Advanced Beginner: Begins to incorporate basic lifestyle questions into history-taking and starts to use validated lifestyle medicine survey tools.

   Competent: Consistently gathers and documents lifestyle vital signs and uses validated tools.

   Proficient: Systematically integrates lifestyle medicine vital signs data into clinical decision-making.

   Expert: Teaches and models comprehensive lifestyle assessment as routine practice.
2. Analyze and implement evidence-based clinical practice guidelines relevant to lifestyle medicine (Practice-Based Learning and Improvement/Patient Care).

   Novice: Identifies evidence-based clinical practice guidelines relevant to lifestyle medicine.

   Advanced Beginner: Applies evidence-based clinical practice guidelines relevant to lifestyle medicine with supervision.

   Competent: Independently interprets and applies evidence-based clinical practice guidelines relevant to lifestyle medicine.

   Proficient: Evaluates and adapts evidence-based clinical practice guidelines relevant to lifestyle medicine for individual patients.

   Expert: Contributes to the development of clinical practice guidelines relevant to lifestyle medicine and actively educates about or researches the use of these guidelines.
3. Describe the treatment of disease with the lifestyle medicine pillars as compared with medication (Medical Knowledge).

   Novice: Names lifestyle medicine pillars and lists how they act as medication.

   Advanced Beginner: Describes fundamental differences between prescriptions for lifestyle medicine pillars and prescriptions for medications.

   Competent: Explains how lifestyle medicine pillars can complement medication for patients.

   Proficient: Integrates lifestyle medicine pillar prescriptions into disease management plans.

   Expert: Leads research or clinical innovation using lifestyle medicine pillar prescriptions alongside medication prescriptions.
4. Demonstrate how to screen, diagnose, treat, and monitor a lifestyle-related disease and provide lifestyle medicine-focused anticipatory guidance (Patient Care and Procedural Skills).

   Novice: Lists common lifestyle-related diseases.

Advanced Beginner: Performs basic screening for lifestyle-related disease and discusses preliminary management.

Competent: Provides evidence-based guidance tailored to lifestyle-related diseases.

Proficient: Manages diagnosis, treatment, and follow-up of lifestyle-related disease independently.

Expert: Develops evidence-based protocols and mentors others in evidence-based comprehensive disease management.

5. Discuss strategies for a practice to access and implement the use of local, national, and global resources (Systems-Based Practice).

   Novice: Identifies available evidence-based resources.

   Advanced Beginner: Initiates engagement with identified evidence-based resources.

   Competent: Integrates evidence-based resources use into clinical workflows.

   Proficient: Develops and leads efforts to optimize evidence-based resource access.

   Expert: Shapes institutional or community evidence-based resource networks and policies.

6. Describe the key strategies for leveraging interprofessional teams to enhance health behavior change interventions (Systems-Based Practice).

   Novice: Recalls the role of the various lifestyle medicine team members.

   Advanced Beginner: Participates in team-based care with guidance.

   Competent: Coordinates with team members to implement interventions independently.

   Proficient: Facilitates interprofessional collaboration for patients with complex medical conditions.

   Expert: Leads team-based models, trains others, and advocates for integrated care for patients.

7. Examine how group visits and telehealth can optimize lifestyle medicine treatment encounters (Practice-Based Learning and Improvement).

   Novice: Identifies requirements to run group visits, shared medical appointments, and telehealth.

   Advanced Beginner: Participates in group visits, shared medical appointments, and telehealth.

   Competent: Conducts or facilitates group visits, shared medical appointments, and/or telehealth visits effectively.

   Proficient: Designs and evaluates group visits, shared medical appointments, and telehealth programs.

   Expert: Innovates scalable models, researches outcomes, and mentors peers to run group visits, shared medical appointments, and telehealth.

8. Create and use data from office systems, like Electronic Medical Records (EMRs), to guide clinical decisions (Systems-Based Practice).

   Novice: Identifies basic functions of electronic health records.

   Advanced Beginner: Retrieves and documents electronic data with guidance.

   Competent: Uses electronic data to inform decisions (e.g., screenings, follow-ups).

   Proficient: Analyzes and reports electronic data to improve the quality of patient care.

   Expert: Develops electronic data-driven workflows and quality metrics for lifestyle medicine.

9. Analyze the evidence for collaborative and chronic care models on improved lifestyle outcomes (Practice-Based Learning and Improvement).

   Novice: Lists the benefits of collaborative and chronic care models and their goals.

   Advanced Beginner: Identifies key research studies and summarizes them.

   Competent: Critically evaluates evidence for specific health outcomes using collaborative and chronic care models.

   Proficient: Applies evidence to optimize multidisciplinary models.

   Expert: Leads or conducts research influencing care models and policies.

10. Discuss successful primary care and office-based models for lifestyle modification (Systems-Based Practice).
    Novice: Names existing models for primary care and office-based lifestyle modification.
    Advanced Beginner: Describes elements of effective models.
    Competent: Analyzes factors contributing to success.
    Proficient: Implements and adapts models tailored to practice settings.
    Expert: Leads development, evaluation, research, and dissemination of innovative, scalable models to improve access and outcomes in lifestyle medicine.
11. Design a quality improvement (QI) project for lifestyle medicine clinical practice, using tools such as Plan-Do-Study-Act (PDSA) cycles (Practice-Based Learning and Improvement).
    Novice: Recalls basic concepts of QI and PDSA.
    Advanced Beginner: Assists in small QI initiatives with supervision with tools such as PDSA.
    Competent: Independently plans and implements simple QI projects with tools such as PDSA.
    Proficient: Uses data to refine and improve QI projects with tools such as PDSA and scales successful interventions.
    Expert: Leads institution-wide QI initiatives with tools such as PDSA, mentors others, and disseminates findings.
12. Explain principles of evidence-based medicine (EBM) and their application to lifestyle medicine (Medical Knowledge/Practice-Based Learning).
    Novice: Describes the basics of EBM.
    Advanced Beginner: Applies EBM principles to answer specific clinical questions.
    Competent: Critically evaluates literature and integrates evidence into patient care.
    Proficient: Guides colleagues in applying EBM and translating evidence into practice.
    Expert: Contributes to guidelines, systematic reviews, or the development of EBM tools.
13. Describe methods of assessing the effectiveness of interventions, such as patient activation measures and therapeutic alliance measures (Medical Knowledge/Practice-Based Learning and Improvement).
    Novice: Identifies concepts of patient activation and alliance.
    Advanced Beginner: Describes basic assessment tools for interventions, such as patient activation measures and therapeutic alliance measures, and their purpose.
    Competent: Implements assessment tools for interventions, such as patient activation measures and therapeutic alliance measures, and interprets results to guide care.
    Proficient: Uses findings from assessment tools to improve patient engagement and therapeutic relationships.
    Expert: Develops and/or validates assessment tools and teaches others how to measure effectiveness of interventions and improve these metrics.

26.10.8 Fundamentals of Health Behavior Change

1. Summarize health behavior change theories, such as the health belief model, social learning theory, and TTM, and their application to lifestyle medicine practice (Medical Knowledge).
   Novice: Names fundamental theories of health behavior change.
   Advanced Beginner: Describes key components of each health behavior change theory.
   Competent: Explains how each behavior change theory applies to lifestyle medicine.
   Proficient: Integrates multiple behavior change theories to tailor patient interventions.
   Expert: Contributes to behavior change theory development or teaches advanced applications.

2. Demonstrate key elements of conducting a patient assessment within the Transtheoretical Model of Change (TTM) and collaborate to develop stage-matched responses (Patient Care and Procedural Skills)

   Novice: Identifies the stages of change in TTM and stage-appropriate counseling.

   Advanced Beginner: Performs basic assessments of stages of change with supervision.

   Competent: Independently assesses stage of change and performs stage-appropriate counseling.

   Proficient: Tailors TTM interventions effectively for complex patients with multiple chronic conditions.

   Expert: Designs advanced assessment protocols for behavior change and trains others.
3. Apply the process of building effective and therapeutic alliances with patients that foster their personal growth (Interpersonal and Communication Skills).

   Novice: Identifies basic empathetic communication skills.

   Advanced Beginner: Demonstrates active listening in patient interactions.

   Competent: Consistently builds trust and rapport during patient encounters.

   Proficient: Facilitates patient self-exploration and growth.

   Expert: Leads in teaching and modeling advanced therapeutic alliance-building skills.
4. Explain how to collaborate with your patients to promote health behavior changes (Medical Knowledge).

   Novice: Recognizes basic collaborative approaches.

   Advanced Beginner: Describes shared decision-making principles.

   Competent: Applies collaboration techniques in clinical encounters.

   Proficient: Facilitates patient engagement and autonomy.

   Expert: Develops models for collaborative behavior change approaches.
5. Apply motivational interviewing, cognitive behavioral, health coaching, and positive psychology techniques (Interpersonal and Communication Skills).

   Novice: Identifies motivational interviewing, cognitive behavioral, health coaching, and positive psychology techniques.

   Advanced Beginner: Demonstrates basic use of motivational interviewing, cognitive behavioral, health coaching, and positive psychology techniques.

   Competent: Uses motivational interviewing, cognitive behavioral, health coaching, and positive psychology techniques effectively in patient encounters.

   Proficient: Integrates multiple motivational interviewing, cognitive behavioral, health coaching, and positive psychology techniques fluently to support change.

   Expert: Coaches others on the application and adaptation of motivational interviewing, cognitive behavioral, health coaching, and positive psychology approaches.
6. Summarize the evidence to support the use of behavior change techniques in clinical practice (Medical Knowledge).

   Novice: Recalls key studies about behavior change techniques.

   Advanced Beginner: Describes the evidence for specific behavior change techniques.

   Competent: Analyzes how behavior change evidence supports clinical use.

   Proficient: Critically evaluates the strength of evidence for behavior change techniques.

   Expert: Contributes to research, systematic reviews, or guideline development for behavior change techniques.
7. Use the skills of open inquiry, reflections, and empathy to develop and maintain a therapeutic alliance (Interpersonal and Communication Skills).

   Novice: Listens actively, mindfully, and deeply.

   Advanced Beginner: Uses open-ended questions and reflections (simple and complex).

   Competent: Maintains active engagement during consultations through empathy.

   Proficient: Facilitates patient-led discussions, fostering trust during patient encounters.

   Expert: Teaches and models advanced communication skills.

8. Describe the impact of positive emotions on the success of health behavior change (Medical Knowledge).

   Novice: Identifies basic concepts of positive emotion and motivation.

   Advanced Beginner: Explains how emotions influence behavior.

   Competent: Employs positive emotions to support stress resilience and helps patients sustain behavior change.

   Proficient: Incorporates emotion management into counseling with complex patients.

   Expert: Develops innovative approaches combining the science of positive emotions and behavior change.
9. Develop patient-centered, written action plans on the basis of the appropriate stage of change of the Transtheoretical Model of Change (TTM) (Patient Care and Procedural Skills).

   Novice: Identifies simple action plans that are appropriate for the patient's stage of change.

   Advanced Beginner: Drafts stage-specific plans with guidance.

   Competent: Independently develops tailored plans.

   Proficient: Adjusts patient care plans based on patient feedback and progress.

   Expert: Creates comprehensive, adaptable plans for complex patients and trains others.
10. Summarize the process of follow-up for ongoing lifestyle change progress, including building self-efficacy and relapse prevention (Medical Knowledge/Patient Care and Procedural Skills).

    Novice: Recognizes that follow-up is essential for lifestyle change.

    Advanced Beginner: Describes basic follow-up strategies and the concept of self-efficacy.

    Competent: Implements follow-up protocols to monitor progress and address relapses.

    Proficient: Uses tailored motivational techniques during follow-up to enhance self-efficacy and relapse prevention.

    Expert: Develops comprehensive follow-up models, trains others, and integrates relapse prevention strategies into standard practice.
11. Describe the factors that support sustained behavior change (Medical Knowledge and Interpersonal and Communication Skills).

    Novice: Lists general factors that sustain behavior change, such as motivation and support.

    Advanced Beginner: Explains the influence of social support, self-efficacy, and readiness to change on sustained behavior change.

    Competent: Analyzes individual and contextual factors affecting maintenance of behavior change.

    Proficient: Incorporates individual and contextual factors into personalized intervention plans.

    Expert: Contributes to research and education on promoting sustained behavior change.
12. Explain the role of family and other support to initiate and maintain health behavior change (Medical Knowledge).

    Novice: Recognizes that social support influences behavior.

    Advanced Beginner: Describes how family and social support networks facilitate change.

    Competent: Integrates family involvement and social support into patient care plans.

    Proficient: Navigates complex social dynamics to optimize support for patients with chronic conditions.

    Expert: Develops community social support and family-based programs and trains others in the use of family and social support to empower patients to change.
13. Manage disruptions to the therapeutic alliance (Interpersonal and Communication Skills).

    Novice: Recognizes that disruptions (e.g., misunderstandings, conflicts) can occur in patient relationships.

Advanced Beginner: Identifies common sources of disruption and demonstrates basic conflict resolution techniques.

Competent: Addresses and resolves minor conflicts and misunderstandings effectively.

Proficient: Uses advanced communication strategies to repair and strengthen the therapeutic alliance after significant disruptions.

Expert: Coaches others in conflict management, leads organizational efforts to foster a resilient patient-provider relationship, and develops strategies to manage and prevent disruptions.

14. Identify patient resources for sustainable behavior change in relation to the pillars of lifestyle medicine (Medical Knowledge).

    Novice: Identifies basic resources like community groups, online evidence-based resources or evidence-based apps.

    Advanced Beginner: Describes evidence-based resources relevant to typical patient needs.

    Competent: Recommends appropriate evidence-based resources tailored to individual patients during clinical encounters.

    Proficient: Collaborates with community organizations and uses evidence-based resources for comprehensive patient support.

    Expert: Leads efforts to develop new patient evidence-based resources, researches outcomes, advocates for evidence-based resource availability, and educates others on the topic.

26.10.9 Emotional and Mental Health Assessment and Interventions

1. Apply screening tools for stress, depression, and anxiety in clinical practice (Patient Care and Procedural Skills).

    Novice: Recognizes the need for mental health screening and names standard tools.

    Advanced Beginner: Administers basic mental health screening tools under supervision during clinical encounters.

    Competent: Performs and interprets mental health screening independently during clinical encounters.

    Proficient: Integrates mental health screenings into routine practice and tailors follow-up based on results.

    Expert: Develops or trains others in efficient mental health screening protocols; advocates for mental health screening policies.

2. Explain the relationship and pathophysiology between emotional and physical health (Medical Knowledge).

    Novice: Lists emotions that can influence physical health.

    Advanced Beginner: Describes basic mechanisms linking emotional states with physiological responses.

    Competent: Explains how stress and emotions modulate bodily systems.

    Proficient: Integrates complex pathophysiological concepts into clinical reasoning to address emotional and physical health.

    Expert: Contributes to research or education that advances understanding of mind-body interactions.

3. Summarize the nature of stress, the role of stressors such as adverse childhood experiences, and manageable elements of pathogenic stress reactions (Medical Knowledge).

    Novice: Identifies basic concepts of stress (acute and chronic) and adversity.

    Advanced Beginner: Describes key stressors throughout the lifespan and their effects.

Competent: Explains the impact of key stressors throughout the lifespan, childhood adversity, and their impacts on mental and physical health.

Proficient: Analyzes individual and systemic factors contributing to pathogenic stress, distress, chronic stress, and strain.

Expert: Develops or promotes interventions and policies addressing stress and adversity.

4. Describe and use evidence-based and patient-centered mental and emotional health self-management and resilience-building techniques (Patient Care and Procedural Skills).

    Novice: Lists common self-management and resilience-building techniques like breathing exercises and positive thinking.

    Advanced Beginner: Demonstrates basic use of self-management and resilience-building techniques.

    Competent: Tailors and teaches self-management and resilience-building techniques based on patient needs.

    Proficient: Incorporates self-management and resilience-building strategies into comprehensive care plans.

    Expert: Leads and/or develops programs to teach self-management and resilience at community or institutional levels.

5. Analyze the clinical relevance and evidence base for mindfulness-based stress reduction and related stress management strategies (Practice-Based Learning and Improvement).

    Novice: Identifies mindfulness-based stress reduction and stress management strategies.

    Advanced Beginner: Describes research supporting mindfulness-based stress reduction and stress management interventions.

    Competent: Critically evaluates medical literature on mindfulness-based stress reduction and stress management interventions.

    Proficient: Implements evidence-based mindfulness-based stress reduction and stress management strategies in clinical practice.

    Expert: Contributes to research, guidelines, or education on mindfulness-based stress reduction and stress management techniques.

6. Manage treatment plans for lifestyle-related mental health diseases, such as depression and anxiety (Patient Care and Procedural Skills).

    Novice: Recognizes basic management principles for mental health conditions such as depression and anxiety.

    Advanced Beginner: Implements initial lifestyle medicine treatment plans for mental health conditions such as depression and anxiety under supervision.

    Competent: Develops and adjusts comprehensive lifestyle medicine management plans for mental health conditions such as depression and anxiety independently.

    Proficient: Coordinates multidisciplinary lifestyle medicine focused care for mental health conditions such as depression and anxiety and monitors outcomes.

    Expert: Researches, leads, or innovates lifestyle medicine mental health management programs.

7. Describe indications for referral to mental health professionals (vs when clinically indicated) (Systems-Based Practice).

    Novice: Recognizes mental health concerns requiring referral to a mental health professional.

    Advanced Beginner: Describes typical referral criteria to a mental health professional.

    Competent: Identifies and initiates referrals to a mental health professional confidently.

    Proficient: Coordinates ongoing care with mental health professionals.

    Expert: Develops system-wide referral protocols for referral to mental health professionals and educates teams.

8. Apply mindfulness skills to enable presence, clarity, and curiosity in the clinical encounter (Patient Care and Procedural Skills/Interpersonal and Communication Skills).
   Novice: Identifies evidence-based mindfulness concepts.
   Advanced Beginner: Practices mindfulness in clinical encounters.
   Competent: Uses mindfulness techniques to enhance patient care during clinical encounters.
   Proficient: Fosters a mindful presence that improves clinical reasoning, empathy and the therapeutic alliance.
   Expert: Teaches and advocates for mindfulness-based approaches in clinical training and practice.

26.10.10 The Role of Connectedness and Positive Psychology

1. Apply positive psychology in health behavior change counseling (Patient Care and Procedural Skills).
   Novice: Recognizes basic concepts of positive psychology and how they influence health behavior change counseling.
   Advanced Beginner: Demonstrates simple application of positive psychology to behavior change efforts.
   Competent: Integrates positive psychology strategies effectively within patient interactions focused on behavior change.
   Proficient: Tailors and adapts positive psychology activities to individual patient needs to promote behavior change.
   Expert: Leads and teaches others in applying positive psychology principles to promote behavior change broadly across practice settings.
2. Describe how positive psychology strategies support achieving and sustaining healthy behaviors (Medical Knowledge).
   Novice: Lists key positive psychology strategies such as PERMA, optimism, and gratitude.
   Advanced Beginner: Explains mechanisms by which these positive psychology strategies support health behaviors.
   Competent: Integrates evidence-based positive psychology techniques into clinical reasoning.
   Proficient: Evaluates the effectiveness of positive psychology strategies for individual patients, group visits, and communities.
   Expert: Contributes to research or education on the long-term impact of positive psychology on behavior change and health.
3. Compare and contrast eudaimonia and hedonia and explain their effects on physical health, including longevity (Medical Knowledge).
   Novice: Defines eudaimonia and hedonia.
   Advanced Beginner: Contrasts the basic effects of eudaimonia and hedonia on well-being.
   Competent: Explains the biology behind how eudaimonia and hedonia influence health outcomes and longevity.
   Proficient: Analyzes complex interactions of eudaimonia and hedonia and applies them to clinical or community health and lifestyle medicine strategies.
   Expert: Develops or advances theories that connect these concepts to health and lifestyle medicine.
4. Describe how social connectedness and social networks affect emotional well-being, physical health, and longevity (Medical Knowledge).
   Novice: Identifies the impact social connectedness has on health outcomes.

Advanced Beginner: Describes physiological and psychological mechanisms by which social connectedness impacts health outcomes.

Competent: Explains research studies linking social connectedness with health outcomes.

Proficient: Applies this understanding of how social connectedness is linked to health outcomes to optimize community or individual health interventions.

Expert: Leads research, education, or policy efforts to enhance social connectedness.

5. Summarize the deleterious and positive effects social media have on emotional well-being and flourishing (Medical Knowledge).

   Novice: Identifies basic positive and negative impacts of social media on emotional well-being and flourishing.

   Advanced Beginner: Explains studies supporting both positive and negative effects of social media use.

   Competent: Critically appraises research studies on the impact of social media on well-being.

   Proficient: Advises patients on healthy social media use.

   Expert: Participates in developing evidence-based guidelines or interventions related to social media use.

6. Explain the relationship among the lifestyle pillars, positive emotions, and flourishing (Medical Knowledge).

   Novice: Lists positive emotion, defines flourishing, and identifies basic links between lifestyle medicine pillars, positive emotions, and flourishing.

   Advanced Beginner: Describes how the lifestyle medicine pillars, physical activity, nutrition, restorative sleep, stress resilience, positive social connections, and avoidance of risky substances relate to positive emotions and flourishing.

   Competent: Integrates the concepts connecting the interactions between lifestyle medicine pillars, positive emotions, and flourishing into patient counseling sessions.

   Proficient: Applies the understanding of the connection among lifestyle medicine pillars, positive emotion, and flourishing to improve health programs and patient outcomes by writing personalized prescriptions for positive psychology activities.

   Expert: Conducts or advances research on the connection between the lifestyle medicine pillars, positive emotions, and flourishing and health optimization.

7. Describe positive psychology activities that can boost emotional well-being and flourishing (Medical Knowledge).

   Novice: Lists common positive psychology and flourishing activities (e.g., expressing gratitude, journaling, performing acts of kindness).

   Advanced Beginner: Explains how these positive psychology and flourishing activities work to improve mental well-being.

   Competent: Guides patients through evidence-based positive psychology and flourishing activities and recommends activities according to specific patient needs and preferences.

   Proficient: Customizes positive psychology and flourishing interventions, recommendations, and prescriptions for diverse populations.

   Expert: Researches, creates, and/or advocates for positive psychology and flourishing interventions and educational curricula.

These proposed milestones will be modified and updated over time. In the meantime, residents, program directors, and others can use them to help residents meet lifestyle medicine competencies, with guideposts along the way. Fellows in lifestyle medicine may also be able to utilize them. An intensivist fellowship in lifestyle medicine will be discussed next.

26.11 LIFESTYLE MEDICINE INTENSIVIST FELLOWSHIP-GME BEYOND RESIDENCY

The Lifestyle Medicine Intensivist Fellowship (LMIF) was first established at Loma Linda University Health. It is designed to meet educational requirements for specialist certification, including 1,200 hours of lifestyle medicine training, clinical practice, group visits, scholarly activity, and case studies demonstrating disease reversal (8,9).

A lifestyle medicine intensivist is different from a physician who is board-certified in lifestyle medicine. The ABLM certifies physicians as lifestyle medicine intensivists. Intensivists must first be board-certified in lifestyle medicine. Then, through their clinical work and documentation of results, they can apply for the special designation of lifestyle medicine intensivist (10). There are specific core competencies for a lifestyle medicine intensivist that are documented in medical journal articles, including Lifestyle Medicine Intensivist Competencies: 2023 Expert Consensus Update, published in the *American Journal of Lifestyle Medicine* (11).

According to the American Board of Lifestyle Medicine, the requirements to be a lifestyle medicine intensivist are as follows (12):

- Certification as a lifestyle medicine physician by ABLM/IBLM
- Submission of an application to the ABLM, using a template provided by
- ABLM upon request, evidencing that:
    - Within a seven-year period, the physician obtained 1,200 hours of combined clinical and scholarly lifestyle medicine activity.
    - There is evidence of chronic disease reversal in the physician's patients by submitting ten separate case studies, with a minimum of three contact points over three months (four of the ten case studies must have three contacts over six months).
    - Payment of the Application Fee

26.11.1 Lifestyle Medicine Fellowship Content

The lifestyle medicine fellowship emphasizes all six pillars: nutrition, physical activity, restorative sleep, stress resilience, positive social connection, and avoidance of risky substances. The 88 lifestyle medicine competencies discussed earlier are central to the lifestyle medicine fellowship. The training focuses on behavioral change techniques and personal health behaviors. Essential educational experiences include clinical practice, teaching (physicians, students, and other providers), developing lifestyle medicine interventions, and health promotion programs, with research and fundraising mentioned as important but perhaps less important than the other components (13,14).

At Loma Linda, fellows spend 40% of their time on lifestyle medicine clinical revenue generation in their primary specialty, 40% on lifestyle medicine clinical activities, and 20% on scholarly activities in lifestyle medicine (9). The Lifestyle Medicine Intensivist Fellowships are necessary for the ABLM to be recognized as a medical subspecialty by the American Board of Medical Specialties (ABMS) (8,9). Although there has been limited uptake of the one Lifestyle Medicine Intensivist Fellowship at Loma Linda, there are plans to create a virtual fellowship and to inspire the development of more fellowships across the country.

There are different core competencies for the Lifestyle Medicine Intensivist. These differ from those included in Chapter 24, which reviews core competencies for medical students, and from those shared earlier in this chapter for the general specialty of lifestyle medicine. These were already mapped to the ACGME six core competencies in this chapter. The 46 lifestyle medicine intensivist core competencies were described in the article titled "Lifestyle Medicine Intensivist Competencies: 2023 Expert Consensus Update" and published in the *American Journal of Lifestyle Medicine* (11). In the article, these were categorized by the ACGME's six core competencies as follows.

26.11.2 Patient Care and Procedural Skills (Eleven Competencies)

1. Demonstrate expertise in the treatment settings in which lifestyle medicine intensivists commonly practice (e.g., a psychologically safe, ethical environment for inpatient, residential, outpatient, or group visits).
2. Apply evidence-based lifestyle medicine guidelines (such as those published by the expert lifestyle medicine panel and other expert panels) to treat lifestyle-related disease to achieve maximal remission and functionality.
3. Implement lifestyle medicine protocols that match the appropriate intervention to pathophysiology severity for treatment, "reversal" (ITLC), and disease prevention.
4. Manage medication adjustments safely and appropriately as a patient adopts a healthier lifestyle, in collaboration with the primary attending clinician as necessary:
    1. Appropriately manage de-escalation of medications and deprescribing.
5. Evaluate the function of relevant body systems and implement lifestyle medicine protocols that appropriately match the intensity of lifestyle treatment dosing needed to arrest and/or reverse disease pathophysiology and mitigate sequelae.
6. Conduct a health history and physical examination specific to lifestyle-related health status, including lifestyle vital signs.
7. Obtain and interpret appropriate tests to screen, diagnose, and guide the arrest and/or reversal of lifestyle-related disease:
    1. Interpret lab values that may be abnormal for those with a typical diet and lifestyle but are appropriate for those on an optimal lifestyle and diet regimen (e.g., low HDL-C [high-density lipoprotein cholesterol] when total cholesterol is low, etc.).
8. Assess the biological, psychological, social, cultural, and spiritual effects of patients' behaviors on associated health outcomes.
9. Evaluate patient and family readiness and ability to make healthful behavioral changes to inform practice decisions by:
    1. Identifying the bio-psycho-social barriers to change as part of the risk assessment workup and subsequent action plan.
    2. Aligning recovery and relapse prevention expectations.
10. Compare and contrast lifestyle medicine guidelines and nationally recognized practice guidelines (such as hypertension and smoking cessation) in order to facilitate informed patient decision-making for self-management of patient health behavior and lifestyle.
11. Collaborate with patients and their families to develop evidence-based, achievable, specific, written action plans such as lifestyle prescriptions.

26.11.3 Systems-Based Practice (Nine Competencies)

1. Describe the structure and function of the health care system as it relates to lifestyle medicine and identify the roles of lifestyle medicine intensivists therein.
2. Advocate for medical system and public health reforms that support and empower evidence-based lifestyle medicine integration into employee health, patient care, and community benefit across the care continuum.
3. Implement business systems and practices to support lifestyle medical care, including decision support technology (computer-based information system that supports clinical decision-making) and appropriate payment mechanisms (e.g., value-based payment, billing for shared medical appointments, etc.).
4. Demonstrate familiarity with appropriate community and professional resources to refer patients for ongoing support of lifestyle changes to support and sustain positive lifestyle changes, particularly in the transition from intensive interventions to less-intensive levels of care.

5. Coordinate and communicate with referring providers.
6. Make appropriate choices to refer patients to other health care resources.
7. Collaborate with key stakeholders and community leaders to reduce health care disparities using lifestyle medicine.
8. Advocate for lifestyle medicine as a solution to achieve the quintuple aim of health care.
9. Articulate and demonstrate the role of lifestyle medicine-based programs in value-based payment systems.

26.11.4 Medical Knowledge (Five Competencies)

1. Evaluate and discuss the scientific evidence that specific intensive lifestyle changes can arrest or reverse chronic disease.
2. Interpret how lifestyle medicine plays a role within basic medical science.
3. Discuss and apply the major components of lifestyle medicine that have determining effects on patients' health outcomes.
4. Describe the benefits of physician engagement with patients and families regarding its effect on patients' health behaviors.
5. Evaluate best applications of prominent conventional, complementary, and/or alternative therapies that may influence the application of lifestyle medicine interventions, including when and how to start, stop, and/or titrate medications, herbs, or other supplements.

26.11.5 Interpersonal and Communication Skills (Eight Competencies)

1. Establish effective relationships across culturally and linguistically diverse patient populations to initiate and sustain behavioral change using evidence-based counseling, educational tools, and appropriate follow-up.
2. Collaborate with patients and their families to develop evidence-based, achievable, specific, written action plans such as lifestyle prescriptions.
3. Collaborate with community, insurance, hospital, and clinical leadership in the integration of lifestyle medicine as a foundation of primary care and a key component of specialty care.
4. Advocate for lifestyle medicine as a unique specialty.
5. Discuss the role of intensive inductive lifestyle medicine interventions in initiating and maintaining remission of lifestyle-related diseases and conditions.
6. Engage with patients and families as a "coach" as well as an "expert," by applying empathy, understanding, and motivational interviewing techniques through a compassionate but firm approach.
7. Display leadership, passion, vitality, and positivity through all channels of communication.
8. Develop positivity resonance in interactions with the health care team and patients to broaden their problem-solving capacity in behavior change and self-management.

26.11.6 Practice-Based Learning and Improvement (Seven Competencies)

1. Monitor treatment processes and outcomes to improve the quality of lifestyle interventions in individuals and groups of patients with a focus on
    a. Lifestyle medicine-specific models of care, policies, and procedures
    b. Patient behavior change (activation) measures
    c. Person-centered care utilizing validated lifestyle vital signs relevant to each pillar
2. Utilize data technology to maximize the treatment effects of lifestyle interventions while tracking changes in individuals and patient populations over time, including:

   a. Lifestyle medicine patient assessment
   b. Chronic disease risk profile assessments
   c. Bio-psycho-social barriers
   d. Lifestyle behavior change (activation) and patient experience measures
   e. Follow-up systems/methods for supporting lifestyle changes
3. Establish continuous quality improvement processes.
4. Demonstrate the ability to collaborate with clinical research related to the key components of lifestyle medicine.
5. Demonstrate the ability to design, utilize, and advocate for financially viable health delivery models by:
   a. Implementing disease-specific shared medical appointment programs (general, programmed, or drop-in)
   b. Deploying intensive therapeutic lifestyle change interventions (ITLC)
   c. Utilizing in-person and virtual telehealth platforms
6. Manage a lifestyle medicine practice or program, including human, financial, and material resources.
7. Establish and lead interdisciplinary teams conducting multifactorial lifestyle change treatment programs to arrest and reverse disease, with attention to:
   a. Team culture
   b. Quality improvement (QI)
   c. Interdisciplinary patient-centered whole-person care, either with onsite practice or external health care providers

26.11.7 Professionalism (Six Competencies)

1. Promote healthful lifestyle choices as foundational to medical care, disease prevention, and health promotion.
2. Educate, inspire, and advance the field of lifestyle medicine as an expert by facilitating opportunities such as seminars, workshops, presentations, and conferences.
3. Model personal healthful lifestyle choices as an individual and as a clinical team.
4. Foster educational, occupational, community, and domestic environments that support healthful lifestyle choices in society.
5. Exhibit cultural proficiency in patient interactions and embrace diversity-based needs of health care colleagues and patients.
6. Engage in lifelong learning and continuous professional development in lifestyle medicine.

26.12 SUMMARY

The ACGME six core competencies guide resident and fellow education. The Lifestyle Medicine Residency Curriculum (LMRC) is available at the ACLM for purchase by residency program sites. There are also residency programs that are integrating the six pillars of lifestyle medicine and behavior change into their training without using the LMRC. Lifestyle medicine is relatively new, as discussed in Chapter 18, which introduces lifestyle medicine education. The LMRC was introduced in 2018. Since that time, the field has grown tremendously, as has the interest in lifestyle medicine education at the resident level.

Six years after the founding of the American College of Lifestyle Medicine, the field's original core competencies were published in JAMA (2). These competencies were updated 12 years later (3). The competencies were first mapped to the ACGME six core competencies in 2024, published in the Mayo Clinic Proceedings: Innovations, Quality, and Outcomes (4). Residency curricula are built around the core competencies of a specialty. Specifically, breaking down competencies into milestones is the recommended process of the ACGME. Lifestyle medicine does not have an ACGME-accredited residency program at this time. Regardless, the education of residents in lifestyle medicine must adhere to the highest academic standards; therefore, milestones have been defined for the first time and are presented in this chapter. These will need to be modified and updated over time, but they are a starting point.

Lifestyle medicine board certification has been available since 2017. There are two pathways to certification: the experiential path and the educational path. The experiential path is open to any ABMS- or AOA-boarded physician who meets eligibility requirements, completes a case study, and passes the written board examination. The educational pathway is through residency education via the LMRC or an equivalency pathway.

The American Board of Lifestyle Medicine administers a Lifestyle Medicine Intensivist designation. There are specific core competencies for this designation. A lifestyle medicine intensivist fellowship was started at Loma Linda, but there have not been many fellows to date. Physicians who are already board-certified in lifestyle medicine and have met all requirements, including hours, case studies, and evidence of disease reversal with lifestyle medicine prescriptions, have been certified as lifestyle medicine intensivists. There are only about two dozen globally. The International Board of Lifestyle Medicine certifies physicians outside the United States.

Each year, interest in lifestyle medicine certification continues to grow. Each year, ACLM's specialty and medical education activities expand. The specialty strives to set an educational standard on par with the most rigorous academic institutions in the country. For this reason, there is a process of continual updates to the competencies, re-evaluation of the areas covered, alignment with ACGME core competencies, and most recently the initial creation of milestones shared in this chapter.

REFERENCES

1. USMLE Content Outline, A Joint Program of the Federation of State Medical Boards and NBME. https://www.usmle.org/sites/default/files/2022-01/USMLE_Content_Outline_0.pdf. Accessed November 23, 2025.
2. Lianov L, Johnson M. Physician competencies for prescribing lifestyle medicine. *JAMA*. 2010;304(2): 202–203. doi: 10.1001/jama.2010.903. PMID: 20628134.
3. Lianov LS, Adamson K, Kelly JH, Matthews S, Palma M, Rea BL. Lifestyle medicine core competencies: 2022 update. *Am J Lifestyle Med.* 2022;16(6):734–739.
4. Frates B, Ortega HA, Freeman KJ, Co JPT, Bernstein M. Lifestyle medicine in medical education: maximizing impact. *Mayo Clin Proc Innov Qual Outcomes.* 2024;8(5):451–474. doi: 10.1016/j.mayocpiqo.2024.07.003. PMID: 39263429; PMCID: PMC11387546.
5. Rea BL, Cheema S, Lanza S, et al. Lifestyle medicine core competencies: 2025 update. *Am J Lifestyle Med.* 2025:15598276251379821. doi: 10.1177/15598276251379821. Epub ahead of print. PMID: 41169934; PMCID: PMC12568558.
6. American Board of Lifestyle Medicine Competencies and Weighting. https://ablm.org/competencies-weighting. Accessed November 23, 2025.
7. American Board of Lifestyle Medicine. www.ablm.org. Accessed November 23, 2025.
8. Rea B, Worthman S, Shetty P, Alexander M, Trilk J. Medical education transformation: lifestyle medicine in undergraduate and graduate medical education, fellowship, and continuing medical education. *Am J Lifestyle Med.* 2021;15:514–525. doi: 10.1177/15598276211006629.
9. Rea B, Wilson A. Creating a lifestyle medicine intensivist fellowship: a replicable and sustainable model. *Am J Lifestyle Med.* 2020;14:278–281. doi: 10.1177/1559827620907552.
10. Kelly J, Karlsen MC, Lianov L. Establishing competencies for physicians who specialize in the practice of lifestyle medicine. *Am J Lifestyle Med.* 2019;14(2):150–154. doi: 10.1177/1559827619856542. PMID: 32231481; PMCID: PMC7092408.
11. Kelly JH, Lianov L, Shurney D, et al. Lifestyle medicine intensivist competencies: 2023 expert consensus update. *Am J Lifestyle Med.* 2023;18(1):141–149. doi: 10.1177/15598276231192846. PMID: 39184278; PMCID: PMC11339762.

12. American Board of Lifestyle Medicine, Prerequisites for Certified Lifestyle Medicine Intensivist https://ablm.org/eligibility-prerequisites/. Accessed November 23, 2025.
13. Polak R, Dacey ML, Keenan H, et al. Bridging the gap – planning lifestyle medicine fellowship curricula: a cross-sectional study. *BMC Med Educ*. 2014;14:1045. doi: 10.1186/s12909-014-0271-4.
14. Bonnet JP, Edshteyn I, Phillips EM, Hull SK, Polak R. Perspectives on a lifestyle medicine fellowship curriculum from interested medical students. *Am J Lifestyle Med*. 2016;13(1):106–110. doi: 10.1177/1559827616681270.

27 Assessment and Feedback for Residents and Residency Programs

27.1 ASSESSING CLINICAL SKILLS

Attendings need to observe residents during their day-to-day interactions with patients to evaluate their performance in a variety of areas such as general counseling skills, clinical judgment, ability to work in teams, communication with patients and family members, patient safety, physical exam skills, history-taking skills, motivational interviewing skills, ability to co-create SMART goals, ability to write prescriptions for all six pillars in an organized framework such as FITT (frequency, intensity, time, and type), proper referral process, performing a workup with labs and diagnostic testing when appropriate, and effective use of assessment tools.

The various methods for assessing residents can be mapped to Miller's Pyramid of Clinical Competence (1). Miller's pyramid of clinical competence has four basic levels: knows, knows how, shows how, and does (2). For example, written exams and multiple-choice questions that require factual recall demonstrate the lowest level of clinical competency: "knows." Examples of lifestyle medicine multiple choice questions were shared earlier in this book in Chapter 25-Evaluations and Assessment for Lifestyle Medicine Courses. "Knows how" can be assessed with written exams, as well as when the multiple choice questions are clinical context-based. "Shows how" can be evaluated with OSCEs, simulated patients or actors, and role-playing. "Does" can be assessed by watching residents in action and reviewing charts or logs. Direct observation of residents during clinical encounters is an excellent way to evaluate their performance in real time. Figure 27.1 shows Miller's Pyramid, with assessments identified at each level (1).

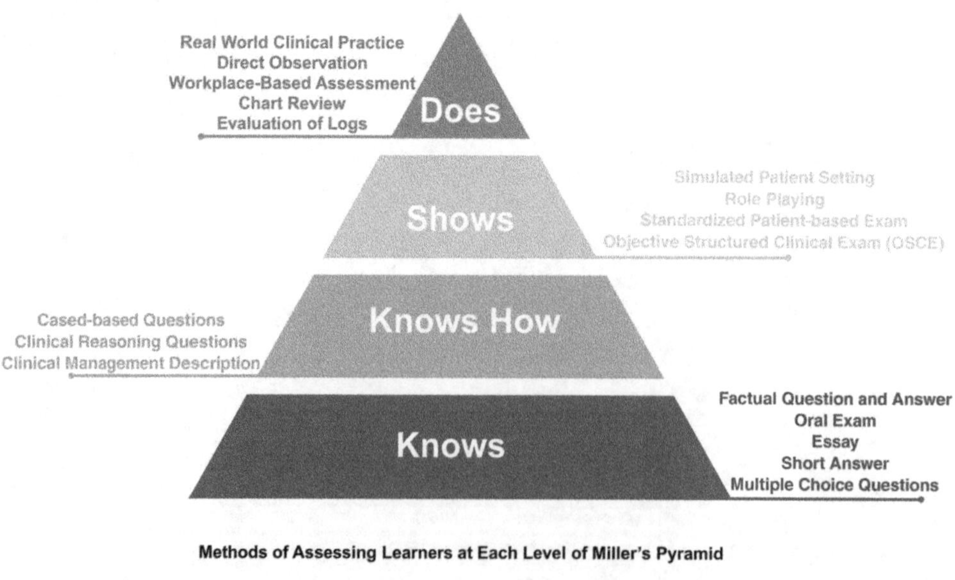

FIGURE 27.1 Miller's pyramid of clinical competence aligned with assessment strategies.

DOI: 10.1201/9781003630043-27

Modifications to Miller's Pyramid of Clinical Competence have been suggested over the years. Cruess and colleagues (3), in an article published in Academic Medicine, proposed adding a component of professional identity formation and a level of "is" to the pyramid. Adding a fifth level or layer to the pyramid that represents "is" or "trust" introduces the element of entrustable professional activities (EPAs) and entrustment. Is the learner trusted? (4) This modification is shown in Figure 27.2.

For this level of entrustment, faculty members identify residents or learners based on five categories: agency, reliability, integrity, capability, and humility, and there is a mnemonic called "A RICH" to help remember these critical attributes and abilities (5). "A RICH" is spelled out by Ten Cate et al. in their article "The Ingredients of a Rich Entrustment Decision," published in Medical Teacher, as follows:

- "Agency (proactive toward work, team, safety, personal development)"
- "Reliability (conscientious, predictable, accountable, responsible)"
- "Integrity (truthful, benevolent, patient-centered)"
- "Capability (task-specific knowledge, skills, experience, situational awareness)"
- "Humility (recognizes limits, asks for help, receptive to feedback)" (5)

This top-tier level of "is," with personal identity and "trust" with entrustment, is a signal of accomplishment beyond does. It also signifies "will do." It implies that the learner is trusted to continue performing at the highest levels with reliability, integrity, and humility, even in the most difficult and unforeseen circumstances (3). Assessing learners at this level requires more than multiple-choice exams (knows), clinical case-scenario questions (knows how), practice patients, simulated patients, OSCEs (shows how), and direct observation in the clinic (does). It is an evaluation or assessment that develops over time as the learner is observed in many different clinical environments. The A RICH attributes and abilities are intangible in many respects (integrity and humility) and need to be experienced and felt by the evaluators.

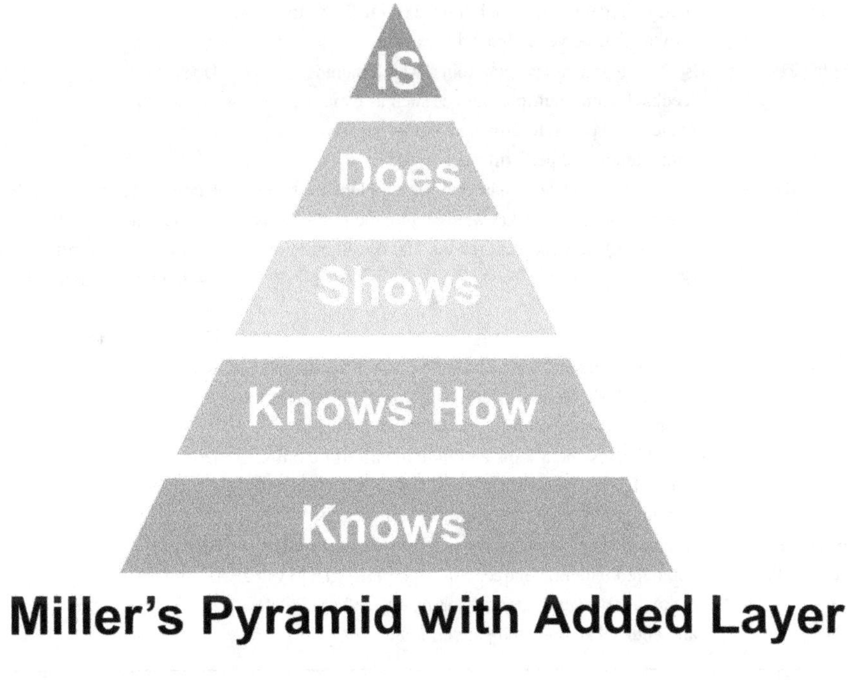

FIGURE 27.2 Miller's pyramid with added layer of "Is."

27.2 METHODS TO ASSESS RESIDENTS

There are several standard methodologies to assess residents in the "knows," "knows how," "shows how," and "does" realms. A description of common assessment strategies used by faculty to assess residents is listed in Table 27.1.

The Mini-Clinical Evaluation Exercise (mini-CEX) is an assessment tool that is used by many residency programs because it is structured, practical, and educational (24,25). As part of the mini-CEX, the faculty member documents the names of the faculty and resident, notes the date, and identifies the resident year (R1, R2, or R3). The patient's problem and diagnosis are listed, along with the visit setting (ambulatory, inpatient, ER, or other), the patient's age and sex, and whether the visit is a follow-up or a new visit. There is a field to indicate the encounter level (low, moderate, or high) and to specify the focus of the visit (data collection, diagnosis, or counseling). The resident is graded on a Likert scale from 1 to 9 (13) across the following areas: medical interviewing skills, physical exam skills, professionalism, clinical judgment, counseling skills, organization/efficiency, and overall clinical competence. The faculty must also note the number of minutes spent assessing and observing the resident, as well as the number of minutes spent on providing feedback to the resident. Both the faculty and the resident rate the overall experience with the mini-CEX direct observation process on a scale of 1–9. There is space for the faculty and the resident to write comments. Both the faculty and resident must sign the mini-CEX form. The whole experience is a shared learning opportunity.

TABLE 27.1
Assessment Tools for Evaluating Residents

Tool	Description	Miller's Pyramid of Clinical Competence
Direct observation (6–9)	Observe the resident during routine clinical encounters, giving formative feedback at the end of a session.	Does
Workplace-based assessments (10–14)	Perform structured direct observation with tools like the mini-Clinical Evaluation Exercise (mini-CEX) to provide formative feedback to residents.	Does
Multi-source feedback (15–17)	Use 360-degree assessment tools, which include feedback from multiple sources such as patients, nurses, and peers, to provide a comprehensive view of competency and performance.	Does
Written exams and record audits (6,7,11,18,19)	In-training exams and chart reviews supplement direct observation to assess knowledge, judgment, proper use of the electronic medical record, and documentation skills.	Knows—Written Examinations testing facts Knows how—Written Examinations with clinical context-based questions Does—Chart reviews
Structured evaluation forms (6,20,21)	Many programs use forms based on ACGME, such as the use of Milestones or other structured competencies, often with Likert scales, to standardize evaluations	Knows How
Self-assessment tools (6,22)	Use self-assessment tools and Individualized Learning Plans (ILPs) to encourage resident self-reflection and encourage resident ownership of their progress	Does
Objective structured clinical exam (OSCE) and simulated patients (23)	Structured timed sessions for residents to visit with a simulated patient, conduct a history, perform a physical exam, analyze and interpret lab results and other data, and counsel a simulated patient or an actor.	Shows How

When completing a mini-CEX, it is essential to use it not only to assess the resident but also to guide their individual learning plan and personal growth. Faculty who plan to use the mini-CEX should undergo training to ensure proper use of the tool (25,26). Faculty who conduct direct observation assessments must view them as formative tools and link them to the residency's core competencies and milestones (6).

Best practices for direct observation and evaluation of residents include selecting faculty observers who are familiar with the competencies being assessed and have clinical skills and experience in those specific areas (27). For lifestyle medicine, it is ideal to select faculty who are board-certified in lifestyle medicine or who have trained in it and are working toward certification. After the observers are selected for appropriateness, they will require training in the evaluation process, whether using mini-CEX or another methodology (27,28). The observers also need to be familiar with the Accreditation Council for Graduate Medical Education (ACGME) and lifestyle medicine core competencies. The observations made and shared with the resident should be relevant to at least one competency area (27,29). Ensuring that residents are aware of the clinical competencies and milestones from the outset of their training will guide development through direct observation and feedback.

The ACGME also recommends the direct observation tools on its website under supporting materials. A downloadable version of the mini-CEX is available on their website for faculty use (30). To make an account on the ACGME site, a faculty member simply inputs an email address and password. Membership or payment is not required. Another ACGME tool available in the supporting materials is the Rater Assessment Form, which invites faculty to observe the resident and complete a specific assessment form. On the form, the faculty is asked to list the things that went well in the encounter, to list the areas of deficiency or errors made by the resident, to prioritize the most crucial areas to address in feedback, to summarize the overall assessment of the resident's skills demonstrated in the encounter, and to rate the resident in terms of overall competence and safety for the specific skill being judged as either: can be an observer, can practice the skill with direct observation, can practice the skill with indirect observation, or can practice unsupervised. In the conclusion section on this ACGME Rater Assessment Form, the faculty is asked to determine the next steps for this resident after this direct observation. Direct observation can be conducted during part of a clinic visit, including the introduction, history and physical, assessment and plan, or wrap-up. The resident can receive feedback on specific sections of the visit if the faculty member does not have time to observe the entire visit. It is best to observe residents multiple times and provide feedback on numerous occasions. This supports residents' training, growth, and development as they learn and practice throughout the program.

The ACGME provides a faculty development toolkit to improve assessment through direct observation (30). The website is excellent and comprehensive, with multiple sections: overview, microlearnings, example workshops, videos, workshops and webinars, supporting materials, and additional resources. The microlearnings include a Facilitator's Guide and PowerPoint slides covering multiple topics. Regarding the direct observation process, the ACGME website offers frameworks in the supporting materials section. One of the frameworks is taking a history. For residents, the framework is broken up into sections: sets the stage, elicits chief concerns/sets agenda, begins with non-focusing questions to help patient express self, uses focusing skills to elicit symptom story, personal, and emotional content, transitions to middle of interview, obtains remainder of history, wraps up history, and uses electronic health record (EHR) appropriately. There are tasks under each category that the resident is meant to complete. The framework is shared with residents and helps them to frame their visits. When faculty observe residents, they can use the same framework to assess the residents.

The American College of Lifestyle Medicine (ACLM) staff members in the education department have been collaborating with the ACGME on lifestyle medicine-focused tools for faculty. They are working on a Lifestyle Medicine: Return Visit in Primary Care handout. A draft was shared at the ACLM annual meeting in Dallas, Texas, in November 2025. In the framework, there were seven sections to the patient encounter assessment: setting the stage; discussion of diagnosis and lifestyle medicine; motivational interviewing skills; knowledge and content of the plan; wrap-up with a patient-centered summary; behaviors throughout the encounter; and use of the electronic health record. The ACGME Framework: Lifestyle Medicine (LM) approach had additional components compared to the general primary care approach.

In the first section of the patient encounter, also called the set-the-stage section, the LM Approach adds a task to orient the patient to the purpose of the visit, using language such as "in this visit" or "in the time we have today," and then asks for the patient's concerns or priorities.

The following section discusses the patient's diagnosis and the application of lifestyle medicine. In this second section, the resident practices (a) assessing the patient's current health behavior patterns and risk factors related to the diagnosis/prognosis, (b) assessing patient understanding of how the diagnosis/prognosis and health behaviors are interconnected, (c) discussing informed consent with all treatment options presented, such as lifestyle medicine pillars with or without medications and surgical interventions based on disease-specific algorithm guidelines, (d) discussing how medication and lifestyle medicine intervention dosing and intensity impact health outcomes, (e) assessing readiness to change, and (f) exploring patient preference/willingness to engage in various lifestyle medicine behavior change plans, dependent on stage of change.

The third section is devoted to motivational interviewing skills, including affirming the patient, asking open-ended questions, using summaries, using the Ask-Provide-Ask technique to share information, using reflections, addressing perceived barriers to change, and using confidence and readiness rulers.

The fourth section is the knowledge and content plan part of the patient encounter. The resident practices providing accurate information about lifestyle medicine, using shared decision-making to co-create a plan with SMART goals, and using appropriate lifestyle prescription strategies.

The fifth section is the wrap-up, with a patient-centered summary that includes summarizing the plan, using teach-back methods, negotiating a follow-up plan, and setting expectations for the next visit, as well as providing patient support before concluding the visit and saying goodbye.

The sixth section of the handout about the lifestyle medicine patient encounter addresses behaviors throughout the encounter, emphasizing speaking plainly, adapting the conversation to the patient's level of understanding, using person-first language, avoiding judgmental language, providing information in small chunks with frequent pauses, encouraging a back-and-forth conversation with the patient doing most of the talking, encouraging the patient to ask questions, and addressing the patient's questions.

The seventh and final section addresses the use of the electronic health record. It is recommended that residents use technology in a way that supports, rather than distracts from, the patient relationship. This handout was in the initial stages of development. More than likely, it will be updated and modified. A document like this can be a valuable tool for residents looking to learn more about lifestyle medicine practice and gain competence in conducting a return visit in primary care.

ACGME provides numerous high-quality open-access resources and tools on its website. In addition, they offer an online course on their website for which you can register free of charge. The course helps learners improve resident assessment skills and use direct observation (30). To access these resources, navigate to Featured Content, then Faculty Development.

27.3 FEEDBACK SESSIONS FOR RESIDENTS

The process by which faculty provide feedback to residents is often an area of weakness and an area for growth in many residency programs (31,32). During the direct observation and feedback sessions, the resident should feel supported. That is a vital component of any evaluation. The focus should be on the resident's behaviors, skills, and performance (27). Comments about personality, personal attributes, or non-behavioral remarks are not part of the direct observation process.

The goal of the direct observation is to foster growth, not to provide harsh judgment (33). Many faculty members trained at a time when feedback was full of harsh judgment. Times are different and much improved for the resident learning environment. The resident should feel inspired to learn and grow after the feedback session, not shamed and hopeless. These direct observations serve the resident best when repeated over time (34), especially when the same faculty member provides multiple points of feedback and fosters a trusted relationship (33). This can be helpful to the resident, but it is not often feasible when faculty members are busy with their own clinics and responsibilities. In fact, they may only serve on inpatient units once or twice a year. Designating a faculty member as the Direct Assessor (DA) for a resident is also an option (32). In this way, faculty trained in direct observation and feedback can focus on this vital task with dedicated time and energy. Long-term relationships built on trust and respect can also support the feedback process (33). Making the experience comfortable and nonintimidating helps residents participate fully and authentically, rather than feeling nervous, reserved, or afraid (33). The observer also needs to feel relaxed and ready to be mindfully present during the session. For this to happen, the observer needs protected time (32–35). If the faculty observer is distracted or rushed, the direct observation process is compromised.

There is no leadership training in most medical schools and residency programs. Thus, faculty members conducting these resident evaluations may not be skilled in delivering feedback. This is a critical skill required of any leader. Faculty members working with residents are mentors and leaders, and they often require guidance for delivering feedback. Training for faculty involved in direct observation is recommended (28,33,35). For example, training faculty members to use a checklist of behaviors as part of the assessment and teaching them how to effectively share the list with residents is useful because it is a valuable way to align the session's goals and provide structure to the feedback session (36). Other programs have used a structured clinical outcomes form to guide residents and faculty in focusing on specific behaviors and clinical skills during direct observation (37).

Reading recommendations on providing feedback, reviewing checklists, and using direct observation tools to prepare for the critical role of assessing residents is advised for all faculty members who are new to the process or even if they are seasoned at the task. Becoming familiar with the concepts and new approaches before a faculty training on the topic can help faculty gain confidence and competence. The suggestions listed in Chapter 22, covering feedback in Lifestyle Medicine for medical students, are also applicable to residents.

As a reminder and to practice repetition in learning while reading this book, Chapter 22 discussed the importance of the positivity ratio, the sandwich technique, growth mindset, the FIT and ABLE mnemonic (F-Frequent, I-Interactive, T-Timely, A-Appropriate for Learner Level, B-Behavior Specific and Balanced, L-Labeled, and E-Empathetic) (38), and Pendleton's Model's five steps (39,40), including a give-and-take with the feedback recipient and provider with (a) recipient going first to share 2–3 points that went well, (b) provider provides 2–3 points that went well, (c) provider asks recipient for 2–3 points that could be improved, (d) provider shares 2–3 improvement areas and discusses strategies to close the gap, and (e) provider or recipient summarizes the most crucial points of the conversation. There is also the ALOBA Model—Agenda-Led Outcome-Based Analysis (41), the "Ask-Tell-Ask" Approach (42), Advocacy-Inquiry Technique (43), and the COACH Approach for feedback (44,45). Putting on the Coach Hat, figuratively, when working with residents on feedback after assessments is useful. Learning the COACH way of being is helpful for this aspect of medical education (46). The COACH mnemonic is curious, open, appreciative, compassionate, and honest.

The ACGME Toolkit for Assessment provides two handouts on additional resources for feedback: the R2C2 model and the Prepare to ADAPT framework (47). The R2C2 Model stands for relationship and reaction for the 2 Rs and content and coaching for the 2 Cs (48). According to the ACGME handout, there are four phases: Phase 1: build relationships; Phase 2: explore reactions and reflections; Phase 3: confirm content; and Phase 4: coach for change and co-create an action plan. This R2C2 Model focuses on connection and collaboration between faculty and residents. The goal is for the resident to feel supported. This can occur only if there is a connection and a respectful relationship between the faculty and the resident, and if there is a foundation of trust. The self-assessment, accompanied by the resident's reactions and reflections, is central to this model. The resident will be more comfortable expressing these freely if there is a good relationship with the faculty. Following this self-assessment, the resident and faculty agree on the content to be covered. Subsequently, the faculty member coaches the resident on the specified content, and then the resident selects a specific goal to work toward, accompanied by an action plan.

The other feedback model shared by the ACGME is the Prepare to ADAPT Feedback Framework (49). ADAPT stands for Ask-Discuss-Ask-Plan Together. This mnemonic speaks for itself as to what it is, what it highlights, and what it values. As mentioned in Chapter 21, teaching is a two-way street. This feedback process is a teaching tool. Thus, the invitation component asks the resident to share their thoughts and reflections. The role of the faculty member, serving as a coach, is to ask thought-provoking questions that invite the resident to reflect deeply and adopt new perspectives. The main asks, or questions, are simple: "What went well with the patient encounter? What did not go so well, in your opinion? And what would you do differently?" Additional prompts include, "Tell me more about that. What do you think was going on at that time? What was your clinical reasoning for that? What were you feeling at that time?" In this part of the process, the faculty member listens deeply without interrupting.

After the first A or first Ask in the ADAPT model for feedback, there is the D which stands for discussion. At this time, the faculty member serving as a coach shares their thoughts. Sharing in a nonjudgmental manner is key. The coach can use the **COACH** mnemonic (50)—**C**urious, **O**pen (non-judgmental), **A**ppreciative for the opportunity to support the resident, appreciative of any positive aspects of the patient encounter or insights the learner shared, **C**ompassionate, remembering the learner is a resident on a learning journey to become a competent and proficient physician, and lastly **H**onest, providing necessary critical appraisal of the interaction to keep patients safe and the resident functioning at the highest level. With this in mind, the faculty coach speaks candidly about their observations in an honest, nonjudgmental, and compassionate manner to maintain a positive and supportive learning environment while providing appropriate guidance for future patient encounters. The goal of the discussion step is to talk in a neutral tone, focus on describing behaviors, skills, and clinical practices, and avoid discussing personal attributes and characteristics.

After the discussion and D in ADAPT, there is another A, or ask step in the process. Again, the faculty coach invites the resident's input. The faculty coach may ask, "What do you make of what I just shared? How do you feel about the feedback I just gave? What surprised you about what I shared just now? Of the information I shared, what resonated with you? Was my feedback useful? If so, in what way?" The resident talks; the faculty listens. During this second ask session, the faculty coach listens deeply to the resident learner again. Listening is a sign of respect, and learners deserve respect.

After the second A, or ask step, comes the PT, which is the plan-together step. After asking, discussing, and asking again, planning begins. This is led by the resident learner, with the faculty coach guiding. The faculty can help the resident prioritize and focus on the critical skills and attitudes required to attain competency and proficiency in the practice of medicine, with particular attention to the program's residency milestones and core competencies. The plan needs to be specific. The resident learner may use the SMART goal framework to make goals concrete—specific, measurable, action-oriented, realistic, and time-bound. Approaching these feedback sessions with a coach approach is recommended (51). In Chapter 21 on teaching strategies for medical students, self-determination theory was reviewed. As a reminder, people need autonomy, competence, and relatedness to stay motivated to pursue goals, and this applies to residents in medical training, especially those who are underperforming (52). This Prepare to ADAPT Feedback framework helps provide the resident with autonomy, competence, and relatedness. The entire process is driven by the connection and relationship between the resident learner and the faculty coach, rooted in mutual respect, trust, and shared goals.

Faculty coaches should remember that when resident learners are struggling, they are not doing so intentionally. Residents are not giving the program a hard time; they are having a hard time themselves. They do not deserve punishment, shaming, or blaming. They deserve respect, compassion, understanding, help, support, and guidance. If the resident's actions are reckless, that is a different scenario, and the residency program director addresses these dangerous circumstances directly. Otherwise, the direct observation sessions are times for formative feedback and guidance.

The faculty coach may use the five-step collaboration cycle described in Chapter 22. As a reminder, the cycle has five distinct and vital steps: (a) express empathy, (b) align motivation, (c) build confidence, (d) set SMART goals, and (e) set accountability in this plan together (44,45). The fifth step, establishing accountability, is significant. This follow-up is essential, as residents require ongoing support and monitoring. One step may be to schedule another direct observation session with the same faculty coach or with a different faculty coach. Making sure to check in with the resident learner before closing the session requires another round of questions, such as "How was this feedback session for you? What could I have done better as a faculty coach? Where do you see things going from here? What was helpful in this process? Before we say goodbye, would you please summarize the next steps? How do you want to be held accountable for this action plan we co-created? How can I be helpful at this point as the faculty coach? What have you learned through this feedback process?" This final check-in with the resident learner helps solidify key lessons from the session and again signals that this was a feedback session. The entire process begins and ends with checking in with the resident learner. This is a learner-centric process (35). Faculty who serve as faculty coaches work to balance their roles as coaches and teachers, a balance that requires practice and experience to master (46).

This quote summarizes the process well and is included in the ACGME handout on the ADAPT Feedback Framework: "Academic coaching focuses on student-centered development, which capitalizes on students' strengths and empowers them to be leaders," said Maya Hammoud, MD, MBA.

As a reminder, the model is called Prepare to ADAPT. The ADAPT part of the model was just covered. However, the Prepare step has not been covered yet. This first step in Prepare to ADAPT is one of the most significant. Preparation is key and sets faculty up for success. How faculty set themselves up for this feedback is critical In this case, the faculty member is serving as a coach and setting the tone of the interaction. In preparation, the faculty coach should take deep breaths, relax, and enter a state of neutral mindfulness. The learner is invited to take deep breaths, remain calm during the direct observation period, and be as natural as possible. This Prepare to ADAPT method is reported in detail in the journal article by Fainstad et al., titled "Feedback Can Be Less Stressful: Medical Trainee Perceptions of Using the Prepare to ADAPT (Ask-Discuss-Ask-Plan Together) Framework" (49).

To begin a feedback session following the direct observation, a recommended methodology is outlined. First, ask if it is a good time for the resident or learner to participate in the feedback session. Even if the feedback session was prearranged and confirmed, it is recommended to check in with the learner. Things may have changed. A resident may need to pick up a child at daycare or take a sick pet to a vet and thus can be distracted or rushing. It is also essential to "signpost" the session by stating, "This is a feedback session," as is recommended in the ACGME handout on the ADAPT Feedback process (47). Holding the session in a private location helps create a quiet, calm environment for the discussion. This takes planning. Reserving a room or using a faculty member's office are good options. It can be hectic to find a quiet space in a hospital or clinic. A rushed approach takes away from the peaceful, empowering, and supportive experience that is optimal for a resident feedback session. It is essential that the resident feels safe during the feedback session (53). This includes physical and psychological safety, the latter of which is exceedingly important and often overlooked (54).

Successful direct observation sessions are the responsibility of faculty and residents. Joint workshops with faculty and residents have been successfully employed (55). The healthcare system and academic institutions also bear responsibility for ensuring there is time and space for resident assessment and feedback (27). The culture of a residency program plays a significant role in the direct observation and feedback processes. If leadership has created a supportive culture for faculty, faculty are more likely to develop a supportive environment for residents. If leadership demonstrates respect, trust, integrity, inclusivity, and humility, faculty are more likely to exhibit these attributes as well. This extends to residents as well. It is with these core attributes of respect, trust, integrity, inclusivity, and humility that high-quality relationships are created in departments and divisions in the hospital. Modeling these high-quality relationships with residents is the key to fostering a supportive and stable environment for residency training and learning.

27.4 ASSESSMENT OF RESIDENCY EDUCATION

27.4.1 Current Research Insights in Lifestyle Medicine Residency Education

Research on lifestyle medicine residencies indicates feasibility, increasing implementation, positive effects on resident skills and behaviors, and ongoing challenges in curriculum integration and evaluation. Most published research on lifestyle medicine residency programs reports outcomes at the lower levels of the Kirkpatrick evaluation model—primarily Levels 1 (engagement/reaction/satisfaction) and 2 (learning/knowledge/skills)—and some studies report Level 3 impact (behavior change, personally or in clinical practice) (56). At this time, there are no readily available medical education articles on lifestyle medicine at Level 4 impact (patient or organizational results).

As an example of Kirkpatrick Level 1 results, the Lifestyle Medicine Residency Curriculum (LMRC) was successfully implemented in the Harvard Medical School Occupational and Environmental Residency, with residents demonstrating interest through attendance and active engagement in didactic sessions and application activities (57). An end-of-the-year survey of the residents revealed, "All seven respondents reported finding the LMRC lectures to be educational, evidence-based, enjoyable, and a value-add to the existing OEMR program. The residents unanimously reported feeling that the LMRC will positively influence their careers, with six of seven residents indicating their intent to pursue certification in lifestyle medicine in the future" (57). These are all Level 1 findings revealing engagement, positive reactions, and satisfaction.

Participation in lifestyle medicine residencies improves residents' knowledge, self-efficacy, and confidence in counseling patients on lifestyle changes. These have an impact at Level 2 in Kirkpatrick's Model. Objective assessments (e.g., OSCEs) and self-reports show increased competence in lifestyle medicine topics and patient discussions, again at Level 2 (58,59). Residents exposed to lifestyle medicine curricula often report improvements in their health behaviors, which fall under Level 3 in the Kirkpatrick Model and have an impact on behavior (58,59). Family medicine residents view lifestyle medicine training as integral to their role, but those without specific training in lifestyle medicine feel less confident and are less knowledgeable than those family medicine residents who were trained in lifestyle medicine (60). Family medicine residents express a strong interest in further lifestyle medicine education and certification (61). Despite this interest, there is currently a lack of training in the six pillars of lifestyle medicine in residency programs (62). The three biggest barriers to including lifestyle medicine into residency programs are (a) limited curricular time, (b) lack of trained faculty, and (c) competing clinical demands (62).

Figure 27.3 demonstrates the amount of research available for each level of the Kirkpatrick Model.

ACLM's LMRC is a packaged product that residency programs can purchase to help address barriers related to a lack of trained faculty to teach the six pillars of lifestyle medicine and the core competencies. An introductory LMRC package is available for residents to try prior to purchasing the full program. To date, there is a dearth of research on the LMRC, which was first offered in 2018. An article published in the American Journal of Lifestyle Medicine in 2024 described the implementation and dissemination of the LMRC over the years (63). The growth of the LMRC was highlighted: 7 programs had access to the LMRC in 2018, 13 in 2019, 29 in 2020, 82 in 2021, 204 in 2022, 304 in 2023, and 368 in 2024 (63). Data on the total number of residents who have sat for the exam and those

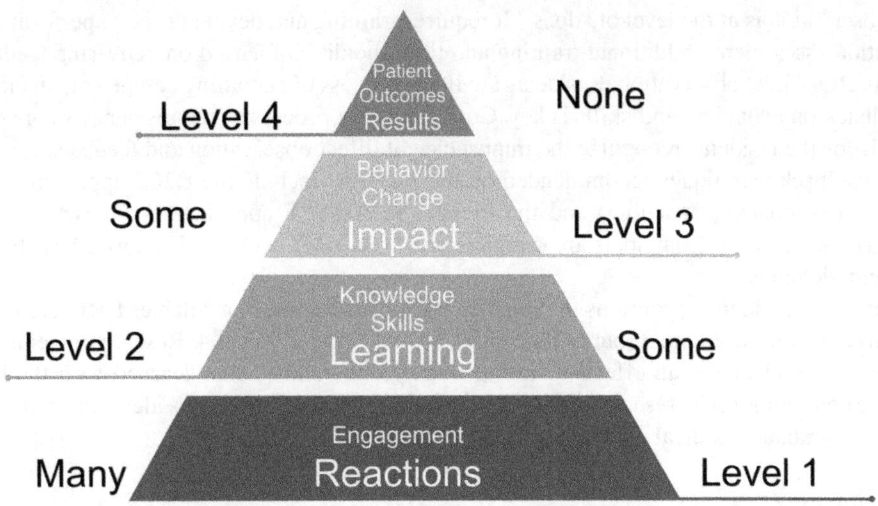

FIGURE 27.3 Kirkpatrick Model with lifestyle medicine research.

who passed were shared. In 2023, 59 residents in the country sat for the exam, and 55 passed on the first attempt, with a first-time pass rate of 93% (63). In 2024, the paper reported that approximately 109 residents sat for the exam and approximately 105 passed on the first attempt, yielding a first-time pass rate of 96% (63). Given that as of 2024, 368 residency programs offer the LMRC, the number of residents taking the board exam is projected to increase substantially in the next few years.

More research on the LMRC is needed. Many questions remain unanswered. What percentage of residents in the 368 programs offering the LMRC are actively using the curriculum? How many complete the program out of those who are enrolled? What percentage of residents enrolled in the LMRC continue to get board-certified in lifestyle medicine by the American Board of Lifestyle Medicine? Do residents who participate in the LMRC counsel more often on the six pillars of lifestyle medicine and counsel more patients on the six pillars compared to residents who do not participate in the LMRC? Are attendings who completed the LMRC during their residency more successful at helping their patients achieve remission of chronic conditions through lifestyle medicine prescriptions compared to those who did not complete the LMRC? Is there an impact on patient outcomes? A more robust evaluation of program outcomes, with a focus on patient results, is needed. This corresponds to Level 4 in the Kirkpatrick Model.

To address the shortage of trained medical school faculty and board-certified physicians who are confident and competent to teach lifestyle medicine to residents, faculty development programs could provide lifestyle medicine education, funding for CME courses in lifestyle medicine, and opportunities for faculty to obtain board certification. The limited curricular time and competing clinical demands during residency must be addressed within each residency program. Ultimately, the goal is to integrate lifestyle medicine across all years of residency training (62). For a resident's continuity clinic, this would include assessing all six pillars of lifestyle medicine and developing treatment plans to address chronic conditions, including lifestyle medicine pillar prescriptions (62). The lifestyle medicine material and teaching may need to be individualized to the program and adjusted to fit program requirements and the current curriculum.

27.5 SUMMARY

Assessing residents' skills is required by all ACGME-accredited residency programs. There are recommended procedures and tools to assist faculty in assessing residents' clinical skills. The mini-CEX is commonly used for direct observation. In Miller's pyramid of clinical competence, direct observation is at the level of "does." It requires training and devoted time to perform a direct observation assessment. Additional training and time should be focused on delivering feedback to residents after direct observation. Residents are in the process of becoming competent, and focusing the feedback on behaviors and skills is key. Connecting the process to the residency's core competencies helps the residents recognize the importance of direct observation and feedback.

Two feedback techniques recommended by the ACGME include the R2C2 approach (relationship, reaction, content, coaching) and the Prepare to ADAPT approach (Ask-Discuss-Ask-Plan Together). Resources and handouts are available on the ACGME website that cover these two feedback methodologies.

Research on residency programs that include lifestyle medicine is available. There are results at Kirkpatrick Levels 1, 2, and 3, but to date, none are available at Level 4. Researching educational endeavors in residency is an effective way to share results and lessons learned with the broader academic community. The research helps shape future programs and sparks ideas for further investigations in graduate medical education.

REFERENCES

1. Wass V, Van der Vleuten C, Shatzer J, Jones R. Assessment of clinical competence. *Lancet.* 2001;357(9260): 945–949. doi: 10.1016/S0140–6736(00)04221-5. PMID: 11289364.
2. Miller GE. The assessment of clinical skills/competence/performance. Acad Med. 1990 Sep;65(9 Suppl):S63-7. doi: 10.1097/00001888-199009000-00045. PMID: 2400509.
3. Cruess RL, Cruess SR, Steinert Y. Amending Miller's pyramid to include professional identity formation. *Acad Med.* 2016;91(2):180–185. doi: 10.1097/ACM.0000000000000913.
4. Ten Cate O, Carraccio C, Damodaran A, et al. Entrustment decision making: extending Miller's pyramid. *Acad Med.* 2021;96(2):199–204. doi: 10.1097/ACM.0000000000003800.
5. Ten Cate O, Chen HC. The ingredients of a rich entrustment decision. *Med Teach.* 2020;42(12):1413–1420. doi: 10.1080/0142159X.2020.1817348.
6. Lee G, Chiu A. Assessment and feedback methods in competency-based medical education. *Ann Allergy Asthma Immunol.* 2021. doi: 10.1016/j.anai.2021.12.010.
7. Danilovich N, Kitto S, Price D, Campbell C, Hodgson A, Hendry P. Implementing competency-based medical education in family medicine: a narrative review of current trends in assessment. *Fam Med.* 2021;53(1):9–22. doi: 10.22454/fammed.2021.453158.
8. Kogan JR, Holmboe ES, Hauer KE. Tools for direct observation and assessment of clinical skills of medical trainees: a systematic review. *JAMA.* 2009;302(12):1316–1326. doi: 10.1001/jama.2009.1365. PMID: 19773567.
9. Phillips DP, Zuckerman JD, Kalet A, Egol KA. Direct observation: assessing orthopaedic trainee competence in the ambulatory setting. *J Am Acad Orthop Surg.* 2016;24(9):591–599. doi: 10.5435/JAAOS-D-15–00401. PMID: 27479831.
10. Mortaz Hejri S, Jalili M, Masoomi R, Shirazi M, Nedjat S, Norcini J. The utility of mini-clinical evaluation exercise in undergraduate and postgraduate medical education: a BEME review: BEME guide No. 59. *Med Teach.* 2020;42(2):125–142. doi: 10.1080/0142159X.2019.1652732. Epub 2019 Sep 15. PMID: 31524016.
11. Holmboe E, Hawkins R. Methods for evaluating the clinical competence of residents in internal medicine: a review. *Ann Intern Med.* 1998;129:42–48. doi: 10.7326/0003-4819-129-1-199807010-00011.
12. Norcini JJ, Blank LL, Arnold GK, Kimball HR. The mini-CEX (clinical evaluation exercise): a preliminary investigation. *Ann Intern Med.* 1995;123(10):795–799.
13. Norcini JJ, Blank LL, Duffy FD, Fortna GS. The mini-CEX: a method for assessing clinical skills. *Ann Intern Med.* 2003;138(6):476–481. doi: 10.7326/0003–4819-138-6–200303180-00012. PMID: 12639081.
14. Johnson NR, Pelletier A, Berkowitz LR. Mini-clinical evaluation exercise in the era of milestones and entrustable professional activities in obstetrics and gynaecology: resume or reform? *J Obstet Gynaecol Can.* 2020;42(6):718–725. doi: 10.1016/j.jogc.2019.10.002. Epub 2019 Dec 25. PMID: 31882285.
15. Joshi R, Ling FW, Jaeger J. Assessment of a 360-degree instrument to evaluate residents' competency in interpersonal and communication skills. *Acad Med.* 2004;79(5):458–463. doi: 10.1097/00001888–200405000-00017. PMID: 15107286.

16. Lewis J, Balaji L, Grossestreuer A, Ullman E, Rosen C, Dubosh N. Correlation of attending and patient assessment of resident communication skills in the emergency department. *AEM Educ Train.* 2021;5. doi: 10.1002/aet2.10629.
17. Hennel EK, Trachsel A, Subotic U, Lörwald AC, Harendza S, Huwendiek S. How does multisource feedback influence residency training? A qualitative case study. *Med Educ.* 2022;56(6):660–669. doi: 10.1111/medu.14798. Epub 2022 Mar 16. PMID: 35263461; PMCID: PMC9314722.
18. Chou S, Lockyer J, Cole G, McLaughlin K. Assessing postgraduate trainees in Canada: are we achieving diversity in methods? *Med Teach.* 2009;31(2):e58–e63. doi: 10.1080/01421590802512938. PMID: 19089723.
19. Hildebrand C, Trowbridge E, Roach MA, Sullivan AG, Broman AT, Vogelman B. Resident self-assessment and self-reflection: University of Wisconsin-Madison's Five-Year Study. *J Gen Intern Med.* 2009;24(3):361–365. doi: 10.1007/s11606-009-0904-1. *Epub* 2009 Jan 21. PMID: 19156469; PMCID: PMC2642556.
20. Holt K, Miller R, Nasca T. Residency programs' evaluations of the competencies: data provided to the ACGME about types of assessments used by programs. *J Grad Med Educ.* 2010;2(4):649–655. doi: 10.4300/jgme-02-04-30.
21. Swing SR. Assessing the ACGME general competencies: general considerations and assessment methods. *Acad Emerg Med.* 2002;9(11):1278–1288. doi: 10.1111/j.1553–2712.2002.tb01588.x. PMID: 12414482.
22. De Fátima Diniz Souza É, Machado A, De Oliveira J, et al. Inventory of self-assessed competences: a tool for identifying training strengths and weaknesses in medical and multiprofessional residency programmes for primary health care. *BMC Med Educ.* 2025;25. doi: 10.1186/s12909-025-07521-z.
23. Epstein RM, Hundert EM. Defining and assessing professional competence. *JAMA.* 2002;287(2):226–235. doi: 10.1001/jama.287.2.226. PMID: 11779266.
24. Batra P, Batra R, Verma N, Bokariya P, Garg S, Yadav S. Mini clinical evaluation exercise (mini-CEX): a tool for assessment of residents in department of surgery. *J Educ Health Promot.* 2022;11:253. Sivaraman G, Lakshmanan J, Alexander A, et al. Use of mini-CEX as formative assessment tool in the training of undergraduate medical students in ENT situation analysis and the way forward. *Indian J Otolaryngol Head Neck Surg.* 2024;76(3):2698–2703.
25. Durrani SF, Hameed A, Rani P, et al. Effect of Mini-CEX as formative learning tool for clinical skills in undergraduate medical students in a private medical university in Karachi, Pakistan. *BMC Med Educ.* 2025;25:1356. doi: 10.1186/s12909-025-07962-6.
26. Liao KC, Pu SJ, Liu MS, Yang CW, Kuo HP. Development and implementation of a mini-clinical evaluation exercise (mini-CEX) program to assess the clinical competencies of internal medicine residents: from faculty development to curriculum evaluation. *BMC Med Educ.* 2013;13:31.
27. Kogan J, Hatala R, Hauer K, Holmboe E. Guidelines: the do's, don'ts and don't knows of direct observation of clinical skills in medical education. *Perspect. Med Educ.* 2017;6:286–305. doi: 10.1007/s40037-017-0376-7.
28. Holmboe E, Hawkins R, Huot S. Effects of training in direct observation of medical residents' clinical competence. *Ann Intern Med.* 2004;140:874–881. doi: 10.7326/0003-4819-140-11-200406010-00008.
29. Berz J, Cheng T, Quintiliani L. Milestones-based direct observation tools in internal medicine resident continuity clinic. *BMC Med Educ.* 2017;17. doi: 10.1186/s12909-017-1077-y.
30. ACGME Faculty Development Tool Kit. https://dl.acgme.org/pages/acgme-faculty-development-toolkit-improving-assessment-using-direct-observation#SupportingMaterials. Accessed November 23, 2025.
31. Shafian S, Ilaghi M, Shahsavani Y, Okhovati M, Soltanizadeh A, Aflatoonian S, Karamoozian A. The feedback dilemma in medical education: insights from medical residents' perspectives. *BMC Med Educ.* 2024;24. doi: 10.1186/s12909-024-05398-y.
32. Acker A, Hawksby E, MacPherson P, Leifso K. Dedicated assessors: description of an innovative education intervention to facilitate direct observation in the clinical setting. *Can Med Educ J.* 2021;12:e69–e73. doi: 10.36834/cmej.69260.
33. Young J, Sugarman R, Schwartz J, O'Sullivan P. Overcoming the challenges of direct observation and feedback programs: a qualitative exploration of resident and faculty experiences. *Teach Learn Med.* 2020;32:541–551. doi: 10.1080/10401334.2020.1767107.
34. Smith J, Jacobs E, Li Z, Vogelman B, Zhao Y, Feldstein D. Successful implementation of a direct observation program in an ambulatory block rotation. *J Grad Med Educ.* 2017;9(1):113–117. doi: 10.4300/jgme-d-16-00167.1.

35. Schlair S, Dyche L, Milan F. Longitudinal faculty development program to promote effective observation and feedback skills in direct clinical observation. *MedEdPORTAL*. 2017;13. doi: 10.15766/mep_2374-8265.10648.
36. Graddy R, Reynolds S, Wright S. Coaching residents in the ambulatory setting: faculty direct observation and resident reflection. *J Grad Med Educ*. 2018;10(4):449–454. doi: 10.4300/jgme-17-00788.1.
37. Hamburger E, Cuzzi S, Coddington D, et al. Observation of resident clinical skills: outcomes of a program of direct observation in the continuity clinic setting. *Acad Pediatr*. 2011;11(5):394–402. doi: 10.1016/j.acap.2011.02.008.
38. Beckman TJ, Lee MC. Proposal for a collaborative approach to clinical teaching. *Mayo Clin Proc*. 2009;84(4):339–344. doi: 10.1016/S0025–6196(11)60543-0. PMID: 19339652; PMCID: PMC2665979.
39. van de Ridder JMM. Pendleton's rules: a mini review of a feedback method. *Am J Biomed Sci Res*. 2023;19(1):19–21. doi: 10.34297/AJBSR.2023.19.002542.
40. Pendleton D, Schofield T, Tate P, Havelock P. *The New Consultation: Developing Doctor-Patient Communication*. Oxford: Oxford University Press, 2003.
41. Orsini C, Rodrigues V, Tricio J, Rosel M. Common models and approaches for the clinical educator to plan effective feedback encounters. *J Educ Eval Health Prof*. 2022;19:35. doi: 10.3352/jeehp.2022.19.35. Epub 2022 Dec 19. PMID: 36537186; PMCID: PMC9842479.
42. Lee GB, Chiu AM. Assessment and feedback methods in competency-based medical education. *Ann Allergy Asthma Immunol*. 2022;128(3):256–262. doi: 10.1016/j.anai.2021.12.010. Epub 2021 Dec 17. PMID: 34929390.
43. Castillo AY, Chan JD, Lynch JB, Bryson-Cahn C. How to disagree better: utilizing advocacy-inquiry techniques to improve communication and spur behavior change. *Antimicrob Steward Healthc Epidemiol*. 2023;3(1):e201. doi: 10.1017/ash.2023.457. PMID: 38028895; PMCID: PMC10654947.
44. Frates EP, Bonnet J. Collaboration and negotiation: the key to therapeutic lifestyle change. *Am J Lifestyle Med*. 2016;10(5):302–312. doi: 10.1177/1559827616638013. PMID: 30202286; PMCID: PMC6125074.
45. Frates EP, Moore MA, Lopez CN, McMahon GT. Coaching for behavior change in physiatry. *Am J Phys Med Rehabil*. 2011;90(12):1074–1082. doi: 10.1097/PHM.0b013e31822dea9a. PMID: 22019966.
46. Armson H, Lockyer J, Zetkulic M, Könings K, Sargeant J. Identifying coaching skills to improve feedback use in postgraduate medical education. *Med Educ*. 2019;53. doi: 10.1111/medu.13818.
47. ACGME Featured Content, Faculty Development Toolkit, Supporting Materials. https://dl.acgme.org/pages/acgme-faculty-development-toolkit-improving-assessment-using-direct-observation#SupportingMaterials. Accessed November 24, 2025.
48. Sargeant J, Mann K, Manos S, Epstein I, Warren A, Shearer C, Boudreau M. R2C2 in action: testing an evidence-based model to facilitate feedback and coaching in residency. *J Grad Med Educ*. 2017;9(2):165–170.
49. Fainstad T, McClintock AA, Van der Ridder MJ, Johnston SS, Patton KK. Feedback can be less stressful: medical trainee perceptions of using the prepare to ADAPT (ask-discuss-ask-plan together) framework. *Cureus*. 2018;10(12):e3718.
50. Frates B, Bonnet J, Joseph R, Peterson J. *The Lifestyle Medicine Handbook* (2nd ed). Monterey, CA: Healthy Learning, Chapter 2, 2021.
51. Brown LE, Rangachari D, Melia M. Beyond the sandwich: from feedback to clinical coaching for residents as teachers. *MedEdPORTAL*. 2017;13:10627.
52. Ajjawi R, Bearman M, Molloy E, Noble C. The role of feedback in supporting trainees who underperform in clinical environments. *Front Med*. 2023;10:1121602.
53. Boileau É, Talbot-Lemaire M, Bélanger M, St-Onge C. "Playing in the big leagues now": exploring feedback receptivity during the transition to residency. *Health Prof Educ*. 2019;5(4):Article 7. doi: 10.1016/j.hpe.2018.09.003.
54. Hitchner L, Yore M, Burk C, Mason J, Sawtelle Vohra S. The resident experience with psychological safety during interprofessional critical event debriefings. *AEM Educ Train*. 2023;7(2):e10864.
55. Kim B, Rajagopalan A, Tabasky E, Reddy S, Topor D. Sharing perspectives on feedback: a combined resident-faculty workshop. *BMC Med Educ*. 2022;22. doi: 10.1186/s12909-022-03253-6.
56. Pasarica M, Boring M, Lessans S. Current practices in the instruction of lifestyle medicine in medical curricula. *Patient Educ Couns*. 2022;105(2):339–345. doi: 10.1016/j.pec.2021.05.042. Epub 2021 Jun 2. PMID: 34116891.
57. Lutchman K, Wan M, Lan F-Y, Kales SN, Frates EP. Integrating the lifestyle medicine residency curriculum into an occupational medicine training program. *J Occup Environ Med*. 2024;66(4):e143–e144. doi: 10.1097/JOM.0000000000003056.

58. Nawaz H, Petraro P, Via C, et al. Lifestyle medicine curriculum for a preventive medicine residency program: implementation and outcomes. *Med Educ Online.* 2016;21. doi: 10.3402/meo.v21.29339.
59. Malatskey L, Zeev B, Tzuk-Onn A, Polak R. Lifestyle medicine course for family medicine residents: preliminary assessment of the impact on knowledge, attitudes, self-efficacy and personal health. *Postgrad Med J.* 2017;93:549–554. doi: 10.1136/postgradmedj-2016-134726.
60. Malatskey L, Zeev B, Polak R, Tzuk-Onn A, Frank E. A nationwide assessment of lifestyle medicine counseling: knowledge, attitudes, and confidence of Israeli senior family medicine residents. *BMC Fam Pract.* 2020;21. doi: 10.1186/s12875-020-01261-3.
61. Veazey E. Lifestyle medicine education: medical school to residency. *Am J Lifestyle Med.* 2022;17:54–55. doi: 10.1177/15598276221114282.
62. Frates B, Ortega H, Freeman K, Co J, Bernstein M. Lifestyle medicine in medical education: maximizing impact. *Mayo Clin Proc Innov Qual Outcomes.* 2024;8:451–474. doi: 10.1016/j.mayocpiqo.2024.07.003.
63. Miller CM, Cramer SR, Aney SJ, et al. The innovation, implementation, and dissemination of the lifestyle medicine residency curriculum (LMRC) in graduate medical education. *Am J Lifestyle Med.* 2025:15598276251393211. doi: 10.1177/15598276251393211.

28 Ways Forward for Medical Education

The first 17 chapters of this book cover the research and science supporting the use of the six pillars of lifestyle medicine and therapeutic lifestyle change for the prevention, treatment, and remission of chronic conditions. The following 11 chapters describe the state of medical education at all levels, from undergraduate to graduate. The details of designing presentations, classes, and complete courses in lifestyle medicine were reviewed. In addition, teaching strategies for medical students and residents were described and discussed. Assessments and feedback for medical students and residents were also covered in previous chapters. The importance of core competencies was highlighted many times. The lifestyle medicine core competencies were mapped to the Accreditation Council for Graduate Medical Education ACGME's six core competencies and listed under each category for easy reference. Courses need to align with the core competencies. ACGME works with milestones for each competency. This book shares the first draft of milestones for each of the 88 lifestyle medicine competencies. The goal of this book is to provide medical school and healthcare professional faculty with the science and art of teaching lifestyle medicine.

There are many resources available to help faculty members teach lifestyle medicine to learners at different levels. Figure 28.1 shows the resources available at various stages of medical education. The figure is from the *Mayo Clinic Proceedings: Innovations, Quality, and Outcomes* article titled "Lifestyle Medicine Education: Maximizing Impact" (1).

There are many barriers to implementing these resources and teaching lifestyle medicine in medical schools or residency programs. Table 28.1 lists the barriers and multiple solutions to these barriers. There are also examples of how to employ the solutions. With creativity and perseverance, faculty members can advance the teaching of lifestyle medicine.

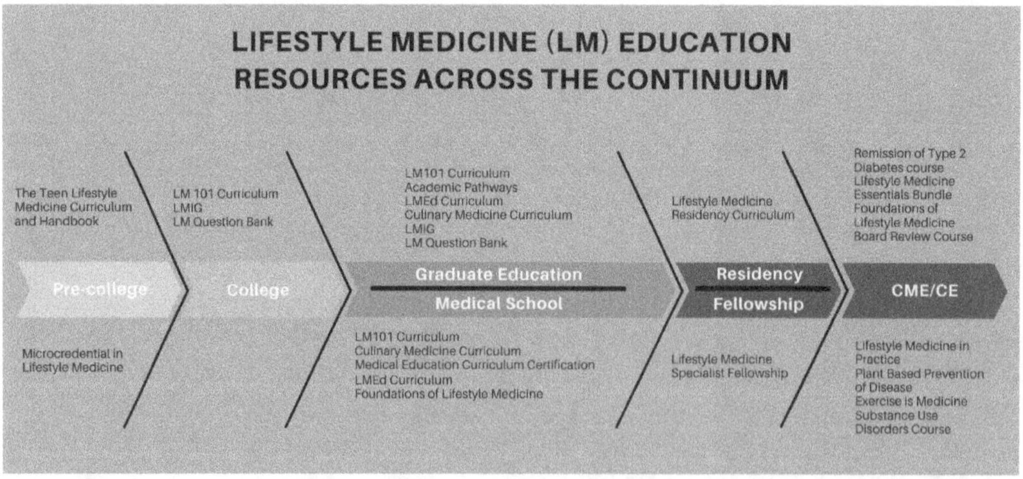

FIGURE 28.1 Lifestyle medicine resources across the curriculum. (Source: Frates B, Ortega HA, Freeman KJ, Co JPT, Bernstein M. Lifestyle medicine in medical education: maximizing impact. *Mayo Clin Proc Innov Qual Outcomes*. 2024;8(5):451–474. doi: 10.1016/j.mayocpiqo.2024.07.003. PMID: 39263429; PMCID: PMC11387546. Used with permission.)

DOI: 10.1201/9781003630043-28

TABLE 28.1
Common Barriers to Including Lifestyle Medicine in Medical and Health Professional Education

Barriers	Solutions	Examples
Core curriculum is full	Offer a separate elective	• Lifestyle medicine elective
	Create optional opportunities for lifestyle medicine education	• Lifestyle medicine distinction • Lifestyle medicine certificate
	Parallel curriculum	• Post-graduate advanced practice provider lifestyle medicine residency programs
	Weave lifestyle medicine into current courses and cases	• LMIG • Lifestyle medicine Theme
	Create a Master's Program	• Master of Science in lifestyle medicine
Not enough trained faculty to teach	Increased training in lifestyle medicine	• Board certification in lifestyle medicine
	Increased knowledge	• Certificate course in lifestyle medicine • Training the trainer
	Bring in experts	• Attend CME courses • Grand rounds • Lectures from DipABLM/IBLM/ACLM certified professionals
	Live or recorded lecture offerings	• Virtual ACLM LMIG • Webinars on ACLM's Connect Platform • LM Summits
Lack of established resources	Complementary resources	• ACLM LM101 Curriculum • LMEd Curriculum • Lifestyle Medicine Foundation Curriculum • ACLM Essentials Bundle • ACLM Culinary Medicine Syllabus • Lifestyle Medicine Question Bank
	Resources with costs associated	• ACLM LMRC • American College of Culinary Medicine Health Meets Food curriculum or Certified Culinary Medical Specialist course • Gaples Institute CME on nutrition • Lifestyle medicine journals such as the *American Journal of Lifestyle Medicine*
	Viewing documentaries	• Code Blue, You Are What You Eat, Forks over Knives, Game Changers, Blue Zones, They're Trying to Kill Us, What the Health? Eating You Alive • *Manual of Lifestyle Medicine* Edited by J Rippe
	Lifestyle Medicine Textbooks	• Rippe Series in Lifestyle Medicine • *The Lifestyle Medicine Handbook* • *The Lifestyle Medicine Pocket Guide* • *Health Promotion and Disease Prevention for Advanced Practice*
Lack of funding	Apply for research grants to study the impact of lifestyle medicine education courses and workshops on medical students, residents, and physicians	• Ardmore Institute of Health has funded lifestyle medicine programs and education efforts • Local funding with grants from the medical school or hospital • Clinical Translational Science Awards, Health Resources and Services Administration, National Institute of Health Grants • Taste of Lifestyle Medicine Micro-grants

(*Continued*)

TABLE 28.1 (*Continued*)
Common Barriers to Including Lifestyle Medicine in Medical and Health Professional Education

Barriers	Solutions	Examples
Lack of understanding of and familiarity with lifestyle medicine	Educate Deans Educate Faculty Educate Students	Give grand rounds on a lifestyle medicine topic at the hospital
Lack of LM questions on licensing exams	Educate medical school course directors and residency program directors	Deliver LM workshop at ACGME and AAMC national meetings
	Publish articles in the medical literature	Create special lifestyle medicine editions in major medical journals
	Bring awareness to current lifestyle medicine research	Run a journal club on lifestyle medicine topics
	Collaborate with STEP 1, 2, and 3 licensing boards	ACLM UME Question Bank and other resources to help jump start question creation

Source: Frates B, Ortega HA, Freeman KJ, Co JPT, Bernstein M. Lifestyle medicine in medical education: maximizing impact. *Mayo Clin Proc Innov Qual Outcomes.* 2024;8(5):451–474. doi: 10.1016/j.mayocpiqo.2024.07.003. PMID: 39263429; PMCID: PMC11387546. Used with Permission.

28.1 INTEGRATING LIFESTYLE MEDICINE WITH MAJOR CHRONIC CONDITIONS IN MEDICAL EDUCATION

Nutrition and the other five pillars of lifestyle medicine are integral to discussions of the major chronic conditions outlined in the first part of this book, including heart disease, diabetes, cancer, obesity, metabolic syndrome, and cognitive decline. They also need to be addressed when medical students learn about aging, women's health, and pediatrics. This book is designed to help faculty easily locate and apply research to develop lectures and educational experiences that support medical students' learning of the six pillars of lifestyle medicine.

Medical schools use different curricular maps that cover the science of healthy organ function, the pathophysiology of disease, the treatment of disease, and the practice of medicine, including professionalism. Schools often follow an organ system approach. With this approach, each pillar of lifestyle medicine can be highlighted as part of the root cause of a condition impacting a system, such as sedentary behavior contributing to cardiovascular disease, diet contributing to diabetes, smoking contributing to cancer, alcohol increasing the risk of atrial fibrillation, or sleep insufficiency contributing to the risk of Alzheimer's disease. In addition, the pillars of lifestyle medicine can be discussed and integrated into the treatment of many common chronic conditions.

For lesson planning purposes, the specific sections of this book that correspond to different organ systems and disease conditions are outlined below.

28.1.1 For the Cardiovascular System: Heart Disease and Hypertension

In this book:

Chapter 2—Physical Activity—Section IV—Physical Activity and Chronic Disease
Chapter 3—Nutrition—Section III—Current Nutritional Recommendations
Chapter 3—Nutrition—Section IV—Healthy Diets

Chapter 4—Weight Management—Section VI—Overweight and Obesity and Chronic Disease
Chapter 6—Sleep—Section VI—Sleep Disordered Breathing (SDB) and Chronic Disease
Chapter 7—Positive Connections—Section VII—Individual Health Outcomes
Chapter 9—Cardiovascular Disease

In the Rippe Series: *Lifestyle Medicine and the Primary Care Provider*
Chapter 14—Lifestyle Medicine Disease-Specific Applications: Cardiovascular Disease

28.1.2 For the Endocrine System: Diabetes, Metabolic Syndrome

In this book:
Chapter 2—Physical Activity—Section V—Physical Activity and Diabetes, Pre-Diabetes, and the Metabolic Syndrome
Chapter 3—Nutrition—Section III—Current Nutritional Recommendations
Chapter 3—Nutrition—Section IV—Healthy Diets
Chapter 4—Weight Management—Section VI—Overweight and Obesity and Chronic Disease
Chapter 5—Substance Use Disorder—Section II—Cigarette Smoking
Chapter 6—Sleep—Section VI—Sleep Disordered Breathing (SDB) and Chronic Disease
Chapter 7—Positive Connections—Section VII—Individual Health Outcomes
Chapter 10—Diabetes
Chapter 13—Metabolic Syndrome

In the Rippe Series: *Lifestyle Medicine and the Primary Care Provider*
Chapter 12—Lifestyle Medicine Disease-Specific Applications: Diabetes

28.1.3 For the Immune System: Autoimmune Diseases, Infections

In this book:
Chapter 6—Sleep—Section VI—Sleep Disordered Breathing (SDB) and Chronic Disease
Chapter 7—Positive Connections—Section VII—Individual Health Outcomes

28.1.4 For the Neurologic System and Psychiatric Conditions: Cognition and Mood

In this book:
Chapter 2—Physical Activity—Section IX—Brain Health and Cognition
Chapter 6—Sleep—Section IV—Short-Term Health Consequences of Sleep Disruption
Chapter 6—Sleep—Section VI—Sleep Disordered Breathing (SDB) and Chronic Disease
Chapter 7—Positive Connections—Section VII—Individual Health Outcomes
Chapter 14—Brain Health, Cognitive Function, Dementia Prevention

In the Rippe Series: *Lifestyle Medicine and the Primary Care Provider*
Chapter 16—Lifestyle Medicine Disease-Specific Applications: Mental Health (Depression and Anxiety)

28.1.5 For the Musculoskeletal System: Arthritis

In this book:
Chapter 4—Weight Management—Section VI—Overweight and Obesity and Chronic Disease
Chapter 6—Sleep—Section VI—Sleep Disordered Breathing (SDB) and Chronic Disease

28.1.6 For Weight Management: Overweight and Obesity

In this book:
Chapter 2—Physical Activity—Section VI—Physical Activity, Weight Gain, and Obesity
Chapter 4—Weight Management

Chapter 6—Sleep—Section VI—Sleep Disordered Breathing (SDB) and Chronic Disease
In the Rippe Series: *Lifestyle Medicine and the Primary Care Provider*
Chapter 13—Lifestyle Medicine Disease-Specific Applications: Obesity

28.1.7 For Oncology

In this book:
Chapter 2—Physical Activity—Section VII—Physical Activity and Cancer
Chapter 3—Nutrition—Section 1—Introduction
Chapter 4—Weight Management—Section VI—Overweight and Obesity and Chronic Disease
Chapter 5—Substance Use Disorder—Section II—Cigarette Smoking.
Chapter 11—Cancer
In the Rippe Series: *Lifestyle Medicine and the Primary Care Provider*
Chapter 15—Lifestyle Medicine Disease-Specific Applications: Cancer

28.1.8 For Behavior Change

In this book:
Chapter 31—Behavior Change
In the Rippe Series: *Empowering Behavior Change in Patients: Practical Strategies for the Healthcare Professional*

28.2 SUMMARY

This book provides the information to empower medical education faculty to teach lifestyle medicine and to integrate it into medical school and residency curricula. With the rigorous research in the first 17 chapters of this book and the teaching, assessment, and feedback strategies in the second 11 chapters, educators can design and develop compelling presentations, practical classes, and powerful courses in lifestyle medicine. There are additional chapters on individual and planetary health, health equity, and behavior change. To teach lifestyle medicine, educators need to know the science of the six pillars and the art of teaching. This book shares both.

REFERENCE

1. Frates B, Ortega HA, Freeman KJ, Co JPT, Bernstein M. Lifestyle medicine in medical education: maximizing impact. *Mayo Clin Proc Innov Qual Outcomes.* 2024;8(5):451–474. doi: 10.1016/j.mayocpiqo.2024.07.003. PMID: 39263429; PMCID: PMC11387546.

29 Individual and Planetary Health

29.1 INTRODUCTION

While most of the chapters in this book and, indeed, the counseling sessions in the embedded curriculum focus largely on individual health, there is also a very important consideration for planetary health in this area.

While this might not be something that is central to counseling sessions with your patients, it is an area where all of us in the medical community should play a very significant role. This is one of the areas where what we recommend to our individual patients also has profound implications for the very health of our planet. This has become critically important as global warming has continued to relentlessly advance.

Physicians generally understand that emissions from automobiles, coal-fired plants, etc. contribute to global warming. Many fewer physicians are aware that the current diet that most individuals consume in the United States, and increasingly around the world, significantly contributes to greenhouse gases (GHG). Moreover, the changes that we have recommended for individual health are profoundly important for the overall health of the planet. Thus, counseling sessions for individual patients should at least mention the role that plant-forward diets play in individual health, which can also be a very important contributor to planetary health.

This concern has become increasingly apparent and is increasingly important to individual patients. In addition, physicians themselves should be very cognizant of the connection between individual and planetary health. We hope that by making this connection strongly in this chapter, we will encourage physicians to think about yet another reason to personally engage in plant-forward nutrition and consistently discuss this with their patients.

A very strong relationship exists between the diet that is consumed around the world and planetary health (1–10). This type of diet and the food system that is required to support it has been increasingly recognized as a major source of adverse environmental impact. For example, the food system is currently estimated to contribute between 19% and 29% of GHG emissions and account for approximately 70% of fresh water usage (11,12). Providing the global population with healthy diets from sustainable food systems represents an immediate and significant challenge (13–21).

Global food production, since World War II, has largely focused on calories and has kept a reasonable pace with population growth. However, more than 820 million people currently have insufficient food, and many more consume low-quality diets that cause micronutrient deficiencies. Low-quality diets contribute in significant ways to the increasing prevalence of obesity and diet-related non-communicable diseases (NCDs).

Sound nutrition is a cornerstone of the World Health Organization (WHO) initiative to combat non-communicable diseases (22). The unhealthy diets consumed around the world contribute to many NCDs, including coronary heart disease (CHD), stroke, and diabetes. Since most of the world's population is poorly nourished and the environmental systems and processes that are utilized to supply the type of food that we are currently eating, a global transformation of the food system is urgently needed.

Numerous prestigious bodies have provided important information in this area. Perhaps the single most important document to read in this area comes from the Lancet Commissions (23). It is entitled "Food in the Anthropocene: The EAT-Lancet Commission on Healthy Diets from

DOI: 10.1201/9781003630043-29

Sustainable Food Systems." Information contained in this extensive, evidence-based document provides the basis for much of what we will discuss in this chapter.

Some of the emerging literature frames the environmental outcomes related to GHG in the broader term of sustainable diets, which also includes social and economic impact (14–21). It is particularly important to understand that dietary strategies to reduce environmental impact must still be nutritionally complete and support long-standing public health and nutrition objectives, which may differ significantly from country to country and region to region. This area is extremely complicated, given the wide variety of cultural differences, the variety of foods eaten, and the diversity of agricultural production methods.

Much of this literature focuses on minimizing animal-sourced foods and largely replacing them with plant-based foods. This is the core concept behind what the EAT-Lancet Commission called "The Great Food Transformation." As outlined in this important document, this transformation of the food system is urgently needed.

It will be a daunting task to make a transformation from a largely meat-based diet to a plant-forward diet. Around the world, it is estimated that two billion people consume primarily a meat-based diet (8). The good news is that an estimated four billion people live primarily on a plant-based diet. This issue is also complicated since the WHO has reported that more than three billion people around the world are malnourished (2,24,25).

Multiple issues are diet-related in the United States. For example, the US population has doubled in the past 60 years and is projected to double again in the next 70 years. The US food production system currently uses 50% of US land area, approximately 80% of fresh water, and consumes 17% of fossil fuel energy in the country (26–29).

These figures all suggest that the US food system is not sustainable. As we have noted in multiple chapters in this book, the diet that is commonly consumed in the United States also creates multiple adverse health consequences. This, of course, is one of the key issues that we focus on both in this book and in the embedded curriculum to provide physicians with specific ways of encouraging their patients and indeed themselves to consume a plant-forward diet.

As noted in the EAT-Lancet Commission report, the global population is expected to reach about ten billion in the year 2050, which makes the current issues related to diet and environmental impact all the more important to urgently address.

The global burden of NCDs, as outlined by the WHO, is predicted to become worse. The effects of food production on greenhouse gas emissions, as well as nitrogen and phosphorus pollution, biodiversity loss, and water and land use, are all issues that will adversely impact the earth. Moreover, transformation to a healthy diet from sustainable food systems is necessary to achieve the UN Sustainable Development Goals as well as the Paris Agreement. Healthy diets have an appropriate caloric intake. They also contain the diversity of plant-based food as well as low amounts of animal sources and unsaturated rather than saturated fats, while reducing refined grains, highly processed foods, and added sugars.

To transform current dietary patterns to healthier patterns by 2050, it will require substantial dietary shifts on a local, national, and international level. These shifts will include a greater than 50% reduction in global consumption of unhealthy foods such as red meat and sugar and a greater than 100% increase in consumption of healthy foods such as fruits and vegetables, nuts, and legumes (23). Changes will vary considerably by region. One great benefit of making these dietary changes is the enormous benefit to human health. It has been estimated that such a transformation will avert between 2.8 and 3.6 million deaths per year, which represents a reduction of 19%–24% in all-cause mortality.

29.2 WHAT CONSTITUTES A HEALTHY DIET?

Defining a healthy diet is important for multiple reasons. Healthy dietary patterns form the basis of dietary guidance to a population and provide the framework for counseling in clinical settings. Healthy diets not only emphasize dietary quality for the individual but also for the population (30,31).

As we have noted in multiple chapters in this book, in the United States, the Dietary Guidelines for Americans 2020–2025 (DGAs 2020–2025) (30), the American Heart Association (32), and the Academy of Nutrition and Dietetics all define healthy diets in very similar ways (33). These diets contain an abundance of fruits and vegetables, whole grains, fish (particularly oily fish), legumes, and nuts. They all minimize red and processed meats, refined grains, tropical oils, and sugar.

The healthy dietary patterns that have been recommended include the Mediterranean (MedDiet) (34), the DASH diet (35), and the Healthy US Style Eating Pattern diet (30). On a global basis, defining a healthy diet is challenging given the diversity of populations around the world. The WHO has defined a healthy diet as one that optimizes factors to create a state of "complete physical, mental, and social well-being and not just the absence of disease" (36).

The EAT-Lancet Commission on healthy diets and sustainable food systems defines a healthy diet as one that uses diverse food groups while taking into consideration nutritional adequacy. The healthy diet pattern prescribed by the EAT-Lancet Commission consists of a range of intake for each food group, which allows for flexible global applications. This also allows for preferences and cultures from different populations. A healthy diet must also have adequate energy and energy balance. The global average per capita energy intake has been estimated at 2,370 kcal/day.

In addition, a healthy diet should contain adequate protein intake for adults, which is considered at 0.8 g/kg body weight or 56 g/day for a 70 kg individual, or about 10% of energy intake (23). It is important to recognize that these protein requirements can be largely met through plants. In many cultures, red meat consumption (mainly beef and pork) is associated with all-cause mortality. Dairy products also fit into this general category. The recommendation in the United States and in Europe has been to consume three servings of low-fat dairy as a means of maintaining bone health and fracture prevention due to its high calcium content. Large amounts of calcium, however, can also be obtained in plant-based diets.

With regard to specific components of a healthy diet, fish intake has been associated with reduced risk of cardiovascular disease largely due to its high content of omega-3 fatty acids. Legumes have also been associated with a lower risk of coronary heart disease and serve as an alternative and healthier source of protein than red meat (37,38). High fruit and vegetable consumption has been shown to result in a lower risk of CVD and cancer.

In the area of fat, added fats from animal sources, such as butter and lard, may comprise up to 30% of total energy in some diets around the world. Most dietary recommendations suggest reducing total fat intake (39,40). Both polyunsaturated and monounsaturated fats have been associated with a lower risk of CVD. For example, in the MedDiet, as reported in the PREDIMED study, extra virgin olive oil, which is a major source of monounsaturated fats, reduced the risk of CVD (41). Sugar and other refined starches have been associated with multiple adverse metabolic effects, including increased triglycerides, weight gain, and increased likelihood of T2DM and increased CVD mortality (42). For this reason, most national recommendations, as well as those from the WHO, recommend that sugar intake be less than 10% of energy (43).

To summarize this complex literature, healthy diets, as defined by multiple sources, feature protein sources primarily from plants, fat from unsaturated plant sources, low intake of saturated fats, carbohydrates primarily from whole grains, less refined grains, and less than 10% of energy from sugar. In addition, five servings of fruits and vegetables per day, as well as moderate dairy consumption, are all components of a healthy diet. These recommendations allow great flexibility and are compatible with a wide variety of food and agricultural systems, cultural traditions, and individual dietary preferences. This type of healthy diet is also associated with significantly less adverse impact on planetary health.

29.3 SUSTAINABLE FOOD PRODUCTION AND DIETS

A key consideration in the transformation of nutrition, both for individuals and for the planet, is the development of sustainable food practices. Many researchers have commented that sustainable food production and human well-being are inextricably intertwined. Farming practices, for example, need to include the reduction of nutrient leakage from fields (particularly nitrogen and phosphorus) (44,45). In addition, enhanced efficiency of water use by crops is critical. Sustainable food production involves lowering GHG emissions, making more efficient land and water use, controlling nitrogen and phosphorus applications, reducing biodiversity loss, and reducing chemical harm from herbicides and pesticides (46). All of these are part of sustainable food production. In addition, it should be noted that over one-third of food produced is lost or wasted.

There is a clear linkage between sustainable food production and a sustainable diet (47). Individual diets represent a good entry point into what individuals can do and ultimately, collectively, to improve food systems (48). The High Level Panel of Experts (HLPE) defined the interface between food security and nutrition as the following: "A food system gathers all the elements (environment, people, inputs, processes, infrastructures, institutions, etc.) and activities that relate to the production, processing, distribution, preparation, and consumption of food and the outputs from these activities, including socio-economic and environmental outcomes" (49). At the center of this definition is a sustainable diet, which HLPE defines as follows: "A sustainable diet is a diet that contributes to food nutritional status and long-term good health of the individual/community, that contributes to and is enabled by sustainable food systems, thus incorporating long-term food security and nutrition."

At the current time, the food system is not fulfilling this sustainability function. Striking evidence for this comes from the high levels of hunger and malnutrition that are evident on a global scale.

29.4 CLIMATE CHANGE

Emissions from human activities drive GHGs, which are the underlying cause of climate change. This, in turn, leads to the disruption of multiple planetary systems, including rising sea levels and increasing frequency of extreme weather events. Systems of food production release GHGs both directly and indirectly by driving land use change, which adds carbon dioxide when forests are cleared, wetlands are drained, and soils are tilled.

Food production is the prime source of methane and nitrous oxide, which have 56 and 280 times more adverse effects contributing to GHG than does carbon dioxide. Methane is produced through the breakdown of manure from livestock, particularly cows and sheep, as well as anaerobic decomposition of organic material in flooded rice paddies (50). Nitrous oxide mainly arises from soil microbes and from crop plants and pastures that are affected by fertilizer application. For all these reasons, it is essential that significant changes occur in food production to lower GHG emissions, which should be a target of healthy diets for the global population in order to help meet the targets from the Paris Agreement.

29.5 FRESH WATER USE

Food production is the world's largest consumer of fresh water. Most farmland uses fresh water from rain (84%), while 16% uses irrigation water (i.e., water from freshwater lakes, rivers, and aquifers). Irrigation is responsible for (50) 70% of all global water withdrawals. It should be noted that countries with advanced technologies may be able to limit water withdrawals to 20% of current levels. This suggests that emerging technologies can be helpful in this area. It will remain a challenge to reduce the consumption of water since plants transpire water to grow, and water evaporates from the soil.

29.6 NITROGEN AND PHOSPHORUS FLOWS

Nitrogen and phosphorus are crucial for plant growth and are the key constituents of virtually every fertilizer (23). Natural availability of these two elements may limit growth in many ecosystems.

Thus, nitrogen and phosphorus fertilizers are utilized to maximize crop yield. Excessive application of nitrogen and phosphorus can raise substantial adverse consequences, particularly through runoff into streams and rivers. It should be noted that human sewage is also an important source of nitrogen.

Nitrogen application can reduce biodiversity and cause acidification of water. Furthermore, nitrous oxide is a potent greenhouse gas and a component of ammonia in the atmosphere. Phosphorus fertilizer comes from a non-renewable source mined from phosphate rock deposits. These deposits are estimated to run out within 50–100 years.

It will be a major challenge that interacts with both human nutrition and farming practices to maximize food production per unit of nitrogen and phosphorus while maintaining losses of these nutrients into the environment at a minimum (51,52).

29.7 BIODIVERSITY LOSS

Biodiversity loss harms the richness of all living organisms and is essential for the stability of ecosystems. The world is currently losing species at a rate of 1,000 times greater than in previous eras.

Multiple human actions contribute to biodiversity loss. These include deforestation as land is appropriated for food production, resulting in diminished habitat. In addition, climate change, chemical pollution, and unsustainable harvest of wild species have further contributed to biodiversity loss.

It has been suggested by some experts in this area that there should be no more than 1–80 extinctions per million species per year, which represents an appropriate goal to achieve (23). The loss of biodiversity is often underestimated when individuals think about negative effects of current agricultural practices; in particular, the widespread adoption of animal product consumption exacerbates biodiversity loss. Livestock currently comprises 1/5 of total terrestrial biomass and also results in the consumption of 1/3 of global cereal production. Thus, animal product consumption by humans is likely the leading cause of species extinctions, since it is not only the major driver for deforestation but also the principal driver of land degradation, pollution, climate change, and overfishing.

29.8 LAND SYSTEM CHANGE

In some areas, such as temperate regions in Europe, Russia, and North America, land areas used for food production have remained relatively constant in the last century (53,54). However, in the tropics, substantial expansion of agricultural land has occurred. This includes countries such as Brazil, the Democratic Republic of Congo, and Indonesia. The increased land-use system contributes to declines in biodiversity and greenhouse gas emissions. About 40% of the terrestrial land mass of the world that is ice-free is dedicated to croplands and grazing lands. Of this 40%, about 23% of the land surface is used for grazing land. It is important to reduce or eliminate increased land use for agricultural purposes, particularly for livestock.

29.9 ACHIEVING HEALTHY DIETS FROM SUSTAINABLE FOOD SYSTEM

It has been estimated that the current food production system is not sustainable for food security for the expanding population of the world in the future (13,23). The capacity to produce enough food in the future is limited by a number of factors, including potentially water, soil fertility, land use, and sewage dispersal in seas and oceans. As already indicated, the current food production system adversely affects a number of natural resources, including the use of more than 70% of fresh water, and also generates 30% of greenhouse gas emissions and results in 80% of deforestation. Food production is the largest source of loss of biodiversity and of both nitrogen and phosphorus flows, which, in turn, can lead to degradation of fresh water and salt water.

Investigators have maintained that the most promising methods for both present and future food needs involve shifting individual and population food choices and patterns. As we have discussed in multiple chapters in this book and emphasized in the embedded curriculum, healthy dietary patterns include the Dietary Approach to Stop Hypertension (DASH) diet, the Mediterranean Dietary Pattern (MedDiet), and the Healthy US Style Eating Pattern, all of which fit into the definition from the WHO of the most healthy diets.

A number of modeling studies have yielded strategies for a substantial decrease in GHG emissions and also lowered the risk of resource use such as water, energy, and land use from adopting plant-forward diets. In one model in the UK, greenhouse gas emissions from meat eaters were two times as high as those for vegans. With regard to personal health issues, the MedDiet reduces the risk of CVD and T2DM as well as cancer mortality and lowers the rate of cognitive decline. The MedDiet also reduces GHG emissions in cropland use compared to the current Western Diet (50,55).

The DASH diet is also associated with lower GHG emissions; however, it should be noted that greater adherence to the DASH diet is associated with higher dietary costs. For many individuals, both in the United States and in lower-income countries, cost represents a considerable consideration. One study from the United Kingdom, however, showed that a sustainable diet that reduced meat and dairy products still resulted in lower GHG emissions and was accomplished without increased cost.

29.10 DIETARY PATTERNS IN RELATION TO HEALTH AND SUSTAINABILITY OUTCOMES

It is important to evaluate dietary patterns both for individual health benefits but also their sustainability for planetary health. The following diets have been demonstrated to yield both individual health benefits and improve sustainability:

- *Vegetarian and Omnivorous Diets*: Various studies have explored variations of vegetarian diets, ranging from vegan to omnivorous, related to associated health and environmental outcomes. Not surprisingly, these studies demonstrated that reduced meat consumption improved both health outcomes and decreased GHG emissions as well as land, energy, and water usage. Similar findings have been generated in the Adventist Health Study II.
- *Mediterranean Diet and DASH Diet*: Studies of both of these diets have demonstrated that in comparison to usual diets such as the Western diet, both of these diets reduce the environmental footprint and reduce GHG emissions (56–58). In the area of sustainability, meat-based diets, when compared to plant-based diets with regard to effects on the environment, have shown that the meat-based system requires more energy, land, and water resources than a lacto-ovo vegetarian diet. Some interest has also been generated in a type of diet called a Flexitarian Diet (59,60), which allows some consumption of meat. Following this type of diet may make the transition easier for many people who may find an abrupt change to a vegetarian diet difficult to follow.

29.11 THE FUTURE OF FOOD IN THE FACE OF CLIMATE CHANGE

A number of reports, including the EAT-Lancet Commission report, have emphasized that current food production is both unsustainable and generates climate change, which will exacerbate this issue in the future. Most studies that have explored this have suggested that climate change will result in a reduction in future agricultural productivity. One study predicted an 8% reduction in the mean yield of all crops across Africa and South Asia by the year 2050 (11). Climate change is also thought to adversely affect fisheries. For example, migration of fish toward either the North or South Pole because of warming of oceans has been estimated to reduce maximum catch potential in some tropical areas by up to 40%.

On all of these issues related to climate change, the effects of agriculture are taken together. One estimate has concluded that climate change will result in decreased agricultural production and cause 500,000 climate-related deaths by the year 2050.

A number of different recommendations have been made to try to lower the potential problems with agriculture and climate change. One analysis from the Food and Agriculture Organization (FAO) of the UN has listed crop diversity as the leading potential adaptation solution. In addition, developing crop varieties that can withstand changes in climate may also have a positive effect.

29.12 THE ROLE OF SEAFOOD IN GLOBAL DIETS

Seafood is an important component of many diets. In fact, seafood provides over three billion people with about 20% of their daily intake of animal protein (23). Seafood consumption is particularly important for the world's poorest regions. Unfortunately, 90% of global wild fish stocks are currently being overfished or fished at capacity. There has been an increase in fish from aquaculture. Seafood may be a viable source of food for the future, but aquaculture alone is insufficient to solve the challenges of feeding over ten billion people with healthy diets. Seafood could, however, help reduce the production of land-based animal-sourced proteins (30).

29.13 FRAMEWORK FOR A GREAT FOOD TRANSFORMATION

The EAT-Lancet Commission report sounded a clarion call to revise the ways that the overall population is fed. This report documents that it will be necessary to move from the current dietary situation to what some experts have called a "great food transformation." This will require cooperation among nations to change the way food is eaten and how it is produced. This will also require a high level of consensus around the world and the political will to accomplish it.

The EAT-Lancet Commission report recommended five potential strategies to assist in this enormous transformation (23). They are the following:

- *Strategy 1*: Seek international and national commitment to shift toward healthy diets.
- *Strategy 2*: Reorient agricultural priorities from producing large quantities of food to producing healthy food.
- *Strategy 3*: Sustainably intensify food production, generating high-quality output.
- *Strategy 4*: Implement strong and coordinated governmental approaches to land and oceans.
- *Strategy 5*: Cut food loss and waste at least in half in line with sustainable dietary goals.

While these recommendations may be beyond the purview of most physicians who are practicing primary care or lifestyle medicine, it is important to have a clear understanding that individual and planetary health are inextricably tied together.

29.14 THE ROLE OF PHYSICIANS AND OTHER HEALTH CARE WORKERS IN PLANETARY HEALTH

Numerous studies have shown that a physician's recommendation is one of the most effective ways of changing individual behavior. Physicians also carry the prestige of being trusted authorities in a variety of areas. Physicians must recognize that the safety of the planet is also a consideration that they can impact in various significant ways. For this reason, we have included the issue of how individual and planetary health are related. This is a topic that we hope and believe physicians can effectively translate into recommendations for their patients and also follow in their own lives.

29.15 CONCLUSIONS/CLINICAL APPLICATIONS

- It is important for clinicians to counsel their patients not only on the individual benefits of a healthy diet, but also to make the link between a healthy diet for individuals and planetary health. Healthy diets consist of increased fruits, vegetables, and whole grains, as opposed to an unhealthy diet, which features more red meat, sugar, and tropical oils.
- Healthy diets exert less adverse impact on the health of the planet than do unhealthy diets.
- Physicians, as opinion leaders, should advocate strongly for healthy diets not only for individual patients but also for the health of the planet.

REFERENCES

1. Willett W, Rockström J, Loken B, et al. Food in the anthropocene: the EAT-Lancet Commission on healthy diets from sustainable food systems. *Lancet.* 2019;393(10170):447–492.
2. Springmann M, Wiebe K, Mason-D'Croz D, et al. Health and nutritional aspects of sustainable diet strategies and their association with environmental impacts: a global modelling analysis with country-level detail. *Lancet Planet Health.* 2018;2(10):e451–e461.
3. Eshel G, Shepon A, Makov T, et al. Land, irrigation water, greenhouse gas, and reactive nitrogen burdens of meat, eggs, and dairy production in the United States. *Proc Natl Acad Sci USA.* 2014;111(33):11996–12001.
4. Eisen M, Brown P. Rapid global phaseout of animal agriculture has the potential to stabilize greenhouse gas levels for 30 years and offset 68 percent of CO_2 emissions this century. *PLOS Climate.* 2022;1(2):e0000010.
5. FAOSTAT. Food and Agriculture Organization of the United Nations. https://www.fao.org/faostat/en/#data. Accessed March 12, 2025.
6. Harwatt H, Sabat J, Eshel G, et al. Substituting beans for beef as a contribution toward US climate change targets. *Climatic Change.* 2017;143(1–2):261–270.
7. Ridoutt B, Hendrie G, Noakes M. Dietary strategies to reduce environmental impact: a critical review of the evidence base. *Adv Nutr.* 2017;15;8(6):933–946.
8. Thompson H, Brick M. Perspective: closing the dietary fiber gap: an ancient solution for a 21st century problem. *Adv Nutr.* 2016;7(4):623–626.
9. Marinova D, Bogueva D. Planetary health and reduction in meat consumption. *Sustain Earth Rev.* 2019;(2):3.
10. Shah U, Merlo G. Personal and planetary health-the connection with dietary choices. *JAMA.* 2023;329(21):1823–1824.
11. Vermeulen S, Campbell B, Ingram J. Climate Change and Food Systems. *Annu Rev Environ Resour.* 2012;37(1):195–222.
12. Whitmee S, Haines A, Beyrer C, et al. Safeguarding human health in the anthropocene epoch: report of The Rockefeller Foundation-Lancet Commission on planetary health. *Lancet.* 2015;14;386 (10007):1973–2028.
13. Meybeck A, Gitz V. Sustainable diets within sustainable food systems. *Proc Nutr Soc.* 2017;76(1):1–11.
14. Malik VS, Willett WC, Hu FB. Global obesity: trends, risk factors and policy implications. *Nat Rev Endocrinol.* 2013;9(1):13–27.
15. World Health Organization. Cardiovascular Diseases. WHO 2017. https://www.who.int/news-room/fact-sheets/detail/cardiovascular-diseases-(cvds). Accessed March 12, 2025.
16. World Health Organization. Diabetes. WHO 2017.https://www.who.int/news-room/fact-sheets/detail/diabetes. Accessed March 12, 2025.
17. Sabaté J, Soret S. Sustainability of plant-based diets: back to the future. *Am J Clin Nutr.* 2014;100(Suppl 1):476S–482S.
18. Pimentel D, Pimentel M. Sustainability of meat-based and plant-based diets and the environment. *Am J Clin Nutr.* 2003;78(3 Suppl):660S–663S.
19. Dietary Guidelines Advisory Committee. Report of the 2015 Dietary Guidelines Advisory Committee. Washington, DC: US Department of Agriculture and US Department of Health and Human Services, 2015.
20. Aune D, Giovannucci E, Boffetta P, et al. Fruit and vegetable intake and the risk of cardiovascular disease, total cancer and all-cause mortality – a systematic review and dose-response meta-analysis of prospective studies. *Int J Epidemiol.* 2017;46(3):1029–1056.

21. Zong G, Gao A, Hu F, et al. Whole grain intake and mortality from all causes, cardiovascular disease, and cancer: a meta-analysis of prospective cohort studies. *Circulation*. 2016;133(24):2370–2380.
22. The World Health Organization. Advancing the global agenda on prevention and control of noncommunicable diseases 2000 to 2020: looking forwards to 2030. WHO, July 2023.
23. Willett W, Rockström J, Loken B, et al. Food in the Anthropocene: the EAT-Lancet Commission on healthy diets from sustainable food systems. *Lancet*. 2019;393(10170):447–492.
24. Tzioumis E, Kay M, Bentley M, et al. Prevalence and trends in the childhood dual burden of malnutrition in low- and middle-income countries, 1990–2012. *Public Health Nutr.* 2016;19(8):1375–1388.
25. Brent K, Santo R, Scatterday A, et al. Country-specific dietary shifts to mitigate climate and water crises. *Global Environ Change.* 2020;62:101926.
26. Sáez-Almendros S, Obrador B, Bach-Faig A, et al. Environmental footprints of Mediterranean versus Western dietary patterns: beyond the health benefits of the Mediterranean diet. *Environ Health.* 2013;12:118.
27. Aleksandrowicz L, Green R, Joy E, et al. The impacts of dietary change on greenhouse gas emissions, land use, water use, and health: a systematic review. *PLoS One.* 2016;11(11):e0165797.
28. FAO/WHO 2015 Second International Conference on Nutrition (ICN2). Report of the Joint FAO/WHO Secretariat on the Conference. The Food and Agricultural Organization of the United States. Rome: FAO.
29. Nelson M, Hamm M, Hu F, et al. Alignment of healthy dietary patterns and environmental sustainability: a systematic review. *Adv Nutr.* 2016;7(6):1005–1025.
30. U.S. Department of Agriculture and U.S. Department of Health and Human Services. U.S. Department of Agriculture and U.S. Department of Health and Human Services. Dietary Guidelines for Americans, 2020–2025 (9th ed). December 2020. Available at DietaryGuidelines.gov. 2020. https://www.dietaryguidelines.gov/resources/2020-2025-dietary-guidelines-online-materials.
31. Bechthold A, Boeing H, Tetens I, et al. Perspective: food-based dietary guidelines in europe-scientific concepts, current status, and perspectives. *Adv Nutr.* 2018;9(5):544–560.
32. Lichtenstein AH, Appel LJ, Vadiveloo M, et al. 2021 Dietary guidance to improve cardiovascular health: a scientific statement from the American Heart Association. *Circulation.* 2021;144(23):e472–e487.
33. Academy of Nutrition and Dietetics Evidence Analysis Library. Adult Weight Management: Executive Summary of Recommendations 2014. Academy of Nutrition and Dietetics. https://www.andeal.org/topic.cfm?menu=5276&cat=4690. Accessed March 18, 2025.
34. Guasch-Ferré M, Salas-Salvadó J, Ros E, et al. The PREDIMED trial, Mediterranean diet and health outcomes: How strong is the evidence? *Nutr Metab Cardiovasc Dis.* 2017;27(7):624–632.
35. Sacks FM, Svetkey LP, Vollmer WM, et al. Effects on blood pressure of reduced dietary sodium and the dietary approaches to stop hypertension (DASH) Diet. *N Engl J Med.* 2001;344(1):3–10.
36. World Food Summit. Rome Declaration World Food Security. 1996. Rome: FAO. https://www.fao.org/3/w3613e/w3613e00.htm. Accessed March 12, 2025.
37. Afshin A, Micha R, Khatibzadeh S, et al. Consumption of nuts and legumes and risk of incident ischemic heart disease, stroke, and diabetes: a systematic review and meta-analysis. *Am J Clin Nutr.* 2014;100(1):278–288.
38. Anderson J, Major A. Pulses and lipaemia, short- and long-term effect: potential in the prevention of cardiovascular disease. *Br J Nutr.* 2002;88(Suppl 3):S263–S271.
39. Wang D, Li Y, Chiuve S, et al. Association of specific dietary fats with total and cause-specific mortality. *JAMA Intern Med.* 2016;176(8):1134–1145.
40. Li Y, Hruby A, Bernstein A, et al. Saturated fats compared with unsaturated fats and sources of carbohydrates in relation to risk of coronary heart disease: a prospective cohort study. *J Am Coll Cardiol.* 2015;66(14):1538–1548.
41. Zong G, Li Y, Sampson L, et al. Monounsaturated fats from plant and animal sources in relation to risk of coronary heart disease among US men and women. *Am J Clin Nutr.* 2018;107(3):445–453.
42. Johnson R, Appel L, Brands M, et al. Dietary sugars intake and cardiovascular health: a scientific statement from the American Heart Association. *Circulation.* 2009;120(11):1011–1020.
43. World Health Organization. WHO Calls on Countries to Reduce Sugars Intake Among Adults and Children. https://www.who.int/news/item/04-03-2015-who-calls-on-countries-to-reduce-sugars-intake-among-adults-and-children/. Accessed March 12, 2025.
44. Sobal J, Khan LK, Bisogni C. A conceptual model of the food and nutrition system. *Soc Sci Med.* 1998;47(7):853–863.
45. FAO. 2015 Presentation by Alexandre Meybeck at the *12th European Nutrition Conference, FENS 2015, Sustainable Diet III: Future and Matter of Debate*, Berlin, October 2015.

46. Ericksen P, Stewart B, Dixon J, et al. *The Value of a Food System Approach. Food Security and Global Environmental Change.* London: Earthscan, 2010.
47. Ericksen P. What is the vulnerability of a food system to global environmental change? *Ecol Soc.* 2008;13(2).
48. Ingram JA. Food systems approach to researching food security and its interactions with global environmental change. *Food Sec.* 2011;3:417–431.
49. HLPE. Food Losses and Waste in the Context of Sustainable Food Systems. A Report by the High Level Panel of Experts on Food Security and Nutrition of the Committee on World Food Security. Rome: FAO, 2014.
50. Xu X, Sharma P, Shu S, et al. Global greenhouse gas emissions from animal-based foods are twice those of plant-based foods. *Nat Food.* 2021;2(9):724–732.
51. Smith Y, Smith A, Seymour C, et al. Response of Avian diversity to habitat modification can be predicted from life-history traits and ecological attributes. *Landscape Ecol.* 2015;(30):1225–1239.
52. Machovina B, Feeley K, Ripple W, et al. Biodiversity conservation: the key is reducing meat consumption. *Sci Total Environ.* 2015;(536):419–431.
53. Mila I Canals, Munoz I, McLaren S. et al. LCA methodology and modelling considerations for vegetable production and consumption. CES Working Paper Published by: Centre for Environmental Strategy, University of Surrey, February 2007.
54. European Commission Joint Research Centre. *ILCD Handbook: Recommendations for Life Cycle Impact Assessment in the European Context Based on Existing Environmental Impact Assessment Models and Factors*, Vol 24571. Luxembourg: Publication Office of the European Union, 2011.
55. Ewing B, Moore D, Goldfinger S. et al. The Ecological Footprint Atlas 2010. Oakland Global Footprint Network. Ecological Footprint Atlas 2010.pdf. Accessed March 17, 2025.
56. Tukker A, Goldbohm R, de Koning A, et al. Environmental impacts of changes to healthier diets in Europe. *Ecol Econ.* 2011;70(10):1776–1788.
57. Milner J, Green R, Dangour A, et al. Health effects of adopting low greenhouse gas emission diets in the UK. *BMJ Open.* 2015;5(4):e007364.
58. van Dooren C, Marinussen M, Blonk H, et al. Exploring dietary guidelines based on ecological and nutritional values: a comparison of six dietary patterns. *Food Policy.* 2014;44:36–46.
59. Pike A. What is the flexitarian diet? International Food Information Council. May 17, 2021.
60. Derbyshire E. Flexitarian diets and health: a review of the evidence-based literature. *Front Nutr.* 2016;3:55.

30 Health Equity

30.1 INTRODUCTION

While this book has focused largely on counseling individuals in the components of lifestyle and lifestyle medicine, it is also important that clinicians take a broader view of what truly impacts people's health. For this reason, it is important to deal with an issue that is not often talked about in clinical medicine, and that is health equity. Health equity has significant interaction with social determinants of health (SDOH) (1–14). Oftentimes, clinicians feel that there is not much they can do about this broader social and economic area. However, it significantly impacts multiple health considerations. Lifestyle medicine modalities can play a critically important role, particularly in individuals who come from disadvantaged groups who often do not have the appropriate levels of medical care and suffer significant adverse health impacts (14).

These issues were brought into stark focus during the COVID-19 pandemic, when individuals who come from disadvantaged backgrounds were found to have three to four times more severe infections and were more likely to die of COVID-19 compared to affluent, advantaged individuals (5). In particular, individuals in lower socioeconomic status (SES) groups had more serious complications from COVID-19 than individuals in higher SES groups. Black and Hispanic populations have been particularly susceptible to severe adverse impacts of COVID-19 compared to more affluent individuals.

Multiple components of lifestyle significantly impacted health outcomes for COVID-19 in individuals who became infected during the pandemic. It is important to understand, however, that health equity impacts multiple conditions other than this severe infection. For example, both children and individuals over the age of 65 who come from disadvantaged groups are particularly prone to suffering from malnutrition (15–22).

For all these reasons, it is important for clinicians to have a firm understanding of health equity and the SDOH, since these issues impact the way individuals are cared for and the health outcomes they achieve.

30.2 WHAT IS MEANT BY HEALTH EQUITY?

Considerable research and discussion about health equity have occurred in medical and public health in the past two decades. Prestigious medical bodies, including the American Heart Association (AHA) (23,24), the American College of Physicians (ACP) (1, 8), and the American College of Lifestyle Medicine (ACLM) (14), have all issued statements on health equity and have offered definitions of the term. The field is complicated and hindered by a variety of definitions that have been put forth.

In 2017, the Robert Wood Johnson Foundation (RWJF) published a report that attempted to clarify various definitions of health equity. This report stated that, in general terms, health equity connotes that everyone "has a fair and just opportunity to be as healthy as possible." It is important to note that the words "fair" and "just" are included in this definition. The RWJF document also stated that, to accomplish a fair and just opportunity, it is essential to remove obstacles to health, such as poverty and discrimination, and their consequences.

Multiple other factors create disparities in health and result in a lack of health equity. These include lack of access to good-paying jobs, quality education, housing, healthcare, and a safe environment. The terms "fairness" and "justice" are attempts to provide broad ethical concepts related to human rights and principles. People often tend to think of justice and fairness in terms of civil and political rights, but equity extends these concepts to the right to avoid obstacles to good health.

DOI: 10.1201/9781003630043-30

Good health is often influenced by SDOH factors such as income, wealth, education, neighborhood characteristics, and social inclusion that people experience in their lives. There is no question that individual responsibility is important, but health equity incorporates concepts that recognize that people who lack opportunities and resources to make healthy choices may have difficulties that personal responsibility cannot overcome. It should be emphasized that health equity does not include issues such as genetic endowment. It is also important to recognize that health equity is not the same as health disparity (25, 26).

Health equity incorporates the concept that an individual should be able to achieve the best health possible for himself or herself. Health disparity, in contrast, may be considered somewhat avoidable based on current scientific understandings, which indicate that better health may be possible or could be provided with adequate political will. Certainly, health equity, in the broadest sense, involves not only health care but also social determinants such as poverty, discrimination, etc., and their consequences (27). Nonetheless, it is critically important that physicians, who are the key gatekeepers in health and also key influencers, recognize health equity as part of the mandate for delivering good health care.

30.3 SOCIAL DETERMINANTS OF HEALTH AND HEALTH EQUITY

Multiple lifestyle-related issues are impacted by SDOH (28–31). The field and concept of SDOH, however, are much broader than just lifestyle-related issues. A recent position paper from the American College of Physicians (ACP) listed six separate barriers that contributed to SDOH (1). These included socioeconomic status, housing, transportation, food and agriculture, the digital divide, and racial and ethnic disparities. All of these contribute in very significant ways to considerations related to health equity. Here are more details from the ACP position paper:

- *Socioeconomic Status*: The primary non-medical factor affecting health is socioeconomic status (SES). The top 1% of earners in the United States earn three times as much as they did in the 1980s, while the bottom 50% are at the same average income as they were in 1980. In addition, excess mortality among African American adults compared to White, non-Latino adults is estimated at 38%.

  To compound the problem of low SES in areas of nutrition, neighborhoods with concentrated poverty often lack grocery stores with fresh food (food deserts), as well as adequate transportation, access to public spaces, and access to health services. Education and employment status also contribute to SES.
- *Housing*: Adequate housing is an essential component of basic needs for humans. Poor housing increases the potential for exposure to lead and asthma triggers such as dust, mold, moisture, and rodents. The COVID-19 pandemic clearly demonstrated that overcrowded living conditions also contribute to the spread of airborne disease (32). Inadequate housing may be further complicated by the fact that people with low SES may spend more than 30% of their income on housing and are at higher risk for potential homelessness following eviction. Multiple diseases are associated with inadequate housing, including tuberculosis and hepatitis C.
- *Transportation*: Automobiles are the primary source of transportation in the United States. Individuals with low SDOH often lack transportation options, which significantly increases barriers to healthcare needs. Low-income persons may rely on active transportation, such as walking or biking, or public transportation. In disadvantaged communities, moreover, the infrastructure for walking or biking, such as sidewalks, street lighting, etc., to make this option safe, is lacking.
- *Food and Agriculture*: As already indicated, an adequate supply of healthy food is necessary for a healthy and productive life. Approximately 11% of households in the United States (25.8 million adults and 12.4 million children) are food insecure. Many people of

low SES live in what have been called "food deserts." Individuals who live in food deserts are at increased risk of obesity and diabetes.
- *The Digital Divide*: The digital divide is defined as the gap between those who have access to technology, such as the internet, and those who do not. This is also associated with low SES. Lack of reliable internet hinders a person's ability to access medical portals. A survey in 2012 showed that 21% of uninsured persons did not use the internet, and 59% of uninsured persons do not report seeking health information online. According to data from the Health and Human Services in 2019, over 16% of poor people have no internet access (33). Access to the internet varies by race and ethnicity, with Asians and Whites having more access than Blacks, Hispanics, and American Indians.
- *Racial and Ethnic Health Disparity* (1): In order to address SDOH, it is essential to improve health equity among racial and ethnic populations. For example, Latino women are more likely than Caucasians to lack health insurance. African Americans have the highest rate of cancer burden of any racial or ethnic group for all types of cancers. All of these considerations, as outlined by the position paper from the ACP, emphasize the need for all physicians to be aware of the multiple and diverse impacts of SDOH on health, particularly for individuals of low SES.

As already indicated, the term "health equity," as defined according to the WHO, involves "giving all people the opportunity to reach their full potential regardless of race, education, gender identity, sexual orientation, job, neighborhood location, or disability." A classic example of disparities that harm health relates to the area of nutrition (13). People with less money, less education, and poor living conditions are more likely to experience food insecurity, have less healthy eating patterns, and develop diet-related diseases such as obesity and diabetes. Medical and nutritional professionals must recognize that health and illness result from broad social, political, and economic realities. Physicians and other health care professionals need to advocate for social justice. Individual practitioners need to acknowledge the presence of structural racism and consider the impact of poverty and other components of SDOH on health.

Physician interactions with patients must start with screening for food insecurity and other determinants of health. There are many options to help address this situation. For example, physicians and/or health care organizations can partner with local food banks and farmers' markets that offer quality produce and groceries to underserved communities at an affordable cost.

The federal government also has been involved with multiple policies related to SDOH and health equity, including the National School Lunch Program, the Supplemental Nutrition Assistance Program (SNAP), and Supplemental Nutrition for Women, Infants, and Children (WIC), in attempts to improve food security and healthy eating patterns by assisting with the purchase of nutritious foods and beverages.

It is also important that professional organizations themselves establish diverse workforces. Currently, for example, there is a distinct minority of Black or Hispanic physicians. Only 5.8% of physicians are Hispanic, and 5.0% are Black or African American (12).

30.4 OTHER LIFESTYLE MEDICINE MODALITIES AND HEALTH EQUITY

While most of the information related to health equity deals with nutrition, multiple other lifestyle medicine modalities exist that are strongly impacted by health equity. For example, in the area of physical activity, inverse relationships exist between habitual physical activity levels and the odds of hospitalizations and deaths associated with COVID-19, particularly in low SES groups (34). In one study published in the *British Medical Journal*, which compared physically active individuals (35) (meeting the PAGA 2018 Guidelines) (36) on all assessments versus consistently inactive individuals (fewer than ten minutes per week of aerobic activity on all assessments) versus inconsistently active individuals (active below the guidelines or meeting the guidelines in only some measurements), inactive individuals were 2.3 times as likely to be hospitalized, 1.7 times as likely to be admitted to intensive care, and 2.5 times as likely to die during the COVID-19 pandemic. Of note, these factors are strongly related to SDOH. Perhaps most startling was that inactive individuals had adjusted odds of death of 2.49, which is greater than those associated with extreme obesity (1.90) and smoking (1.20). Thus, physical activity carries strong benefits that may be very difficult for people in lower SES categories to accomplish.

In addition, both nutrition and physical activity relate to sleep. We know that disordered eating can adversely impact sleep, as can a sedentary lifestyle. Clearly, practitioners of lifestyle medicine should focus on the interrelationship between these lifestyle factors and health equity.

As already indicated, issues related to stress and interpersonal relationships also interact with nutrition and can further exacerbate adverse consequences related to health equity.

30.5 EQUITY-RELATED BURDENS ON THE HEALTH CARE SYSTEM

Equity-related differences create problems for the health care system in addition to individuals' health problems. Among the burdens to the health care system are the impacts of equity on obesity and related conditions. In addition, SDOH can result in insufficient nutrition knowledge among health care providers. This, in turn, may adversely impact whether individuals in low SES groups participate in important health-promoting activities such as healthy nutrition, regular physical activity, adequate sleep, and stress reduction (37–40).

These deficiencies are prevalent among older adults, particularly among those in disadvantaged populations.

30.6 MALNUTRITION AND FOOD INSECURITY

Despite being the most affluent country in the world, the United States still carries a significant burden of food insecurity and malnutrition (41–44). These conditions are often neglected or underestimated by clinicians.

It has been estimated that 10% of all households in the United States experience food insecurity, meaning that they do not have an adequate amount to eat (45,46). The COVID-19 pandemic underscored the relationship between health disparities and nutrition (47,48). Over 21% of Black families and 17% of Latinx families experienced food insecurity during the pandemic. This is more than double that of White households (7.1%). Poor nutritional habits are often related to food insecurity, and, in turn, these habits are related to obesity, diabetes, hypertension, and heart failure. For all of these reasons, it is important for clinicians to assess whether or not their patients are experiencing food insecurity or other manifestations of malnutrition.

The USDA estimates that poor nutrition is the leading cause of chronic illness in the United States and is responsible for more than 600,000 deaths per year (49). This represents 50,000 deaths per month from poor nutrition. Poor nutrition also exerts an impact on academic achievement and increases financial stress. Individuals in disadvantaged groups often feel anxious about their ability to provide adequate food and have been shown to increase consumption of energy-dense but nutritionally poor foods. In a typical week, US adults living in food-insecure families consume significantly fewer servings of fruits, vegetables, and milk/dairy products compared to individuals who live in food-secure environments (50).

Malnutrition is particularly common in individuals over the age of 65. A detailed assessment of whether or not an individual suffers from malnutrition is beyond the scope of this chapter. However, there are validated scales and indicators of malnutrition (51). Malnutrition is an area that clinicians should pay careful attention to because of the broad adverse health implications that food insecurity and malnutrition carry (52–56).

Malnutrition represents a particularly prominent issue in individuals over the age of 65, who account for approximately 9% of all food-insecure homes in the United States (53, 54). Elderly food-insecure individuals may adopt various strategies to ensure adequate food during times of reduced food access. For example, they may restrict personal intake of food, overeat when food is available, and consume primarily low-cost foods or eat the same foods regularly, which can contribute to an overall decline in essential nutrient intake.

In addition to financial barriers to achieving food security, there are other issues in the elderly population that can restrict access to food, including inadequate transportation, physical limitations, and cognitive decline. Thus, a careful history of food intake in individuals over the age of 65 should be undertaken at all clinic visits. The diagnosis and management of malnutrition are often overlooked. To address this issue, the Academy of Nutrition and Dietetics and multiple other stakeholders developed a malnutrition toolkit for hospitals called the "MQii" toolkit, which is now in use in over 50 hospitals around the United States (57).

30.7 HEALTH EQUITY AND PUBLIC POLICY

Recent attention has been given at the level of the federal government of the United States to deal with issues related to health equity and food insecurity (58–61). Several key pieces of food and nutrition legislation have been passed, including the reauthorization of the Farm Bill. A recent White House Conference on Hunger, Nutrition, and Health, held in September 2022, concluded that the United States has a once-in-a-generation opportunity to address food insecurity and health equity (62). This conference articulated three general strategies. They are the following:

- Reduce poverty as an integral step to reducing hunger
- Create more accessible and affordable food production and distribution systems
- Address the impact of climate change and improve market competition to ensure long-term food stability for all.

30.8 FOOD INSECURITY, NUTRITION, AND OBESITY

Health equity is particularly important in the area of obesity. Individuals in lower SES circumstances often experience worse health outcomes than their higher SES counterparts (12). While there are many contributing factors to this, determinants of food choice and access play important roles. Therefore, equity-oriented social policies that target these determinants are important. It is clear that there is a higher prevalence of obesity in lower SES groups. It is important for clinicians to understand the impact of SDOH on obesity and not view this as a problem of individual choice or lack of discipline.

30.9 IMPROVING FRUIT AND VEGETABLE ACCESSIBILITY TO ADVANCE NUTRITIONAL SECURITY AND HEALTH EQUITY

Nutritional security and health equity are inextricably bound together. Food and vegetable (FV) consumption is central to obtaining and sustaining a healthy diet. The Dietary Guidelines for Americans 2020–2025 (DGAs) recommend that Americans consume a minimum of 1.5–2 cups per day of fruit and 2.5 cups per day of vegetables as components of a healthy diet (63). Unfortunately, the CDC estimates that only 12% of adults meet the fruit requirement, and only 9% of adults meet the vegetable requirement. In addition, FV consumption has been demonstrated to show inequalities by sex, race, ethnicity, and SES. A number of initiatives are in progress from the federal government, including the reauthorized Farm Bill, which aims to better align with the DGAs 2025 by increasing supplemental dollars to households to purchase FVs. This represents another area where clinicians can play an active role by seeking ways to assess FV consumption, particularly in disadvantaged patients.

30.10 FOOD INSECURITY AND FOOD ADDICTION SYMPTOMS

Several studies have suggested that there is an association between food insecurity and symptoms of food addiction. These studies have suggested that individuals in lower SES classes who experience food insecurity may experience disordered eating. In addition, they may choose less expensive, highly processed food, which may in turn activate reward system responses that are associated with behavioral patterns that may, in fact, mirror substance use disorders. These represent very preliminary data, but clinicians should be cognizant of this potential.

30.11 HEALTH EQUITY IN THE HEALTH PEOPLE 2030 DOCUMENT

The issues of health equity comprise one of the overarching goals of Healthy People 2030 (64). This document states a goal to "reduce health disparity, achieve health equity, and attain health literacy to improve the health and well-being of all." Multiple issues related to SDOH are included in the Healthy People 2030 document. Multiple lifestyle medicine issues are embedded in this document. The Healthy People 2030 document reflects that health equity has assumed a very prominent place in discussions about health in the United States moving forward.

30.12 NIH NUTRITION HEALTH DISPARITIES FRAMEWORK: A MODEL TO ADVANCE HEALTH EQUITY

Since nutrition plays such a significant role in health equity, the National Institutes of Health (NIH) has developed a framework related to multiple health outcomes linked to poor nutrition, including obesity, Type 2 diabetes (T2DM), cardiovascular disease (CVD), and diet-related cancers. The goal of the NIH framework is to make health equity considerations central to discussions about how diet-related disparities are perpetuated among disadvantaged populations. This framework is designed to be a resource for both health care professionals and nutritional professionals, with the goal of improving health outcomes and increasing health equity in diverse populations (65).

30.13 UNITED NATIONS INITIATIVE ON SUSTAINABLE DEVELOPMENT GOALS AND HEALTH EQUITY

In 2012, the United Nations launched a global consultation on Sustainable Development Goals (SDGs). Under the rubric "The World We Want," the UN General Assembly agreed to 17 sustainable goals (66). Goals 1 and 2 are directly related to nutrition and health equity. Goal 1 is to end poverty in all forms everywhere. Goal 2 is to end hunger, achieve food security, improve nutrition, and promote sustainable agriculture. (These issues are discussed in more detail in Chapter 26 on Individual Health and Planetary Health.) Improving health equity for Americans will involve affordable health care with a strong emphasis on preventive care. The COVID-19 epidemic underscored the understanding that SDOH can have a major impact on people's health. This further underscores the fact that SDOH are intrinsically linked to health equity. This is particularly true for individuals over the age of 60. This understandably also reflects that poor health and multiple disparities reflect SES. Many of the national initiatives related to this are incorporated in the Healthy People 2030 initiative. These issues are particularly important for addressing nutritional security and malnutrition in older adults.

30.14 NATIONAL NUTRITIONAL POLICIES AND HEALTH EQUITY

Health equity-oriented policy actions represent a key public health principle. Multiple issues are reflected in these principles, which have been discussed previously in this chapter, including daily living conditions (67), lack of transportation, food prices, and school food environments. These issues ultimately reflect on nutrition equity and overall health equity, which are particularly relevant to underserved or less affluent populations (68).

It is important to understand that health equity issues have often been framed in the past as a behavioral problem requiring individual response. A prominent example of this is in the area of obesity. This incorrect framing has the potential to hinder government involvement related to upstream problems that lead to inequities and health problems. It is important that national policies reflect equitable health care priorities and focus on population-wide behavioral issues related to nutrition and other lifestyle issues.

30.15 THE ROLE OF PHYSICIANS IN HEALTH EQUITY

As emphasized throughout this chapter, health equity is critically important to overall individual health. Clinicians must understand that significant disparities exist in health in the United States population, which has created an enormous gap between more affluent and less affluent individuals. This creates a significant problem in the area of health equity. Physicians need to be sensitive to how SDOH issues may reflect on the overall health of their patients, particularly those in lower SES. This is an area where multiple lifestyle issues, such as healthy nutrition, regular physical activity, weight management, stress reduction, avoidance of risky substances such as alcohol and cigarettes, and positive relations with others, all play significant roles. These lifestyle factors can provide keys moving forward, not only for individual health but also for overall public health.

One benefit of these lifestyle factors is that they are low-cost and have the potential to yield significant health benefits, helping to address the current significant problems in the area of health equity.

30.16 CONCLUSIONS/CLINICAL APPLICATIONS

In the United States, health equity has recently been recognized as a significant mandate for overall health for individuals and the country. Clinicians need to be tuned in to the fact that SDOH considerations can lead to considerable health disparities and exacerbate the gap between more affluent and less affluent individuals when it comes to their overall health. The goal in this chapter has been to provide background information, definitions, and some specific information related to the field of health equity. We applaud the AHA, the ACP, and the ACLM for their leadership in bringing health equity to the front of our national discussion of overall health. We hope that the information in this chapter will encourage physicians to take a careful look at health equity when they evaluate patients, particularly those in lower SES. There is no question that our view of health must be expanded to understand the significant relationship between overall health and SDOH. It is our hope that expanded understanding and sensitivity to this issue will help not only individual physicians but also public policy makers in the United States create initiatives to help ease the enormous health issues related to health equity.

REFERENCES

1. Daniel H, Bornstein S, Kane GC, et al. Addressing social determinants to improve patient care and promote health equity: an American College of Physicians Position Paper. *Ann Intern Med.* 2018;168(8):577–578.
2. Braveman P, Arkin E, Orleans T, et al. What is health equity? *Behav Sci Policy.* 2018;4(1):1–14.
3. Braveman P, Egerter S, Williams DR. The social determinants of health: coming of age. *Annu Rev Public Health.* 2011;32:381–398.
4. Healthy People 2030. Heath Equity in Healthy People 2030. https://odphp.health.gov/healthypeople. Accessed January 12, 2024.
5. Belanger M, Hill M, Angelidi A, et al. COVID-19 and disparities in nutrition and obesity. *N Engl J Med.* 2020;383(11):e69.
6. Whitehead M. The concepts and principles of equity and health. *Health Promot Int.* 1991;6:217–228.

7. Braveman P, Gruskin S. Defining equity in health. *J Epidemiol Community Health.* 2003;57:254–258.
8. American College of Physicians. Racial and Ethnic Disparities in Health Care. Philadelphia, PA: American College of Physicians, 2010.
9. Williams DR, Priest N, Anderson NB. Understanding associations among race, socioeconomic status, and health: patterns and prospects. *Health Psychol.* 2016;35(4):407–411.
10. McLoughlin G, McCarthy J, McGuirt J, et al. Addressing food insecurity through a health equity lens: a case study of large urban school districts during the COVID-19 pandemic. *J Urban Health.* 2020;97:759–775.
11. Asada Y, Hughes A, Chriqui J. Insights on the intersection of health equity and school nutrition policy implementation: an exploratory qualitative secondary analysis. *Health Educ Behav.* 2017;44(5):685–695.
12. Kumanyika SK. A framework for increasing equity impact in obesity prevention. *Am J Public Health.* 2019;109(10):1350–1357.
13. World Health Organization. Social Determinants of Health. 2018. https://www.who.int/health-topics/social-determinants-of-health. Accessed April 9, 2025.
14. Cassoobhoy A, Sardana JJ, Benigas S, et al. Building health equity: action steps from the American College of Lifestyle Medicine's health disparities solutions summit (HDSS) 2020. *Am J Lifestyle Med.* 2021;16(1):61–75.
15. Parnarouskis L, Gearhardt A, Mason A, et al. Association of food insecurity and food addiction symptoms: a secondary analysis of two samples of low-income female adults. *J Acad Nutr Diet.* 2022; 122(10):1885–1892.
16. Houghtaling B, Greene M, Parab KV, et al. Improving fruit and vegetable accessibility, purchasing, and consumption to advance nutrition security and health equity in the United States. *Int J Environ Res Public Health.* 2022;19(18):11220.
17. Harris J, Tan W, Mitchell B, et al. Equity in agriculture-nutrition-health research: a scoping review. *Nutr Rev.* 2021;80(1):78–90.
18. Leung CW, Parnarouskis L, Slotnick MJ, et al. Food insecurity and food addiction in a large, national sample of lower-income adults. *Curr Dev Nutr.* 2023;7(12):102036.
19. Galea S, Tracy M, Hoggatt KJ, et al. Estimated deaths attributable to social factors in the United States. *Am J Public Health.* 2011;101(8):1456–1465.
20. Chetty R, Stepner M, Abraham S, et al. The association between income and life expectancy in the United States, 2001–2014. *JAMA.* 2016;315(16):1750–1766.
21. Ubri P, Artiga A. Disparities in Health and Health Care: Five Key Questions. The Henry J. Kaiser Family Foundation. August 2016. https://collections.nlm.nih.gov/catalog/nlm:nlmuid-101694257-pdf. Accessed January 16, 2024.
22. Taylor LA, Tan AX, Coyle CE, et al. Leveraging the social determinants of health: what works? *PLoS One.* 2016;11(8):e0160217.
23. Lloyd-Jones D, Adams RJ, Brown TM, et al. Executive summary: heart disease and stroke statistics – 2010 update: a report from the American Heart Association. *Circulation.* 2010;121(7):948–954.
24. Lloyd-Jones DM, Hong Y, Labarthe D, et al. Defining and setting national goals for cardiovascular health promotion and disease reduction: the American Heart Association's strategic Impact Goal through 2020 and beyond. *Circulation.* 2010;121(4):586–613.
25. Braveman P, Barclay C. Health disparities beginning in childhood: a life-course perspective. *Pediatrics.* 2009;124(Suppl 3):S163–S175.
26. Braveman PA, Egerter SA, Mockenhaupt RE. Broadening the focus: the need to address the social determinants of health. *Am J Prev Med.* 2011;40(1 Suppl 1):S4–S18.
27. Adler NE, Stewart J. Preface to the biology of disadvantage: socioeconomic status and health. *Ann NY Acad Sci.* 2010;1186:1–4.
28. Braveman P, Egerter S, Woolf SH, Marks JS. Do we know enough to recommend action on the social determinants of health? *Am J Prev Med.* 2011;40(1 Suppl 1):S58–S66.
29. Braveman PA, Cubbin C, Egerter S, et al. Socioeconomic status in health research: one size does not fit all. *J Am Med Assoc.* 2025;294:2879–2888.
30. Braveman PA, Cubbin C, Egerter S, et al. Socioeconomic disparities in health in the United States: what the patterns tell us. *Am J Public Health.* 2010;14:20–35.
31. Brennan-Ramirez LK, Baker EA, Metzler M. *Promoting Health Equity: A Resource to Help Communities Address Social Determinants of Health.* Atlanta, GA: U.S. Department of Health and Human Services Center for Disease Control Prevention, 2008.
32. Hasson R, Sallis JF, Coleman N, Kaushal N, Nocera VG, Keith N. COVID-19: implications for physical activity, health disparities, and health equity. *Am J Lifestyle Med.* 2021;16(4):420–433.

33. Department of Health and Human Services. Persons in Low-Income Households Have Less Access to Internet Services. https://aspe.hhs.gov/reports/low-income-internet-access. Accessed April 9, 2025.
34. Rippe JM. COVID-19 and health equity. *Am J Lifestyle Med.* 2022;16(4):416–419.
35. Webb P, Stordalen GA, Singh S, et al. Hunger and malnutrition in the 21st Century. *BMJ* 2018;361:k2238.
36. Physical Activity Guidelines Advisory Committee. 2018 Physical Activity Guidelines Advisory Committee. 2018 Physical Activity Guidelines Advisory Committee Scientific Report. Washington, DC: U.S. Department of Health and Human Services, 2018.
37. Ansell DA, Fruin K, Holman R, et al. The anchor strategy – a place-based business approach for health equity. *N Engl J Med.* 2023;388(2):97–99.
38. Saha S, McPhee G, Salazar S, et al. Integrating community health workers in Rhode Island – a roadmap toward health equity. *N Engl J Med.* 2024;391(19):1768–1769.
39. Larson NI, Story MT, Nelson MC. Neighborhood environments: disparities in access to healthy foods in the U.S. *Am J Prev Med.* 2009;36(1):74–81.e10.
40. Healthy People 2020. National Center for Health Statistics. Public Health Service, U.S. Department of Health and Human Services, 2020.
41. High Level and Emerging Issues for Food Security and Nutrition. Panel of Experts. Second Note on Critical High Level Panel of Experts on Food Security and Nutrition of the Committee on World Food Security. Rome, Italy. 2017 Nutrition and Food Systems. A Report by the High Level Panel of Experts on Food Security and Nutrition of the Committee on World Food Security. September 2017. fao.org. Accessed April 9, 2025.
42. Food and Agriculture Organization of the United Nations. International Fund for Agricultural Development. World Food Programme. Rome: The State of Food Security and Nutrition in the World. 2017. docs.wfp.org/api/documents/WFP-0000022419/download/?_ga=2.91393434.1221853846.1698945941-1391691674.1698945941. Accessed April 9, 2025.
43. Pangaribowo E, Evita H, Gerber N, et al. Food and nutrition security indicators: a review (February 1, 2013). SSRN. 2013(ZEF Working Paper No 108). Food and Nutrition Security Indicators. Accessed April 9, 2025.
44. Feeding America. U.S. Hunger Relief Organization | Feeding America. www.feedingamerica.org/. Accessed April 9, 2025.
45. U.S. Department of Agriculture Economic Research Service. Trends in food insecurity and very low food security by race and ethnicity, 2000–2014. 2016.
46. No Kid Hungry. End Child Hunger in America | No Kid Hungry. www.nokidhungry.org. Accessed April 9, 2025.
47. Kurtz A, Grant K, Marano R, et al. Long-term effects of malnutrition on severity of COVID-19. *Sci Rep.* 2021;11(1):14974.
48. Bedock D, Bel Lassen P, Mathian A, et al. Prevalence and severity of malnutrition in hospitalized COVID-19 patients. *Clin Nutr ESPEN.* 2020;40:214–219.
49. Centers for Disease Control and Prevention. National Center for Health Statistics. Leading Causes of Death. FastStats – Leading Causes of Death. cdc.gov. Accessed April 9, 2025.
50. Leung CW, Ding EL, Catalano PJ, et al. Dietary intake and dietary quality of low-income adults in the Supplemental Nutrition Assistance Program. *Am J Clin Nutr.* 2012;96(5):977–988.
51. Anderson SA. Core indicators of nutritional state for difficult-to-sample populations. *J Nutr.* 1990;120:1555–1598.
52. Kvamme J, Olsen J, Florholmen J, et al. Risk of malnutrition and health-related quality of life in community-living elderly men and women: the Tromso study. *Qual Life Res.* 2011;20(4):575–582.
53. Wellman N, Weddle D, Kranz S, et al. Elder insecurities: poverty, hunger, and malnutrition. *J Am Diet Assoc.* 1997;97(10 Suppl 2):S120–S122.
54. Swinburn B, Kraak V, Allender S, et al. The global syndemic of obesity, undernutrition, and climate change: the Lancet Commission report. *Lancet.* 2019;393(10173):791–846.
55. Wells JC, Sawaya AL, Wibaek R, et al. The double burden of malnutrition: aetiological pathways and consequences for health. *Lancet.* 2020;395(10217):75–88.
56. Ghattas H, Acharya Y, Jamaluddine Z, et al. Child-level double burden of malnutrition in the MENA and LAC regions: prevalence and social determinants. *Matern Child Nutr.* 2020;16(2):e12923.
57. Malnutrition Quality Improvement Initiative. 2025. https://malnutritionquality.org/mqii-toolkit/. Accessed April 9, 2025.
58. Mozaffarian D, Angell SY, Lang T, Rivera JA. Role of government policy in nutrition-barriers to and opportunities for healthier eating. *BMJ.* 2018;361:k2426.
59. Social Determinants of Health at CDC. Centers for Disease Control and Prevention. December 8, 2022. Washington, DC. Accessed April 14, 2025.

60. National Academies of Sciences, Engineering, and Medicine; Health and Medicine Division; Board on Population Health and Public Health Practice; Committee on Applying Neurobiological and Socio-Behavioral Sciences from Prenatal Through Early Childhood Development: A Health Equity Approach. Vibrant and Healthy Kids: Aligning Science, Practice, and Policy to Advance Health Equity. Negussie Y, Geller A, DeVoe JE (eds.). Washington, DC: National Academies Press (US), 2019. PMID: 31855338.
61. Zorbas C, Browne J, Chung A, et al. National nutrition policy in high-income countries: is health equity on the agenda? *Nutr Rev.* 2021;79(10):1100–1113.
62. The White House Conference on Hunger, Nutrition and Health. September 22, 2022. Washington, DC: USDA. Accessed April 14, 2025.
63. Department of Agriculture and U.S. Department of Health and Human Services. U.S. Department of Agriculture and U.S. Department of Health and Human Services. Dietary Guidelines for Americans, 2020–2025 (9th ed). December 2020. Available at DietaryGuidelines.gov. 2020. https://www.dietaryguidelines.gov/resources/2020-2025-dietary-guidelines-online-materials.
64. Healthy People 2030. Office of Disease Prevention and Health Promotion. Office of the Assistant Secretary for Health, Office of the Secretary, U.S. Department of Health and Human Services, 2024.
65. Agurs-Collins T, Alvidrez J, El Shourbagy et al. Perspective: nutrition health disparities framework: a model to advance health equity. *Adv Nutr.* 2024;15(4):100194.
66. Baker P, Hawkes C, Wingrove K, et al. What drives political commitment for nutrition? A review and framework synthesis to inform the United Nations Decade of Action on Nutrition. *BMJ Glob Health.* 2018;3(1):e000485.
67. Fang Zhang F, Liu J, Rehm CD, et al. Trends and disparities in diet quality among US adults by supplemental nutrition assistance program participation status. *JAMA Netw Open.* 2018;1(2):e180237.
68. Isaacs SL, Schroeder SA. Class – the ignored determinant of the nation's health. *N Engl J Med.* 2004;351(11):1137–1142.

31 Behavior Change[1]

31.1 INTRODUCTION

Empowering people to change is an essential element of practicing lifestyle medicine, whether in one-on-one clinic visits with patients or in group consultations, in person or virtually. Lifestyle medicine is a burgeoning new field of medicine that uses six pillars, including physical activity, a whole food plant predominant eating pattern, restorative sleep, stress resiliency techniques, positive social connections, and avoidance of risky substances, to help patients prevent, treat, and in some cases even reverse conditions considered chronic diseases, such as heart disease, diabetes, obesity, metabolic syndrome, hypertension, and high cholesterol, to name a few. With these lifestyle-related conditions on the rise, there is an increasing need for counseling on behavior change that empowers people to adopt and sustain change. How health care professionals talk about change influences how people receive the information and whether they absorb, digest, and ultimately use it.

Behavior change is critical to reducing the risk of chronic diseases. It is also an essential part of the academic curriculum embedded in this book. For this reason, we dedicate a separate chapter to behavior change, with the hope that academic medical professionals will use this information not only in their own clinical practice but also as a central component of teaching their students how to help patients in the process of changing behaviors toward healthier ones.

Behavior change is also central to the work that both Dr. Rippe and Dr. Frates have performed for many years. Dr. Frates has written numerous articles and book chapters on this topic and, indeed, is the first editor of a textbook in the *Lifestyle Medicine Series* entitled "*Empowering Behavior Change in Patients: Practical Strategies for Healthcare Professional.*" She has also served as the Section Editor for large sections on behavior change in both the third and fourth editions of Dr. Rippe's academic textbook, Lifestyle Medicine. Dr. Rippe has emphasized the process of behavior change as a key component of every edition of his *Lifestyle Medicine* textbook.

There is a large academic field devoted to behavioral medicine. We will highlight a few theories of change, with the hope that academic lifestyle medicine professionals will use the references we cite at the end of this chapter to deepen their knowledge and background in the theoretical constructs that underlie the academic discipline of behavioral change.

"No man walks in the same river twice," Heraclitus once said. This quote underscores that change is part of life. We grow from child to adult. A river moves water and silt minute by minute. Our epithelial cells change daily (1). Nothing remains the same. We are aging day by day. Some changes are beyond our control, and others are within our control. What's out of our control? The COVID pandemic, hurricanes, waves, global wars, rain, other cars on the highway, jealousy of others, and other people's behaviors, for example. What is in our control? Our actions, our words, the speed of the car we drive, our use of an umbrella, and our responses to others' behavior are all within our control. One of the first things to identify is what is in our control and what is not. In behavior change, we focus on what is within our control.

31.2 CHANGE IS CONSTANT

What is behavior change? The American Psychological Association defines behavior change as:

1. A systematic approach to changing behavior through the use of operant conditioning.
2. Any alteration or adjustment of behavior that affects a patient's functioning, brought about by psychotherapeutic or other interventions or occurring spontaneously (2).

DOI: 10.1201/9781003630043-31

In lifestyle medicine, the focus is on addressing lifestyle behaviors, patterns, and practices. Lifestyle behaviors include physical activity, nutrition, sleep, stress management, social support, and the use of risky substances. Even the way we list these pillars and describe them can make a world of difference. For example, we can discuss joyous movement, delicious and nutritious foods, restorative sleep, positive social connections, and the avoidance of risky substances. Research indicates that unhealthy behaviors play a role in the development of chronic conditions. Genetics also plays a role in some diseases, such as cancer, heart disease, stroke, obesity, and dementia. Even in cases of genetic susceptibility to a particular condition, healthy lifestyle behaviors can help mitigate disease development and progression. This phrase, or a similar one, has been said by many people: "Genetics loads the gun, and lifestyle behaviors pull the trigger." Lifestyle is that powerful.

In some cases, lifestyle changes can prevent, treat, and even reverse certain chronic conditions, including type 2 diabetes, high blood pressure, and obesity (3,4). For this reason, behavior change is a critical component of lifestyle medicine. The American College of Lifestyle Medicine (ACLM) revised its definition of lifestyle medicine in the spring of 2022 to the following:

> Lifestyle medicine is a medical specialty that uses therapeutic lifestyle interventions as a primary modality to treat chronic conditions, including, but not limited to, cardiovascular diseases, type 2 diabetes, and obesity. Lifestyle medicine certified clinicians are trained to apply evidence-based, whole-person, prescriptive lifestyle change to treat and, when used intensively, often reverse such conditions. Applying the six pillars of lifestyle medicine—a whole-food, plant-predominant eating pattern, physical activity, restorative sleep, stress management, avoidance of risky substances and positive social connections—also provides effective prevention for these conditions (5).

31.3 WHAT IS THE AMERICAN COLLEGE OF LIFESTYLE MEDICINE

According to their website https://lifestylemedicine.org,

> ACLM is the medical professional society for physicians and other professionals dedicated to clinical and worksite practice of lifestyle medicine as the foundation of a transformed and sustainable health care system.

Lifestyle medicine research, education, and practice are all rapidly growing. As of 2025, the ACLM had over 15,000 members. To be certified in lifestyle medicine, physicians and other health care professionals must demonstrate proficiency in exercise prescription, nutrition, sleep, social connection, stress management, and avoidance of high-risk substance use. In addition, they need to know about behavior change. Questions on the board exam for certification in lifestyle medicine focus on behavior change theories and counseling strategies. That's because knowledge is powerful, but it's not powerful enough to instill lasting behavior change. Clinicians need to know the facts and figures, the data and the results of research studies, and they need to master the skills of empowering people to change behaviors. The American Board of Lifestyle Medicine (ABLM) is responsible for administering and grading the exam and issuing certificates to MDs and DOs (https://ablm.org). The ACLM certifies other health care professionals after they pass the ABLM exam.

It is not just health care professionals who are interested in behavior change. Behavior change is often on the minds of people when they are patients, parents, clinicians, teachers, pet owners, people who have loved ones who smoke, drink in excess, or have substance use disorder, managers in companies, or partners in a relationship. In other words, the topic of behavior change applies to everyone.

In this chapter, key aspects of behavior change will be covered, including the transtheoretical model of change, motivational interviewing, group consultations, self-efficacy, the behavioral-intention gap, and health coaching. This chapter will summarize key behavior change theories, health coaching information, research on health coaching and the process of motivational interviewing.

To be proficient in delivering behavior change, people spend years reading research, performing experiments, and writing papers before earning their PhDs in behavior change. There are

TABLE 31.1
The 13 Keys to Behavior Change

The 13 Keys to Behavior Change
The Patient's Agenda is the Guide
Work with the Patient's Stage of Change
Build Self-efficacy and confidence
Tap into the Patient's Motivation
Honor the Patient's Autonomy
Appreciate the Positive and what is working well
Co-create Goals with the Patient
Maintain Motivation
Overcome Obstacles
Identify and use the Patient's Strengths
Set Accountability
Enjoy the Process and five-step cycle of Collaboration for Behavior Change
Use Group Intervention and Social Support to Power Behavior Change

Source: From Table 1.1, page 4 in *Empowering Behavior Change in Patients: Practical Strategies for Healthcare Professional*, Edition 1, 2024, CRC Press, Taylor and Francis Group. Used with permission.

master's degrees in psychology that focus on behavior change. Health and wellness coaches are educated in and become proficient in behavior change during their training and certification. Medical schools often include lectures and workshops on motivational interviewing in the pre-clinical and clinical years. Nurses have behavior change as part of their education as well. Parents often work to better understand behavior change and take courses to help their children behave in a respectful, honest, and compassionate manner. Many people can benefit from learning more about behavior change.

Behavior change is a hot topic for researchers. In one research study exploring behavior change theories, it was determined that these theories focus on five main areas: (a) motives, (b) self-regulation, (c) resources, (d) habits, and (e) environmental and social influences (6). In another study, 82 different theories of behavior change were identified. Most were described over two decades ago, and some as early as 1941 with Miller's Social Learning Theory, 1947 with Sutherland's Differential Association Theory, 1956 with Skinner's Operant Conditioning Theory, 1968 with Locke's Goal Setting Theory, 1977 with Bandura's Social Cognitive Theory, 1977 with Bandura's Self-Efficacy Theory, 1983 with Prochaska's Transtheoretical Model of Change, 1985 with Ajzen's Theory of Planned Behavior/Reasoned Action, 2000 with Deci's Self-Determination Theory, and 2006 with Panter-Brick's Social Ecological Model of Behavior Change (7). Interestingly, many of these theories still guide behavior counseling efforts to this day. A 2021 review of behavior change techniques used to help oral health professionals with tobacco cessation counseling with their patients identified effective strategies, including goal setting, providing written materials, using readiness-to-quit and ability assessment, tobacco-use assessment, providing self-efficacy boosts, listing reasons for quitting, action planning, and environmental restructuring (8).

There are 13 keys to behavior change. They are listed in Table 31.1.

31.4 REVIEW OF MAJOR BEHAVIORAL CHANGE THEORIES

31.4.1 The Transtheoretical Model

The Transtheoretical Model of Change, developed by Dr. James Prochaska and colleagues, is a critical theory to understand and use effectively. This is an important way for health care professionals to tailor their counseling and coaching to the individual patient in front of them, whether in person or via Zoom, Microsoft Teams, or another virtual platform. In some counseling sessions, the patient may be on a treadmill alongside the clinician. Alternatively, counseling may take place one-on-one outdoors during a quiet, private nature walk. There are times when counseling takes place in a group setting, and the individual's stage of change may differ from that of other group members. In this group setting, it is vital to tailor conversations to the individual receiving one-on-one attention at that time. Group discussion can include strategies at multiple stages of change. As a reminder, there are five stages: pre-contemplation, contemplation, preparation, action, and maintenance. Table 31.2 may be useful to consult during a clinic visit with a patient or during group visits. It reviews the five stages of change and provides a summary of feelings patients commonly report in those specific stages.

TABLE 31.2
The Five Stages of Change and Patients' Feelings

	Precontemplation	Contemplation	Preparation	Action	Maintenance
Patient's feelings	Confusing	Considering	Getting ready	In motion	Steady
Patients' expressions	I won't I can't No way. Leave me alone.	I may. It's a good idea.	I'm ready. I need a plan.	I'm doing it.	I've been doing it, and I will keep doing it.
Practitioner's feelings	Frustrated	Hopeful	Excited	Satisfied	Inspired
Practitioner's expressions and questions	I hear you. You are not ready. I am here for you when you are ready. Would you be interested in reading articles or watching videos on the topic of exercise and heart disease? Would you be interested in hearing about a patient who was just like you and made some major changes that improved her well-being?	I hear some ambivalence. What are the pros and cons of change for you? How important is this for you right now? How would your life be different if you did start this new healthy habit?	What needs to be in place for you to get started? What are some of the barriers in your way?	Congratulations on your progress. How do you feel? What seems different to you? What benefits are you noticing? What are your plans to continue?	Congratulations on your continued progress and commitment to this healthy habit! What are you doing that keeps you going? What's your motivation for maintaining this habit? What are your plans for the next month or two? How can I help you to keep going?

Source: From Table 1.2, Page 5 in *Empowering Behavior Change in Patients: Practical Strategies for Healthcare Professionals*, Edition 1, 2024, CRC Press, Taylor and Francis Group. Used with permission.

31.4.2 Social Cognitive Theory

What we witness impacts our thoughts, feelings, and development. Dr. Albert Bandura's social cognitive theory examines how social influences affect personality development and behavior (9,10).

The three areas of focus in social cognitive theory are as follows:

1. A person's cognition
2. Their external environment
3. A person's behavior

A person's social experience throughout their life shapes much of who they are. What others do and say around a person helps the individual learn and grow without going through those experiences themselves. If an individual witnesses a sibling, cousin, or friend get in trouble for stealing or cheating, they may retain that memory and use it when a similar situation arises in their own lives. In group interventions, patients listen to one another's strategies, successes, and failures, and they learn together.

31.4.3 Self-Efficacy

People are more apt to change when they believe they can be successful. Self-efficacy is an individual's belief that they can be successful at a particular task. Confidence is an overarching sense of empowerment and strength, whereas self-efficacy is task-specific. Someone can be confident but lack self-efficacy in their ability to ballroom dance or fix a broken pipe. In managing chronic conditions, an individual may be confident at work but lack self-efficacy in exercising regularly or following a healthy eating pattern.

Self-efficacy is essential to Bandura's social cognitive theory (9). He first described self-efficacy in the 1970s (10). According to his theory, one can develop self-efficacy through four primary sources:

1. *Mastery Experiences*: Having opportunities to try new things, practice, and master them.
2. *Vicarious Experiences*: Interactions with others and watching others' success.
3. *Social Persuasion*: listening to the stories and suggestions of others.
4. *Emotional States*: experiencing anxiety and depression impacts one's ability to feel that they are capable of performing a specific task and being successful.

Self-efficacy is essential for behavior change because it facilitates successful goal setting and goal attainment. People with high self-efficacy make progress toward their healthy lifestyle behavior goals.

Dr. James Prochaska describes how dramatic relief can help individuals in the precontemplation stage. Listening to someone else's story, either another participant in a group setting, hearing about a patient who had a similar problem and overcame obstacles, or watching a powerful movie about someone else's change process, all allow for these vicarious experiences, social persuasion, and emotional states. Goal setting helps to highlight how mastery experiences are essential for sustained change.

During the behavior change consultation, the clinician asks numerous open-ended questions to learn more about the patient. Motivational interviewing will be covered later in this chapter. These open-ended questions are a critical part of motivational interviewing, as they invite the patient to reflect and to dive into the recesses of their brains to think about circumstances, experiences, and thoughts with a fresh perspective. In fact, examining their own self-perception is an integral part of the process. Evaluating the patient's social connections and social interactions will help them to understand how people and past activities or events work to shape who they are today. How patients talk about their past to the clinicians and to themselves also shapes their reality. Self-talk is powerful. It can serve to build people up or tear them down. Someone's self-talk is a reflection of their own beliefs about themselves and their self-efficacy.

Self-talk can lead to insecurity or build confidence. Confidence is built by previous successes. It is also created by rising from a fall and realizing that one mishap is not going to lead to perpetual failure. Confidence brings energy and empowerment. Self-talk can bolster both confidence and self-efficacy. If a person is constantly telling themselves, "I can't do that. I won't do that. That's impossible for me," they are keeping themselves in the pre-contemplative stage. This self-talk is often expressed to others in conversations. Asking someone about how confident they are about reaching a specific goal helps gauge their self-efficacy for that action step.

31.4.4 Self-Determination Theory

Deci and Ryan first described Self-Determination Theory in 1985 (11). According to this theory, the three main components of volitional, sustained motivation are autonomy, competence, and relatedness (12). When these three essential factors are in place, performance, creativity, and productivity improve. When working to help people adopt and sustain healthy patterns of living, it is crucial to make sure they have autonomy. Providing people with choices and allowing them to choose the best fit for them is an effective way to gain buy-in and engagement. People want a sense of control, and they want a sense of competence. When people feel competent, they are motivated to try new tasks and make progress. This helps people get out of their comfort zone. Self-efficacy, which was described earlier as the belief that one can be successful at a task, is linked to the competence aspect of Self-Determination Theory. These theories build on each other and often support one another. The last component of Self-Determination Theory is relatedness. Maslow's hierarchy of Needs emphasizes this same concept in the third level of his hierarchy of needs (13). Maslow explains that, first, people need a sense of belonging. People need people. Individuals long to belong. Providing people with positive, supportive social connections facilitates behavior change and motivation to stay on track.

31.4.5 Social Ecological Model of Change

Initially, in the behavior change process, the focus is on the individual: their beliefs, lifestyle behaviors, strengths, goals, dreams, visions, past successes, past failures, fears, desires, wants, needs, self-efficacy, insecurity, obstacles, motivators, and attitudes. If behavior change counselors or coaches focused solely on the individual, their ability to help people adopt and sustain healthy lifestyle behaviors would be limited. People exist in communities, not in vacuums. It is a rare individual who is not associated with, living with, working with, or connected to another human being in some way. Most people live in apartments, condominiums, or houses in neighborhoods or other communities. There are laws and policies at the local and national levels that people must follow. And there are cultural norms that people adhere to or, in some cases, rebel against. In all cases, the external environment influences each individual, their options, choices, and experiences.

The closest ecological model to the home is the kitchen. What is in the kitchen, and who is shopping for food? This question will affect a person's ability to maintain a healthy eating pattern. Who is cooking the food? A great question to ask in an interview is, "What is in your refrigerator right now?" and "What is in your kitchen cabinetry?" These questions help the clinician better understand the person's home life and its influence. In addition, identify who the person lives with, what their lifestyle patterns entail, and what daily exposures they experience.

In some cases, family members may purchase and bring into the kitchen cookies, cakes, or ice cream. Understanding the people and food items in the home equips the patient with the tools needed to navigate challenging conversations and make difficult choices. Marking foods with red, yellow, or green with a pen, tape, or sticky note can be a first step toward a better understanding of the kitchen. Red would indicate danger. Yellow would indicate caution. And green would indicate go for it!

Many people spend the majority of their days at work, at least from 8 a.m. to 5 p.m. However, COVID-19 also changed this for many people. Some people are still working from home. However, some people are resuming daily commutes, and they may spend more time outside the house than inside on weekdays. And, for some, work events and dinners after hours are part of the job. In these cases, exploring the work environment is key. Is there a refrigerator or microwave available at the office? Taking dinner leftovers to work for lunch is a great idea and saves money as well. When people can batch-cook on Sundays and freeze food, they can bring homemade, healthy lunch options to work and microwave them if a microwave is available. In some workplaces, unfortunately, there are still candy jars on desks, and work meetings involve pizza delivery and soda or juice. In addition to these nutrition issues, there are physical activity issues.

In addition to food options at the office, checking the desk setup at work is also useful. Encouraging people to use stand-up workstations, treadmill workstations, and stationary bike workstations can help people increase the number of minutes of physical activity they accumulate. Using a physio ball as a desk chair is another option that can engage a person's core as they work. There are also portable peddlers that people can use at work under their desks. Setting timers every hour to take standing or walking breaks will help break up sedentary behavior.

A person's culture impacts their daily life and decisions. When growing up with parents who practice specific eating patterns and prefer certain dishes, one may become accustomed to that way of eating, healthy or not. As a child, there is not much choice. When people grow up and live on their own, they often fall back on what they knew as children. In addition, they may still participate in family meals. Understanding how to make healthy food while honoring diverse cultures is key. A recent review article on healthy eating noted that the Mediterranean, Japanese, Okinawan, and Nordic eating patterns can all be healthy (14). Understanding the components of a healthy diet is the place to start. In this article, the authors noted the healthful similarities in these diets from different cultures, including the use of herbs, spices, and other natural seasonings. Protein intake was moderate, primarily from plants, lean meats, and fish; red or processed meat was consumed rarely; and intake of processed foods, sugar, and alcohol was minimal or avoided.

On the other hand, these healthful diets encouraged the intake of mono- and polyunsaturated fats, such as olive oil and nuts (14). In some cultures, people commonly jog on sidewalks; in others, jogging is rare. It is critical to understand a person's culture while working on behavior change. Along these lines, it may not be safe to walk in certain neighborhoods worldwide. Walking is a good form of physical activity, and being outside in nature is healthy as well. However, this recommendation may not be feasible for some due to dangerous or violent surroundings, excessive heat, or extreme cold.

A person's physical environment is an essential factor in behavior change counseling. For example, when discussing the obesity epidemic, we do not simply speak of willpower and individual choices. We must address the food environment in which they live. Some people live in food deserts, where it is nearly impossible to buy fresh produce, or in food swamps, where there are fast-food restaurants on every corner. The food industry has created food products that may be multicolored, dye-laden, chemically laden, sugar-laden, fat-laden, and excessively salty. These hyperpalatable foods interact with the brain's dopamine system in a way that leads the person who eats them to crave the same food and the same reward. Helping people understand the healthy options is one part of the journey to nutritious eating; providing ample opportunities to obtain these options is another. Even food pantries are now stocking their shelves with whole-food, plant-predominant options, recognizing the importance of plants for optimal health.

Knowing a person's background and current circumstances enables a clinician to co-create a plan tailored to that individual. Behavior change does not work if the clinician simply provides the guidelines for exercise, nutrition, sleep, social connections, stress reduction, and avoidance of risky substances without knowing the whole person, their home environment, work environment, neighborhood, culture, and social values (Figure 31.1).

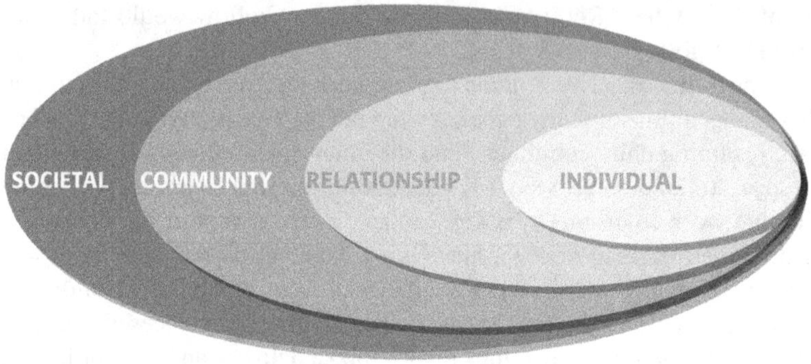

FIGURE 31.1 The social ecological model of change in enclosure circles ("societal," "community," "relationship" "individual"). (Used with permission from: Frates B, Bonnet JP, Joseph R, Peterson JA. *Lifestyle Medicine Handbook: An Introduction to the Power of Healthy Habits* (2nd ed). Monterey, CA: Healthy Learning, 2021. Chapter 3 on page 100.)

31.5 SOCIAL DETERMINANTS OF HEALTH (SDOH)

There has been a shift in focus not only to the individual but also to the environment and to how multiple forces affect an individual's lifestyle patterns and practices. In a 2021 article, the authors recommended using terms such as "eating practices and patterns" rather than "food choices and decisions" to better capture the intricate interconnectedness between individuals' diets and their environments (15). Food availability, local grocery store inventory, whether someone can have their own garden, food advertising, the marketing of hyperpalatable foods that are high in sugar, fat, and salt, the number of fast food chains in the vicinity of someone's home, a person's income, a person's understanding of the impact of food on their health, and whether or not the person has a primary care physician or access to a nutritionist or health coach can all impact their food intake, patterns, and practices. Factors such as race, ethnicity, and age can also influence the quality and variety of available food (16). Those in underserved communities have less access to nutritious food and greater odds of experiencing food insecurity (16).

Behavior change is not just a matter of willpower. How is a person going to take a walk outside if there are gangs, drug deals, and shootings in their neighborhoods? They will need to find solutions for movement that work for them. A person's education level, economic status, family background, and neighborhood all influence a person's available options, decisions, and choices (17). The social determinants of health are essential to consider when counseling a patient about behavior change (18). These are depicted in Figure 31.2 and include economic stability, education access and quality, health care access and quality, neighborhood and built environment, and social and community context.

Many of the studies in behavior change have a homogeneous subject pool. Including many more people of color, immigrants, and individuals who live in underserved areas will be necessary for future investigations. The more information collected about current practices, patterns, and problems, the better equipped health care professionals will be to meet the needs of these populations. Encouraging people of color and populations living in under-resourced areas to seek education and employment in the health care field will also help. In many cases, this will take funding and extra support. It was noted that during the COVID-19 pandemic, some populations avoided hospitals because they felt a lack of trust, fear, and a disconnect with health care professionals (19). This was experienced by people of color, minorities, immigrants, different genders, and people from economically challenged areas. Counseling on behavior change may open the door for individuals who are resistant or hesitant to seek medical attention and encourage them to take the step toward clinicians that they can relate to and may be able to trust more readily (17).

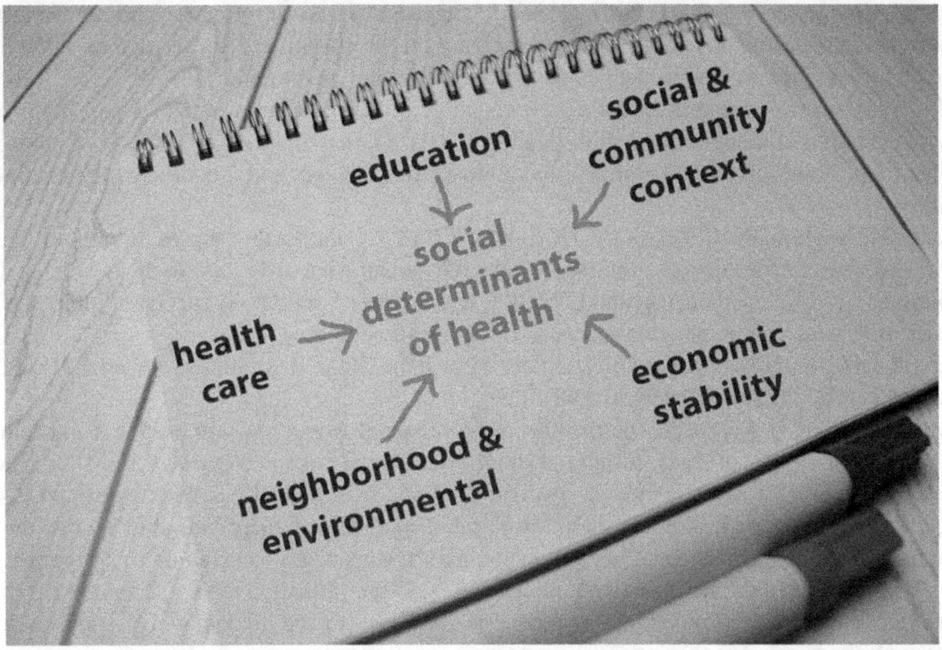

FIGURE 31.2 The social determinants of health (SDOH).

Shutterstock number. Asset id: 1699249525

31.6 WHAT IS HEALTH COACHING?

Health coaching is a profession that focuses on behavior change. There is a National Board of Health and Wellness Coaching (20), which certifies individuals in health coaching after they take an exam, submit a case study, and provide a log of client interactions. Getting certified is one step in the process of learning how to coach, but the learning and growing do not end there. The key is the doing and practicing of health coaching day to day with patients. Practicing coaching is key to becoming an effective coach. One does not need to be a certified health and wellness coach to use coaching strategies and to practice counseling patients in this way.

Many healthcare professionals are used to using the "EXPERT Approach" and telling people what to do. However, this tell-and-sell approach does not work for sustained behavior change. Every individual is different and requires a unique approach that suits their needs. Some people are concerned about their pre-diabetes. They may have BMIs in the obese range, carry extra adipose tissue in their abdomen, have a high waist circumference, and are worried about the plethora of conditions associated with obesity, such as high blood pressure, heart disease, metabolic syndrome, sleep apnea, diabetes, and some cancers, while others are struggling to quit smoking or drinking. Many individuals wrestle with the same unhealthy lifestyle patterns, like eating fast food that is cheap and easy to acquire, skimping on sleep, drinking four to five glasses of wine, forgoing any exercise, and spending so much time working that their social relationships are suffering.

Though the unhealthy lifestyles people are following may be similar, each individual will require a different approach. They may be in different stages of change for their behaviors. They may have tried several different strategies already. They may have a home environment that demands attention with a mother who has dementia or a child with Down syndrome. No matter what the situation is or what the individual's personal struggles may be, a health coach can work with that person to adopt and sustain healthy behaviors by taking into account the person's personality, preferences, attitudes, educational level, home environment, past successes and failures, their neighborhood, work environment, cultural influences, and more. A health coach helps co-create small goals that are compelling to the individual, doable, specific, measurable, action-oriented, and time-sensitive. It is through counseling, listening, and collaborating that the health coach can partner with clients to create powerful plans that propel people to take action and maintain it.

If you are a trained and certified health coach or a health care professional looking to help empower patients to adopt and sustain healthy lifestyle behaviors, taking a COACH Approach will help. Dr. Frates created this mnemonic almost a decade ago, and it continues to help people to this day.

Table 31.3 reviews the Frates COACH Approach™ (21). Contrast this approach to the EXPERT Mnemonic when the health care professional tells the patient what to do, how to do it, when to do it, and why to do it. In emergencies, this EXPERT Approach is essential for survival (Table 31.4). In the case of chronic conditions, this approach can build resistance.

Five specific domains of communication distinguish the COACH Approach™ from the EXPERT Approach™ (22). These are listed in Table 31.5.

With the COACH Approach, the healthcare professional works to share pertinent information with the patient in front of them. Instead of simply sharing research and knowledge that healthcare professionals consider essential for the patient, they check in with the patient, assess what they already know, ask for permission to share information, and let the patient's responses guide the trajectory of the clinical encounter. They follow the patient's agenda. It is essential to ask permission because patients need the same three components of self-determination theory as any other type of adult in order to sustain motivation—relatedness, competence, and autonomy. By asking permission, the clinician respects the patient's autonomy.

TABLE 31.3
Frates COACH Approach™

C-Curiosity
O-Openness
A-Appreciation
C-Compassion
H-Honesty

Source: Frates B, Bonnet J, Joseph R, et al. *Lifestyle Medicine Handbook: An Introduction to the Power of Healthy Habits.* Monterey, CA: Healthy Learning, 2020. Used with Permission.

TABLE 31.4
EXPERT Mnemonic

E = Examine the patient
X = X-ray and other imaging to diagnose the problem
P = Plan the resolution of the problem
E = Explain the problem, the solution, and the strategy
R = Repeat what you said multiple times
T = Tell the patient what to do. The "Tell-and-Sell" approach

Source: Frates B, Bonnet J, Joseph R, et al. *Lifestyle Medicine Handbook: An Introduction to the Power of Healthy Habits.* Monterey, CA: Healthy Learning, 2020. Used with Permission.

TABLE 31.5
Frates' Five Specific Domains of Communication for Coaching

Sharing knowledge
Listening
Asking questions
Addressing problems
Taking Responsibility

Source: Frates EP, Bonnet J. Collaboration and negotiation: the key to therapeutic lifestyle change. *Am J Lifestyle Med.* 2016;10(5):302–312. Used with Permission.

In a behavior change counseling session focused on coaching, the patient talks more than the healthcare professional. The healthcare professional works hard to listen deeply. This generous listening means the patient does most of the talking in response to carefully crafted open-ended questions posed by the healthcare professional. Listening is a skill that needs practice.

Asking powerful questions is also a skill that requires practice. The importance of open-ended questions will be discussed again in the Motivational Interviewing (MI) section of the chapter. A simple analogy is that an open-ended question is like a rotary or roundabout on the road. There are multiple directions to choose from. A closed-ended question is like a dead-end road. There is only one way to go. There is a one-word answer that ends the conversation until the next question is asked. Keep this in mind while reading the section on MI and Open-ended questions, Affirmations, Reflections, and Summaries (OARS) in this chapter.

When problems arise, the healthcare professional often resorts to "fix-it" mode and "solve-it" strategies. In the EXPERT approach, the healthcare professional is trained to have all the answers and to find all the solutions they possibly can. However, in a coaching encounter, the issues of concern are lifestyle behaviors, and the solutions are often specific to the patient's circumstances, environment, abilities, past attempts to change, needs, desires, cultural preferences, and social determinants of health. These are the areas in which the patient is an expert. They often have ideas about potential solutions and sharing them with a trusted healthcare professional can be the step they need to complete to put their solutions into action.

With a coaching model, the healthcare professional does not take full responsibility for the clinical encounter or the outcomes. Instead, the patient takes responsibility for setting goals and meeting those goals. The SMART goal framework is used (Specific, Measurable, Action-Oriented, Realistic, and Time-Sensitive). The clinician and patient work to develop strategies for success and a plan that is challenging enough but not out of reach. The coaching encounter is a collaboration, and the patient is ultimately responsible for their lifestyle behaviors.

31.7 LANDMARK STUDIES IN COACHING AND BEHAVIOR CHANGE

The results of research demonstrate that health and wellness coaching is a promising intervention for individuals seeking to adopt and sustain healthy lifestyles. Some small randomized clinical trials demonstrate improvements in health outcomes with health coaching. Early studies about two decades ago showed positive effects in the areas of cardiovascular disease, diabetes, cancer pain, and asthma. Table 31.6 highlights some of the seminal studies that were randomized controlled trials (RCTs).

In 2003, Vale and colleagues studied 792 patients with cardiac disease to determine the impact of a coaching intervention, Coaching on Achieving Cardiovascular Health (COACH) (23). After five telephone coaching sessions over a six-month period, subjects in the intervention group had a greater drop in cholesterol, lost more weight, reduced their fat intake, and walked more than patients in the control group.

TABLE 31.6
Landmark Studies Chart

Study	Number of Participants	Primary Outcomes
Vale et al. (23)	Study on 792 patients with cardiac disease	Cholesterol lowered 21 vs. 7 mg/dL ($p<.0001$)
Whittemore et al. (24)	Study on 53 women with type 2 diabetes	Better diet self-management, less diabetes related distress, higher satisfaction with care
Wolever et al. (25)	Study on 56 patients with type 2 diabetes subjects ≥7	Significant reduction in Hemoglobin A1C among subjects with baseline A1C >=7
Fisher et al. (26)	Asthma outcomes in 191 children (parents and children coached)	Decreased re-hospitalization rates compared to controls 35.6% vs. 59.1% ($p<.01$)
Oliver et al. (27)	Study on 67 patients with cancer	Improved pain severity compared to controls ($p=.014$)

Source: *"Empowering Behavior Change in Patients: Practical Strategies for the Healthcare Professional"* [Frates B, Faries M. CRC Press (Boca Raton, FL), 2023], which is a volume in the *Lifestyle Medicine Series* edited by Dr. Rippe. Used with Permission.

In 2004, Whittemore and colleagues studied 53 women with type 2 diabetes (24). They participated in six coaching sessions delivered by nurses. Results showed that those in the coaching group who were better able to manage their diets had less diabetes-related distress, improved exercise management, lowered BMI, and reported greater satisfaction with their medical care than those in the usual care group.

In 2010, Wolever and colleagues studied the effects of coaching on 56 patients with type 2 diabetes who were randomly assigned to integrative care coaching for six months or usual care (25). The coaching intervention included 14 sessions of telephonic coaching, each lasting 30 minutes. The subjects in the coaching group had lower hemoglobin A1C when compared to those in the usual care group. In addition, those in the coaching group had less stress, better perceptions of their health, and better exercise adherence.

In 2009, Fisher and colleagues investigated children with asthma and their parents (26). The subjects included 191 children and their parents, who were randomly assigned to the coaching or usual care group. The coaching included telephone and in-person coaching to parents, followed by bi-weekly calls for three months and monthly calls for two years. Children in the families who were coached had fewer hospitalizations (35.6%) than children whose families did not receive the coaching intervention (59.1%).

In 2001, Oliver and colleagues researched pain and coaching (27). The study included 67 cancer patients with moderate pain. The subjects were randomly assigned to receive one 20-minute coaching session before their oncologist visit, or they were assigned to an education session, which was usual care. The coach reviewed the World Health Organization pain control guidelines with the subject. They also discussed techniques for talking to and asking their oncologist questions about the treatment plan. Two weeks after the intervention, in a follow-up phone interview, the subjects in the coach group reported significantly less pain than the usual care group.

31.8 REVIEW STUDIES IN COACHING AND BEHAVIOR CHANGE

Interest and research in coaching have grown significantly since the landmark studies were published in the early 2000s. Several reviews looked at between 2 and 284 studies. They examined outcomes of patients with cardiovascular disease, chronic obstructive pulmonary disease, cancer, rehabilitation medicine, and those in retirement. The overall findings revealed that coaching is effective in these settings. There are gaps in the research, including long-term effectiveness, that need to be addressed in future studies. Table 31.7 highlights more recent studies in coaching.

TABLE 31.7
Review Studies Chart

Study	Number of Participants	Primary Outcomes
An and Song (28)	15 studies of adults with Cardiovascular risk	Significant effects on physical activity, dietary behaviors, management of stress, health responsibility
Stara et al. (29)	Two studies with aging workers	Improved well-being based on physical criteria
Obro et al. (30)	Review of nine studies on chronic disease coaching	Patients prefer face-to-face coaching
Singh et al. (31)	12 studies on pharmacist coaching	Improved clinical and non-clinical outcomes
Long et al. (32)	Meta-analysis with ten RCTs on COPD	Improved QOL and reduced COPD hospital admissions (p=.0001)
Dejonghe et al. (33)	14 studies in preventive and rehab settings	Improved outcomes in three studies in each group
Barakat et al. (34)	12 studies including 1,038 cancer survivors	Improved physical activity, mood, and QOL
Kivelä et al. (35)	13 studies on adults with chronic disease	Improved weight management, increased physical activity, improved health status (physical and mental)
Wolever et al. (36)	Review of 284 studies	Coaching operationalization of articles: Patient-centered 86%. Self-discovery/active learning 63%. Provides education and coaching 91%. Encourages accountability for behaviors 86%. Consistent ongoing relationship 78%

Source: *"Empowering Behavior Change in Patients: Practical Strategies for the Healthcare Professional"* [Frates B, Faries M. CRC Press (Boca Raton, FL), 2023], which is a volume in the *Lifestyle Medicine Series* edited by Dr. Rippe. Used with Permission.

31.9 RECENT COACHING INTERVENTION STUDIES

In 2020, An and colleagues conducted a meta-analysis on the effects of health coaching on behavior in patients at risk for cardiovascular disease (28). Fifteen randomized studies were included in the review. The review evaluated how coaching impacts patient responsibility, physical activity, dietary decisions, stress management, and smoking behaviors. Effect sizes of the coaching interventions were small but significant for four of the categories examined, including physical activity, patient responsibility, stress management, and dietary decisions. Smoking behaviors did not reveal significance.

Stara and colleagues conducted a systematic review examining the use of digital health coaching for aging workers to help them adopt healthy behaviors and extend their time in the workforce (29). The review consisted of examining only two studies that met the inclusion criteria out of 1,931 identified. The digital health programs improved physical well-being among older workers, but social and psychological well-being were not addressed.

Obro and colleagues focused on the use of mobile health to help patients self-manage chronic diseases with health coaching. In this literature review, nine studies were included (30). The authors found that an important factor in developing self-management skills was patient engagement. According to the findings in this review, patients preferred face-to-face coaching. Mobile health may be more efficient when it is used to assist the coach with telecommunication and to monitor disease.

Singh and colleagues examined the literature from 2000 to 2009 to identify studies investigating health coaching techniques utilized by pharmacists (31). Twelve studies were included in this systematic review. The authors sought to determine whether face-to-face, telephone, or electronic communication was used to coach patients and assess coaching training and health outcomes. Of the 12 studies selected, most used a combination of communication techniques, but four were just face-to-face, and one was just by telephone. Review of the literature revealed that coaching by the pharmacist improved clinical outcomes for subjects diagnosed with diabetes, hypertension, high cholesterol, and depression. There were also improved non-clinical outcomes, including medication adherence, attitudes toward drug therapy, medical costs, and patient satisfaction with the service.

Long and colleagues performed a meta-analysis on the use of health coaching to improve health-related quality of life (HRQoL) and reduce hospital admissions in patients with chronic obstructive pulmonary disease (COPD) (32). Ten RCTs that used motivational interviewing, goal setting, and health education for COPD were included in this review. Coaching was found to decrease hospital admissions related to COPD and to enhance the quality of life in this population.

Dejonghe and colleagues reviewed the long-term effects of health coaching on healthy individuals and patients with chronic disease in a systematic review (33). Fourteen studies were included in the review: seven focused on prevention and seven focused on rehabilitation. The authors evaluated health coaching for the prevention of disease and also for rehabilitation to assess how coaching influenced health outcomes. Three out of the seven studies in each group demonstrated a positive long-term effect of coaching on health outcomes at 24 weeks.

Barakat and colleagues performed a systematic review on the use of health coaching to build capacity to support cancer survivors (34). Six randomized trials and six pre-post quasi-experimental studies were included, yielding a total of 1,038 cancer survivors. Research showed that coaching for patients with cancer increased quality of life, physical activity, social connections, and decreased pain and fatigue. Five out of the six studies included in the review revealed that coaching can improve mental health (depression/anxiety) outcomes. The authors identified future research topics as how coaching can improve self-efficacy and influence patient environments.

Kivela and colleagues conducted a systematic review examining the impact of health coaching on patients with chronic disease (35). Thirteen articles were included in the review out of the 1,696 articles published between 2009 and 2013. The authors reported that coaching improved chronic disease management by promoting positive psychological, behavioral, and physiological outcomes. Specifically, it was noted that coaching patients with chronic conditions helped improve weight management, increased physical activity, and improved mental health.

Wolever and colleagues performed a systematic review of 284 articles on health and wellness coaching available in 2014 (36). The goal of the review was to create a concrete definition of coaching. The authors identified health coaching as a process performed by a health professional using behavior change theory and education in 91% of the studies. Coaching was considered a patient-centered process in 86% of the studies. In 71% of the studies, coaching was offered to help patients set their own goals. Self-discovery was considered a component of coaching used to help patients explore new ways to achieve their goals in 63% of papers. Seventy-eight percent of the reviewed research studies defined coaching as a reliable and consistent relationship between a patient and a clinician.

31.10 RESEARCH ON EFFECTIVE BEHAVIOR CHANGE TECHNIQUES AND STRATEGIES FOR SPECIFIC POPULATIONS

31.10.1 Retirement Age, Nutrition, and Physical Activity

According to a paper by Lara and colleagues, clinicians can help aging adults adopt healthy eating patterns and increase their physical activity by educating them about the benefits of these behaviors (37). These benefits may include disease prevention. Following an assessment of the patient's readiness to change, the clinician can help them identify goals and perceived barriers to success. This involves identifying potential barriers to adopting healthy lifestyle behaviors and coaching patients to explore solutions. Using a patient-centric approach to brainstorming allows patients to decide how they may use social support to achieve their goals. This approach enables them to plan solutions with the support of friends, family, or social groups. This may entail changing social settings or selecting new group activities. The use of clinician follow-up prompts supports patient accountability and improves self-care. Providing feedback on performance helps build and maintain a responsive clinician-patient relationship.

31.10.2 Adults with Obesity

The literature on coaching for adult obesity has examined specific behaviors and strategies to increase self-efficacy and physical activity. Coaching to improve the patient's self-efficacy includes action planning for specific physical activity (38). Remember, small successes build confidence for later success. This requires time management and self-monitoring of outcomes. The use of social support includes supervised and group activities or connecting with professional support, such as a registered dietitian (RD).

Coaching to increase healthy behavior prompts the patient to self-monitor. Clinicians teach patients to use prompts and cues. Coaching allows the patient to reflect on what they did right and either replicate the behavior or self-correct to ensure future success. Rewards that match the effort or progress are used to self-motivate.

Effective behavior change techniques to increase activity in obese adults address short- and long-term goals. Both short- and long-term behavior changes rely upon goal setting and self-monitoring of behavior. Long-term behavior change includes feedback on outcomes. In the long term, clinicians may implement graded tasks with increasing levels of difficulty and add aids to the environment, such as step counters or smartwatches.

Effective counseling strategies for behavior change in adults who are overweight change over time. Strategies that do not change include maintaining support for the patient's autonomy, adopting a patient-centered approach, and using motivational interviewing.

31.11 BEHAVIOR AND WEIGHT CHANGE IN ADULTS

Several predictors of beneficial weight and behavior change have been identified in the literature (39). Patients who successfully increased their physical activity had higher intrinsic motivation, self-efficacy, and self-regulation. Those who were better at weight control had positive body image and were more flexible with eating constraints.

31.12 CHILDHOOD OBESITY

Coaching to change physical activity and eating in children who have a BMI that puts them in the obesity category relies upon management and prevention interventions (40). Management interventions are structured to provide information on the consequences of unhealthy behavior to the child and family. Families are prompted to restructure the environment to help the child adopt new behaviors. Prompting new behaviors is practiced with the family. Identification of family members as role models for healthy behavior creates an environment that supports the child's success. Family training on managing emotional and stress eating is part of the coaching process, as is training in communication skills. Prevention intervention also includes prompting the family to generalize the behavior.

31.13 DIABETES AND BEHAVIOR CHANGE

A literature review on behavior change techniques for people with diabetes looked at 14 RCTs between 1975 and 2015 (41). This review found 4 out of 46 behavior change techniques to be effective: (a) instructions to carry out a behavior, (b) demonstration of the behavior, (c) behavior rehearsal, and (d) action planning. Strategies that worked for patients included supervised physical activity, group exercise, and connecting with an exercise physiologist and a dietitian. Studies that used increased frequency and intensity of physical activity had better patient outcomes.

31.14 TEN TAKEAWAYS FROM THE BEHAVIOR CHANGE SECTION

1. Empowering patients to change involves behavior change theories, processes, and strategies that are evidence-based.
2. There are psychological theories that are foundational to behavior change.
3. The COACH Approach™ is a way of being that embodies and utilizes curiosity, openness, appreciation, compassion, and honesty.
4. The EXPERT Approach™ is a way of being that puts the responsibility of the outcome on the clinician. The clinician uses examining, X-raying, planning, explaining, repeating, and telling as a way to interact with the patient and solve the patient's problem.
5. Most healthcare clinicians were taught the EXPERT Approach™ in their healthcare professional schools and training.
6. To move from the EXPERT to the COACH Approach™ way of being, the clinician needs to focus on five main areas: the way they share knowledge, listen, ask questions, address problems, and take responsibility.
7. Health and wellness coaching is a healthcare profession focused on behavior change.
8. There is research from randomized controlled studies that supports the use of health and wellness coaching interventions with patients experiencing chronic conditions.
9. Asking questions is key to the behavior change process and empowering patients to change.
10. Behavior change takes time and patience on the part of the patient and the clinician.

31.15 MOTIVATIONAL INTERVIEWING (MI)*

*This section is taken from the chapter "Motivational Interviewing" by Peter Fifield and Joji Suzuki in the book *Empowering Behavior Change in Patients: Practical Strategies for the Healthcare Professional* [Frates B, Faries M., CRC Press (Boca Raton), 2023], which is a volume in the *Lifestyle Medicine Series* edited by Dr. Rippe.

31.15.1 Importance of Motivational Interviewing

Motivational Interviewing is one of the most powerful tools for helping individual patients achieve behavioral change. Motivational interviewing involves a collaborative and goal-oriented style of communication. It requires that the clinician abandon the "expert" model and adopt a collaborative approach, working as an equal with the individual patient. As indicated in this chapter, motivational interviewing (MI) combines two entities: the clinician brings expertise in *health*, and the client brings expertise in *self*. There is a large body of academic literature supporting the efficacy of motivational interviewing. This will become clear by the end of this chapter.

31.15.2 What Is Motivational Interviewing?

Working Definition: "Motivational interviewing is a collaborative goal-oriented style of communication with particular attention to the language of change. It is designed to strengthen personal motivation for and commitment to a specific goal by eliciting and exploring the person's own reasons for change within an atmosphere of acceptance and compassion (42)."

MI was first conceived during a clinical trial comparing treatment approaches for individuals who reported problem drinking. Initially, the researchers noted that empathic statements made by the clinicians had a stronger effect on reducing problem drinking behaviors than other interventions, such as directive comments. Although this was only the beginning, it led to Miller creating the structural framework that would later become MI. The first edition of MI was published in 1999. Now in its third edition, this communication model continues to focus on the intentional application of specific techniques, designed to increase change talk and decrease sustain talk.

MI is very useful in navigating ambivalence — a phase in which a person may feel two ways about something — they could change, or they could not change and stay the same — both could be equally acceptable. Most likely, MI would not be used when a person is in the action phase because excessive processing, talking, and contemplation may just reverse their current level of motivation and action. However, MI is most effective in negotiating this ambivalence within the individual and is often present during the pre-contemplative or contemplative phases of change.

The Four Processes: MI has four processes — engaging, focusing, evoking, and planning — all of which are fluid and intertwined. Although clinicians do not always complete every stage, the processes tend to unfold in a general order, each building on the one before while remaining free to overlap and recur. Typically, clinicians using MI first engage with the individual, then focus on changing behavior, and finally evoke the change talk that will bring about the process of creating a plan. In practice, behavior change often requires repeating these processes over weeks, months, or even years!

MI revolves around building a therapeutic alliance by using OARS to understand the patient/client better. OARS stands for open-ended questions, affirmations, reflections, and summaries. Open-ended questions are those for which the patient/client needs to provide an expanded answer. In contrast, a closed-ended question requires a one-word answer: yes or no, true or false, a number like 120 minutes or 7 hours, etc. Affirmations are words that congratulate and acknowledge a patient's/client's efforts toward healthy change. Reflections are opportunities for the clinician to demonstrate their empathy and their listening skills by repeating or paraphrasing the patient's/client's words. Simple reflections involve simple re-sharing of what the clinician heard. Amplified reflections exaggerate an aspect of what the patient/client shared in order to evoke change talk, as mentioned above. Change talk is one of the main goals of MI. It is the words the patient/client uses themselves to express the importance of changing their own behavior. Double-sided reflections can also evoke change talk. This is a reflection that demonstrates to the patient/client their own ambivalence. On one hand, the patient/client wants to start exercising to feel better mentally, but on the other hand, the patient/client says they have no time to exercise. The last letter in OARS is S for summaries. This involves listening to the patient/client carefully and mindfully throughout the encounter and remembering the words the patient/client used, the emotions expressed, and the main points covered during the time spent together. Using OARS also helps to build therapeutic rapport.

Using compassion is critical for building therapeutic rapport. Listening more and talking less is a hallmark of MI. Compassionately guiding patients/clients to focus on the positive aspects of change and engage in change talk is a skill. The opposite of change talk is sustain talk. Patients/clients use sustain talk to fight against change. Sustain talk is often used by patients/clients when a clinician tries to convince or force change by emphasizing all the risks of the unhealthy behavior, the threats of possible cancer, heart attack, or death as a result of certain behaviors, or the sharing of statistics and data that prove the healthy behavior is, indeed, healthy. When clinicians are using the EXPERT Approach, they can evoke sustain talk. Most patients/clients know that smoking is unhealthy or drinking causes liver damage and potentially cancer, and they don't need to be told again or scolded. Judging and shaming patients is not compassionate care, and patients/clients do not respond well to that approach. Evoking change talk with the OARS of MI is the alternative and a more effective approach.

31.15.3 The Need for Motivational Interviewing in Lifestyle Medicine

Clinicians forget that they often ask their patients/clients to change—take that medication, lose that weight, do this exercise, go to this referral—clinicians are constantly requesting a "next step" or behavior change from their clients. For some, change is easy; however, for others, making changes requires a level of vulnerability, humility, and acceptance that we are entering the unknown but are willing to go there anyway. Clinicians may not remember what it feels like to be vulnerable—to commit to something when they don't *know* the outcome or to act when they don't really *want to.* The act of being vulnerable allows clinicians to balance the interaction with their patients/clients, knowing that clinicians are the experts in a certain field, and the patients/clients are the experts in themselves. The key to Motivational Interviewing (MI) is to combine these two entities—the clinicians are bringing their expertise in *health,* and the patients/clients are bringing their expertise in themselves.

In general, managing complex chronic medical concerns could be called "wicked problems" (43), problems that are so complex that they have no straightforward solution, only better or worse strategies. There is no one-size-fits-all approach. For years, we relied on the directive approach, where the clinicians would tell clients what to do, and the motivated client would follow those instructions. The clinicians would play the expert role and the client would play the novice, the empty vessel, awaiting the clinician to impart upon them their infinite wisdom. Often, these seemingly straightforward plans were not successful, and subsequently, the client was seen as non-compliant or unmotivated. Providing different solutions to the same problem is a version of first-order change. This approach is linear and incremental; if you do "A," then "B" will happen. Management of behavioral changes, however, is too complex to generally be approached in such a linear fashion. Another option is to use a non-linear approach and attempt what some System Theorists would call second-order change (44), abandoning a transactional or incremental approach in favor of a radical, transformational one. Creating therapeutic rapport is key to the motivational interviewing process.

MI can facilitate second-order change, for it allows us to see change through a transformational lens as a non-linear process. Clinicians recognize they can expect with some regularity that a standard prescription for one patient/client will not work for another. We also know that patients/clients approach behavioral change with different levels of readiness. MI (42) is a clinical tool that offers a shift in focus; a view into the patient's/client's world that the clinician has not seen before. It offers an approach that is evidence-based, client-centered, and proven to be effective in getting clients closer to and planning for change (42). Clinicians can use MI as a more effective strategy to address these *complex problems* in hopes of increasing the odds of successfully assisting the client in the process of change.

This process involves working with the client to investigate options for increasing intrinsic motivation. It also includes facing the challenge of sitting in the discomfort of not being the expert in what may work best for the client—fighting the reflex to fix the problem. A common pearl of wisdom in the MI world is to "be responsible for the interaction and not the outcome." This acceptance is rooted in the fundamental truism that clinicians can do very little to **make** their clients implement sustained behavior change unless they want to do so. Clinicians can, however, assist them in increasing and strengthening their internal motivation and preparedness for change. As Miller and Rollnick (42) put it, MI "involves a collaborative partnership with clients, a respectful evoking of their own motivation and wisdom and a radical acceptance recognizing that ultimately whether change happens is each person's own choice, an autonomy that cannot be taken away no matter how much one might wish to at times."

31.15.4 Evidence Base in Support of Motivational Interviewing

Since the time that MI was adopted in clinical settings as a tool to help patients change behavior, the rigor with which this intervention was both implemented and evaluated stands out among many of the psychotherapeutic approaches currently in use in health care settings. There have been hundreds of controlled and uncontrolled trials of MI for a wide range of target behaviors, such as unhealthy substance use, exercise, diabetes management, weight-related outcomes, physical activity, diet, medication adherence, and self-care. Of note, both males and females in adult and adolescent populations are well represented in these trials, as are diverse racial and ethnic patient populations. Given the enormous volume of research that has been conducted over the decades, a review of all the evidence base is beyond the scope of this chapter.

Nevertheless, we can summarize the available evidence by reviewing published systematic reviews and meta-analyses. In 2018, the most comprehensive systematic review of reviews was published, which included 104 systematic reviews and 38 meta-analyses of MI (45). The overall quality of the evidence was rated as low, but the authors concluded that MI appears to be most effective in stopping or reducing unhealthy behaviors such as unhealthy alcohol use, smoking, and other substance use. The results also indicated that evidence to support MI in helping to reduce weight among obese and overweight adults is generally lacking, although the evidence does point to MI helping to increase physical activity.

Since then, additional reviews of a variety of target behaviors have been published to further clarify MI's role in helping patients improve health-related behaviors and outcomes. These studies now confirm that MI has robust empirical support in improving medication adherence (46), weight-related outcomes in adolescents (47), diabetes management (48), physical activity (49), and self-care among individuals with heart failure (50). In contrast to the conclusion in the 2018 systematic review of reviews, the most recent systematic review of MI for adult obesity failed to show a statistically significant impact on weight-related outcomes such as weight or BMI among adults. Taken together, the most up-to-date evidence base suggests that MI is effective in influencing a wide range of target behaviors with a particular impact on reducing and preventing unhealthy behaviors, but MI may be more challenging when improving weight-related outcomes for adults who are obese or overweight. Therefore, clinicians need to recognize that MI alone will not be the most effective strategy in impacting weight-related outcomes in overweight adults.

31.15.5 Key Points for Motivational Interviewing

- MI is a strengths-based approach that focuses on evoking the client's inherent strengths and capabilities to successfully navigate lifestyle changes.
- MI recognizes and accepts the fact that every client enters the process of lifestyle changes at different levels of readiness and willingness to change their behavior.
- Ambivalence is normal behavior that should be expected when anyone considers making a change in their lives. The client can see both the reasons for and against change.
- Before discussing the next steps or "plans," clinicians should first focus their attention on creating a therapeutic rapport with the client, then increasing change talk and decreasing sustain talk.

31.16 FURTHER RESOURCES

In addition to the book edited by Frates and Faries (51), there are a number of other resources that have been published in the *Lifestyle Medicine Series,* which contain useful information for the clinician in the area of behavioral change. These include the book by Fagundes C, Merlo G. *Lifestyle Psychiatry: Through the Lens of Behavioral Medicine*. Boca Raton, FL: CRC Press, 2024 (52), as well as the book by Stout R, Reichert D, Kelly R: *Lifestyle Medicine and the Primary Care Provider: A Practical Guide to Enabling Whole Person Care*. Boca Raton, FL: CRC Press, 2025 (53). In the former book, Merlo and Fagundes introduce the important concept of lifestyle psychiatry and elaborate on how psychiatry can move toward assisting behavior change. In the book by Stout et al., the concept of how trained mental health professionals, mental health counselors, and psychologists can make significant contributions to assist in the process of behavior change is discussed.

31.17 SUMMARY

Behavior change is a science and an art. Many scientific journal articles have experimented with different methods to help people change their behavior, adopt healthy lifestyle behaviors, and sustain them. Reviewing the science is essential. Many important psychological theories serve as the guiding principles for strategies and techniques used in behavior change counseling. These include, but are not limited to, the Transtheoretical Model of Change, the Social Cognitive Theory, the Self-Determination Theory, and the Social Ecological Model of Change. In addition to these theories, the social determinants of health are essential to consider when counseling individuals to adopt and sustain healthy lifestyle behaviors. Motivational Interviewing is a powerful technique for working with patients/clients with lifestyle-related chronic conditions and those seeking to prevent such conditions.

NOTE

1 Much of the content of this section of the chapter has been drawn from the chapter entitled "Introduction to Behavior Change" in the academic textbook *"Empowering Behavior Change in Patients: Practical Strategies for the Healthcare Professional"* [Frates B, Faries M. CRC Press (Boca Raton, FL), 2023], which is a volume in the *Lifestyle Medicine Series* edited by Dr. Rippe.

REFERENCES

1. Duszyk K, Gomez GA, Schroder K, et al. In life there is death: how epithelial tissue barriers are preserved despite the challenge of apoptosis. *Tissue Barriers.* 2017;5(4):e1345533. doi: 10.1080/21688370.2017.1345533.
2. American Psychological Association. APA Dictionary of Psychology. 2022. https://dictionary.apa.org/behavior-change.
3. Ozemek C, Tiwari S, Sabbahi A, et al. Impact of therapeutic lifestyle changes in resistant hypertension. *Prog Cardiovasc Dis.* 2020;63(1):4–9. doi: 10.1016/j.pcad.2019.11.012.
4. Almutairi N, Hosseinzadeh H, Gopaldasani V. The effectiveness of patient activation intervention on type 2 diabetes mellitus glycemic control and self-management behaviors: a systematic review of RCTs. *Prim Care Diabetes.* 2020;14(1):2–20. doi: 10.1016/j.pcd.2019.08.009.
5. American College of Lifestyle Medicine. https://lifestylemedicine.org/overview/. Accessed October 1, 2025.
6. Kwasnicka D, Dombrowski SU, White M, et al. Theoretical explanations for maintenance of behaviour change: a systematic review of behaviour theories. *Health Psychol Rev.* 2016;10(3):277–296. doi: 10.1080/17437199.2016.1151372.
7. Michie S. Theories of behaviour and behaviour change across the social and behavioural sciences: a scoping review. *Health Psychol Rev.* 2015;9(3):323–344. doi: 10.1080/17437199.2014.941722.
8. Moafa I, Hoving C, van den Borne B, et al. Identifying behavior change techniques used in tobacco cessation interventions by oral health professionals and their relation to intervention effects – a review of systematic literature. *Int J Environ Res Public Health.* 2021;18(14):7481. doi: 10.3390/ijerph18147481.
9. Bandura A. *Social Foundations of Thought and Action: A Social Cognitive Theory.* Englewood Cliffs, NJ: Prentice-Hall, 1986.
10. Bandura A. *Self-Efficacy: The Exercise of Control.* New York: W H Freeman/Times Books/Henry Holt & Co, 1997.
11. Deci EL, Ryan R. *Intrinsic Motivation and Self-Determination in Human Behavior.* New York: Plenum, 1985.
12. The Center for Self-Determination Theory (CSDT). https://selfdeterminationtheory.org/theory/.
13. Maslow AH. *Motivation and Personality* (2nd ed). New York: Harper & Row, 1970.
14. Dominguez LJ, Veronese N, Baiamonte E, et al. Healthy aging and dietary patterns. *Nutrients.* 2022;14(4):889. doi: 10.3390/nu14040889.
15. Olstad DL, Kirkpatrick SI. Planting seeds of change: reconceptualizing what people eat as eating practices and patterns. *Int J Behav Nutr Phys Act.* 2021;18(1):32. https://doi.org/10.1186/s12966-021-01102-1.
16. Banks AR, Bell BA, Ngendahimana D, et al. Identification of factors related to food insecurity and inadequate access to the determinants of health services. *BMC Public Health.* 2021;21(1):1440. doi: 10.1186/s12889-021-11465-6.
17. Magnan S, Fisher CV, Cosenzo LG, et al. Social determinants as moderators of the effectiveness of health behavior change interventions: scientific gaps and *opportunities. Health Psychol Rev.* 2020;14(1):132–144. doi: 10.1080/17437199.2020.1718527.

18. U.S. Department of Health and Human Services, Office of Disease Prevention and Health Promotion. Social Determinants of Health. https://odphp.health.gov/healthypeople/priority-areas/social-determinants-health.
19. Kumar V, Encinosa W. Racial disparities in the perceived risk of COVID-19 and in getting needed medical care. *J Racial Ethn Health Disparities*. 2023;10(1):4–13. doi: 10.1007/s40615-021-01191-5.
20. National Board for Health and Wellness Coaching. https://nbhwc.org.
21. Frates B, Bonnet J, Joseph R, et al. *Lifestyle Medicine Handbook: An Introduction to the Power of Healthy Habits* (2nd ed). Monterey, CA: Healthy Learning, 2021.
22. Frates EP, Bonnet J. Collaboration and negotiation: the key to therapeutic lifestyle change. *Am J Lifestyle Med*. 2016;10(5):302–312.
23. Vale MJ, Jelinek MV, Best JD, et al. Coaching patients on achieving cardiovascular health (COACH): a multicenter randomized trial in patients with coronary heart disease. *Arch Int Med*. 2003;163(22):2775–2783. doi: 10.1001/archinte.163.22.2775.
24. Whittemore R, Melkus GD, Sullivan A, et al. Nurse-coaching intervention for women with type 2 diabetes. *Diabetes Educ*. 2004;30(5):795–804. doi: 10.1177/014572170403000515.
25. Wolever RQ, Dreusicke M, Fikkan J, et al. Integrative health coaching for patients with type 2 diabetes: a randomized clinical trial. *Diabetes Educ*. 2010;36(4):629–639. doi: 10.1177/0145721710371523.
26. Fisher EB, Strunk RC, Highstein GR, et al. A randomized controlled evaluation of the effect of community health workers on hospitalization for asthma: The asthma coach. [published correction appears in *Arch Pediatr Adolesc Med*. 2009;163(5):483]. *Arch Pediatr Adolesc Med*. 2009;163(3):225–232. doi: 10.1001/archpediatrics.2008.577.
27. Oliver JW, Kravitz RL, Kaplan SH, et al. Individualized patient education and coaching to improve pain control among cancer outpatients. *J Clin Oncol*. 2001;19(8):2206–2212. doi: 10.1200/JCO.2001.19.8.2206.
28. An S, Song R. Effects of health coaching on behavioral modification among adults with cardiovascular risk factors: systematic review and meta-analysis. *Patient Educ Couns*. 2020;103(10):2029–2038. doi: 10.1016/j.pec.2020.04.029.
29. Stara V, Santini S, Kropf J, et al. Digital health coaching programs among older employees in transition to retirement: systematic literature review [published correction appears in *J Med Internet Res*. 2020;22(12):e5065]. *J Med Internet Res*. 2020;22(9):e17809. doi: 10.2196/17809.
30. Obro LF, Heiselberg K, Krogh PG, et al. Combining mHealth and health-coaching for improving self-management in chronic care: A scoping review [published correction appears in *Patient Educ Couns*. 2021;104(10):2601]. *Patient Educ Couns*. 2021;104(4):680–688. doi: 10.1016/j.pec.2020.10.026.
31. Singh H, Kennedy GA, Stupans I. Does the modality used in health coaching matter? A systematic review of health coaching outcomes. *Patient Prefer Adherence*. 2020;14:1477–1492. doi: 10.2147/PPA.S265958.
32. Long H, Howells K, Peters S, et al. Does health coaching improve health-related quality of life and reduce hospital admissions in people with chronic obstructive pulmonary disease? A systematic review and meta-analysis. *Br J Health Psychol*. 2021;26(2):372–397. doi: 10.1111/bjhp.12366.
33. Dejonghe LAL, Becker J, Froboses I, Schaller A. Long-term effectiveness of health coaching in rehabilitation and prevention: a systematic review. *Patient Educ Couns*. 2017;100(9):1643–1653. doi: 10.1016/j.pec.2017.04.012
34. Barakat S, Boehmer K, Abdelrahim M. et al. Does health coaching grow capacity in cancer survivors? A systematic review. *Popul Health Manag*. 2018;21(1):63–81. doi: 10.1089/pop.2017.0040.
35. Kivelä K, Elo S, Kyngäs H, Kääriäinen M. The effects of health coaching on adult patients with chronic diseases: a systematic review. *Patient Educ Couns*. 2014;97(2):147–157. doi: 10.1016/j.pec.2014.07.026.
36. Wolever RQ, Simmons LA, Sforzo GA, et al. A systematic review of the literature on health and wellness coaching: defining a key behavioral intervention in healthcare. *Glob Adv Health Med*. 2013;2(4):38–57. doi: 10.7453/gahmj.2013.042.
37. Lara J, Evans EH, O'Brien N, et al. Association of behaviour change techniques with effectiveness of dietary interventions among adults of retirement age: a systematic review and meta-analysis of randomised controlled trials. *BMC Med*. 2014;12:177. doi: 10.1186/s12916-014-0177-3.
38. Samdal GB, Eide GE, Barth T, et al. Effective behaviour change techniques for physical activity and healthy eating in overweight and obese adults; systematic review and meta-regression analyses. *Int J Behav Nutr Phys Act*. 2017;14(1):42. doi: 10.1186/s12966-017-0494-y.
39. Teixeira PJ, Carraça EV, Marques MM, et al. Successful behavior change in obesity interventions in adults: a systematic review of self-regulation mediators. *BMC Med*. 2015;13:84. doi: 10.1186/s12916-015-0323–6.

40. Martin J, Chater A, Lorencatto F. Effective behaviour change techniques in the prevention and management of childhood obesity. *Int J Obes.* 2013;37(10):1287–1294. doi: 10.1038/ijo.2013.107.
41. Cradock KA, ÓLaighin G, Finucane FM, et al. Behaviour change techniques targeting both diet and physical activity in type 2 diabetes: a systematic review and meta-analysis. *Int J Behav Nutr Phys Act.* 2017;14(1):18. doi: 10.1186/s12966-016-0436-0.
42. Miller WR, Rollnick S. *Motivational Interviewing: Helping People Change* (3rd ed). New York: The Guilford Press, 2013.
43. Rozario, D. Burnout, resilience and moral injury: how the wicked problems of health care defy solutions, yet require innovative strategies in the modern era. *Can J Surg.* 2019;62(4):E6–E8. https://doi.org/10.1503/cjs.002819.
44. Watzlawick P, Weakland J, Fisch R. *Change; Principles of Problem Formation and Problem Resolution.* New York: W.W. Norton & Co, 2021.
45. Frost H, Campbell P, Maxwell M, et al. Effectiveness of motivational interviewing on adult behaviour change in health and social care settings: a systematic review of reviews. *PLoS One.* 2018;13(10):e0204890. doi: 10.1371/journal.pone.0204890. PMID: 30335780; PMCID: PMC6193639.
46. Aubeeluck E, Al-Arkee S, Finlay K, Jalal Z. The impact of pharmacy care and motivational interviewing on improving medication adherence in patients with cardiovascular diseases: a systematic review of randomised controlled trials. *Int J Clin Pract.* 2021;75(11):e14457. doi: 10.1111/ijcp.14457. Epub 2021 Jul 1. PMID: 34105858.
47. Amiri P, Mansouri-Tehrani MM, Khalili-Chelik A, et al. Does motivational interviewing improve the weight management process in adolescents? A systematic review and meta-analysis. *Int J Behav Med.* 2022;29(1):78–103. doi: 10.1007/s12529-021-09994-w. Epub 2021 Jul 15. PMID: 34268708.
48. McDaniel CC, Kavookjian J, Whitley HP. Telehealth delivery of motivational interviewing for diabetes management: a systematic review of randomized controlled trials. *Patient Educ Couns.* 2022;105(4):805–820. doi: 10.1016/j.pec.2021.07.036. Epub 2021 Jul 24. PMID: 34366228; PMCID: PMC8912910.
49. Nuss K, Moore K, Nelson T, Li K. Effects of motivational interviewing and wearable fitness trackers on motivation and physical activity: a systematic review. *Am J Health Promot.* 2021;35(2):226–235. doi: 10.1177/0890117120939030. Epub 2020 Jul 14. PMID: 32662277.
50. Ghizzardi G, Arrigoni C, Dellafiore F, et al. Efficacy of motivational interviewing on enhancing self-care behaviors among patients with chronic heart failure: a systematic review and meta-analysis of randomized controlled trials. *Heart Fail Rev.* 2022;27(4):1029–1041. doi: 10.1007/s10741-021-10110-z. Epub 2021 Apr 17. PMID: 33866487.
51. Frates B, Faries M. *Empowering Behavior Change in Patients: Practical Strategies for the Healthcare Professional.* Boca Raton, FL: CRC Press, 2023.
52. Fagundes C, Merlo G. *Lifestyle Psychiatry: Through the Lens of Behavioral Medicine.* Boca Raton, FL: CRC Press, 2024.
53. Stout R, Reichert D, Kelly R. *Lifestyle Medicine and the Primary Care Provider: A Practical Guide to Enabling Whole Person Care.* Boca Raton, FL: CRC Press, 2025.

Appendix A
Recommended Nutrition Plan

Throughout this book, we have emphasized that plant-forward nutrition plans have been repeatedly demonstrated to lower the risk of various chronic diseases. Broad consensus exists among major medical organizations including the American Heart Association, the Dietary Guidelines for Americans, the Academy of Nutrition and Dietetics, and many others that recommend plant-forward nutritional plans. We strongly support this concept.

One excellent plant-forward nutrition plan that we can highly recommend is the Full Plate Living Core Program. This is a program you can confidently recommend to your patients. The Full Plate Living Program is one of the few programs certified by the American College of Lifestyle Medicine. A long list of employers, including hospitals and universities, have recommended the Full Plate Living Program for their employees. The results have been very impressive. Indeed, in one article published by the American Journal of Health Promotion, it was found that "employees lost weight, reported increased energy, and improved confidence in making healthy food choices."

If you choose to recommend the Full Plate Living Program, you can get started by clicking on: https://www.fullplateliving.org/.

We have also listed the Table of Contents for the Full Plate Living Core Program below:

A.1 FULL PLATE LIVING CORE PROGRAM TABLE OF CONTENTS

Orientation

- Welcome
- Success Stories and Your Health Vision
- Download Your Workbook
- Fiber Inventory
- How Did You Do?
- Moving Forward

Module 1: The Basics

- Welcome to Module 1
- *Lesson 1*: All About Fiber
- *Lesson 2*: The 75/25 Plate
- *Lesson 3*: Fiber and Water – A Secure Couple
- *Lesson 4*: Easy Does It
- *Lesson 5*: Fiber First Challenge
- What You Learned in Module 1
- Moving Forward
- You've Completed Module 1!

Module 2: Your 75/25 Plate

- Welcome to Module 2
- *Lesson 1*: The Plate

- *Lesson 2*: What's in the 75%?
- *Lesson 3*: What's in the 25%?
- *Lesson 4*: Finding Your Core Values and Preparing for Change
- What You Learned in Module 2
- Moving Forward
- You've Completed Module 2!

Module 3: Starting Your Day With Healthy Habits

- Welcome to Module 3
- *Lesson 1*: How Do You Build a Habit?
- *Lesson 1*: Continued
- *Lesson 2*: Your Relationship With Your Kitchen
- *Lesson 2*: Continued
- *Lesson 3*: Breakfast
- What You Learned in Module 3
- Moving Forward
- You've Completed Module 3!

Module 4: Getting Social, Finding Support, and Navigating Family Meals

- Welcome to Module 4
- *Lesson 1*: Drum Up Support
- *Lesson 2*: Dinners and Family Meals
- *Lesson 3*: Navigating Social Situations
- *Lesson 4*: The Power of Community and Connection
- What You Learned in Module 4
- Moving Forward
- You've Completed Module 4!

Module 5: Meal Prep and Dining Out

- Welcome to Module 5
- *Lesson 1*: Eating Out
- *Lesson 2*: Lunch
- *Lesson 3*: Setting Yourself Up for Success
- What You Learned in Module 5
- Moving Forward
- You've Completed Module 5!

Module 6: Snacking, Satisfaction and Emotional Eating

- Welcome to Module 6
- *Lesson 1*: Finding Your Satisfaction Point
- *Lesson 2*: Mindful Eating
- *Lesson 3*: Eating for Reasons Other Than Hunger
- *Lesson 4*: Snacking
- What You Learned in Module 6
- Moving Forward
- You've Completed Module 6!

Module 7: Setting Yourself Up for a Lifetime of Health

- Welcome to Module 7
- *Lesson 1*: Staying on Track
- *Lesson 2*: Other Lifestyle Factors to Explore
- Move "More" Daily
- Stress Less
- Embrace Healthy Relationships
- Get Enough Restful Sleep
- Avoid Risky Substances
- Fiber Inventory Re-Check
- Moving Forward
- Congratulations! What now?

One reason why we are enthusiastic about the Full Plate Living Program is that it not only provides evidence-based, healthy nutrition but it is also motivational and easy to follow.

The Full Plate Living Program has been provided by the Ardmore Institute for Health. This is a non-profit organization that has played a very significant role in advancing the evidence base for lifestyle medicine. The Full Plate Living Program was developed by physicians, nutritionists, and exercise physiologists.

Appendix B
RLI Fitness Walking Programs

Blue Program

Week	**1–2**	**3–4**	**5**	**6**	**7–8**	**9**	**10**	**11**	**12–13**	**14**	**15–16**	**17–18**	**19–20**
Warm-up (mins. before walk stretches)	5–7	5–7	5–7	5–7	5–7	5–7	5–7	5–7	5–7	5–7	5–7	5–7	5–7
Mileage	1.0	1.25	1.5	1.5	1.75	2.0	2.0	2.0	2.25	2.5	2.5	2.75	3.0
Steps	2,000	2,500	3,000	3,000	3,250	4,000	4,000	4,000	4,500	5,000	5,000	5,500	6,000
Pace (mph)	3.0	3.0	3.0	3.5	3.5	3.5	3.75	3.75	3.75	3.75	4.0	4.0	4.0
Heart rate (% of max)	60	60	60	60–70	60–70	60–70	60–70	70	70	70	70	70–80	70–80
Cool down (mins. after walk stretches)	5–7	5–7	5–7	5–7	5–7	5–7	5–7	5–7	5–7	5–7	5–7	5–7	5–7
Frequency (times per week)	5	5	5	5	5	5	5	5	5	5	5	5	5

Green Program

Week	1–2	3–4	5–6	7	8–9	10–12	13	14	15–16	17–18	19–20
Warm-up (mins. before walk stretches)	5–7	5–7	5–7	5–7	5–7	5–7	5–7	5–7	5–7	5–7	5–7
Mileage	1.5	1.75	2.0	2.0	2.25	2.5	2.75	2.75	3.0	3.25	3.5
Steps	3,000	3,500	4,000	4,000	4,500	5,000	5,500	5,500	6,000	6,500	6,500
Pace (mph)	3.0	3.0	3.0	3.5	3.5	3.5	3.5	4.0	4.0	4.0	4.0
Heart rate (% of max)	60–70	60–70	60–70	70	70	70	70	70–80	70–80	70–80	70–80
Cool-down (mins. after walk stretches)	5–7	5–7	5–7	5–7	5–7	5–7	5–7	5–7	5–7	5–7	5–7
Frequency (times per week)	5	5	5	5	5	5	5	5	5	5	5

Yellow Program

Week	1	2	3–4	5	6–8	9–10	11–12	13–14	15	16–17	18–20
Warm-up (mins. before walk stretches)	5–7	5–7	5–7	5–7	5–7	5–7	5–7	5–7	5–7	5–7	5–7
Mileage	2.0	2.25	2.5	2.75	2.75	3.0	3.0	3.25	3.5	3.5	4.0
Steps	4,000	4,500	5,000	5,500	5,500	6,000	6,000	6,500	7,000	7,000	8,000
Pace (mph)	3.0	3.0	3.0	3.0	3.5	3.5	4.0	4.0	4.0	4.5	4.5
Heart rate (% of max)	70	70	70	70	70	70	70–80	70–80	70–80	70–80	70–80
Cool-down (mins. after walk stretches)	5–7	5–7	5–7	5–7	5–7	5–7	5–7	5–7	5–7	5–7	5–7
Frequency (times per week)	5	5	5	5	5	5	5	5	5	5	5

Orange Program*

Week	1	2	3–4	5	6	7	8	9–10	11–14	15–20
Warm-up (mins. before walk stretches)	5–7	5–7	5–7	5–7	5–7	5–7	5–7	5–7	5–7	5–7
Mileage	2.5	2.75	3.0	3.25	3.25	3.5	3.75	4.0	4.0	4.0
Steps	5,000	5,500	6,000	6,500	6,500	7,000	7,500	8,000	8,000	8,000
Pace (mph)	3.5	3.5	3.5	3.5	4.0	4.0	4.0	4.0	4.5	4.5
Incline/weight +**										
Heart rate (% of max)	50–70	50–70	50–70	50–70	50–70	50–70	50–70	50–70	50–70	
Cool-down (mins. after walk stretches)	5–7	5–7	5–7	5–7	5–7	5–7	5–7	5–7	5–7	5–7
Frequency (times per week)	5	5	5	5	5	5	5	5	5	3

* *At the end of the 20-week fitness protocol, follow the Orange/Red Maintenance Program for a lifetime of fitness walking.*

** *During weeks 15–20, arm weights or incline may be added to increase intensity.*

Red Program*

Week	1	2	3	4	5	6	7–20
Warm-up (mins. before walk stretches)	5–7	5–7	5–7	5–7	5–7	5–7	5–7
Mileage	3.0	3.25	3.5	3.5	3.75	4.0	4.0
Steps	6,000	6,500	7,000	7,000	7,500	8,000	8,000
Pace (mph)	4.0	4.0	4.0	4.5	4.5	4.5	4.5
Incline/weight +**							
Heart rate (% of max)	70	70	70	70–80	70–80	70–80	70–80
Cool-down (mins. after walk stretches)	5–7	5–7	5–7	5–7	5–7	5–7	5–7
Frequency (times per week)	5	5	5	5	5	5	3

* *At the end of the 20-week fitness protocol, follow the Orange/Red Maintenance Program for a lifetime of fitness walking.*

** *During weeks 15–20, arm weights or incline may be added to increase intensity.*

Yellow Maintenance Program

Warm-up	5–7 minutes before walk stretches
Aerobic work out	Mileage: 4.0; pace: 4.5 mph
Heart rate	70%–80% of maximum
Cool-down	5–7 minutes after walk stretches
Frequency	3–5 times per week
Weekly mileage	12–20 minutes
Weekly steps	24,000–40,000

Orange/Red Maintenance Program

Warm-up	5–7 minutes before walk stretches
Aerobic work out	Mileage: 4.0; pace: 4.5 mph weight/incline: Add weights to upper body or add hill walking as needed to keep heart rate in target zone (70%–80% of predicted maximum)
Heart rate	70%–80% of maximum
Cool-down	5–7 minutes after walk stretches
Frequency	3–5 times per week
Weekly mileage	12–20 minutes
Weekly steps	24,000–40,000

Sources: Charts taken from Rippe JM, *Increasing Physical Activity*, CRC Press, Boca Raton, 2021. Adapted from Rippe JM, *Ward A: The Rockport Walking Program*, Prentice Hall Press, New York, 1989.

GETTING STARTED ON FITNESS WALKING PROGRAMS

In this Appendix, we have provided five different Fitness Walking Programs. Our hope is that physicians who utilize this book, if they have not been physically active, will find these programs useful in their own lives. They are also geared toward use for your patients.

The programs are color-coded. The Blue Program is the least intense and is for people who have been sedentary. The Green and Yellow Programs are for people who have been intermittently active and who want to start at a little bit higher level with more distance.

The Orange and Red Programs are for individuals who are already engaged in fitness walking and want to slowly progress to the point where they are obtaining 150 minutes of moderate-intensity physical activity per week.

These walking programs were developed by Dr. Rippe and his research laboratory and were updated in his physical activity book in 2021 (*Increasing Physical Activity: A Practical Guide*, CRC Press, 2021).

Appendix C

Recent Books, Articles, and Position Papers Supporting Academic Lifestyle Medicine

C.1 ACADEMIC TEXTBOOKS

1. Rippe JM. *Lifestyle Medicine* (4th ed). Boca Raton, FL: CRC Press, 2024.

C.2 BOOKS IN THE LIFESTYLE MEDICINE SERIES[1]

1. Rippe JM. *Increasing Physical Activity: A Practical Guide*. Boca Raton, FL: CRC Press, 2020.
2. Tollefson M, Eriksen N, Pathak N. *Improving Women's Health Across the Lifespan*. Boca Raton, FL: CRC Press, 2021.
3. Rippe JM. *Manual of Lifestyle Medicine*. Boca Raton, FL: CRC Press, 2021.
4. Rippe JM, Foreyt J. *Obesity Prevention and Treatment. A Practical Guide*. Boca Raton, FL: CRC Press, 2021.
5. Merlo G, Berra K. *Lifestyle Nursing*. Boca Raton, FL: CRC Press, 2022.
6. Rippe JM. *Integrating Lifestyle Medicine in Cardiovascular Health and Disease Prevention*. Boca Raton, FL: CRC Press, 2022.
7. Via M, Mechanic J. *Lifestyle Medicine and Diabetes, Pre-Diabetes and the Metabolic Syndrome*. Boca Raton, FL: CRC Press, 2023.
8. Frates B, Faries M. *Empowering Behavior Change in Patients: Practical Strategies for the Healthcare Professional*. Boca Raton, FL: CRC Press, 2023.
9. Merlo G, Fagundes C. *Lifestyle Psychiatry: Through the Lens of Behavioral Medicine*. Boca Raton, FL: CRC Press, 2024.
10. Rippe J. *Lifestyle Nutrition: Eating for Good Health by Lowering the Risk of Chronic Diseases*. Boca Raton, FL: CRC Press, 2024.
11. Stout R, Reichert D, Kelly R. *Lifestyle Medicine and the Primary Care Provider: A Practical Guide to Enabling Whole Person Care*. Boca Raton, FL: CRC Press, 2025.
12. Friedman S. *Geriatrics, Lifestyle Medicine and Healthy Aging*. Boca Raton, FL: CRC Press, 2025.
13. Rippe JM, Frates B. *Academic Lifestyle Medicine: A Curriculum for Medical Educators*. Boca Raton, FL: CRC Press, 2026 (in press).
14. Brothers J, Daniels S. *Lifestyle Medicine and Pediatrics*. Boca Raton, FL: CRC Press, 2026 (in press).
15. Ali Q, Bowman D, Nyong F. *Achieving Health Equity with Lifestyle Medicine*. Boca Raton, FL: CRC Press, 2026 (in press).
16. Frates B, Kin C, Lillemoe K, Suk M. *Lifestyle Medicine and Surgery: A Guide for Surgeons and Providers Caring for Surgical Patients*. Boca Raton, FL: CRC Press, 2026 (in press).
17. Pathak N. *Lifestyle Medicine for Human and Planetary Health*. Boca Raton, FL: CRC Press, 2026 (in press).

18. Joy L, Macintyre J. *Musculoskeletal Failure: A Lifestyle Approach to Prevention and Management.* Boca Raton, FL: CRC Press, 2026 (in press).

C.3 ARTICLES

1. Rippe J. Lifestyle medicine: the health promoting power of daily habits and practices. *Am J Lifestyle Med.* 2018;13(6).
2. Rippe J. Are we ready to practice lifestyle medicine? *Am J Med.* 2019;132(1):6–8.
3. Rippe J. Lifestyle strategies for risk reduction, prevention and treatment of cardiovascular disease. *Am J Lifestyle Med.* 2018;13(2):204–212.
4. Merlo G, Rippe J. Physician burnout: a lifestyle medicine perspective. *Am J Lifestyle Med.* 2020;15(2):148–157.
5. Rippe J. Lifestyle medicine and cardiovascular health. *Am J Lifestyle Med.* 2026;26 (in press).
6. Rippe JM, Frates B. Academic lifestyle medicine and physician education. *Am J Lifestyle Med.* 2025:15598276251355163. doi: 10.1177/15598276251355163. Epub ahead of print. PMID: 40584608; PMCID: PMC12204994.
7. Merlo G, Snellman L, Sugden S. Connectedness: the updated and expanded pillar of lifestyle psychiatry and lifestyle medicine. *Am J Lifestyle Med.* 2025:15598276251345455. doi: 10.1177/15598276251345455. Epub ahead of print. PMID: 40469950; PMCID: PMC12129969.
8. Rippe J. Social interactions and health: new insights into the role of connectedness. *Am J Lifestyle Med.* 2025;19(8):1125–1126. doi:10.1177/15598276251355177.
9. Williams K, Ikram M, Frates B, et al. Dietary and lifestyle habits of cardiologists: perception vs practice. *J Am Coll Cardiol.* 2025;86(9):673–675. doi:10.1016/j.jacc.2025.06.021.
10. Mauro S, Eller M, Stout R. Lifestyle medicine and behavioral health: a time for deeper integration. *Am J Lifestyle Med.* 2025. doi:10.1177/15598276251381252.
11. Rippe J. Lifestyle medicine and behavioral health: synergies, opportunities and challenges. *Am J Lifestyle Med.* 2025. doi:10.1177/15598276251382106.
12. Karlsen M, Merlo G, Sugden S, et al. Lifestyle interventions for major depressive disorder (MDD): an expert consensus statement from the American College of Lifestyle Medicine. *Am J Lifestyle Med.* 2026 (in press).
13. Marshall S, Patel P, Anand R, et al. Lifestyle medicine as a framework for high-value care: a position statement from the American College of Lifestyle Medicine. *Am J Lifestyle Med.* 2025:15598276251390437. doi: 10.1177/15598276251390437. Epub ahead of print. PMID: 41246049; PMCID: PMC12611736.
14. Rippe J. Value in lifestyle medicine: the final challenge. *Am J Lifestyle Med.* 2026 (in press).
15. Godfrey EM, Kim ES, Frates B. Lifestyle medicine: the case for using educational frameworks and instructional approaches that meet adult learning needs. *Am J Lifestyle Med.* 2025. doi:10.1177/15598276251393587.
16. Hooker SA, Lianov L, Billock C, et al. Meaning, purpose and spirituality in lifestyle medicine (supplement). *Am J Lifestyle Med.* 2026 (in press).
17. Rippe J. Meaning, purpose and spirituality: the 800 pound bear for behavior change in lifestyle medicine and indeed, for American health care. *Am J Lifestyle Med.* 2026 (in press).
18. Stout R. The foundation of lifestyle medicine: meaning, purpose, and spirituality. *Am J Lifestyle Med.* 2026 (in press).
19. Sleet D, Scarbrough W, Brown C, et al. Alcohol harms, injuries, and health: clinical implications for lifestyle medicine. *Am J Lifestyle Med.* 2025. doi:10.1177/15598276251350863.

20. Rippe J. Alcohol consumption and health: the plot thickens. *Am J Lifestyle Med.* 2025:15598276251355851. doi: 10.1177/15598276251355851. Epub ahead of print. PMID: 40584609; PMCID: PMC12202373.
21. Rosenfeld R, Grega M, Karlsen M, et al. Executive summary of lifestyle interventions for treatment and remission of type 2 diabetes and prediabetes in adults: a clinical practice guideline from the American College of Lifestyle Medicine. *Am J Lifestyle Med.* 2025;19(2_suppl):132S–154S. doi:10.1177/15598276251325485.
22. Mozaffarian D, Agarwal M, Aggarwal M, et al. Nutritional priorities to support GLP-1 therapy for obesity: a joint Advisory from the American College of Lifestyle Medicine, the American Society for Nutrition, the Obesity Medicine Association, and The Obesity Society. *Obesity* 2025;33(8):1475–1503. doi: 10.1002/oby.24336. Epub 2025 May 30. PMID: 40445127; PMCID: PMC12304835.
23. Rippe J. Lifestyle medicine and GLP-1 therapy for obesity: time to get real. *Am J Lifestyle Med.* 2025. doi:10.1177/15598276251336677.
24. Rippe JM. The heart of whole health: articles based on presentations at the 2024 National Meeting of the American College of Lifestyle Medicine. *Am J Lifestyle Med.* 2025;19(7):940–945. doi:10.1177/15598276251333330.
25. Rippe, JM. Translating lifestyle medicine education into practice (supplement). *Am J Lifestyle Med.* 2025. Published First online: December 15, 2025.
26. Rippe J. Translating lifestyle medicine education into practice. *Am J Lifestyle Med.* 2025;19(3 Suppl):4S–5S. doi: 10.1177/15598276251346218. PMID: 41409772; PMCID: PMC12705962.
27. Miller CM. From education to implementation: the expanding role of lifestyle medicine training. *Am J Lifestyle Med.* 2025;19(3 Suppl):6S–9S. doi: 10.1177/15598276251396695. PMID: 41409774; PMCID: PMC12705965.
28. Rippe JM. American Journal of Lifestyle Medicine 2025: continued progress, expanded mandate. *Am J Lifestyle Med.* 2024;19(1):4–5. doi:10.1177/15598276241263791.
29. Eisenberg D, Cole A, Maile E, et al. Proposed nutrition competencies for medical students and physician trainees: a consensus statement. *JAMA Netw Open.* 2024;7(9):e2435425. doi: 10.1001/jamanetworkopen.2024.35425.

NOTE

1 Dr. Rippe serves as Editor-in-Chief of the *Lifestyle Medicine Series.*

Index

Note: **Bold** page numbers refer to tables and *italic* page numbers refer to figures.

www.ingramcontent.com/pod-product-compliance
Lightning Source LLC
LaVergne TN
LVHW061154180826
845923LV00032B/447

* 9 7 8 1 0 4 1 0 3 7 9 5 8 *